*Pediatric Neuropsychology
in the Medical Setting*

Pediatric Neuropsychology in the Medical Setting

IDA SUE BARON, Ph.D.

EILEEN B. FENNELL, Ph.D.

KYTJA K. S. VOELLER, M.D.

New York   Oxford   OXFORD UNIVERSITY PRESS   1995

Oxford University Press

Oxford   New York
Athens   Auckland   Bangkok   Bombay
Calcutta   Cape Town   Dar es Salaam   Delhi
Florence   Hong Kong   Istanbul   Karachi
Kuala Lumpur   Madras   Madrid   Melbourne
Mexico City   Nairobi   Paris   Singapore
Taipei   Tokyo   Toronto

and associated companies in
Berlin   Ibadan

Library of Congress Cataloging-in-Publication Data
Baron, Ida Sue.
Pediatric neuropsychology in the medical setting / Ida Sue Baron,
Eileen B. Fennell, Kytja K.S. Voeller.
p. cm.   Includes bibliographical references and index.
ISBN 0-19-506345-7
1. Pediatric neuropsychology.
I. Fennell, Eileen B.
II. Voeller, Kytja K. S.
III. Title.
    [DNLM: 1. Neuropsychology—in infancy & childhood.
  2. Pediatrics.
  3. Neuropsychological Tests—in infancy & childhood.
  WS 350.6   B265p   1995]
  RJ486.5.B37   1995
  618.92'8—dc20   DNLM/DLC
  for Library of Congress   94-26424

9 8 7 6 5 4 3 2 1

Printed in the United States of America
on acid-free paper

To Peter, David, and Cara

*My family and to the graduate students
at the University of Florida, Gainesville,
who encouraged us to write this book*

John, Bonnie, Sue, Chris, and Jan

Preface

The assessment of brain function in pediatric patients with varying medical conditions holds interest for many practitioners in psychology and the health professions. We have witnessed and participated in the growth of pediatric neuropsychology as a field of investigation and practice, yet we have been unable to identify a volume that answers many of the questions raised by students, by child psychology colleagues, by medical and allied health staff within our own medical settings, and by adult neuropsychology colleagues interested in the neuropsychological evaluation of children. Further, while neurological populations have been our main focus for more than two decades each, our experience with nonneurological patients has made us aware that references to the broader applications of neuropsychology and to pediatric nonneurological populations are scarce. This volume was written in an attempt to bridge these gaps.

It is not our intent to provide an in-depth review of the existing literature, although we cite sufficient relevant literature to guide the interested reader toward more specific sources for further review. We concentrate on practical matters, try to sharpen the delineation of clinical concerns, and aim to expand knowledge about the neuropsychological aspects of specific medical conditions. Since some fundamental information has been incorporated into existing child and adult texts, we encourage readers to refer to these books, which include resources for neuroanatomy, neuropsychology, and psychopathology:

Brodal, A. 1981. *Neurological Anatomy in Relation to Clinical Medicine*, 3d ed. New York: Oxford University Press.

Heilman, K. M., and Valenstein, E. (eds.). 1993. *Clinical Neuropsychology*, 3d ed. New York: Oxford University Press.

Kolb, B., and Whishaw, I. Q. 1990. 3d ed. *Fundamentals of Human Neuropsychology*. San Francisco: W. H. Freeman.

Menkes, J. H. 1990. *Textbook of Child Neurology*. Philadelphia: Lea & Febiger.

Nieuwenhuys, R.; Voogd, J.; and van Huijzen, C. 1988. *The Human Central Nervous System*, 3d ed. New York: Springer-Verlag.

Reynolds, C. R., and Fletcher-Janzen, E. (eds.). 1989. *Handbook of Clinical Child Neuropsychology*. New York: Plenum Press.

Rourke, B. P.; Bakker, D. J.; Fisk, J. L.; and Strang, J. D. 1983. *Child Neuropsychology: An Introduction to Theory, Research, and Clinical Practice*. New York: Guilford Press.

Rutter, M. (ed.). 1983. *Developmental Neuropsychiatry.* New York: Guilford Press.

Schwartz, S., and Johnson, J. H. 1985. *Psychopathology of Childhood: A Clinical-Experimental Approach,* 2d ed. New York: Pergamon Press.

Spreen, O.; Risser, A. T.; & Edgell, D. 1995. *Developmental Neuropsychology.* New York: Oxford University Press.

We do not advocate applying a unitary test battery, since we prefer a flexible approach to assessment. The test instruments we select in practice depend heavily on the variables that emerge during the course of an evaluation. Many reference works discuss battery versus flexible testing strategies; and various individual chapters outline specific test selection and test availability for adults and/or children. The reader is encouraged to consult these, including the following volumes:

Lezak, M. 1995. *Neuropsychological Assessment,* 3d ed. New York: Oxford University Press.

Spreen, O., and Strauss, E. 1991. *A Compendium of Neuropsychological Tests: Administration, Norms and Commentary.* New York: Oxford University Press.

Our objective is to provide the reader with a useful, practical guide and source book that can support responsible assessment of the medically ill child. Chapter 1 offers an introduction to pediatric neuropsychology and its applications within the medical environment. Thereafter, the text is divided into three major parts.

Part I covers normal and abnormal brain development. Chapter 2 provides a brief summary of current theory and knowledge about normal and abnormal brain development, derived from animal and human studies. Chapter 3 describes common neurodevelopmental anomalies and genetic syndromes.

Part II has a more practical orientation. Chapter 4 describes the pediatric neurological evaluation, with emphasis on the neurobehavioral perspective. Chapter 5 describes methods of evaluating the child and the adolescent, including interviewing, observational techniques, ways of encouraging test taking, and strategies for coping with less compliant children. Chapter 6 describes ways to communicate results orally (in the interpretive session) and in writing (in a formal report).

Part III emphasizes the medical and neuropsychological knowledge a neuropsychologist must possess to evaluate children with various common medical diseases and conditions. It focuses on patient populations that are commonly encountered within the pediatric medical setting. We review diagnostic considerations, assessment techniques, and treatments specific for each population; and we summarize knowledge about cognitive and neuropsychological function and dysfunction. Included are hydrocephalus and myelomeningocele, seizure disorders, head trauma, cancer, cardiovascular disease, renal disease, and neuropsychiatric disorders.

We have deliberately excluded diagnoses and issues that are commonly treated on an outpatient basis. Therefore, we do not discuss (except tangentially) broad categories of diagnoses for which pediatric neuropsychologists are often consulted—learning disability, attentional deficit disorder, developmental immaturity, and so on. In the interest of brevity, we have also had to omit illnesses and conditions that have received scant attention in the neuropsychology literature. We certainly recognize that a pediatric neuropsychologist may be consulted in other inpatient populations and settings. But our intent has been to focus on the more common pediatric diagnostic groups and the contributions of the neuropsychologist to the care and treatment of these medically ill children. Finally, as we were encouraged to work in these settings by our own mentors, we hope that this volume will encourage others to apply a child neuropsychological approach to hospital-based consultations.

Potomac, Md.   I.S.B.
Gainesville, Fla.   E.F.
August 1994   K.V.

Acknowledgments

We would like to acknowledge the contributions of colleagues who provided helpful critical comments and expertise. We gratefully thank Pim Brouwers, Ph.D.; Regina Bussing, M.D.; Robert S. Fennell, III, M.D.; Gerard Gioia, Ph.D.; Ellen Goldberger, Ph.D.; Kathleen McKay, B.S.; Lowell W. Perry, M.D.; Elsa Shapiro, Ph.D.; Stephen R. Shapiro, M.D.; and Peter Starke, M.D. We also especially appreciate the support, advice, and editorial assistance provided by Jeffrey House of Oxford University Press. Finally, we express our gratitude to Jack Fletcher, Ph.D. whose reviews of working versions of many chapters were invaluable.

Contents

Pediatric Neuropsychology in the Medical Setting

1

Introduction to Pediatric Neuropsychology

Pediatric neuropsychologists have diverse educational backgrounds, training, and employment experiences. Professionals trained in clinical child psychology, educational psychology, adult neuropsychology, neurology and behavioral neurology, psychobiology, cognitive psychology, developmental psychology, neurolinguistics, and other disciplines have brought diversity to the field, combining differing clinical perspectives and theoretical approaches. They share a common desire to contribute to the understanding of brain–behavior relationships in the developing child.

ROLE OF THE PEDIATRIC NEUROPSYCHOLOGIST

Neuropsychologists have been called upon to play an expanded role in the care of children within medical settings. Understandably, early interest focused on children diagnosed with specific neurological, neurosurgical, or psychiatric disorders, such as epilepsy, hydrocephalus, or schizophrenia. The early emphasis on assessment of broadly defined groups of children and adolescents with abnormal neurological development gave the discipline a strong foundation, but it has since evolved from this early role in assessing the effects of brain injury or disease.

Advances in pediatric neuropsychology occurred simultaneously with developments in allied neuroscience fields. New neurodiagnostic technology, a more sophisticated range of neuropathological techniques, and refinements in methodological approaches all had a direct impact on the field. A greatly enhanced understanding of brain growth and development resulted (see Chapter 2). Questions about developmental brain pathology and behavioral abnormalities became more specific. In response, practitioners were stimulated to expand the existing base of assessment approaches and instrumentation. Cumulative medical data about the impact of physical disease on the developing nervous system led to a greater variety of treatment regimens. The resources of pediatric neuropsychology increasingly became applicable to these treatment protocols. As innovative medical treatments improved the outcome of many childhood illnesses, the associated morbidity received greater attention. Often, neuropsychological data proved necessary for understanding the long-term consequences of medical decisions. For example, neuropsychological data were incorporated into clinical trials designed to prolong the lives of children with leukemia. As survival rates improved, negative effects of the treatment on cognition became evident and protocols were modified accordingly. The initiation of rehabilitative strategies and programs was a natural development for a discipline whose evaluations permit precise delineation of cognitive strengths and weaknesses.

The pediatric neuropsychologist plays an increasingly important role within the multidisciplinary team approach to patient care in many pediatric medical settings. This approach combines the efforts of multiple medical and allied health professionals to provide a child and family with integrated care. Neuropsychologists bring to the team an orientation that combines psychological and medical concerns. For example, one of us (I. S. B.) was a guest observer at a team session about a young boy with learning problems. Team members included a pediatrician, a clinical psychologist, a speech and language therapist, an occupational therapist, a physical therapist, a social worker, and an educational diagnostician. In turn, the professionals addressed salient features of their examinations. Psychological test data documented average IQ but revealed subtest score variability. High scores on measures of expressive vocabulary and verbal reasoning contrasted with low scores on number sequence recall, picture arrangement, and picture completion. The psychologist's discussion of the personality test responses did not mention certain qualitative features that are distinctive to neurological disorder and were present in the data—for instance, idiosyncratic "dripping," "dropping," and "falling" responses on the Rorschach inkblot test; off-balance, dehumanized, asymmetrical figure drawing; inconsistent behavior within and between staff visits. The patient's characteristic "in and out," "good moment, bad moment" attention profile—one that is associated with neurological disorder—was likewise not highlighted. The team's diagnostic formulation of learning disability with associated poor self-image lacked specificity. The neuropsychologist, after explaining how these responses were typical for a child who experiences out-of-control episodes, formulated a presumptive diagnosis of petit mal seizure disorder and recommended that a pediatric neurologist be consulted. An electroencephalogram confirmed the presumptive diagnosis. The clinician's recognition of an aberrant clinical profile permitted diagnosis of an unrecognized and treatable neurological disorder.

Neuropsychology is emerging as an essential discipline within the pediatric medical setting. The traditional referral populations of early years have now broadened to include children with a wide variety of childhood conditions, including systemic disorders that may affect the brain secondarily. The extension of pediatric neuropsychology into new areas of medical disorder is only possible when the essential elements of brain development and maturation are well understood. Pediatric neuropsychology is distinctly different from adult neuropsychology. Understanding the differences between the two is an essential aspect of preparing for professional practice.

DIFFERENCES BETWEEN ADULT AND CHILD
NEUROPSYCHOLOGY

Children are not merely small adults. Early attempts to extend knowledge of brain–behavior relationships to children on the basis of knowledge established in adult neuropsychology proved inadequate and inappropriate. Brain–behavior relationships differ in children and adults, with or without brain injury (Aram 1988; Thal et al. 1991; Vargha-Khadem, O'Gorman & Watters 1985). The relationships between brain function and behavior in the developing child are both qualitatively and quantitatively different from those in the adult. The pediatric neuropsychologist should be familiar with concepts of normal variation as these apply to each developmental stage, and with levels of expected skill acquisition at different age levels. This knowledge is necessary to understand the relationship between a neurological insult and behavioral sequelae that vary at different developmental stages and in response to critical influences encountered at each stage. While such knowledge may be acquired both didactically and through direct clinical experience, rarely does one or the other alone suffice. Both hands-on experience and textbook knowledge of normal physical, cognitive, emotional, and social development are needed. Experienced neuropsychologists in adult settings who want to transfer their knowledge to a pediatric population are at a great disadvantage if they lack knowledge of normal child development.

Knowledge from adult neuropsychology cannot be applied directly to child neuropsychology for several reasons. These include the specific maturational changes that complicate the pediatric assessment process, the "behavioral plasticity" or capacity for reorganization of an immature brain, the differing diagnostic considerations in adult and child neurology, the potential for great variability in test-taking behavior at younger ages, the limited applicability of brain–behavior function rules in children, and the important impact of environmental and social factors on the developing organism.

Maturational Change

Maturation is a complex variable. Deficits in adulthood are commonly apparent as loss of function in a fully developed organism—for example, a Broca's (expressive) aphasia following left posterior frontal lobe infarction. Pediatric dysfunction is not always as easily recognized, since disorder may not be evidenced as a functional loss. For example, a child may not have matured sufficiently to attain expressive language skill, which would have been affected by a focal insult. The behavioral effect may therefore seem to be absent or may remain undetected until the child is older.

Dynamic, step-by-step transitions from one developmental level to another characterize normal child development. Interference in the normal acquisition of behaviors affects outcome variably. A child may fail to develop an ability, thenceforth no longer progressing normally along the developmental continuum. A child may experience an altered rate of development while in the process of acquiring a behavior. For example, a 15-month-old who has begun to combine two words may show slowed or temporarily halted language development following an infectious process. A child may regress from developmental milestones. For example, a child may slowly lose motor milestones achieved before the onset of a degenerative lipid storage disorder. Interruption, or cessation, of normal development is generally the earliest indication of disorder. While delayed development is an expected occurrence, normal development following early brain insult may reflect absence of damage or natural compensatory activity (St. James-Roberts 1979).

Maturational level affects every aspect of neuropsychological evaluation: the range of behaviors that can be assessed; the choice of test instruments; the evaluation of success or failure on any one behavioral measure; the evaluation of a child's test performance, independent of group considerations; and the choice of therapeutic options. Maturational level also complicates the assessment of treatment outcome, since one must attempt to ascertain whether a positive outcome is due solely to an effective intervention or is confounded by normal age-appropriate maturational changes occurring during the treatment period. Evaluating a changing, developing nervous system is an intricate endeavor. But the dynamic change associated with maturation is what makes clinical evaluation so interesting. "The art in child assessment is to separate effects due to cognitive impairment from those that reflect normal but immature function" (Dennis 1979, p. 575).

Children vary widely in the age at which they achieve developmental milestones. Variability across age ranges may therefore be quite difficult to interpret. Skill acquisition late in the normal range of development may be perfectly appropriate, or it may be a marker of pathological delay. In clinical evaluation, one must consider each skill separately and in relation to the child's acquisition of other skills. For example, while one child may walk independently at 9 months of age, another may not take independent steps until 15 months. One child's first word may be spoken at 10 months of age, while another may not clearly utter a single word until 14 months of age. In these examples, all four children fall within normal limits. More importantly, it would be erroneous to conclude, based on these single observations, that the later-maturing child is developmentally delayed.

To distinguish normal from abnormal development, one must often assess a wide range of behaviors. A behavioral screening carries the risk of omitting essential data, especially since loss of function may not be present. The range of normal variation, in context with behavioral variables (such as interest, attention, or fatigue), may render extensive behavioral sampling necessary. Additionally, a test that reliably assesses one type of psychological process in adults may not assess the same process in a child (Reed 1984). For example, the presence of a moderate number of left-sided tactile imperception errors may suffice to implicate right parietal lobe dysfunction in an adult. On the other hand, this error profile may occur in some normal children, or it may indicate momentary attentional lapses, anxiety about being touched while eyes are closed, general resistance to the testing process, or fatigue. By administering additional measures to "back up" brain function hypotheses, one may more confidently draw conclusions about the significance of a single result.

It may be difficult to conclude that a child's behavior is abnormal. For example, an adult's failure to inhibit perseveratory responses is a classic sign of abnormality. Yet the ability to inhibit attention to irrelevant stimuli and perseveratory responses is not completed until nearly 10 years of age, with mastery generally achieved by 12 years (Passler, Isaac & Hynd 1985). The boundaries of acceptable responding may be difficult to clarify in a child whose chronological age matches the outside age limit for normal specific skill maturation. Moreover, statistical boundaries of normality are often wider for children than for adults, as reflected by large standard deviations for particular test scores.

Cognitive skills evolve with maturity, resulting in age-linked strategic differences in the way a person accomplishes a behavior. For example, at different ages children have different strategies for encoding and retrieving information to be remembered (Kail 1984; Schneider & Pressley 1988). It is not until about age 11 years that children utilize mnemonic strategies such as semantic grouping in rehearsal or recall (Kail 1984). Therefore, failure to encode information semantically is a normal finding in younger children, but it may be evidence of disorder in adolescents and adults.

Potential for Brain Reorganization

Behavioral plasticity and the capacity for brain reorganization following childhood lesions are unparalleled. Various explanations for this have been proposed. One early psychological theory emphasized the capacity for the formation or substitution of new strategies to enable successful accomplishment of a task (Hebb 1949; Kennard 1942). Physiological explanations have also been offered. These include reinnervation of denervated neurons by regenerating axons or by the proliferation of axon collaterals; development of supersensitivity of deafferentated neurons, which compensates for the loss of presynaptic elements; and *diaschisis*—the finding of depressed functioning in related (but intact) neural regions distal from a lesion site, which eventually recover and return to normality (Goldman & Lewis 1978).

One interesting explanation of the capacity for plasticity is offered by Bjorklund and Green (1992). They suggest that children's immature cognitive systems demand more effortful, rather than automatic, mental processing. In their view, this inefficient processing may be the most important factor in intellectual plasticity. Reduced automaticity of processing protects the child from acquiring cognitive patterns that may be disadvantageous when the child grows older. Cognitive flexibility is maintained by an immature nervous system, which with age develops more automatic mental operations. In this way, "lessons learned as a young child will not interfere with the qualitatively different tasks required of the adult" (p. 50).

Children do have an enormous capacity for preserving function in the face of catastrophic brain injury. It may be a mistake, however, to assume that early brain damage is less impairing than later damage or that intact areas are always capable of taking over functions from damaged areas in the young brain (Isaacson 1975). Major neurological insult in childhood may be followed by considerable (and often rapid) but not necessarily complete cognitive recovery. The effects of brain damage may not become fixed or static until years after an injury (Stein, Finger & Hart 1983). Although it has been suggested that, with comparable site, type, and severity of injury, an adult and a child suffer equally (Robinson 1981), parallel improvement for an adult with a similar neurological insult is unexpected, and resulting patterns of impairment are less consistent in children than in adults (Thal et al. 1991). For example, milder linguistic deficits rather than frank aphasic clinical syndromes may result after early brain injury (Aram 1988), and lesion size may have an insignificant effect on linguistic development (Thal et al. 1991).

Cognitive deficits associated with lateralized brain insult are generally less specific in children than in adults (Rutter 1982). Actual expression of deficit may therefore be very different (St. James-Roberts 1979) or may be a transient occurrence. For example, acute aphasia following head injury is unusual in children and resolves rapidly when present. It is therefore rarely witnessed. Lateralized lesions involving cortical language areas may result in relatively minor impairment or no impairment at all (Stein, Finger & Hart 1983). They may only be manifested as poorer functioning on general tests, such as on IQ measures. Milner (1974) suggested that this is due to "crowding" of verbal and nonverbal functions in the unaffected (that is, right) hemisphere.

Judgments about integrity must be made for all aspects of a child's behavioral repertoire. Childhood brain damage may be expressed in a wide spectrum of behavior, however, ranging from subtle delay to overt abnormality. Such variability complicates efforts to determine etiology and to assess deficits. Symptoms of childhood brain injury often do not fall readily within classically defined categories of impairment, and they may differ from expectations based on adult models. For example, left posterior cortical lesions suffered prenatally or within the first 6 months of life resulted in slower rates of recovery from expressive delays but did not affect lexical comprehension when the children were between 12 and 35 months of age (Thal et al. 1991). Aphasia symptoms may appear as a generalized inability to speak rather than as a circumscribed language deficit (Isaacson 1975). A child may exhibit delayed speech development rather than a classic aphasic disorder as a consequence of a brain insult (Woods & Carey 1979), but similar speech delay may be noted in children for whom there is no identifiable etiology. Therefore, one must consider the possibility that the child's speech represents normal variability in rate of development.

Deficit detection may require timely, astute observation. For example, the presence of neglect may be missed unless very early post-injury evaluation occurs (Ferro & Martins 1990). Recovery may follow a radically different clinical course in children than in adults. Children with severe head trauma and prolonged coma may make significant recovery (Mahoney et al. 1983). Hemispherectomy or lobectomy in childhood is associated with fewer behavioral manifestations than in adults (Dennis 1980b; Dennis, Lovett & Weigel-Crump 1981; Gott 1973; Smith & Sugar 1975). Inferences about the functional plasticity of the remaining hemisphere remain tentative, however, since it may not be anatomically intact (Strauss & Verity 1983).

Evidence of full or nearly full recovery after early left hemisphere damage supports hypotheses of neural plasticity of the young brain. Thal et al. (1991) studied infants with focal brain injury and found delayed lexical development in comprehension and production, supporting the left hemisphere's role in language acquisition at the very earliest ages. A "holistic" approach to language learning—one often associated with a slower rate of language learning—was also documented and was interpreted as suggesting a right hemispheric learning style. While it is believed that the right hemisphere can (albeit less efficiently) mediate language in a young child who has sustained left hemisphere damage, the circumstances under which this adaptation of the young brain may occur are not yet well understood.

Differences in Diagnosis and Clinical Presentation

Differences in diagnosis and in the clinical presentation of neurological insult in children and adults are readily apparent. For example, cortical brain tumors are less common and posterior fossa tumors are more common in children. While gradual cognitive or psychiatric changes may be an early indication of brain tumors in adults, childhood brain tumors are more likely to present acutely—for example, with sudden headache, nausea, and vomiting. Seizure disorders in childhood often exist in isolation from other pathology, whereas adult onset seizures are generally an early symptom of another pathological process, although they occasionally are idiopathic. The seizure type may change with increasing chronological age in childhood, but adult onset seizures are generally unchanging. Cognitive deterioration is less likely to be a stated reason for referral in childhood, as compared to adult-initiated complaints of memory and cognitive change, although children do lose or fail to develop abilities as a result of progressive conditions such as hydrocephalus and degenerative storage diseases. Developmental delay, learning difficulties, or social immaturity may be the first indication of a neurological problem in a child, rather than symptom self-report as is common in adults.

Behavioral Variability in Assessment

There is potential for extreme intraindividual behavioral variability in pediatric assessment. A child may be emotionally ill-equipped to face the many fearful circumstances associated with the medical setting. Attentional capacity may be quite variable. The timing of an assessment may affect results, since many children respond best early in the day. Fatigue may complicate later performances. The results of tests conducted close to the usual nap time may also be affected. Multiple test sessions are often necessary. Different time samples often reveal different facets of a child's behavior, and these may differ in the home, at school, and in the hospital.

A lack of premorbid data is limiting. Oral birth and developmental histories may be the only information available for infants and toddlers, while academic records may be helpful with school-age children. Children should be encouraged to describe changes from premorbid functioning in their own words. Even young children who have suffered a neurologic insult may be able to offer valuable anecdotes. Pediatric assessment and behavioral sampling methods are discussed in Chapter 5.

Limitations of Brain–Behavior Rules

Prediction rules based on adult models often fail to transfer successfully to the pediatric population because of the additional dynamic aspects of change with maturation, the potential for cerebral reorganization following neurological insult, and the potential for delayed expression of effects. Delayed expression of an insult is well documented in animal research (Goldman & Galkin 1978) and is particularly relevant in pediatric neuropsychology (Eslinger et al. 1992; Grattan & Eslinger 1991) (see Chapter 2). Abnormal development may not be clinically manifested until the child must engage in a behavior that depends on the affected neurological substrate. The elapsed time from insult to behavioral expression may be lengthy. For example, injury to prefrontal regions may not be expressed until those brain systems are in ascendancy.

Since sophisticated brain-imaging techniques have reduced the role of neuropsychology in brain lesion localization, and since rules for localizing cerebral function in adults are generally not applicable to children, it is often better to focus on the child's behavior than on the presumptive brain region involved. Emphasis is best placed on more meaningful data collection, to understand the child's profile of strengths and weaknesses and to plan for needed treatment interventions. For example, conceptual sorting performance is highly correlated with anterior cerebral function in adults (Drewe 1974; Milner 1963; Nelson 1976), although this correlation is not exclusive (Anderson et al. 1991) and may not apply to children. While the performance of a child as young as 10 years of age parallels that of a normal adult (Chelune & Baer 1986), one cannot infer that a young child's inability to respond to this measure adequately is proof of frontal lobe pathology, nor would such a distinction be a necessary antecedent to planning appropriate intervention. The behaviors of concern— failure to shift ideas in response to feedback, and failure to generate new hypotheses—may require additional evaluation to permit finer partitioning of the reason for failure on this executive function measure.

To understand brain–behavior relationships in children, one must also critically consider variables that do not complicate the interpretation of test performance by adults. For example, a conclusion of impairment in a 3-year-old who stutters may be erroneous, since this symptom can be merely a developmental phenomenon. Stuttering is known to be a developmentally normal occurrence between the ages of $1\frac{1}{2}$ to 6 years (Guitar 1988). Similarly, expectations about impulsivity or attentional variability change with chronological age. Behaviors considered normal for a 2-year-old are considered abnormal in a 6-year-old.

Environmental, Personality, and Psychosocial Factors

The influences of environmental, psychosocial, and personality factors require consideration. Recovery of function following early brain injury may depend on opportunities for environmental stimulation (Goldman & Lewis 1978). Isaacson (1975) noted that "the behavior of the individual is not specifiable unless the factors of the immediate environment are taken into consideration" (p. 15). The influence of social and environmental factors on cognitive function may be stronger in children than in adults (Plomin 1989), and it may confound the assessment of sequelae of brain insult (Taylor et al. 1991). Important environmental and social factors include exposure to a wide range of stimulating circumstances and educational opportunities (Cahan & Cohen 1989), the presence of siblings (Breslau & Prabucki 1987; Sines 1987), socioeconomic status (Taylor et al. 1990; Waber et al. 1981; Waber et al. 1984), and cultural influences and psychosocial stressors (Breslau 1990; Perrott, Taylor & Montes 1991). As Fletcher and Taylor (1984) pointed out, "failure to carefully acknowledge the social context in which a child performs as well as other factors influencing test performance and behavior may lead to simplistic hypotheses concerning the relationship between behavior and the CNS" (p. 48).

RECENT DEVELOPMENTS IN PEDIATRIC NEUROPSYCHOLOGY

Psychological measurement and evaluation techniques for children have changed considerably in a relatively brief period of time. At one time, global measures or single psychological constructs such as intelligence were relied upon as indications of a child's capacity (Gardner 1983); later, a core battery approach emerged. In early child studies, a single test score proved less reliable as a discriminator between normal and brain-injured children than scores combined from a battery of tests (Ernhart et al. 1963). Strict proponents of the latter approach advocated administering a specific group of tests to each child, independent of observations made during the course of the test session. Unfortunately, this approach often proved insensitive to the individualized concerns raised in referral (Hammeke, Golden & Purisch 1978). The limitations of a strict battery approach became more evident over time. Issues arose in clinical practice in relation to specific children or to groups of children diagnosed with a particular medical condition, and these rendered continued exclusive reliance on batteries unproductive. For example, head-injured children were seriously underaddressed by test batteries that did not sample new learning and memory sufficiently. Modifications to include more diverse tests and to allow procedural variations helped neuropsychologists explore how and when a child could demonstrate accomplishment. This flexible approach is much more practical and efficient in the medical setting.

New Instrumentation

Areas of neuropsychological functioning that were not regularly investigated in the early years of pediatric neuropsychology are now more likely to be considered. For example, measures of attention and vigilance, sensory processing, executive functioning, new learning, memory, social skills, and affective recognition are now available. These instruments permit exploration of more diverse aspects of behavior. They were developed and incorporated in response to the need to explain a child's behavior more fully in order to make appropriate management recommendations. Of course, the current armamentarium of tests still may not fully measure the diverse ways brain disease or injury can affect a child's cognitive capacities (Taylor & Schatschneider 1992; Welsh & Pennington 1988). Nor can we be entirely confident of our ability to analyze existing data fully for all that they might reveal about the brain's development and functioning.

Neuroradiological Advances

Newer brain-imaging and psychophysiological techniques have expanded our knowledge about anatomy and metabolic functioning, thereby directly affecting pediatric neuropsychology. Recourse to subgroups defined by neuroradiological examinations may lead to better understanding of an observed deficit or absence of deficit. For example, the identification of localized pre- or perinatal left cerebral hemisphere lesions allows for prospective longitudinal study of language development (Thal et al. 1991). Computed tomography and magnetic resonance imaging, positron emission tomography, single-photon emission computed tomography, ultrasound for newborns, brain mapping techniques, video electroencephalograms, Wada testing for presurgical language dominance determination, cerebral blood flow studies, and other state-of-the-art medical diagnostic techniques are now available for children. Given the costs, risks, and procedural limitations associated with many of these techniques (for instance, sedation), however, some newer technologies have not been systematically applied to childhood diagnosis. While laboratory techniques may help to define better the presence, location, and extent or type of lesion, neuropsychological data remain the best source of information about the effects of lesions on behavior.

Data Profiles and Error Analysis

The evolution away from rigid testing strategies has favored approaches that emphasize flexibility, maximize opportunity in time-limited behavioral sampling, and focus on specific behaviors of concern. The analysis of test profiles permits more sophisticated descriptions of function and dysfunction, with both quantitative and qualitative features of performance considered. Profiles are being elaborated for more discrete aspects of neuropsychological function and more homogeneous clinical subgroups.

For example, the classical neuropsychological profile of a child with hydrocephalus includes lower-than-average overall general intelligence, weaker visuoperceptual/visuospatial functioning than verbal functioning, pronounced motor and tactual-motor deficiency, variable ability to encode and store factual information normally, variable attentional skills, poor self-image, and social immaturity. This classical profile fails to delineate fully the qualitative features in motor control that affect nonverbal test performance—for instance, the ability to respond rapidly and to manipulate stimuli actively. Conclusions about a global nonverbal, visuospatial deficit are best deferred until pure motor function has been evaluated independent of visuoconceptual, motor planning, and visuospatial skill and until time constraints are adjusted. Such delineation aids in planning rehabilitative strategies (Baron & Goldberger 1993; see Chapter 7).

Questions about what function a test measures, whether a test measures similar functions in adults and children, and when one may conclude that a difference in performances on the same test taken at different times indicates a deficit are beginning to be answered. For example, Halperin et al. (1989) gave children aged 6 to 12 years old the Peabody Picture Vocabulary Test—Revised (PPVT-R) and collected developmental normative data on tests of verbal naming, retrieval, and memory—that is, on the Boston Naming Test (BNT), on paired associate learning (PAL), and on verbal fluency. They found three distinct cognitive or linguistic functions. They found fluency minimally related to vocabulary and verbal memory. Children's PAL performance was comparable to that of adults by 9 years of age, and the test assessed verbal memory with little variance accounted for by linguistic abilities. A high correlation between BNT and PPVT-R scores suggested that word knowledge—not retrieval or fluency, as in adults—was the critical basis for a child's inability to respond well to BNT phonemic cues. Their data suggest that a discrepancy between these two tests may usefully identify a learning-disability subtype.

Error analysis provides sensitive descriptions of neurobehavioral functioning. Knowledge of normal child development is necessary to utilize an error analysis approach. Errors may be categorized initially as belonging to one of two types. The first type is developmental error indicative of immaturity of function. Errors of this type are part of normal performance for a younger child. For example, a child may draw small circles in place of dots until the child's fine motor development becomes sufficiently mature to permit the production of discrete dots. This error differs substantially from errors of the second type: those suggestive of neurological abnormality, independent of age. Errors of the second type are unlikely to be made by a normally developing child, even at a younger age; their very presence, therefore, suggests neurologic impairment. For example, a child may draw a row of dots accurately, but in 90-degree rotation. This response is not a typical immature performance and thus suggests neuropsychological dysfunction. As a "red flag" for perceptual dysfunction, it should signal the need for further exploration to determine its significance and the extent and nature of any nonverbal impairment.

Such distinctions may be made in all behavioral domains. For example, certain language errors are typically observed in younger children—for example, the "baby talk" common to young children. Omission of articles, substitution of incorrect sounds, and omission or substitution of phonemes generally lessen in frequency and eventually disappear with maturation. But persistence of immature speech beyond the uppermost ages acceptable for acquiring mature language use should not be attributed to developmental immaturity, since it may be a significant neurological marker; the situation demands further investigation. Indeed, one must remain hesitant to accept aberrant behavioral patterns as instances of developmental variation.

Since developmental errors may indicate pathology, one must know the age at which a specific behavior ceases to be developmentally appropriate and to fall within normal limits, and at which that behavior may instead indicate dysfunction, exceeding the bounds of developmental variability. Tables or charts of normative data are helpful for distinguishing normality from pathology, as is the internal sense of normal variability that the clinician develops over time. Nonetheless, adjustments must be made for individual circumstances related to environment, growth, and development. Tables may fall short when these variables interact. For example, in assessing a child from a bilingual home environment, one may have to reconsider the boundaries of acceptable linguistic acquisition—for instance, when a language delay is noted for a language spoken only minimally in the home.

Qualitative features may suggest brain function hypotheses that would not have been made on the basis of quantitative data alone. Tests that evolve from clinical experience but do not meet criteria for standardized assessment may yield critical information. Informal measures designed to test a specific hypothesis may be very useful when they are repeated over multiple test sessions. For example, consider a child with surgically corrected hydrocephalus who has maintained stable IQ scores over time, has demonstrated age-appropriate academic progress, and has an unchanged MRI scan, suggesting physiological and developmental stability. Nonetheless, motor changes have been detected recently on nonstandardized instruments: compared to results of prior testing, handwriting was enlarged, letters were less well-formed, and clumsiness and balance problems were evident; sporadic headaches, more days of inexplicable behavioral variability, and greater difficulty retaining new information have also been reported. A possibility of shunt failure had to be considered, notwithstanding the stability noted on global tests with solid psychometric properties (Baron et al. 1983).

Expanded Medical Populations

Certain populations of children have been of interest to pediatric neuropsychologists in medical settings because their conditions have a direct impact on neurological and neuropsychological functioning. Research on children with neurological disorders initially focused on intelligence and academic achievement, but it has gradually expanded to include more comprehensive neuropsychological assessment. Often referred by neurologists and neurosurgeons, these cases include epilepsy (Hermann & Seidenberg 1989; see Chapter 8), head trauma (Chadwick et al. 1981; Ewing-Cobbs et al. 1987; Goldstein & Levin 1985; Levin et al. 1982; see Chapter 9), hydrocephalus (Dennis et al. 1987; Donders, Rourke & Canady 1991; Fletcher et al. 1992; Hammock, Milhorat & Baron 1976; Prigatano et al. 1983; Zeiner & Prigatano 1982; see Chapter 7), cerebral neoplasms (Ellenberg et al. 1987; see Chapter 10), cerebral palsy (see Chapter 3), meningitis (Taylor et al. 1990), and vascular accidents (Dennis 1980*a*).

Research on certain childhood populations referred mainly by psychiatrists has also been extensive. Children diagnosed as having autism, conduct disorder, attention deficit disorder, and somatoform disorders often are considered appropriate referrals to a neuropsychology service (see Chapter 13).

More recently, interest in the neuropsychological problems of other inpatient populations has grown. These referrals do not originate primarily from neurological, neurosurgical, or psychiatric units. Rather, an increasing awareness of the impact of systemic illness on the developing central nervous system has led to the delineation of neuropsychological concomitants of diseases that do not primarily involve the central nervous system. The effects of these medical illnesses and their treatment regimens have been an important new focus. Children with malnutrition (Hoorweg & Stanfield 1976); chronic medical illnesses, including metabolic, endocrine, cardiac (see Chapter 11), infectious, pulmonary, and renal disorders (see Chapter 12); neurotoxic conditions, including in utero exposures (Pérez-Arce et al. 1989); low birthweight (Vohr & Garcia Coll 1985; see Chapter 3); and conditions requiring extracorporeal membrane oxygenation (ECMO) (Culbert et al. 1989) or organ transplantation (Stewart et al. 1991) are populations of growing interest to researchers.

Studies that have increased our understanding of the neurobehavioral effects of nonneurological conditions and treatments are multiplying. These conditions include phenylketonuria (Brunner et al. 1983; Welsh et al. 1990), hypothyroidism (Rovet 1992), hormone insufficiency (Gearing et al. 1992), asthma (Bender 1992), diabetes (Northam et al. 1992; Rovet et al. 1988; Ryan et al. 1984), renal failure (Davidovicz et al. 1981; Fennell et al. 1984; Morris et al. 1985), human immunodeficiency virus (Brouwers et al. 1992), leukemia (Copeland et al. 1985; Eiser 1978; Eiser & Lansdown 1977; Brouwers et al. 1984), Duchenne muscular dystrophy (Sollee et al. 1985), lead exposure (de la Burdé & Choate 1975; Needleman et al. 1979; Needleman & Gatsonis 1990), and bone marrow transplantation for CNS degenerative storage diseases (Shapiro et al. 1992).

Prospective Study

Prospective, longitudinal assessment may provide the best opportunity to understand the developmental course in the presence of congenital or acquired brain dysfunction. Serial study enables one to monitor the developmental impact of an illness and of medical, rehabilitative, and educational interventions. Early studies of head-injured children (Klonoff & Paris 1974) and of groups of medically ill children, such as those with leukemia and other cancers (see review by Fletcher & Copeland 1988) had a strong impact on medical and surgical treatment protocols. These studies helped establish the usefulness of longitudinal neuropsychological evaluations for the medical and psychological management of a child.

Although it is a valuable traditional approach, retrospective data collection may not hold the most promise for the study of the developing brain. Prospective studies are likely to yield greater understanding of the outcome parameters related to early neurological insult. Nevertheless, there are important differences between experimental and clinical neuropsychological longitudinal studies of children. Many longitudinal studies have a particular investigative focus and consequently explore some but not all possible clinical variables of interest—for example, memory (Levin et al. 1988) or language development (Aram et al. 1985). In contrast, the clinician who follows a child longitudinally may change tests in order to sharpen the examination of problems that emerge over time. Thus, there may be limits to the clinical utility of data derived from either approach. The first uses test protocols with restricted batteries and, therefore, produces restricted information; the second has a changing database, which complicates comparisons across tests. The pediatric neuropsychologist must be familiar with these differences in sources of clinical information when predicting outcome for a child with medical illness.

CONCLUSION

The neuropsychology of normally and abnormally developing brains is a rapidly expanding field. The pediatric neuropsychologist in the medical setting has a unique opportunity to contribute to children's overall well-being and care, as well as to research. A medically ill child represents a special challenge for neuropsychological assessment. To meet this challenge, the pediatric neuropsychologist must assume multiple roles within the medical setting: evaluator, teacher, advocate, caregiver, researcher, community resources liaison, and medical team member.

REFERENCES

Anderson, S. W.; Damasio, H.; Jones, R. D.; and Tranel, D. 1991. Wisconsin Card Sorting Test performance as a measure of frontal lobe damage. *Journal of Clinical and Experimental Neuropsychology* 13: 909–22.

Aram, D. 1988. Language sequelae of unilateral brain lesions in children. In F. Plum (ed.), *Language, Communication, and the Brain* (New York: Raven Press), pp. 171–97.

Aram, D.; Ekelman, B.; Rose, D.; and Whitaker, H. 1985. Verbal and cognitive sequelae following unilateral lesions acquired in early childhood. *Journal of Clinical and Experimental Neuropsychology* 7: 55–78.

Baron, I. S., and Goldberger, E. 1993. Neuropsychological disturbances of hydrocephalic children with implications for special education and rehabilitation. *Neuropsychological Rehabilitation* 3: 389–410.

Baron, I. S.; Hammock, M. K.; Milhorat, T. H.; and McCullough, D. C. 1983. Neuropsychological evaluation following surgical intervention for ventriculomegaly in childhood. Paper presented at the Sixth European Meeting of the International Neuropsychological Society, Lisbon, Portugal.

Bender, B. G. 1992. Neuropsychological change associated with Theophylline treatment of asthmatic children. *Journal of Clinical and Experimental Neuropsychology* 14: 112.

Bjorklund, D. F., and Green, B. L. 1992. The adaptive nature of cognitive immaturity. *American Psychologist* 47: 46–54.

Bornstein, R. A.; King, G.; and Carroll, A. 1983. Neuropsychological abnormalities in Gilles de la Tourette's syndrome. *Journal of Nervous and Mental Disease* 171: 497–502.

Breslau, N. 1990. Does brain dysfunction increase children's vulnerability to environmental stress? *Archives of General Psychiatry* 47: 15–20.

Breslau, N., and Prabucki, K. 1987. Siblings of disabled children. *Archives of General Psychiatry* 44: 1040–46.

Brouwers, P.; Moss, H.; Wolters, P.; El-Amin, D.; Tassone, E.; and Pizzo, P. 1992. Neurobehavioral typology of school-age children with symptomatic HIV disease. *Journal of Clinical and Experimental Neuropsychology* 14: 113.

Brouwers, P.; Riccardi, R.; Poplack, D.; and Fedio, P. 1984. Attentional deficits in long-term survivors of childhood acute lymphoblastic leukemia. *Journal of Clinical Neuropsychology* 6: 325–36.

Brunner, R. L.; Jordan, M. K.; and Berry, H. K. 1983. Early-treated phenylketonuria: Neuropsychologic consequences. *Journal of Pediatrics* 102: 831–35.

Cahan, S., and Cohen, N. 1989. Age versus schooling effects on intelligence development. *Child Development* 60: 1239–49.

Chadwick, O.; Rutter, M.; Brown, G.; Shaffer, D.; and Traub, M. 1981. A prospective study of children with head injuries: II. Cognitive sequelae. *Psychological Medicine* 11: 49–61.

Chelune, G. J., and Baer, R. A. 1986. Developmental norms for the Wisconsin Card Sorting Test. *Journal of Clinical and Experimental Neuropsychology* 8: 219–28.

Copeland, D. R.; Fletcher, J. M.; Pfefferbaum-Levine, B.; Jaffe, N.; Ried, H.; and Maor, M. 1985. Neuropsychological sequelae of childhood cancer in long-term survivors. *Pediatrics* 75: 745–53.

Culbert, J. P.; Mueller, D.; & Hamer, R.; 1989. Long-term neuropsychological assessment following right carotid artery ligation in the neonate. Paper presented at the Seventeenth Annual Meeting of the International Neuropsychological Society, Vancover, Canada.

Davidovicz, H.; Iacoviello, J.; and McVicar, M. 1981. Cognitive functions in children on chronic intermittent hemodialysis. *Pediatric Research* 15: 692.

de la Burdé, B., and Choate, M. S. 1975. Early asymptomatic lead exposure and development at school age. *Journal of Pediatrics* 87: 638–42.

Dennis, M. 1979. Neuropsychological assessment. In J. Noshpitz et al. (eds.), *Basic Handbook of Child Psychiatry*, vol. 1 (New York: Basic Books), pp. 574–83.

Dennis, M. 1980a. Strokes in childhood: I. Communication intent, expression, and comprehension after left hemisphere arteriopathy in a right-handed nine-year-old. In R. W. Rieber (ed.), *Language Development and Aphasia in Children* (New York: Academic Press), pp. 45–67.

———. 1980b. Capacity and strategy for syntactic comprehension after left or right hemidecortication. *Brain and Language* 10: 287–317.

Dennis, M.; Hendrick, E. B.; Hoffman, H. J.; and Humphreys, R. P. 1987. Language of hydrocephalic children and adolescents. *Journal of Clinical and Experimental Neuropsychology* 9: 593–621.

Dennis, M.; Lovett, M.; and Wiegel-Crump, C. A. 1981. Written language acquisition after left or right hemidecortication in infancy. *Brain and Language* 12: 54–91.

Dennis, M., and Whitaker, H. A. 1976. Language acquisition following hemidecortication: Linguistic superiority of the left over the right hemisphere. *Brain and Language* 3: 404–33.

Donders, J.; Rourke, B. P.; and Canady, A. I. 1991. Neuropsychological functioning of hydrocephalic children. *Journal of Clinical and Experimental Neuropsychology* 13: 607–13.

Drewe, E. A. 1974. The effect of type and area of brain lesion on Wisconsin Card Sorting Test performance. *Cortex* 10: 159–70.

Eiser, C. 1978. Intellectual abilities among survivors of childhood leukemia as a function of CNS irradiation. *Archives of Disease in Childhood* 55: 766–70.

Eiser, C., and Lansdown, R. 1977. Retrospective study of intellectual development in children treated for acute lymphoblastic leukemia. *Archives of Disease in Childhood* 52: 525–29.

Ellenberg, L.; McComb, J. G.; Siegel, S. E.; and Stowe, S. 1987. Factors affecting cognitive outcome in pediatric brain tumor patients. *Neurosurgery* 21: 638–44.

Ernhart, C. B.; Graham, F. K.; Eichman, P. L.; Marshall, J. M.; and Thurstone, D. 1963. Brain injury in the preschool child: Some developmental considerations: II. Comparison of brain-injured and normal children. *Psychological Monographs* 11: 17–33.

Eslinger, P. J.; Grattan, L. M.; Damasio, H.; and Damasio, A. R. 1992. Developmental consequences of childhood frontal lobe damage. *Archives of Neurology* 49: 764–69.

Ewing-Cobbs, L.; Levin, H. S.; Eisenberg, H. M.; and Fletcher, J. M. 1987. Language functions following closed-head injury in children and adolescents. *Journal of Clinical and Experimental Neuropsychology* 9: 593–621.

Fennell, R. S.; Rasbury, W. C.; Fennell, E. B.; and Morris, M. K. 1984. The effects of kidney transplantation on cognitive performance in a pediatric population. *Pediatrics* 74: 273–78.

Ferro, J. M., and Martins, I. P. 1990. Some new aspects of neglect in children. *Behavioural Neurology* 3: 1–6.

Fletcher, J. M., and Copeland, D. R. 1988. Neurobehavioral effects of central nervous system prophylactic treatment of cancer in children. *Journal of Clinical and Experimental Neuropsychology* 10: 495–538.

Fletcher, J.; Francis, D. J.; Thompson, N. M.; Brookshire, B. L.; Bohan, T. P.; Landry, S. H.; Davidson, K. C.; and Miner, M. E. 1992. Verbal and nonverbal skill discrepancies in hydrocephalic children. *Journal of Clinical and Experimental Neuropsychology* 14: 593–609.

Fletcher, J. M., and Taylor, H. G. 1984. Neuropsychological approaches to children:

Towards a developmental neuropsychology. *Journal of Clinical Neuropsychology* 6: 39–56.

Gardner, H. 1983. *Frames of Mind: The Theory of Multiple Intelligences.* New York: Basic Books.

Gearing, M. A.; Kalin, G.; Rose, S.; Small, B.; Kamp, G.; and Mohr, E. 1992. Neuropsychological consequences of insufficient sex hormone exposure at adolescence. *Journal of Clinical and Experimental Neuropsychology* 14: 113.

Goldman, P. S., and Galkin, T. W. 1978. Prenatal removal of frontal association cortex in the rhesus monkey: Anatomical and functional consequences in postnatal life. *Brain Research* 152: 451–85.

Goldman, P. S., and Lewis, M. 1978. Developmental biology of brain damage and experience. In C. W. Cotman (ed.), *Neuronal Plasticity* (New York: Raven Press), pp. 291–310.

Goldstein, F., and Levin, H. S. 1985. Intellectual and academic outcome following closed head injury in children and adolescents: Research strategies and empirical findings. *Developmental Neuropsychology* 1: 195–214.

Gott, P. S. 1973. Cognitive abilities following right and left hemispherectomy. *Cortex* 9: 266–74.

Grattan, L. M., and Eslinger, P. J. 1991. Frontal lobe damage in children and adults: A comparative review. *Developmental Neuropsychology* 7: 283–326.

Guitar, B. E., 1988. Is it stuttering or just normal language development? *Contemporary Pediatrics* 2: 109–25

Halperin, J. M.; Healey, J. M.; Zeitchik, E.; Ludman, W. L.; and Weinstein, L. 1989. Developmental aspects of linguistic and mnestic abilities in normal children. *Journal of Clinical and Experimental Neuropsychology* 11: 518–28.

Hammeke, T. A.; Golden, C. J.; and Purisch, A. D. 1978. A standardized, short, and comprehensive neuropsychological test battery based on the Luria neuropsychological evaluation. *International Journal of Neuroscience* 8: 135–41.

Hammock, M. K.; Milhorat, T. H.; and Baron, I. S. 1976. Normal pressure hydrocephalus in patients with myelomeningocele. *Developmental Medicine and Child Neurology* Suppl. 37: 55–68.

Hebb, D. O. 1949. *The Organization of Behavior.* New York: Wiley.

Hermann, B. P., and Seidenberg, M., eds. 1989. *Childhood Epilepsies: Neuropsychological, Psychosocial and Intervention Aspects.* New York: Wiley.

Hoorweg, J., and Stanfield, J. P. 1976. The effects of protein energy malnutrition in early childhood on intellectual and motor abilities in later childhood and adolescence. *Developmental Medicine and Child Neurology* 18: 330–50.

Incagnoli, T., and Kane, R. 1981. Neuropsychological functioning in Gilles de la Tourette's syndrome. *Journal of Clinical Neuropsychology* 3: 165–69.

Isaacson, R. L. 1975. The myth of recovery from early brain damage. In N. E. Ellis (ed.), *Aberrant Development in Infancy* (New York: Wiley), pp. 1–26.

Kail, R. V. 1984. *The Development of Memory in Children,* 2d ed. San Francisco: Freeman.

Kennard, M. 1942. Cortical reorganization of motor function: Studies on a series of monkeys of various ages from infancy to maturity. *Archives of Neurology and Psychiatry* 48: 227–40.

Klonoff, H.; Low, M.; and Clark, C. 1977. Head injuries in children with a prospective five-year follow-up. *Journal of Neurology, Neurosurgery and Psychiatry* 40: 1211–19.

Klonoff, H., and Paris, R. 1974. Immediate, short-term and residual effects of acute head injuries in children: Neuropsychological and neurological correlates. In R. M. Reitan and L. A. Davison (eds.), *Clinical Neuropsychology: Current Status and Applications* (Washington, D.C.: V. H. Winston), pp. 179–210.

Levin, H. S.; Eisenberg, H. M.; Wigg, N. R.; and Kobayashi, K. 1982. Memory and intellectual ability after head injury in children and adolescents. *Neurosurgery* 11: 668–73.

Levin, H. S.; High, W. M. Jr.; Ewing-Cobbs, L.; Fletcher, J. M.; Eisenberg, H. M.; Miner, M. C.; and Goldstein, F. C. 1988. Memory functioning during the first year after closed head injury in children and adolescents. *Neurosurgery* 22: 1043–52.

Mahoney, W. J.; D'Souza, B. J.; Haller, J. A.; Rogers, M. C.; Epstein, M. H.; and Freeman, J. M. 1983. Long-term outcome of children with severe head trauma and prolonged coma. *Pediatrics* 71: 756–62.

Milner, B. 1963. Effects of different brain lesions on card sorting. *Archives of Neurology* 9: 90–100.

———. 1974. Hemispheric specialization: Scope and limits. In F. O. Schmitt and F. G. Worden (eds.), *The Neurosciences: Third Study Program* (Cambridge, Mass.: MIT Press), pp. 75–89.

Morris, M. K.; Fennell, E. B.; Fennell, R. S.; and Rasbury, W. C. 1985. A case study of identical twins discordant for renal failure: Long-term neuropsychological deficits. *Developmental Neuropsychology* 1: 81–92.

Needleman, H. L., and Gatsonis, C. A. 1990. Low-level lead exposure and the IQ of children. *Journal of the American Medical Association* 263: 673–78.

Needleman, H. L.; Gummoe, C.; Leviton, A.; Reed, R.; Peresie, H.; Maher, C.; and Barrett, P. 1979. Deficits in psychologic and classroom performance of children with elevated dentine lead levels. *New England Journal of Medicine* 300: 689–95.

Nelson, H. E. 1976. A modified card sorting test sensitive to frontal lobe deficits. *Cortex* 12: 313–24.

Northam, E.; Bowden, S.; Anderson, V.; and Court, J. 1992. Neuropsychological functioning in adolescents with diabetes. *Journal of Clinical and Experimental Neuropsychology* 14: 884–900.

Passler, M.; Isaac, W.; and Hynd, G. W. 1985. Neuropsychological development of behavior attributed to frontal lobe functioning in children. *Developmental Neuropsychology* 4: 349–70.

Pérez-Arce, P.; Johnson, C. B.; Rauch, S.; Bowler, R. M.; and Mergler, D. 1989. Neuropsychological screening of 6- to 15-year-old children exposed to neurotoxins while in-utero. *Clinical Neuropsychologist* 3: 280.

Perrott, S. B.; Taylor, H. G.; and Montes, J. L. 1991. Neuropsychological sequelae, family stress, and environmental adaptation following pediatric head injury. *Developmental Neuropsychology* 7: 69–86.

Plomin, R. 1989. Environment and genes: Determinants of behavior. *American Psychologist* 44: 105–11.

Prigatano, G. P.; Zeiner, H.; Pollay, M.; and Kaplan, R. J. 1983. Neuropsychological functioning in children with shunted uncomplicated hydrocephalus. *Child's Brain* 10: 112–20.

Quart, E. J.; Buchtel, H. A.; and Sarnaik, A. P. 1988. Long-lasting memory deficits in children recovered from Reye's syndrome. *Journal of Clinical and Experimental Neuropsychology* 10: 409–20.

Reed, H. B. C. 1984. Pediatric Neuropsychology. In W. J. Burns & J. V. Lavigne (eds.), *Progress in Pediatric Psychology* (New York: Grune & Stratton), pp. 103–34.

Robinson, R. O. 1981. Equal recovery in child and adult brain? *Developmental Medicine and Child Neurology* 23: 379–82.

Rovet, J. 1992. The effect of neonatal thyroid hormone deficiency on motor development. *Journal of Clinical and Experimental Neuropsychology* 14: 113.

Rovet, J.; Ehrlich, R.; and Hoppe, M. 1988. Specific intellectual deficits in children with early onset diabetes mellitis. *Child Development* 59: 226–34.

Rutter, M. 1982. Developmental neuropsychiatry: Concepts, issues, and prospects. *Journal of Clinical Neuropsychology* 4: 91–115.

Ryan, C. M.; Vega, A.; Longstreet, C.; and Drash, A. 1984. Neuropsychological changes in adolescents with insulin-dependent diabetes. *Journal of Consulting and Clinical Psychology* 52: 335–42.

Schneider, W., and Pressley, M. 1988. *Memory Development Between 2 and 20.* New York: Springer-Verlag.

Shapiro, E. G., and Krivit, W. 1992. Adrenoleukodystrophy, a white matter degenerative disease of childhood: Neuropsychological characteristics and treatment with bone marrow transplantation. *Journal of Clinical and Experimental Neuropsychology* 14: 69.

Sines, J. O. 1987. Influence of the home and family environment on childhood dysfunction. In B. B. Lahey and A. E. Kazdin (eds.), *Advances in Clinical Child Psychology* (New York: Plenum Press), pp. 1–54.

Smith, A., and Sugar, O. 1975. Development of above normal language and intelligence 21 years after left hemispherectomy. *Neurology* 25: 813–18.

Sollee, N. D.; Latham, E. E.; Kindlon, D. J.; and Bresnan, M. J. 1985. Neuropsychological impairment in Duchenne Muscular Dystrophy. *Journal of Clinical and Experimental Neuropsychology* 7: 486–96.

Stein, D. G.; Finger, S.; and Hart, T. 1983. Brain damage and recovery: Problems and perspectives. *Behavioral and Neural Biology* 37: 185–222.

Stewart, S. M.; Silver, C. H.; Nici, J.; Waller, D.; Campbell, R.; Uauy, R.; and Andrews, W. S. 1991. Neuropsychological function in young children who have undergone liver transplantation. *Journal of Pediatric Psychology* 16: 569–83.

St. James-Roberts, I. 1979. Neurological plasticity, recovery from brain insult and child development. In H. W. Reese and L. Lipsett (eds.), *Advances in Child Development and Behavior* (New York: Academic Press), pp. 253–319.

Strauss, E., and Verity C. 1983. Effects of hemispherectomy in infantile hemiplegics. *Brain and Language* 20: 1–11.

Taylor, H. G.; Mills, E. L.; Ciampi, A.; DuBerger, R.; Watters, G. V.; Gold, R.; McDonald, N.; and Michaels, R. H. 1990. The sequelae of Haemophilus influenzae for school-age children. *New England Journal of Medicine* 323: 1657–63.

Taylor, H. G., and Schatschneider, C. 1992. Child neuropsychological assessment: A test of basic assumptions. *Clinical Neuropsychologist* 6: 259–75.

Taylor, H. G.; Schatschneider, C.; and Rich, D. 1991. Sequelae of Haemophilus Influenzae meningitis: Implications for the study of brain disease and development. In M. Tramontana and S. Hooper (eds.), *Advances in Child Neuropsychology*, vol. 1 (New York: Springer-Verlag), pp. 50–108.

Thal, D. J.; Marchman, V.; Stiles, J.; Aram, D.; Trauner, D.; Nass, R.; and Bates, E.

1991. Early lexical development in children with focal brain injury. *Brain and Language* 40: 491–527.

Vargha-Khadem, F.; O'Gorman, A.; and Watters, G. 1985. Aphasia and handedness in relation to hemispheric side, age at injury, and severity of cerebral lesion during childhood. *Brain* 108: 677–96.

Vohr, B. R., and Garcia Coll, C. T. 1985. Neurodevelopmental and school performance of very low-birth weight infants: A seven year longitudinal study. *Pediatrics* 76: 345–50.

Waber, D. P.; Bauermeister, M.; Cohen, C.; Ferber, R.; and Wolff, P. 1981. Behavioral correlates of physical and neuromotor maturity in adolescents from different environments. *Developmental Psychobiology* 14: 513–22.

Waber, D. P.; Carlson, D.; Mann, M.; Merola, J.; and Moylan, P. 1984. SES-related aspects of neuropsychological performance. *Child Development* 55: 1878–86.

Welsh, M. C., and Pennington, B. F. 1988. Assessing frontal lobe functioning in children: Views from developmental psychology. *Developmental Neuropsychology* 4: 199–230.

Welsh, M. C.; Pennington, B. F.; Ozonoff, S.; Rouse, B.; and McCabe, E. R. B. 1990. Neuropsychology of early-treated phenylketonuria: Specific executive function deficits. *Child Development* 61: 1697–1713.

Woods, B. T., and Carey, S. 1979. Language deficits after apparent clinical recovery from childhood aphasia. *Annals of Neurology* 6: 405–9.

Yeates, K. O., and Bornstein, R. A. 1992. Attention deficit disorder and neuropsychological performance in children with Tourette's syndrome. *Journal of Clinical and Experimental Neuropsychology* 14: 109.

Zeiner, H. K., and Prigatano, G. P. 1982. Information processing deficits in hydrocephalic and letter reversal children. *Neuropsychologia* 20: 483–92.

I
Normal and Abnormal Brain Development

2

The Developing Brain

Three aspects of brain development are of central interest to investigators who study cognitive development: the normal sequences of brain development (how the neuronal networks subserving various aspects of behavior and cognition are assembled); the processes of aberrant brain development (how genetic factors, brain lesions, and environmental insult result in neurocognitive deficit); and the influence of ancillary circumstances (how other factors, such as timing of insult, sex hormone differences, and experience, enhance or limit the plasticity of the developing brain). These issues will be explored in this chapter in a broad context of current knowledge about brain development. Much of this information comes from advances in developmental neurobiology and from the experimental laboratory, so both animal and human studies will be discussed.

ADVANCES IN NEUROANATOMIC METHODS

Recent advances in neuroanatomical methods, combined with sophisticated behavioral studies, have contributed to our understanding of normal and aberrant brain development. Classical gold and silver staining techniques that have enabled anatomists to map neuronal processes under the light microscope are now supplemented with other techniques, such as electron microscopy of tissues stained with special cytochemical stains, methods of tracing degenerating neuronal processes, and computerized cell counting. RNA retrovirus-mediated gene transfer permits the experimenter to mark a specific cell and to identify all cells that subsequently develop from that cell, even after it has migrated to a new location (Luskin, Pearlman & Sanes 1988). Neuroblasts can be removed from the developing brain, labeled with retrovirus, and either returned to the original location or placed in a different area. Radioactive tracers and horseradish peroxidase (HRP) labeling make it possible to trace developing neuronal projections. Fluorescent dyes can be used in combination to detect *double-labeling* of neurons (that is, to determine when a neuron receives input from two different projections). Different anterograde tracers are simultaneously injected into two different but interconnected areas (A and B), and these structures are then examined for connectivity. Questions such as "do areas A and B send convergent input to other areas (D and E)?" and "does a projection from area A to area D exclude input from area B?" may be answered with this labeling technique (Selemon & Goldman-Rakic 1988). Special surgical techniques provide important information about the response of the developing brain to lesions. Pieces of cortex from one area can be transplanted into another area so that the researcher can study the effect of a specific neuronal environment. The development of fetal surgery makes it possible to operate on a specific brain area and return the fetus to the uterus to develop to term (Rakic & Goldman-Rakic 1984). As a result of these technical advances, our understanding of the development of the nervous system is advancing at a very rapid pace.

EXPERIMENTS IN THE ANIMAL LABORATORY

Experimental studies of other species, particularly primates, provide information that complements our understanding of human brain development. Each species has a distinct timetable for brain development. It is possible to infer from research on other species how events at specific times and places are likely to affect the development of the human nervous system.

Macaca mulatta, the rhesus monkey, is the primate that most closely resembles the human being genetically. These two species share 90% to 94% of genetic material (Sarich 1985; Wilson, Carlson & White 1977). Macaque and human adult brains bear a strong resemblance both structurally and functionally. For example, the human cerebral cortex can be divided into areas with distinctive structural features (Brodmann 1909) that reflect functional properties (Posner et al. 1988). Similar structural and functional differentiation is also seen in the macaque brain.

The brain of the macaque develops prenatally, as does the human brain. Experimental studies of the macaque are therefore especially relevant to understanding human brain development. Macaque gestation lasts 165 days, in contrast to 280 days for humans. Conception day is known accurately for laboratory macaques. Embryo age is recorded as "E [*embryonic day*]." For example, a 100-day-old fetus is designated E100. Postnatal days are also designated, using the prefix P. Thus, P40 represents postnatal day 40.

Newborn macaques are altricial; that is, they have immature nervous systems that develop after birth, and (like humans) they require tender maternal care to survive. Like human infants, baby rhesus monkeys are born with their eyes open, but their development progresses more rapidly. By $1\frac{1}{2}$ to 2 months, they track visually and reach under visual guidance. Visual object discrimination emerges by 2 months (Boothe, Dobson & Teller 1985). At 2 months, infantile motor reflexes regress and voluntary motor control emerges, implying developing maturation of corticalspinal tracts and frontal functions (Hines 1942). Macaques become adept at manipulating objects with their fingers at around 4 months; and by 7 to 8 months, mature finger skill emerges (Lawrence & Hopkins 1976). They show increasing skill on memory tasks between 2 and 4 months (Bachevalier & Mishkin 1984). Competence on delayed-response-type tasks develops between 2 and 4 months of age (Diamond & Goldman-Rakic 1986). Puberty occurs at around 36 months.

In contrast, some other species (for example, rodents such as rats, mice, and hamsters) are born with closed eyes, and considerable neuronal development takes place after birth. For example, the rat brain reaches maturity at 120 days postnatally. The choice of species for an experiment will vary. For example, studies of the auditory system often use owls and bats. It is helpful to be well-informed about the species under investigation in an experiment, since substantial differences in patterns of connectivity and timing exist between species.

STAGES OF BRAIN DEVELOPMENT

Brain development can be divided into four general stages: cell division, migration, proliferation, and pruning or segregation (see the review in Rakic 1991). This is a remarkable process, because 1 million neurons must be generated and must arrive at the correct location, with the correct connections. As Williams and Herrup (1988) noted, this is "an odd situation for an organ system designed to deal with the environment . . . the production and deployment of neurons has to be done the right way the first time, not an easy job given the extraordinary complexity of the nervous system" (p. 432).

Cell Division

Cortical neuronogenesis starts around E40 in the macaque and, depending on the area, continues until E70 to E100 (Rakic 1988a). No cerebral cortical neurons are generated afterward (Rakic 1985). However, some cerebellar and hippocampal granule cells continue to divide until several months after birth. In humans, cortical neuronogenesis also begins at E40, but it continues until E125. The cortical neurons generated up to the seventeenth gestational week in the human represent the maximum number of cortical neurons possible for the rest of the individual's life!

Where do the neurons that ultimately make up the cortex come from? They are generated in the germinal matrix, in a region called the *ventricular proliferative zone* (Rakic 1975), and migrate from there to their final cortical position. Before macaque E40, the neurons are in active mitosis, each producing two similar daughter cells, which in turn divide to produce other neuronal daughters—a symmetrical division. The number of daughter cells produced is under tight genetic control (Williams & Herrup 1988). At E40, the division becomes asymmetrical: each neuronal progenitor produces one neuron that migrates to the cortex and another neuron that remains in the proliferative zone (Rakic 1988). The neurons arising from this group of common cells are arranged in a vertical array called an *ontogenetic* or *embryonic* column. Different types of neurons, which come to reside in different cortical layers, are produced at different times during neuronogenesis by the same clone (Luskin, Pearlman & Sanes 1988). A correlation exists between neuron number and duration of neuronogenesis in an area: the longer the period of neuronogenesis, the greater the number of neurons in the embryonic column (Rakic 1988*a*).

Migration

Once "born," a neuron moves from the periventricular region through a series of zones to the cortical surface. Each of these zones—the intermediate, sub-plate, cortical plate, and marginal zones—serves a different function. It has been suggested that the transient subplate zone serves as a waiting compart-ment, where neuronal afferents from other areas—brainstem, thalamus, and the ipsi- and contralateral hemisphere—remain until they can form connections with migrating neurons of that region (Rakic 1977; Kostovic & Rakic 1990). Kostovic and Rakic (1990) noted that the subplate zone is the largest in the human fetus, particularly in the human association cortex, possibly related to the evolving cortico-cortical fiber systems (Kostovic, Lukinovic et al. 1989). Kostovic and Rakic (1990) noted that the subplate zone is thicker under so-matosensory cortex, which contains many association fibers, than under visual cortex. After the appropriate connections have been formed, the subplate zone disappears. The cortical plate is laid down during the first stage of neocortical development (E38 to E48) in the human.

Neurons travel up *radial glia,* which consist of one or two glial fibers ex-tending from the ventricular proliferative zone into the cortex. Several neurons migrate up a given radial glia; and when the migratory phase concludes, these neurons (from common mother progenitor cells) are lined up in a single vertical column. Later in development, when cortical infolding starts, and sulci and gyri appear, radial glia curve to accommodate the cortical infolding and provide a curvilinear path for the migrating neuron to follow to its ultimate cortical target. Radial glia vary in length and may become very long, for example, in parts of the occipital lobe. Once migration is completed, in the early post-natal period, radial glia are transformed into astrocytes (Schmechel & Rakic 1979a).

The time taken to complete the migrational process depends on a number of factors: intrinsic characteristics of the neuron; the point in development at which the neuron embarks on migration; the distance from the ventricular or subventricular zones to the cortex; and the thickness of the particular cortical region involved. Some cells are fast and synchronous, while others are slow and asynchronous in their migratory behavior (Rakic 1975). Slow-moving neu-rons attain a more superficial position than do rapidly moving neurons, even though they may have been generated simultaneously. The earliest neurons take up positions deep within the cerebral hemispheres and differentiate earlier than do neurons closer to the surface. Thus, at macaque E63, all neurons destined for the deepest layer (layer VI) have been generated and have completed migra-tion; and about half of the neurons destined for layer V have been generated but are still migrating (Rakic 1974, 1975, 1977). Late-migrating neurons pro-ceed up the radial glia, past already migrated neurons and ultimately come to reside at a more superficial point in the cortex. There is a close relationship between the time of a neuron's "birth" and its eventual cortical layer position (McConnell 1985, 1988a, 1989).

The distance a cell must traverse is relatively short early in development (only about 100 μm, taking less than 3 days). Later in development, the distance can exceed 5000 μm and may take longer than 7 days. Although most neurons follow a strictly radial course, retroviral marker studies have shown that some neurons migrate tangentially across the cortex rather than vertically (Walsh & Cepko 1992; O'Rourke et al. 1992).

The tip of the neuron (the growth cone) guides the young neuron through a combination of chemical attraction and repulsion (Pini 1993). Several types of molecules (predominantly glycoproteins) provide a path with high binding affinity that the growth cone preferentially follows (Chuong 1990). These cell adhesion molecules, as well as extracellular connective tissue components (for instance, laminin) and an array of proteolytic enzymes interact at different phases of migration (Edelman 1983; Rakic 1981b). Some migrational abnormalities may be intrinsic to the migrating neuron and others to the glia. Genetic defects of cell adhesion molecules have been linked to certain neurological deficits in experimental animals, as (for example) in the case of the weaver mouse mutation (Gao & Hatten 1993). A human example is Kallman's syndrome—a disturbance of neuronal migration secondary to the deletion of a DNA segment that codes for an adhesion molecule mapped to chromosome Xp22.3 (Franco et al. 1991; Legouis et al. 1991). Clinically, these patients have hypogonadotropic hypogonadism, anosmia, cerebellar and ocular–motor disturbances, and mirror movements (Danek, Heye & Schroedter 1992).

Proliferation

A period of exuberant neuronal growth characterizes the developing mammalian brain. As opposed to the concept of hierarchical development—according to which areas develop in sequence, with the most complex associational areas developing last—a marked increase in axonal number, synapses, and dendritic spines occurs *simultaneously* across many different cortical areas. In the macaque, a rapid increase in synaptic density was noted in all five major cortical areas studied, starting at E105 and peaking between 2 and 4 months, with subsequent decrease to adult levels (Rakic et al. 1986). The pattern of cortical development is also seen in humans, with exuberant synaptic growth reaching a maximum between the ages of 12 and 24 months before declining to adult levels (Huttenlocher 1979, 1984). A similar pattern is seen in subcortical structures, although these structures typically reach adult levels of maturation earlier than does the cortex (Goldman-Rakic 1987).

During the proliferation phase, in many different species, cortical neurons that have restricted outputs in the adult (for example, pyramidal tract neurons or cortical tectal tract neurons) have a more widespread distribution in the developing brain (O'Leary 1989). Gradually, by the process of segregation and selective cell death, neurons reach their final adult pattern of brain distribution.

Pruning (Segregation)

Regulation of neuronal number by pruning characterizes mammalian brain development; it is rare in invertebrates, fish, and reptiles (Williams & Herrup 1988). Pruning results in readjustment of patterns of connectivity between neurons. Without this remodeling, an abnormally large brain with atypical patterns of connectivity would result, and in many cases would be associated with severe cognitive dysfunction in humans. During the pruning phase, synaptic density declines markedly, to adult levels.

What factors determine which neurons survive and which die? Evidence exists that neurons have specific patterns of connectivity, and trophic stimulation may determine those that survive. In rat striatal neurons, which face a 30% cell death rate, neurons with established connections to the substantia nigra are selectively spared. These neurons tend to be born earlier and to connect earlier than do neurons that later die back (Fishell & van der Kooy 1991).

It is likely that each specific cortical neural circuit follows its own individual pattern of proliferation and pruning within the broader scheme just described. For example, in macaque visual cortex, during the first 3 years of postnatal life, excitatory synapses proliferate and refine their connections in advance of the inhibitory synapses (Lund, Holbach & Chung 1991; Lund & Holbach 1991; Lund & Harper 1991). The alpha (excitatory) neuron synapses peak at from 5 to 8 weeks postnatally, whereas the beta (inhibitory) neuron synapses peak at between 8 and 24 weeks postnatally. Depending on the timing of these developmental events, different patterns of clinical symptoms can result from differences in timing during the various phases of development.

DEVELOPMENT OF SPECIFIC BRAIN REGIONS

Neuronogenesis starts earlier in the brainstem than in either the diencephalic structures or the cortex. In the macaque, brainstem neurons appear at between E30 and E45 (Levitt & Rakic 1982). This section summarizes the development of the following brain regions: thalamus, basal ganglia, neocortex, corpus callosum, non-callosal corticocortical connections, sulci and gyri, temporal lobe, hippocampus, and cerebellum.

Thalamus

Thalamic neurons are present in the macaque by E38 to E43 (Dekker & Rakic 1980), and thalamic nuclei become recognizable at around E142. In the human, axons from the thalamus ascend through the ganglionic eminence (an embryonic structure in the fetal cerebrum) to the outermost area of the wall of the hemisphere (His 1904).

The pulvinar (see Note 1) has been particularly well studied from a developmental perspective. In the human, the pulvinar grows rapidly between the 16th and 37th gestational weeks. Rakic and Sidman (1969) suggested that pulvinar neurons are derived from the ganglionic eminence. The neurons migrate from there through the corpus gangliothalamicum, a fetal structure that exists only while it guides migrating neurons.

Thalamocortical afferents can be identified as early as E82 in prefrontal cortex (Schwartz & Goldman-Rakic 1991; Schwartz, Rakic & Goldman-Rakic 1991). These afferents are sparse in number and mostly ipsilateral. Thalamocortical afferents start to invade occipital cortex around E91 (Rakic 1976a). By E145 to E150, a relatively mature pattern of thalamocortical projections exists, but the branching pattern is more extensive than in the adult. Axons extend into territories far beyond the range they will occupy in the adult. For example, the newborn macaque has extensive projections from the anterior pulvinar to the precentral, motor, premotor, postarcuate cortex, and supplementary motor areas. By 6 months after birth, the more restricted adult thalamocortical pattern is seen. By adulthood, only the precentral projection remains (Darian-Smith, Darian-Smith & Cheema 1990b).

Recent studies have indicated that the structure and function of the thalamic reticular nucleus can be understood much more clearly when viewed from a developmental perspective (Mitrofanis & Guillery 1993). The thalamic reticular nucleus is a conduit for all axons between the dorsal thalamus and the cortex. Initially, the reticular nucleus was viewed as being a diffuse system that was not topographically defined (Jones 1975); but recent studies have shown that there indeed are two-way topographic projections (Harting, van Lieshout & Feig 1991) and that the reticular cells are generally modality-specific. In both the adult and the developing animal, a small perireticular nucleus lies adjacent to the reticular nucleus. Both nuclei shrink in size in the adult; they are considerably larger in the young animal. Mitrofanis (1992) has shown that, in the rat, both the perireticular cells (E13) and reticular cells (E13 to E15) are generated very early. The reticular cells send an axon into the thalamus at around E14— even before thalamocortical connections are established—and these cells are thought to guide the developing neurons. Neurons from the cortex fall into two groups: those that proceed into the brainstem, to form the corticobulbar and corticospinal tracts; and those that take a sharp bend when they encounter the perireticular cells, suggesting that these cells serve to sort the two types of fibers. Mitrofanis and Guillery (1993) suggest that the more immature diffuse projections are replaced during maturation by more somatotopically precise connections.

Basal Ganglia

Knowledge about basal ganglia structure and function has increased considerably over the last decade, based mostly on adult clinical and experimental studies (see Note 2). There have been few developmental studies.

Neostriatal neurons are generated between E36 and E80 in the macaque (Brand & Rakic 1979b). In both macaques and humans (Zecevic & Kostovic 1980), the putamen develops at a faster pace than does the caudate for the first $4\frac{1}{2}$ gestational months. The first synapses are seen in the putamen at E60, and not until E65 in the head of the caudate (macaque) (around the 12th fetal week in the human) (Zecevic & Kostovic 1980). In the macaque, synaptic density increases slowly until E112; then, between E112 and E134, there is a marked acceleration, with a sixfold increase in synapse number. The rate of synaptogenesis levels off to adult levels in the second postnatal month. However, the striatum continues to increase in total volume. Brand and Rakic (1984) suggest that, since synaptic density remains the same between the second postnatal month and adulthood, synaptogenesis must continue during this period to maintain the density-to-size ratio.

Other incoming fiber systems are those from the brainstem (generated between E30 and E45 in the macaque) (Levitt & Rakic 1982), and those from the thalamus (generated between E38 and E43) (Dekker & Rakic 1980). Inputs from the substantia nigra to the putamen are in place by E60 and take longer to reach the caudate. These do not form synaptic contacts with their neostriatal targets until mid-gestation. By birth, the four afferent fiber systems are established (DiFiglia, Pasik & Pasik 1980).

Corticostriatal connections from the motor cortex (layer V) arrive at the putamen around E60 in the macaque (Kunzle 1975; Goldman & Nauta 1977a), and inputs from prefrontal cortex to the head of the caudate appear around E69. Projections from motor cortex are bilateral; those from somatosensory cortex are predominately ipsilateral; and those from prefrontal cortex are ipsilateral with a minor contralateral component (Goldman 1978; Fallon & Ziegler 1979). Up until E95, the corticostriatal terminals are distributed diffusely in the striatum. At E104 to E105, there is evidence of segregation; and by E133, corticostriatal neurons segregate and surround central cores that are relatively free of such processes, adopting the "fenestrated" adult pattern (Goldman-Rakic 1981a). By the 16th fetal week in humans, the caudate nucleus and putamen are well defined, with patch-matrix compartments clearly visible (Kordower & Mufson 1993).

There is considerable remodeling of synaptic contacts, with shifts in proportions of types and locations of synapses. These probably reflect shifts in populations of neurotransmitters (DiFiglia, Pasik & Pasik 1980; Brand & Rakic 1984). Temporary synaptic contacts may be formed as place holders until final synapses have formed (Brand & Rakic 1984). It is likely that projections from the cortex and other regions shape the structure of the neostriatum, although specifics of this process are not yet well understood.

The anlage (precursor) of the globus pallidus and subthalamic nucleus is seen at the 6th gestational week in the human, appearing as a longitudinal bulge on the lateral aspect of the diencephalon. The globus pallidus is formed by dragging this cell mass into the telencephalon, rather than by cell migration (Richter 1912).

Dopamine-containing neurons (of the substantia nigra) are generated in the ventricular zone of the caudal mesencephalon at between 6.5 and 10 weeks in the human. The nigrostriatal pathway was first observed at week 8, and it entered the region out of which the putamen would arise at 9 to 10 gestational weeks (Freeman et al. 1991).

Neocortex

The human cerebral cortex has a complex, laminar structure, with characteristic regional differences in the adult brain, as described by Brodmann (1909) and von Economo (1927). Underlying these regional differences are substantial similarities: the cerebral cortex has six layers, modular processing, intralaminar connections, and region-to-region connections (Creutzfeldt 1977). All cortical areas receive excitatory thalamic input terminating in layers III and IV, and these in turn make excitatory monosynaptic contact with pyramidal cells in layers V and VI. There is a distinct "topographic orderliness" to these projections. A single thalamocortical fiber may drive a number of cortical neurons. Cells of layer VI send projections back to the thalamic projection nucleus; cells from layer V send projections back to the brainstem or spinal nuclei. Association fibers arise from cells in layers II (corticocortical) and III (callosal). Neuronal columns that receive information from the thalamus are interdigitated in some areas with columns that receive information via the corpus callosum from homologous cortical areas of the other hemisphere, and also from other cortical areas (Bugbee & Goldman-Rakic 1983). Creutzfeldt (1977) maintains that the morphologic differences between cortical areas result from different afferent/efferent patterns of connectivity, rather than from task-specific internal wiring, and that all neocortical areas adhere to this basic structure.

Neocortical neurons are categorized into two basic types: *local circuit neurons* and *projection neurons*. These differ in several important respects: appearance, the cortical layers in which they are located, neurotransmitters, their response properties, and (most importantly) their patterns of axonal connectivity (Jones 1986; Rakic 1976b). Retrovirus-mediated gene transfer studies suggest that both of these neuronal types arise from the same clone (Luskin, Pearlman & Sanes 1988), although some neurons (e.g., pyramidal and nonpyramidal cells) may come from different precursor cells.

The basic physiologic units of the cortex are the vertical *neuronal columns*. These columns arise from the same neuronal progenitor in the ventricular proliferative zone, and they all respond to a specific modality and receptive field of stimulation (Mountcastle 1957; Jones, Burton & Porter 1975; Hubel & Wiesel 1977; Goldman & Nauta 1977b; Goldman-Rakic & Schwartz 1982; Goldman-Rakic 1987). In the course of evolution, larger, more complex brains are constructed by adding neuronal columns rather than by expanding the width of these columns or by increasing neuronal packing (Bugbee & Goldman-Rakic 1983).

There are two major viewpoints about how the regional specification of the cerebral cortex develops. One is that the basic structure is genetically programmed—in other words, that it is intrinsic. The other viewpoint proposes that structure is modeled by neuronal activity—that is, by extrinsic or environmental factors. These are not mutually exclusive. The neocortex is programmed or specified as to laminated structure, cortical cell types, and common local circuitry; but epigenetic factors program the actual topography of the area (Schlaggar & O'Leary 1991). Certain factors are common to all areas, while others are specific to a given sensory cortical area (Gilbert & Wiesel 1983; Rockland & Lund 1982; Matsubara & Phillips 1988).

The first evidence of neocortical development in the human fetus is a narrow layer of neuroblasts lying beneath the marginal zone in the lateral wall of the hemisphere dorsolateral to the ganglionic eminence (His 1904). Very few synapses are found at 8.5 weeks; but by 15 weeks they are numerous, and it is possible to identify a marginal zone, a cell-dense cortical plate, and an intermediate zone (Molliver, Kostovic & Van der Loos 1973). In the prefrontal region, the basal dendrites of layers 3 and 5 rapidly increase, timed with the ingrowth of thalamocortical neurons, at around 26 to 27 weeks (Mrzljak et al. 1992). In sensory neocortex, laminar identity emerges first, followed by thalamocortical connections, and then by the intracortical circuitry, which determines neurophysiological response patterns.

The Protomap Hypothesis

It has been postulated that genetic codes contain the blueprints for the cytoarchitectonic map of the cerebral cortex in the ependymal layer of the embryonic cerebral ventricle (Rakic 1988b, 1990). Two sets of controlling genes are postulated: one coding for individual and species-specific characteristics; and the other coding for cell production in the proliferative units. The latter genes are thought to control the length of the cell cycle and to code for cell class-specific molecules and for the adhesion molecules that operate during neuronal migration. As such they each affect different aspects of brain development: formation of proliferative units, of ontogenetic columns, and of cytoarchitectonic areas.

Certain protein (that is, genetically programmed) products are distributed in a spatially restricted manner in the vertebrate brain and are responsible for inducing differentiation of postmitotic cells (Cooper & Steindler 1986; Steindler et al. 1989; Johnston & van der Kooy 1989; Schambra et al. 1989). These biochemical factors serve to define different CNS functional units during early postnatal development. They specify cortical laminar patterns, subcortical nuclear borders, and individual functional units in somatosensory cortex, as well as neostriatal striosomes (Steindler et al. 1989).

The protomap hypothesis is appealing because it explains both the expansion of cortical surface area and the regional specificity seen during evolution. Only a brief prolongation of the proliferative phase and a few more rounds of cell division would be needed to increase the number of ontogenetic columns and, thus, the amount of cortical surface (Rakic 1991). In the course of evolution, individuals that underwent more rounds of cell division would have a selective advantage.

An experimental paradigm that involves removing neurons prior to migration, labeling them, and replacing them in the ventricular zone of a host has been developed (McConnell 1990). Since a neuron contains information that determines its "birthday," which in turn determines its cortical layer, it migrates accordingly and is not substantially influenced by the host neuronal environment. Neurons thus labeled and transplanted to a same-age host follow the normal migration pattern. In an older host, in which the major migration is into layers II and III, neurons whose "birthday" has destined them for layers V and VI end up in layers V and VI, although some also end up in layers II and III. Interestingly, those in layers V and VI even generate lengthy axons typical of neurons in the deeper layer (McConnell 1988a, 1988b). This experiment suggests that neurons contain genetic information that plays an important role in their migratory behavior, although the influence of other factors cannot be excluded.

Corpus Callosum

The corpus callosum is a band of white matter that connects homologous areas of both cerebral hemispheres (Pandya, Karol & Heilbronn 1971). The pattern of connections is highly specific in adults: different areas have different patterns of connectivity and are not continuous. Evidence exists that callosal projections vary from region to region in extent, pattern, and developmental timetable (see Note 3).

In most species, except for the human and the macaque, callosal projections are distributed widely across the neocortex in the developing brain, even in regions that end up being devoid of callosal projections in the mature animal (Innocenti, Fiore & Caminiti 1977; Ivy & Killackey 1981; Innocenti 1981; Feng & Brugge 1983). Moreover, the corpus callosum of an immature animal has many more axons than does that of the adult (Koppel & Innocenti 1983; LaMantia & Rakic 1984, 1990a, 1990b). It has been hypothesized that these two processes are related—that is, that the restricted adult pattern emerges as a result of the pruning of axon collaterals and may depend on postnatal experience (Innocenti 1981; O'Leary, Stanfield & Cowan 1981; Ivy & Killackey 1982).

The situation is quite different in the macaque, and probably in the human as well. In the macaque, callosal fibers develop in a highly specific pattern and manifest the pattern of adult connectivity in fetal life. The loss of callosal axons occurs later, during the early postnatal period. For example, in macaque prefrontal cortex, neurons with axons projecting to the contralateral hemisphere first appear at E82 and increase in number between E89 and E111. Many of these axons simply sit in the white matter of the other hemisphere until around E104, however, waiting for other fiber systems and migrating neurons to reach the appropriate cortical laminar destinations. By E111, the callosal neurons manifest the specific pattern of connectivity seen in the adult (Schwartz & Goldman-Rakic 1991). Young callosal neurons send axons to the other hemisphere during the period when migration to layer 3 is still in process, suggesting that the pattern of connectivity is already specified (Schwartz, Rakic & Goldman-Rakic 1991). This sequence of events is also noted in primary visual cortex (Dehay et al 1988; Chalupa et al. 1989) and somatosensory cortices (Killackey & Chalupa 1986). The pattern of connectivity does not depend on processing environmental visual or somatic sensory information, and it occurs in callosal systems linking complex association areas (Killackey & Chalupa 1986). Thus, the adult pattern of connectivity is well established at birth. The decline in axonal number occurs in the early postnatal period (LaMantia & Rakic 1984, 1990, 1990b).

Like thalamocortical afferents, callosal afferents remain in the "waiting compartment" beneath the neocortex while cell proliferation and migration continue. Callosal afferents enter the cortex considerably later than does the thalamocortical system, and already appear to have anticipated their ultimate pattern of connectivity (Killackey & Chalupa 1986). These authors also noted an inverse relationship between callosal and ventroposterior thalamic projections: callosal projections occur in areas that possess relatively few thalamic projections. The callosal projection neurons are eliminated from areas that contain highly specialized tactile receptors (such as on the monkey's digits).

Another small class of neurons—a callosal-associational hybrid—has been described (Schwartz & Goldman-Rakic, 1982). There are two types of such hybrids: *homotopic callosal neurons,* which have an axon projecting to the homologous area of the other hemisphere; and *heterotopic callosal neurons,* which send a second axon to a remote area of the ipsilateral hemisphere and to a nonhomologous area of the contralateral hemisphere (for example, a cingulate neuron projects to frontal cortex of one hemisphere and to parietal cortex of the other). These were seen in fetal (E132 to E137), infant (P4 to P12), and adult monkeys.

Noncallosal Corticocortical (Associational) Connections

Corticocortical connections also occur within the same hemisphere, with various patterns of connectivity. These circuits were anatomically defined on the basis of single cases, large lesions, and a limited neuroanatomical methodologic repertoire. One was described as *alternating* (Goldman-Rakic 1988b); that is, the callosal and ipsilateral inputs were organized as interdigitating columns. An area of the principal sulcus (frontal lobe) received both ipsilateral parietal cortical and contralateral homologous frontal cortical area input (Goldman-Rakic & Schwartz 1982). Another involved *complementary layers;* in this case, prefrontal and parietal inputs terminated in alternating layers in the superior temporal sulcus (Goldman-Rakic 1988b). Corticocortical fibers are well established in the macaque at birth (Goldman & Nauta 1977b).

Sulci and Gyri

The mature cortex has a characteristic pattern of gyri and sulci, whereas the young fetus has a smooth (lissencephalic) surface. Gyri markedly increase available neocortical surface: two-thirds of neocortex lies within sulci. Gyri and sulci have different patterns of connectivity. For instance, gyri have more extensive thalamic projections than do sulci. In addition, major gyri have more projections from distant body regions than do sulci, which receive corticocortical connections (Goldman-Rakic & Schwartz 1982). And monoaminergic input is more intense to sulci than to the gyri (Levitt, Rakic & Goldman-Rakic 1984).

The timetable for gyral and sulcal development in the human fetus has been described (Chi, Dooling & Gilles 1977). The interhemispheric and transverse cerebral fissures appear at the 10th gestational week, followed by the callosal sulcus and sylvian fissure at 14 weeks. The calcarine fissure appears at 16 weeks. (For comparison, in the macaque, the first hint of the calcarine fissure is seen at E100.) The parietooccipital fissure appears at 16 weeks. The cingulate sulcus arises at 18 weeks. By 20 weeks, the rolandic sulcus is apparent. The postrolandic sulcus and superior frontal sulcus emerge at 25 weeks. The interparietal sulcus and middle temporal sulcus are noted at 26 weeks; the inferior frontal sulcus at 28 weeks; and the inferior temporal sulcus at 30 weeks. The gyrus rectus of the frontal lobe appears around 16 weeks, and the anterior and posterior orbital gyri appear at 36 weeks. The temporal lobe gyri develop at between 23 and 31 weeks. The gyri over the lateral aspect of the parietal lobe develop at between 25 and 35 weeks, and the occipital gyri emerge at between 27 and 30 weeks.

Gyral and sulcal patterns appear after cortical neurons have been generated and at around the time that thalamocortical and corticocortical axons ascend into the cortex (Goldman-Rakic & Rakic 1984). The transient subplate zone is related in some way to the process of modeling the cortical surface, since its size and the length of time it remains are correlated with the number of afferent fiber systems. Thus, the subplate zone remains in the region of the human frontal cortex while modeling of the tertiary gyri is proceeding (Kostovic, Lukinovic et al. 1989).

A series of experiments in which macaque frontal cortex was removed at variable times between E102 and E119 (Goldman & Galkin 1978) demonstrated that marked alterations of sucal and gyral development could be induced. Although thalamic neurons were relatively spared at E106, the gyral/sulcal pattern of remote cortical regions was dramatically affected. For example, unilateral prefrontal lesions resulted in numerous anomalous sulci *bilaterally* in many areas of the cortex—and in remote locations such as the temporal and occipital lobes—at E102 and E106. The younger the animal was at the time of surgery, the more marked were the cortical gyri and sulci anomalies. Gyri and sulci that were forming or had already formed were unaffected. In an animal operated on at E119, few abnormalities in sulcal/gyral patterns were noted; but late-appearing fissures in the frontal, parietal, and occipital lobes were distinctly atypical. Not surprisingly, dramatic changes were noted in the prefrontal region close to the lesion.

In a Golgi study of the development of motor speech areas and adjacent orofacial zones in the right and left hemispheres of humans aged 3 to 72 months of age, Simonds & Scheibel (1989) noted that, when the total length of the basilar dendrite systems and the proximal order dendritic changes were compared at 3 months, the orofacial motor zones surpassed the motor speech areas, and the right hemisphere had a larger area than the left. Over the first 6 years of life, a gradual and by no means monotonic shift to preminence of the left motor speech area occurred.

Temporal Lobe

Less well-studied is the development of the temporal lobe. In the inferior and medial temporal lobe in the young animal, connections not seen in adult macaques were noted (Webster, Ungergleider & Bachevalier 1991). For example, the output from a circumscribed area TE to perirhinal cortex became much more restricted in the adult. Moreover, in the immature animal, a fairly symmetrical input/output ratio exists between areas TEO and TE; but in the adult, the outputs again become more restricted. In monkeys that sustained TE removal during infancy, the projection from TEO to area LB of the amygdala and the parahippocampal cortex was maintained, providing a possible explanation for the sparing of memory (Webster, Ungerleider & Bachevalier 1990).

Hippocampus

Hippocampal development begins at around E38 in the macaque and is almost simultaneous across all areas of the hippocampal formation (entorhinal neurons appear at E36). Generation of neurons ceases at between E56 and E75, depending on the specific area (Rakic & Nowakowski 1981). Except for granule cells, all neurons of the hippocampal region in the macaque are generated over a 6-week period, during the first half of gestation. By E80, only neurons destined for the stratum granulosum of the dentate gyrus are still being generated, and this development continues even after birth. There is an inside-to-outside gradient for neurons of the parahippocampal formation, subiculum, and areas CA1, CA2, and CA3; in contrast, there is an outside-to-inside gradient in the stratum granulosum of the dentate gyrus, and a suprapyramidal-to-infrapyramidal gradient in the stratum granulosum of the dentate gyrus. The subiculum, which is phylogenetically older, has a shorter period of development. The human fetus resembles the macaque in that the general patterns described here hold true. The pattern of development differs from that of the neocortex; that is, synapses are within the marginal zone rather than within the subplate zone. Hippocampal cortex also shows well-differentiated postsynaptic elements and afferent pathways in the second half of gestation. This area has a thin subplate zone and receives a comparatively small number of thalamic and commissural inputs (Kostovic, Seress et al. 1989). It is likely that the entorhinal area and/or subiculum provides input to the hippocampus early in human development (Kostovic, Seress et al. 1989).

Cerebellum

The cerebellum has developed considerably in terms of intricacy of structure, the presence of new structural features, and expansion of these phylogenetically new structures. Thus, the cerebellar hemispheres are enlarged 15.2 times in humans compared to monkeys, whereas the vermis is enlarged only 4.2 times. The dentate nucleus, (which is related to the hemispheres) shows a parallel enlargement, in contrast to the nuclei related to the vermis. Recent studies have indicated that, in humans, the cerebellum serves an important role in cognitive functioning, thus making it a structure of unique interest to neuropsychologists (Leiner, Leiner & Dow 1986; Bracke-Tolkmitt et al. 1989; Schmahmann 1991).

Cerebellar neurons follow the same general migratory principles that were discussed with regard to the cerebral cortex. However, whereas neurons from the cerebral hemisphere neurons migrate from the germinal matrix to the cortical surface along radial glides, cerebellar granule cells are generated in the external granular layer (a derivative of the subventricular zone) and migrate inward along glides formed by Bergmann glial fibers (Rakic 1971). The sequence of development of the human cerebellum parallels that seen in the monkey.

In the macaque, the cerebellar cortex and nuclei develop from the median and lateral migratory zones. At approximately E56, there are two cerebellar laminae; by about E70, the embryonic granular layer appears. By E112, the cortical lamina is well developed in all areas of the cerebellum, but it varies from a six-layered structure in the dorsomedian area to a four-layered cortex in the dorsolateral cortex and flocculus. At this point, the cerebellar nuclei are quite prominent (Verbitskaya 1969).

Early in the 5th gestational month in the human, a six-layered cortex is noted in the area of the vermis, flocculus, and median areas of the cerebellar hemispheres, with the lateral aspects of the hemispheres developing more slowly (about $1\frac{1}{2}$ to 2 months behind. The flocculus and vermis tend to develop in parallel. By 6 gestational months, all areas of the cerebellum have six layers. At birth the three-layered cortex seen in the adult is present, although the embryonic granular layers do not completely disappear until at least 7 to 8 months postnatally (Borovski 1937). Although different lobules of the cerebellum mature at different rates in the human, they reach a pattern of fully mature cellularity in the external and internal granular layers and in the molecular layer by 1 year of age (Verbitskaya 1969). Radiological studies in the child indicate that the rate of growth of the cerebellum as a whole increases rapidly up to the 2nd year of life (12 to 24 months) and then continues at a slower rate, attaining adult size at 6 to 9 years of age (Hayakawa, Konishi & Matsuda 1989).

In the human fetus, cerebellar nuclei first become apparent in the middle of the 2nd month (6 gestational weeks) and then gradually differentiate into a median cluster (the globose, emboliform, and fastigial nuclei) and the lateral group (the dentate nucleus). By 7 months, the appearance of the nuclei is essentially the same as that in adults (Verbitskaya 1969).

In terms of the relationships with other neuronal systems, the olivary climbing fibers form early synapses with cerebellar nuclei. Prior to forming connections with Purkinje cells (at around 30 weeks in the human), the olivary climbing fibers synapse in the lamina dissecans—a transitory zone beneath the Purkinje cells. In the human, the lamina dissecans disappears by 30 to 32 weeks of gestation (Rakic & Sidman 1970).

Autism represents a human example of a disorder that may result from atypical development of the cerebellum as well as of limbic structures. A number of investigators have reported a loss of Purkinje cells without gliosis (Bauman & Kemper 1989; Ritvo et al. 1986). Cells in the fastigial, globose, and emboliform nuclei and olivary neurons were 30% enlarged in younger subjects; in young adults, there was a 30% decrease in cell size in these structures (Anderson et al. 1993). This suggests that the disturbance in neuronogenesis occurred prior to 30 weeks gestational age, and that a neuronal circuit usually seen only in the fetus (between the inferior olivary nucleus and the deep nuclei) may have persisted. Anderson et al. postulate that this persistent fetal circuitry may result in increased loss of Purkinje cells (see Chapter 13).

DEVELOPMENT OF NEUROTRANSMITTER SYSTEMS

In addition to the development of the neuronal systems in the developing brain, complex changes occur in different neurotransmitter systems. Neurotransmitters are found in many primitive organisms, where they function as growth regulators. In vertebrates they regulate early stages of embryonic growth, morphogenesis, and cell migration, both in the nervous system and in other nonneural systems (Lauder 1993). Neurotransmitters, by influencing second-messenger pathways, also affect development of specific neuronal systems. For instance, altered levels of serotonin may adversely affect the development of serotonergic raphe neurons; dopamine concentrations influence striatal development, and acetylcholine affects cortical development. GABA appears to play a role as a trophic factor and may protect cortical neurons from excitotoxic amino acids (Lauder 1993).

With regard to the timetable of development, observations in a number of species suggest that monoaminergic systems are the first to arrive (at E36 to E41, in macaques) (Levitt, Rakic & Goldman-Rakic 1984); then cholinergic afferents, which originate from the basal forebrain, appear (at 15 to 18 weeks in the human in the occipital lobe) (Kostovic & Rakic 1990); and this is followed by the appearance of thalamocortical afferents (Rakic 1977; Kostovic & Rakic 1984). The neurotransmitter characteristics of a neuron are specified even before the cell has completed its migration. Thus, neurons of the substantia nigra contain dopamine, and cholinergic neurons of the basal forebrain display choline acetyltransferase while in the ventricular zone (Schambra et al. 1989).

Postnatally, both the concentration and the rate of synthesis of neurotransmitters appear to be influenced by the specific region involved. This pattern differs from the synchronous development of receptor sites, which mirrors the general pattern of synaptogenesis: there is a rapid increase, followed by a short plateau, and then a slow decrease in synaptic contacts, which occurs simultaneously across many different cortical areas and cortical layers. Various neurotransmitter receptor types (dopaminergic, serotonergic, adrenergic, muscarinic cholinergic, and GABAergic) were studied across several different cortical areas in macaques ranging from birth to 60 months of age, using in vitro binding autoradiography (Lidow, Goldman-Rakic & Rakic 1991).

MYELINATION

Classically, myelination has been viewed as one of the crucial factors in brain development. Initially, brain development was viewed as being hierarchical—that is, as proceeding from sensory to motor to complex associational structures and underlying function. The hierarchichal theory was based in part on Flechsig's (1920) observation that higher association areas (for example, parieto-temporal and frontal) did not stain as intensely with myelin-specific dyes as did primary sensory cortices (for example, visual and somatosensory). The concept also received support from early studies of cerebral metabolic activity (Kennedy et al. 1982) and has had considerable impact on the way researchers interested in development conceptualized their findings (e.g., Ellingson & Willcott 1960; Friedman & Sigman 1981). Regional myelination in the human has been extensively studied by Yakovlev and Lecours (1967).

Current information regarding brain development, however, suggests that the hierarchical theory does not entirely capture the true state of affairs. Hierarchical development does occur in the sense that neuronal systems at a brainstem and subcortical level appear and mature in advance of cortical neurons. But the findings of simultaneous synaptic development across all cortical regions and layers studied to date suggest that the cerebral cortex is not developing in a regional fashion. Rakic and colleagues also point out that there are inconsistencies in and different interpretations of the myelination data: the pyramidal tract is actually the last to myelinate, and areas that are poorly myelinated in the infant are also poorly myelinated in the adult (Lidow, Goldman-Rakic & Rakic 1991; LaMantia & Rakic 1990b). In addition, recent PET scan studies in infants support the idea of simultaneous increase in metabolic activity across different cortical regions (Chugani & Phelps 1986).

RELEVANCE FOR THE NEUROPSYCHOLOGIST

A major aim of this chapter is to provide a theoretical neurobiological foundation for looking at how the developing brain of the human infant responds to injury, prepartory to the clinical perspective presented in Chapter 3. Clinicians recognize that some children emerge relatively unscathed after brain injury, whereas others have severe neurocognitive deficits. Consequently, clinicians have grappled with the issue of neural plasticity.

For instance, the concept of *equipotentiality*—asserting that the right cerebral hemisphere can take over language functions until late childhood—was promulgated by Lennenberg (1967), who based his theory on the series of cases reported by Basser (1962). As discussed in Chapter 1, the situation in brain-injured children is considerably more complicated. From the point of view of the neurobiologist, the issue revolves around *plasticity:* to what extent can the developing brain sustain an injury and yet maintain function? Another way of asking this question is, can neurodevelopmental processes that are controlled by genetic factors be separated from ones that are affected primarily by nongenetic factors? Such a distinction can be made between cell division and migration versus synaptic proliferation and remodeling of connections.

FACTORS THAT AFFECT NEURONAL CONNECTIVITY

At the level of the neuron, *pre*synaptic factors can be distinguished from *post*-synaptic factors. Presynaptic factors determine the functional properties of neurons, whereas postsynaptic factors determine the structural properties of neurons and their connectivity. For example, neurons of different types can make synaptic contacts with the same structural features on a given class of target neuron. (Thus, mossy fibers, which arise from several different regions, make the same type of synaptic ending on cerebellar granule cells.) Alternatively, the same neuron can make different types of synaptic connections on different targets.

EXPERIMENTAL NEUROBIOLOGICAL PARADIGMS

Seven experimental paradigms that tease apart some of the processes underlying plasticity are briefly summarized in the following subsections. These paradigms enable the neuroscientist to discriminate among lesions that disrupt incoming neuronal populations, their synaptic targets, and the interactive response of the developing brain to normal environmental stimulation.

Ablation of an Incoming Population of Neurons

At a thalamic level, removal of an eye at a very early stage of development results in loss of the normal laminar pattern of the lateral geniculate. Rakic (1976*a*, 1977, 1981*a*) suggested that competitive elimination of inappropriately connected axons required the presence of input from both retinae. Casagrande and Condo (1988), suggested that the sorting of axons occurs due to functional differences or retinal location.

Another example involves rodent parietal cortex, which contains characteristic clusters of layer-IV neurons called *barrels* that are innervated by afferents from the ventrobasal thalamus; these in turn correspond to the whisker follicles on the mouse's snout. When whisker follicles are injured at birth, barrels never develop. If damage is inflicted at a later point (for instance, at P7), however, barrels are present and cortical appearance does not change (Woolsey & Wann 1976).

This suggests that ablation of an incoming neuronal population prior to a certain point in development results in the failure of normal structure to develop. However, this is restricted to a temporal window.

Ablating the Usual Target for an Incoming Neuronal Population (A) and Providing a New Target (B) for These Neurons by Ablating the Neurons Destined for (B)

After lesioning the superior colliculus in the golden hamster, Schneider (1973) created neuronal space by ablating neurons destined for the medial geniculate nucleus. The retinal fibers formed synapses on the medial geniculate rather than on the lateral geniculate (Kalil & Schneider 1975). A variant of this experiment involved rerouting the visual fibers to the somatosensory system (e.g., Campbell & Frost 1987). The resulting synapses between the retinal ganglion cells and the ventrobasal nucleus of the thalamus more closely resembled the synapses seen in the somatosensory system than those in the visual system (Campbell & Frost 1987).

Similar experiments done at a cortical level involved diverting retinal neurons destined for visual cortex to auditory cortex instead. In this case, the one-dimensional map of auditory cortex is converted into a two-dimensional visual field map. The auditory map is less precisely organized in these animals (Sur, Pallas & Roe 1990), and both the physiological response pattern and the cortical representation in rewired animals change; but there were no changes in external connectivity patterns of the auditory and visual cortices and only minor alterations in the thalamic-cortical projection pattern (Sur, Garraghty & Roe 1988; Pallas, Roe & Sur 1990; Roe et al. 1990). This suggests that the subplate neurons ("pioneers") may already have specified the cortical efferent pathways and the laminar arrangement.

These experiments suggest that early stages of development are characterized by considerable plasticity and a lack of modality-specificity. Cortical neurons that would normally process one modality are capable of taking over the processing of another.

Transplantation of Fetal Cortex from One Cortical Area into Another

In newborn rats, O'Leary and Stanfield (1989) transplanted rostral cortex from rats (aged E17) to the occipital area, or occipital cortex to the rostral area. The transplanted neurons behaved like the other neurons in the host area rather than resembling neurons from the donor site. Schlagger and O'Leary (1991) transplanted pieces of occipital cortex to the parietal somatosensory cortex of newborn rats, after layer-IV neurons were generated (Lund & Mustari 1977) but before the geniculocortical fibers entered the occipital cortical plate. The occipital cortical transplants developed barrellike structures that resembled those usually seen in parietal somatosensory cortex.

This suggests that the development of these specific cytoarchitectural features, rather than being intrinsic or unique to parietal cortex, is programmed by the incoming ventrobasal thalamocortical afferents.

Altering Intrinsic Neuronal Activity

Even before birth, developing neurons in sensory systems are exposed to rhythmic bursts of activity that contribute to the development of topographic maps. For instance, neighboring retinal ganglion cells tend to fire within a few seconds of each other, so that bursts of activity sweep across the retina rehearsing the kind of stimulation patterns to which the visual system will be exposed in real life. This activity plays a role in refining the eye-specific layers in the lateral geniculate (Meister et al. 1991). When this spontaneous firing is silenced, the normal neuronal structure is profoundly altered (Dubin, Stark & Archer 1986; Stryker & Harris 1986).

Impact of Alteration of One Sensory System on Another

A series of experiments in different species (owls, ferrets, and guinea pigs) has shown that altering visual input affects the formation of auditory maps in the superior colliculus (Knudsen 1988; Knudsen & Knudsen 1990: Knudsen & Brainard 1991; King et al. 1988; Withington-Wray et al. 1990). These experiments suggest that alterations in the nervous system should not be viewed only in terms of the affected modality; that is, since auditory, visual, and tactile systems are interrelated at numerous levels of the neuraxis, altering one system may have profound effects on sensory maps in other systems.

Altering Normal Environmental Stimulation

After birth, brain development proceeds in the context of interaction with the environment (Kaas, Merzenich & Killackey 1983; Sherman & Spear 1982). Classical experiments were performed on the visual system of the cat by Hubel and Wiesel in a series of studies that ultimately won them the Nobel Prize (Hubel & Wiesel 1962, 1963, 1970; Wiesel & Hubel 1963, 1965a, 1965b). These scientists demonstrated that occluding one eye of a kitten during the first month of postnatal development, and thus depriving the animal of form vision, resulted in permanent loss of vision in that eye. The kitten behaved as though it were blind when forced to use the previously occluded eye. Moreover, the connections into the lateral geniculate were dominated by the nonoccluded eye, so the normal laminated pattern of the lateral geniculate did not develop, resembling instead the lateral geniculate of the enucleated fetal monkey. In contrast, the cortex appeared structurally normal but manifested an atypical physiological response.

These studies were later replicated and expanded in experiments with a number of other species. Evidently, no single sensitive period applied to the whole visual system; rather, the different anatomical and functional aspects of the system each had a specific sensitive period. For instance, the macaque visual system has multiple sensitive periods, depending on which aspect of vision is studied (for instance, cone and rod vision, spatial vision, or binocular vision) (Harwerth et al. 1986). Translated into the context of human development, if factors that impair visual acuity occur any time before age 8, they can result in loss of binocular vision and stereopsis.

The maps of other sensory systems have also been shown to have considerable plasticity (Udin & Fawcett 1988). The basic topography of the central auditory system is laid out early, and cochlear frequency organization (which probably occurs before birth in humans) is refined postnatally—as are connections at the collicular and cortical levels. When guinea pigs were raised in omnidirectional white noise, an auditory map was not formed (Withington-Wray et al. 1990). The impact on map formation of introducing such white noise declined as the animal matured, and the noise had no effect on the adult's auditory map. It is possible that, in humans, failure of normal environmental stimulation—for instance, lack of exposure to language during critical periods when the cortex is developing (Simonds & Scheibel 1989)—can significantly alter the person's ability to process linguistic information (Curtiss 1977).

Specific Training and "Rehabilitation"

Early life experiences or training on a task affects the subject's ability to learn to perform a task, even in the context of brain lesions. For example, Goldman (1975) lesioned infant monkeys and then either waited 2 years with no training, or trained on the task at age 1 year. Early exposure to the task (age 1) led to near-normal performance, whereas monkeys first exposed to the task at age 2 years were never able to learn the task. She suggested that "recovery from brain injury is greatly facilitated by experiences, and, indeed, experience was more significant for the operated animals than it was for the unoperated cases . . . unsuccessful training would appear to be better than no training at all" (Goldman 1975, p. 389). These differences in training effects also vary as a function of lesion site (orbitofrontal versus dorsolateral), including some subcortical areas.

FACTORS THAT AFFECT THE OUTCOME OF LESIONS

Timing of Lesion: The Critical Period

As can be seen in the preceding examples, for each species, each sensory system, and each subsystem, there is a *critical period*—a point during development when both normal neuronal connectivity and environmental stimulation are required for development to proceed. If any perturbation occurs during this period, permanent behavioral deficits may result. Subsequent deprivation of normal environmental stimulation can never have the same massive effect once this critical period has ended. Even in the adult brain, rapid changes at a neurophysiological level occur after sensory input is disrupted (Merzenich & Kaas, 1982; Kaas et al. 1990; King & Moore 1991; Kaas 1991). In the developing brain, these changes are often reflected in permanent alterations in structure.

Age at Which the Affected Neuronal System Becomes Functional

Various brain regions become functional at different times, and superficially similar behaviors may be subserved by different brain areas at different points of development. Very early lesions in the fetus may produce no deficits, even after prolonged observation. Goldman and Galkin (1978) reported on a series of studies on macaques with early lesions of the orbital and dorsolateral prefrontal cortex on delayed alternation tasks. Monkeys underwent surgery to dorsolateral prefrontal surgery at E102, E104, E106, and E119. Monkeys that underwent operations prior to E106 had considerable remodeling of the cortical sulcal/gyral surface, exhibited no changes in the mediodorsal thalamic nucleus, and did not manifest any cognitive deficits in later life. In contrast, monkeys that underwent operations at P50 showed a regression on delayed alternation tasks that did not appear until 15 to 24 months of age (Goldman & Galkin 1978). In the immature brain, circuits different from those used in the adult animal may be used to carry out similar behaviors. Infant monkeys that sustained lesions of the head of the caudate between 48 and 54 days of age showed significant deficits on frontal tasks 10 months later (Goldman & Rosvold 1972). According to Kling (1966), animals that underwent amygdalectomy in infancy began to manifest changes in social behaviors at puberty. It is likely that subcortical lesions at critical stages may result in severe deficits. Moreover, evidence suggests that the cortex comes on line later than do subcortical structures. Macaque frontal cortex is not really functional until close to puberty (Alexander & Goldman 1978). In a study in which dorsolateral prefrontal cortex was reversibly cooled, no decrement in performance was observed in monkeys age 9 to 16 months, but substantial deficits were seen at 36 months (Goldman & Alexander 1977).

Thus, to determine the full impact of an early lesion, one must continue observation until well into adulthood, at which time the brain area in question comes on-line. For example, in the motor system, spasticity and rigidity may be nonexistent or minimal in infancy, but may worsen with increasing age (Kennard 1942).

In humans, many neuropsychiatric syndromes (which are genetically programmed) emerge at characteristic ages, suggesting that the underlying neuronal circuitry comes on-line at a specific age. For instance, obsessive compulsive disorder and Tourette's syndrome often do not appear until 7 or 8 years. Schizophrenia—which may be related to aberrant development of the entorhinal cortex, with resulting abnormality in limbic–prefrontal connectivity—is typically manifested by unevenness in early development, coupled with mildly atypical social behaviors in childhood. Full-blown schizophrenia appears for the first time in late adolescence or early adulthood (see Chapter 13).

Gender

In addition to affecting the development of certain cognitive processes that are lateralized in adults (such as spatial processing) (Witelson 1976), gender may have a profound impact on the expression of a specific lesion. Gonadal hormones affect the development of cortical synaptic networks, although the precise mechanisms are not yet known. Goldman (1975) suggested that orbital frontal cortex develops earlier in males than in females, based on the observation that male monkeys made fewer reversal errors on object reversal tasks when tested at P75 (Clark & Goldman-Rakic 1989), but not after 18 months (Goldman et al. 1974). Orbital frontal lesions produced deficits on the object reversal task in males at P75, and in females of the same age that had been treated with androgen, but not in normal females at P75 (Clark & Goldman-Rakic 1989). This holds true for other areas of the brain. There is also likely to be an age-by-sex interaction, with sex-dependent sensitivity to certain pathologic processes. The critical period for hormonal effects extends into the early postnatal period in the macaque (Clark & Goldman-Rakic 1989).

Clearly, multiple factors are involved in the response of the developing brain to lesions. In fact, the concept of lesion itself must be considered in a very broad context, ranging from genetic factors (e.g., disruption of neural adhesion molecules) to disturbances in the intrauterine metabolic environment (as in the case of fetal alcohol syndrome or atypical hormonal levels) to frank lesions. The effect of these insults must be viewed in terms of the age at which they occurred; where they occurred; the sex of the child; what the neuronal developmental context was (that is, were thalamocortical projection systems in place?); what other, more remote systems might be affected; at what age the individual was examined; and what tasks were used. Approached from this detailed perspective, it may become possible to predict more accurately the outcome of events affecting the brain of the child.

CONCLUSION

This chapter undertook to present a broad outline of information about brain development. Recent studies of the closest primate relative of man, the rhesus monkey or macaque, have provided a rich supply of information about this development, in both normal and anomalous brains. It now remains for the clinician to integrate information from the laboratory setting with information from the clinical setting, to identify appropriate clinical models and analogs, and to attempt to enhance further our understanding of this complex evolution. We are only beginning to understand how a child's brain develops normally and how, in the presence of disruption—whether through damage to a specific region or by environmental, sensory, or other stressors—the impact of failure to develop may be demonstrated.

NOTES

1. The pulvinar is a large nucleus located in the posterior thalamus. It has reciprocal connections with visual areas 17 and 18 (Ogren & Hendrickson 1977); posterior parietal areas 5, 7a, and 7b (Asanuma, Anderson & Cowan 1985; Burton & Jones 1976); post-

central somatosensory areas 2 (Pons & Kaas 1985), 1, and 3b (Darian-Smith, Darian-Smith & Cheema 1990*a*); the second somatosensory area and the superior temporal gyrus (Burton & Jones 1976); temporal pole (Markowitsch et al. 1985); and areas of prefrontal cortex (Asanuma, Anderson & Cowan 1985; Goldman-Rakic 1988*a;* 1988*b*). The best-defined subcortical input arises from the ipsilateral superior colliculus.

2. The neostriatum is composed of the *caudate* and *putamen,* the *nucleus accumbens* (or ventral striatum), and the olfactory tubercle. The neostriatum appeared later in evolution than did the globus pallidus, and it increased in size in proportion to the development of the cerebral cortex [neostriatal volume has increased 91 times from rat to human (Johnston et al. 1990)]. The main inputs come from the cerebral cortex, thalamus, and substantia nigra pars compacta, with lesser inputs from the globus pallidus, subthalamic nucleus, dorsal raphe nucleus, and pedunculopontine tegmental nucleus. The major output goes to the substantia nigra and globus pallidus. Three different functional regions of the neostriatum can be identified: the sensorimotor (sensorimotor cortex to putamen); the associative (prefrontal, temporal, parietal, and cingulate to caudate); and the limbic (limbic and paralimbic cortical areas, hippocampus, and amygdala to ventral striatum). The neostriatum is currently conceptualized as consisting of multiple cortico-striato-nigro-thalamocortical parallel circuits that are exquisitely somatotopically organized. Hoover and Strick (1993) showed that, even within a given circuit (in this case, the motor circuit), pallidal output innervates multiple cortical areas as a series of discrete, parallel circuits.

The striatum consists of two different neuronal compartments: patches (also known as striosomes), which are rich in enkephalin, substance-P, and somatostain, but poor in acetylcholinesterase; and acetylcholinesterase-rich matrix, which has distinctive neurotransmitter populations and connectivity. Although much remains to be learned about striatal connections, the patches receive afferents from deep cortical layers V and VI (whereas the matrix receives afferents from superficial layers II and III) (Gerfen 1989), as well as the centromedian parafascicular complex of the thalamus (Herkenham & Pert 1981) and a preponderance of limbic projections. In contrast, the matrix receives projections from sensory motor cortical areas (Gerfen 1984). Both project to the substantia nigra, but the patch neurons send preferentially to the pars compacta, whereas the matrix neurons send efferents to the pars reticulata, in the rat (Gerfen 1989). The ratio of 15% patch to 85% matrix remains relatively constant in the rat, the macaque, and the human; and the average number of patches does not increase, although the area of the individual patch does. This is a strategy quite different from that seen in the expansion of the number of columns in the neocortex, but not of column width (Johnston et al. 1990). In addition, a close relationship appears to exist between cortical layers V and VI and patch neurons, and between cortical layers II and III and matrix neurons, in terms of birthdates, adhesiveness, and corticostriatal connections (Gerfen 1989; van der Kooy et al. 1987; Krushel & van der Kooy 1988; McConnell 1988*a,* 1988*b*). Moreover, the previously accepted anterior–posterior organization of corticostriatal terminal fields has given way to a pattern of longitudinal bands, with interdigitation of corticostriatal terminal fields (Selemon & Goldman-Rakic 1985). For a detailed review of this area, consult *Trends in Neuroscience* volume 13 (July 1990), edited by P. S. Goldman-Rakic & L. D. Selemon.

3. Three areas (3b, 1, and 2) in the postcentral gyrus of the adult macaque each have a complete and separate representation of body surface [area 5 also contains a complex map of the body surface]. These areas are linked in such a way as to suggest that somatosensory information is processed in a hierarchical, front-to-back fashion. The callosal connections of the postcentral gyrus are most dense caudally (area 5) and least

dense anteriorly (3b). Callosal connections are most dense in the areas with maps of the proximal limbs, trunk, and head, and least dense on the distal areas mapping the limbs.

REFERENCES

Alexander, G. E., and Goldman, P. 1978. Functional development of the dorsolateral prefrontal cortex: An analysis utilizing reversible cryogenic depression. *Brain Research* 143: 233–49.

Anderson, J. M.; Bauman, M. L.; Kemper, T. L.; and Arin, D. M. 1993. On the connection of the inferior olive with the cerebellum in early infantile autism. *Neurology* 43: A250.

Asanuma, C.; Anderson, R. A.; and Cowan, W. M. 1985. The thalamic relations of the caudal inferior parietal lobule and the lateral prefrontal cortex in monkeys: Divergent cortical projections from cell clusters in the medial pulvinar nucleus. *Journal of Comparative Neurology* 241: 357–81.

Bachevalier, J., and Mishkin, M. 1984. An early and a late developing system for learning and retention in infant monkeys. *Behavioral Neuroscience* 98: 770–78.

Basser, L. S. 1962. Hemiplegia of early onset and the faculty of speech with special reference to the effects of hemispherectomy. *Brain* 85: 427–60.

Bauman, M. L., and Kemper, T. L. 1989. Abnormal cerebellar circuitry in autism? *Neurology* 39 (Suppl. 1): 186.

Boothe, R. G.; Dobson, V.; and Teller, D. Y. 1985. Postnatal development of vision in human and nonhuman primates. *Annual Review of Neuroscience* 8: 495–545.

Boothe, R., and Sackett G. 1975. Perception and learning in infant rhesus monkeys. In G. H. Bourne (ed.), *The Rhesus Monkey,* vol. VI: *Anatomy and Physiology* (New York; Academic Press), pp. 343–63.

Borovski, M. L. 1937. The postnatal development of the cerebellar cortex of man. In *Jubilee Edition Marking 40th Anniversary of the Scientific Activity of V. J. Tenkov* (Moscow: State Publisher of Medical Literature), pp. 381–412.

Bracke-Tolkmitt, R.; Linden, A.; Canavan, A. G. M.; Rockstroh, B.; Scholz, E.; Wessel, K.; and Diener, H.-C. 1989. The cerebellum contributes to mental skills. *Behavioral Neuroscience* 103: 442–46.

Brand, S., and Rakic, P. 1979a. Synaptogenesis in the caudate nucleus of pre- and postnatal rhesus monkeys. *Anatomical Record* 193: 490.

———. 1979b. Genesis of the primate neostriatum: A [³H] thymidine autoradiographic analysis of the time of neuron origin in the rhesus monkey. *Neuroscience* 4: 767–78.

———. 1984. Cytodifferentiation and synaptogenesis in the neostriatum of fetal and neonatal rhesus monkeys. *Anatomy and Embryology* 169: 21–34.

Brodmann, K. 1909. *Lokalisationslehre der Grosshirnrinde in ihren Principen dargestellt uu Grun des Zellenbaue.* Leipzig: J. A. Barth.

Brunquell, P. J.; Papale, J. H.; Horton, J. C.; Williams, R. S.; Zgrabik, M. J.; Albert, D. M.; and Hedley-Whyte, E. T. 1984. Sex-linked hereditary bilateral anophthalmos: Pathologic and radiologic correlation. *Archives of Ophthalmology* 102: 108–13.

Bugbee, N. M., and Goldman-Rakic, P. S. 1983. Columnar organization of corticocortical projections in squirrel and rhesus monkeys: Similarity of column width in species differing in cortical volume. *Journal of Comparative Neurology* 220: 355–64.

Burton, H., and Jones, E. G. 1976. The posterior thalamic region and its cortical projection in New World and Old World monkeys. *Journal of Comparative Neurology* 168: 249–301.

Campbell, G., and Frost, D. O. 1987. Target-controlled differentiation of axon terminals and synaptic organization. *Proceedings of National Academy of Science, USA* 84: 6929–33.

Carlson, M. 1984. Development of tactile discrimination capacity in Macaca Mulatta: I. Normal infants. *Brain Research* 318: 69–82.

Casagrande, V. A., and Condo, G. J. 1988. Is binocular competition essential for layer formation in the lateral geniculate nucleus? *Brain, Behavior and Evolution* 31: 198–208.

Caviness, V. S., Jr. 1976. Patterns of cell and fiber distribution in the neocortex of the reeler mutant mouse. *Journal of Comparative Neurology* 170: 435–48.

———. 1982. Neocortical histogenesis in normal and reeler mouse: A developmental study based on [^{3}H] thymidine autoradiography. *Brain Research* 256: 293–302.

Caviness, V. S., Jr., and Rakic, P. 1978. Mechanisms of cortical development: A view from mutations in mice. *Annual Review of Neuroscience* 1: 297–326.

Chalupa, L. M.; Killackey, H. P.; Snider, C. J.; and Lia, B. 1989. Callosal projection neurons in area 17 of the fetal rhesus monkey. *Developmental Brain Research* 46: 303–8.

Chi, J. G.; Dooling, E. C.; and Gilles, F. H. 1977. Gyral development of the human brain. *Annals of Neurology* 1: 86–93.

Chugani, H. T., and Phelps, M. E. 1986. Maturational changes in cerebral function in infants determined by ^{18}FDG positron emission tomography. *Science* 231: 840–43.

Chun, J. J. M., and Shatz, C. J. 1989. The earliest-generated neurons of the cat cerebral cortex: Characterization by MAP2 and neurotransmitter immunohistochemistry during fetal life. *Journal of Neuroscience* 9: 1648–67.

Chuong, C. M., 1990. Differential roles of multiple adhesion molecules in cell migration: Granule cell migration in cerebellum. *Experientia* 46: 892–99.

Clark, A. S., and Goldman-Rakic, P. S. 1989. Gonadal hormones influence the emergence of cortical function in nonhuman primates. *Behavioral Neuroscience* 103: 1287–95.

Code, R. A., and Winer, J. A. 1986. Columnar organization and reciprocity of commissural connections in cat primary auditory cortex (AI). *Hearing Research* 23: 205–22.

Connolly, C. J. 1940. Development of cerebral sulci. *American Journal of Physical Anthropology* 26: 113–49.

Cooper, M. L., and Rakic, P. 1981. Neurogenetic gradients in the superior and inferior colliculi of the rhesus monkey. *Journal of Comparative Neurology* 202: 309–34.

———. 1983. Gradients of cellular maturation and synaptogenesis in the superior colliculus of the fetal rhesus monkey. *Journal of Comparative Neurology* 215: 165–86.

Cooper, N. G. F., and Steindler, D. A. 1986. Lectins demarcate the barrel subfield in the somatosensory cortex of the early postnatal mouse. *Journal of Comparative Neurology* 249: 157–69.

Creutzfeldt, O. D. 1977. Generality of the functional structure of the neocortex. *Naturwissenschaften* 64: 507–17.

Curtiss, S. 1977. *Genie: A Psycholinguistic Study of a Modern-day "Wild Child."* New York: Academic Press.

Danek, A.; Heye, B.; and Schroedter, R. 1992. Cortically evoked motor responses in patients with Xp22.3-linked Kallmann's syndrome and in female gene carriers. *Annals of Neurology* 31: 299–304.

Darian-Smith, C.; Darian-Smith, I.; and Cheema, S. S. 1990*a*. Thalamic projections to sensorimotor cortex in the macaque monkey: Use of multiple retrograde fluorescent tracers. *Journal of Comparative Neurology* 299: 17–46.

―――. 1990*b*. Thalamic projections to sensorimotor cortex in the newborn macaque. *Journal of Comparative Neurology* 299: 47–63.

Dehay, C., and Kennedy, H. 1988. The maturational status of thalamocortical and callosal connections of visual areas V1 and V2 in the newborn monkey. *Behavioral Brain Research* 29: 237–44.

Dehay, C.; Kennedy, H.; and Bullier, J. 1986. Callosal connectivity of areas V1 and V2 in the newborn monkey. *Journal of Comparative Neurology* 254: 20–33.

Dehay, C.; Kennedy, H.; Bullier, J. & Berland, M. 1988. Absence of interhemispheric connections of area 17 during development in the monkey. *Nature* 331: 348–50.

Dekker, J. J., and Rakic, P. 1980. Genesis of the neurons in the motor cortex and VA-VL thalamic complex in rhesus monkey. *Society of Neuroscience Abstracts* 6: 205.

de Lacoste, M. C., and Woodward, D. J. 1988. The corpus callosum in nonhuman primates: Determinants of size. *Brain, Behavior and Evolution* 31: 318–23.

Diamond, A., and Goldman-Rakic, P. S. 1986. Comparative development of human infants and infant rhesus monkey on cognitive functions that depend on prefrontal cortex. *Society of Neuroscience Abstracts* 12: 274.

DiFiglia M.; Pasik, P.; and Pasik, T. 1980. Early postnatal development of the monkey neostriatum: A Golgi and ultrastructural study. *Journal of Comparative Neurology* 190: 303–31.

Dubin, M. W.; Stark, L. A.; and Archer, S. M. 1986. A role for action-potential activity in the development of neuronal connections in the kitten retinogeniculate pathway. *Journal of Neuroscience* 6: 1021–36.

Easter, S. S.; Jr.; Purves, D.; Rakic, P.; and Spitzer, N. C. 1985. The changing view of neural specificity. *Science* 230: 507–11.

Edelman, G. M. 1983. Cell adhesion molecules. *Science* 219: 450–57.

Ellingson, R. J., and Willcott, R. C. 1960. Development of evoked responses in visual and auditory cortices of kittens. *Journal of Neurophysiology* 23: 363–75.

Erzurumlu, R. S., and Jhaveri, S. 1990. Thalamic axons confer a blueprint of the sensory periphery onto the developing rat somatosensory cortex. *Developmental Brain Research* 56: 229–34.

Fallon, J. H., and Ziegler, B. T. S. 1979. The crossed cortico-caudate projection in the rhesus monkey. *Neuroscience Letters* 15: 29–32.

Feng, J. Z., and Brugge, J. F. 1983. Postnatal development of auditory callosal connections in the kitten. *Journal of Comparative Neurology* 214: 416–26.

Fishell, G., and van der Kooy, D. 1991. Pattern formation in the striatum: Neurons with early projections to the substantia nigra survive the cell death period. *Journal of Comparative Neurology* 312: 33–42.

Flechsig, P. 1920. *Anatomie des menschlichen Gehirns und Rückenmarks auf myelogenetischer Grundlage.* Leipzig: Thieme.

Franco, B.; Guioli, S.; Pragliola, A.; Incerti, B.; Bardoni, B.; Tonlorenzi, R.; Carrozzo, R.; Maestrini, E.; Pieretti, M.; Taillon-Miller, P.; Brown, C. J.; Willard, H. F.; Lawrence, C.; Persico, M. G.; Camerino, G.; and Ballabio, A. 1991. A gene deleted in Kallmann's syndrome shares homology with neural cell adhesion and axonal path-finding molecules. *Nature* 353: 529–36.

Freeman, T. B.; Spence, M. S.; Boss, B. D.; Spector, D. H.; Strecker, R. E.; Olanow, C. W.; and Kordower, J. H. 1991. Development of dopaminergic neurons in the human substantia nigra. *Experimental Neurology* 113: 344–53.

Friedman, S. L., and Sigman, M. 1981. *Preterm Birth and Psychological Development.* New York: Academic Press.

Frost, D. O., and Metin, C. 1985. Induction of functional retinal projections to the somatosensory system. *Nature* 317: 162–64.

Gadson, D. R., and Emery, J. L. 1976. Some quantitative morphological aspects of post-natal human cerebellar growth. *Journal of Neurological Science* 29: 137–48.

Gao, W-Q., and Hatten, M. E. 1993. Neuronal differentiation rescued by implantation of *weaver* gradule cell precursors into wild-type cerebellar cortex. *Science* 260: 367–69.

Gerfen, C. R. 1984. The neostriatal mosaic: Compartmentalization of corticostrial input and striatonigral output systems. *Nature* 311: 461–64.

———. 1989. The neostriatal mosaic: Striatal patch-matrix organization is related to cortical lamination. *Science* 246: 385–88.

Gilbert, C. D. 1983. Microcircuitry of the visual cortex. *Annual Review of Neuroscience* 6: 217–47.

Gilbert, C. D., and Wiesel, T. N. 1983. Clustered intrinsic connections in cat visual cortex. *Journal of Neuroscience* 3: 1116–33.

Goldman, P. S. 1974. An alternative to developmental plasticity: Heterology of CNS structures in infants and adults. In D. G. Stein, J. J. Rosen and N. Butters (eds.), *Plasticity and Recovery of Function in the Central Nervous System* (New York: Academic Press), pp. 149–74.

———. 1975. Age, sex, and experience as related to the neural basis of cognitive development. In N. A. Buchwald and M. A. B. Brazier (eds.), *Brain Mechanisms and Mental Retardation* (New York: Academic Press), pp. 379–82.

———. 1976a. The role of experience in recovery of function following orbital prefrontal lesions in infant monkeys. *Neuropsychologia* 14: 401–12.

———. 1976b. Maturation of the mammalian nervous system and the ontogeny of behavior. In J. S. Rosenblatt, R. A. Hinde, E. Shaw, and C. Beer (eds.), *Advances in the Study of Behavior,* vol. 7 (New York: Academic Press), pp. 1–90.

———. 1978. Neuronal plasticity in primate telencephalon: Anomalous projections induced by prenatal removal of frontal cortex. *Science* 202: 768–70.

Goldman, P. S. and Alexander, G. E. 1977. Maturation of prefrontal cortex in the monkey revealed by local reversible cryogenic depression. *Nature* 267: 613–15.

Goldman, P. S.; Crawford, H. T.; Stokes, L. P.; Galkin T. W.; and Rosvold, H. E. 1974. Sex-dependent behavioral effects of cerebral cortical lesions in the developing rhesus monkey. *Science* 186: 540–42.

Goldman, P. S., and Galkin T. W. 1978. Prenatal removal of frontal association cortex in the rhesus monkey: Anatomical and functional consequences in postnatal life. *Brain Research* 152: 451–85.

Goldman, P. S., and Mendelson, M. J. 1977. Salutary effects of early experience on deficits caused by lesions of frontal association cortex in developing rhesus monkeys. *Experimental Neurology* 57: 588–602.

Goldman, P. S., and Nauta, W. J. H. 1977a. An intricately patterned prefronto-caudate projection in the rhesus monkey. *Journal of Comparative Neurology* 171: 369–86.

———. 1977*b*. Columnar distribution of cortico-cortical fibers in the frontal association, limbic, and motor cortex of the developing rhesus monkey. *Brain Research* 122: 393–413.

Goldman, P. S., and Rosvold, H. E. 1970. Localization of function within the dorsolateral prefrontal cortex of the rhesus monkey. *Experimental Neurology* 27: 291–304.

———. 1972. The effects of selective caudate lesions in infant and juvenile rhesus monkeys. *Brain Research* 43: 53–66.

Goldman-Rakic, P. S. 1981*a*. Prenatal formation of cortical input and development of cytoarchitectonic compartments in the neostriatum of the rhesus monkey. *Journal of Neuroscience* 1: 721–35.

———. 1981*b*. Development and plasticity of primate frontal association cortex. In F. O. Schmitt, F. G. Worden, G. Adelman, and S. G. Dennis (eds.), *The Organization of the Cerebral Cortex* (Cambridge: MIT Press), pp. 69–97.

———. 1982*a*. Cytoarchitectonic heterogeneity of the primate neostriatum: Subdivision into "island" and "matrix" cellular compartments. *Journal of Comparative Neurology* 205: 398–413.

———. 1982*b*. Neuronal development and plasticity of association cortex in primates. *Neurosciences Research Program Bulletin* 20: 520–40.

———. 1987. Development of cortical circuitry and cognitive function. *Child Development* 58: 601–22.

———. 1988*a*. Changing concepts of cortical connectivity: Parallel distributed cortical networks. In P. Rakic and W. Singer (eds.), *Neurobiology of Neocortex* (Chichester: Wiley), pp. 177–202.

———. 1988*b*. Topography of cognition: Parallel distributed networks in primate association cortex. *Annual Review of Neuroscience* 11: 137–56.

Goldman-Rakic, P. S., and Rakic, P. 1984. Experimental modification of gyral patterns. In N. Geschwind and A. M. Galaburda (eds.), *Cerebral Dominance: The Biological Foundations* (Cambridge: Harvard University Press), pp. 179–92.

Goldman-Rakic, P. S., and Schwartz, M. L. 1982. Interdigitation of contralateral and ipsilateral columnar projections to frontal association cortex in primates. *Science* 216: 755–57.

Goldman-Rakic, P. S., and Selemon, L. D. 1990. New frontiers in basal ganglia research. *Trends in Neurosciences* 13: 241–44.

Grigonis, A. M., and Murphy, E. H. 1991. Organization of callosal connections in the visual cortex of the rabbit following neonatal enucleation, dark rearing, and strobe rearing. *Journal of Comparative Neurology* 312: 561–72.

Grumet, M.; Hoffman, S.; Crossin, K. L.; and Edelman, G. M. 1985. Cytotactin, an extracellular matrix protein of neural and non-neural tissues that mediates glia-neuron interaction. *Proceedings of National Academy of Science, USA* 82: 8075–79.

Harting, J. K.; van Lieshout, D. P.; and Feig, S. 1991. Connectional studies of the primate lateral geniculate nucleus: Distribution of axons arising from the thalamic reticular nucleus of *Galago crassicaudatus*. *Journal of Comparative Neurology* 310: 411–27.

Harwerth, R. S.; Smith E. L., III; Duncan, G. C.; Crawford, M. L. J.; and von Noorden, G. K. 1986. Multiple sensitive periods in the development of the primate visual system. *Science* 232: 235–38.

Hatten, M. E.; Liem, R. K. H.; and Mason, C. A. 1986. Two forms of cerebellar glial cells interact differently with neurons in vitro. *Journal of Cell Biology* 98: 193–204.

Hayakawa, K.; Konishi, Y.; Matsuda, T. Kuriyama, M.; Konishi, K.; Yamashita, K.; Okumura, R., and Hamanaka, D. 1989. Development and aging of brain midline structures: Assessment with MR imaging. *Radiology* 172: 171–77.

Heffner, C. D.; Lumsden, A. G. S.; and O'Leary, D. D. M. 1990. Target control of collateral extension and directional axon growth in the mammalian brain. *Science* 247: 217–20.

Hendrickson, A., and Rakic, P. 1977. Histogenesis and synaptogenesis in the dorsal lateral geniculate nucleus (LGd) of the fetal monkey brain. *Anatomical Record* 187: 602.

Herkenham, M. and Pert, C. B. 1981. Mosaic distribution of opiate receptors, parafascicular projections and acetylcholinesterase in rat striatum. *Nature* 291: 415–18.

Hines, M. 1942. The development and regression of reflexes, postures, and progression in the young macaque. *Contributions to Embryology: Carnegie Institute,* 30: 153–211.

His, W. 1904. *Die Entwickelung des menschlichen Gehirns wahrend der ersten Monate.* Leipzig: S. Hirzel.

Hogan, D., and Berman, N. E. J. 1990. Growth cone morphology, axon trajectory and branching patterns in the neonatal rat corpus callosum. *Developmental Brain Research* 53: 283–87.

Hoover, J. E., and Strick, P. L. 1993. Multiple output channels in the basal ganglia. *Science* 259: 819–21.

Hubel, D. H., and Wiesel, T. N. 1962. Receptive fields, binocular interaction and functional architecture in the cat's visual cortex. *Journal of Physiology* (London) 160: 106–54.

————. 1963. Receptive fields of striate cortex of very young, visually inexperienced kittens. *Journal of Physiology* (London) 26: 994–1002.

————. 1970. The period of susceptibility to the physiological effects of unilateral eye closure in kittens. *Journal of Physiology* (London) 206: 419–36.

————. 1977. Ferrier lecture: Functional architecture of macaque monkey visual cortex. *Proceedings of the Royal Society of London, Series B* 198: 1–59.

Huttenlocher, P. R. 1979. Synaptic density in human frontal cortex—Developmental changes and effects of aging. *Brain Research* 163: 195–205.

————. 1984. Synapse elimination and plasticity in developing human cerebral cortex. *American Journal of Mental Deficiency* 88: 488–96.

————. 1990. Morphometric study of human cerebral cortex development. *Neuropsychologia* 28: 517–27.

————. 1991. Dendritic and synaptic pathology in mental retardation. *Pediatric Neurology* 7: 79–85.

Innocenti, G. M. 1981. Growth and reshaping of axons in the establishment of visual callosal connections. *Science* 212: 824–27.

Innocenti, G. M.; Fiore, L.; and Caminiti, R. 1977. Exuberant projection into the corpus callosum from the visual cortex of newborn cats. *Neuroscience Letters* 4: 237–42.

Innocenti, G. M., and Frost, D. O. 1979. Effects of visual experience on the maturation of the efferent system to the corpus callosum. *Nature* 280: 231–34.

Innocenti, G. M.; Frost, D. O. and Illes, J. 1985. Maturation of visual callosal connections in visually deprived kittens: A challenging critical period. *Journal of Neuroscience* 5: 255–67.

Ivy, G. O., and Killackey, H. P. 1981. The ontogeny of the distribution of callosal projection neurons in the rat parietal cortex. *Journal of Comparative Neurology* 195: 367–89.

———. 1982. Ontogenetic changes in the projections of neocortical neurons. *Journal of Neuroscience* 2: 735–43.

Jay, V.; Chan, F.-W.; and Becker, L. E. 1990. Dendritic arborization in the human fetus and infant with the trisomy 18 syndrome. *Developmental Brain Research* 54: 291–94.

Jeanmonod, D.; Rice, F. L.; and Van der Loos, H. 1981. Mouse somatosensory cortex: Alterations in the barrelfield following receptor injury at different early postnatal ages. *Neuroscience* 6: 1503–35.

Johnson, P. B.; Angelucci, A.; Ziparo, R. M.; Minciacchi, D.; Bentivoglio, M.; and Caminiti, R. 1989. Segregation and overlap of callosal and association neurons in frontal and parietal cortices of primates: A spectral and coherency analysis. *Journal of Neuroscience* 9: 2313–26.

Johnston, J. G.; Gerfen, C. R.; Haber, S. N.; and van der Kooy, D. 1990. Mechanisms of striatal pattern formation: Conservation of mammalian compartmentalization. *Developmental Brain Research* 57: 93–102.

Johnston, J. G., and van der Kooy, D. 1989. Protooncogene expression identifies a transient columnar organization of the forebrain within the late embryonic ventricular zone. *Proceedings of National Academy of Science, USA* 86: 1066–70.

Jones, E. G. 1975. Some aspects of organization of the thalamic reticular complex. *Journal of Comparative Neurology* 162: 285–308.

———. 1986. Connectivity of the primate sensory-motor cortex. In E. G. Jones and A. Peters (eds.), *Cerebral Cortex,* vol. 5 (New York: Plenum), pp. 113–84.

Jones, E. G.; Burton, H.; and Porter, R. 1975. Commissural and corticocortical "columns" in the somatic sensory cortex of primates. *Science* 190: 572–74.

Kaas, J. H. 1991. Plasticity of sensory and motor maps in adult mammals. *Annual Review of Neuroscience* 14: 137–67.

Kaas, J. H.; Krubitzer, L. A.; Chino, Y. M.; Langston, A. L.; Polley, E. H.; and Blair, N. 1990. Reorganization of retinotopic cortical maps in adult mammals after lesions of the retina. *Science* 248: 229–31.

Kaas, J. H.; Merzenich, M. M.; and Killackey, H. P. 1983. The reorganization of somatosensory cortex following peripheral nerve damage in adult and developing mammals. *Annual Review of Neuroscience* 6: 325–56.

Kahle, V. W. 1966. Zur ontogenetischen Entwicklung der Brodmannschen Rindenfelder. In R. Hassler and H. Stephan (eds.), *Evolution of the Forebrain* (Stuttgart: Georg Thieme Verlag), pp. 305–15.

Kalil, R. E., and Schneider, G. E. 1975. Abnormal synaptic connections of the optic tract in the thalamus after midbrain lesions in newborn hamsters. *Brain Research* 100: 690–98.

Kennard, M. A. 1942. Cortical reorganization of motor function: Studies on series of monkeys of various ages from infancy to maturity. *Archives of Neurology and Psychiatry* 47: 227–40.

Kenne, M. F. L., and Hewer E. E. 1931. Some observations on myelination in the human central nervous system. *Journal of Anatomy* 66: 1–13.

Kennedy, C.; Sakurada, O.; Shinohara, M.; and Miyaoka M. 1982. Local cerebral glucose utilization in the newborn macaque monkey. *Annals of Neurology* 12: 333–40.

Killackey, H. P. 1990. Neocortical expansion: An attempt toward relating phylogeny and ontogeny. *Journal of Cognitive Neuroscience* 2: 1–17.

Killackey, H. P., and Chalupa, L. M. 1986. Ontogenetic change in the distribution of callosal projection neurons in the postcentral gyrus of the fetal rhesus monkey. *Journal of Comparative Neurology* 244: 331–48.

King, A. J.; Hutchings, M. E.; Moore, D. R.; and Blakemore, C. 1988. Developmental plasticity in the visual and auditory representations in the mammalian superior colliculus. *Nature* 332: 73–76.

King, A. J., and Moore, D. R. 1991. Plasticity of auditory maps in the brain. *Trends in Neurosciences* 14: 31–37.

Kling, A. 1966. Ontogenetic and phylogenetic studies on the amygdaloid nuclei. *Psychosomatic Medicine* 28: 155–61.

Kling, A., and Tucker, T. J. 1967. Effects of combined lesions of frontal granular cortex and caudate nucleus in the neonatal monkey. *Brain Research* 6: 428–39.

Knudsen, E. I. 1985. Experience alters the spatial tuning of auditory units in the optic tectum during a sensitive period in the barn owl. *Journal of Neuroscience* 5: 3094–109.

———. 1988. Early blindness results in a degraded auditory map of space in the optic tectum of the barn owl. *Proceedings of National Academy of Science USA* 85: 6211–14.

Knudsen, E. I., and Brainard, M. S. 1991. Visual instruction of the neural map of auditory space in the developing optic tectum. *Science* 253: 85–87.

Knudsen, E. I., and Knudsen, P. F. 1990. Sensitive and critical periods for visual calibration of sound localization by barn owls. *Journal of Neuroscience* 10: 222–32.

Koppel, H., and Innocenti, G. M. 1983. Is there a genuine exuberancy of callosal projections in development? A quantitative electron microscopic study in the cat. *Neuroscience Letters* 41, 33–40.

Kordower, J. H., and Mufson, E. J. 1993. NGF receptor (p75)—immunoreactivity in the developing primate basal ganglia. *Journal of Comparative Neurology* 327: 359–75.

Kostovic, I.; Lukinovic, N.; Judas, M.; Bogdanovic, N.; Mrzljak, L.; Zecevic, N.; and Kubat, M. 1989. Structural basis of the developmental plasticity in the human cerebral cortex: The role of the transient subplate zone. *Metabolic Brain Disease* 4: 17–23.

Kostovic, I., and Rakic, P. (1984) Development of prestriate visual projections in the monkey and human fetal cerebrum revealed by transient cholinesterase staining. *Journal of Neuroscience* 4: 25–42.

———. 1990. Developmental history of the transient subplate zone in the visual and somatosensory cortex of the macaque monkey and human brain. *Journal of Comparative Neurology* 297: 441–70.

Kostovic, I.; Seress, L.; Mrzljak, L.; and Judas, M. 1989. Early onset of synapse formation in the human hippocampus: A correlation with Nissl-Golgi architectonics in 15- and 16.5-week-old fetuses. *Neuroscience* 30: 105–16.

Krushel, L. A., and van der Kooy, D. 1988. Birthdate is more important than tissue type for the in vitro reassociation of early postmitotic cortical and striatal neurons. *Society of Neuroscience Abstracts* 14: 91.

Künzle, H. 1975. Bilateral projections from precentral motor cortex to the putamen and other parts of the basal ganglia: An autoradiographic study in Macaca fascicularis. *Brain Research* 88: 195–209.

LaMantia, A. S., and Rakic, P. 1984. The number, size, myelination and regional variation of axons in the corpus callosum and anterior commissure of the developing rhesus monkey. *Society of Neuroscience Abstracts* 10: 1081.

———. 1990a. Cytological and quantitative characteristics of four cerebral commissures in the rhesus monkey. *Journal of Comparative Neurology* 291: 520–37.

———. 1990b. Axon overproduction and elimination in the corpus callosum of the developing rhesus monkey. *Journal of Neuroscience* 10: 2156–75.

Lauder, J. M. 1993. Neurotransmitters as growth regulatory signals: Role of receptors and second messengers. *Trends in Neurosciences* 16: 233–39.

LaVail M. M.; Rapaport, D. H.; and Rakic, P. 1991. Cytogenesis in the monkey retina. *Journal of Comparative Neurology* 309: 86–114.

Lawrence D. G., and Hopkins, D. A. 1976. The development of motor control in the rhesus monkey: Evidence concerning the role of corticomotoneuronal connections. *Brain* 99: 235–54.

Legouis, R.; Hardelin, J. P.; Levilliers, J.; Claverie, J. M.; Compain, S.; Wunderle, V.; Millasseau, P.; Le Paslier, D.; Cohen, D.; Caterina, D.; Bougueleret, L.; Delemarre-Van de Waal, H.; Lutfalla, G.; Weissenbach, J.; and Petit, C. 1991. The candidate gene for the X-linked Kallmann syndrome encodes a protein related to adhesion molecules. *Cell* 67: 423–35.

Leiner, H. C.; Leiner, A. L.; and Dow, R. S. 1986. Does the cerebellum contribute to mental skills? *Behavioral Neuroscience* 103: 998–1008.

Lennenberg, E. 1967. *Biological Foundations of Language.* New York: Wiley.

Levitt, P., and Rakic, P. 1982. The time of genesis, embryonic origin and differentiation of the brainstem monoamine neurons in the rhesus monkey. *Brain Research* 256: 35–57.

Levitt, P.; Rakic, P.; and Goldman-Rakic, P. S. 1984. Region-specific distribution of catecholamine afferents in primate cerebral cortex: A fluoresence histochemical analysis. *Journal of Comparative Neurology* 227: 23–36.

Lidow, M. S.; Goldman-Rakic, P. S.; and Rakic, P. 1991. Synchronized overproduction of neurotransmitter receptors in diverse regions of the primate cerebral cortex. *Proceedings of National Academy of Science, USA* 88: 10218–21.

Linden, D. C.; Guillery, R. W.; Cucchiaro, J. 1981. The dorsal lateral geniculate nucleus of the normal ferret and its postnatal development. *Journal of Comparative Neurology* 203: 189–211.

Lund, J. S.; and Harper, T. R. 1991. Postnatal development of thalamic recipient neurons in the monkey striate cortex: III. Somatic inhibitory synapse acquisition by spiny stellate neurons of layer 4C. *Journal of Comparative Neurology* 309: 141–49.

Lund, J. S., and Holbach, S. M. 1991. Postnatal development of thalamic recipient neurons in monkey striate cortex: I. Comparison of spine acquisition and dendritic growth of layer 4C alpha and beta spiny stellate neurons. *Journal of Comparative Neurology* 309: 115–28.

Lund, J. S.; Holbach, S. M.; and Chung, W. W. 1991. Postnatal development of thalamic recipient neurons in monkey striate cortex: II. Influence of afferent driving on spine acquisition and dendritic growth of layer 4C spiny stellate neurons. *Journal of Comparative Neurology* 309: 129–40.

Lund, R. D.; Mitchell, D. E.; and Henry, G. H. 1978. Squint-induced modification of callosal connections in cats. *Brain Research* 144: 169–72.

Lund, R. D.; and Mustari, M. J. 1977. Development of the geniculocortical pathway in rats. *Journal of Comparative Neurology* 173: 289–306.

Luskin, M. B.; Pearlman, A. L.; and Sanes, J. R. 1988. Cell lineage in the cerebral cortex of the mouse studied in vivo and in vitro with a recombinant retrovirus. *Neuron* 1: 635–47.

Markowitsch, H. J.; Emmans, D.; Irle, E.; Streicher, M.; and Preilowski, B. 1985. Cortical and subcortical afferent connections of the primate's temporal pole: A study of rhesus monkeys, squirrel monkeys, and marmosets. *Journal of Comparative Neurology* 242: 425–58.

Matsubara, J. A., and Phillips, D. P. 1988. Intracortical connections and their physiological correlates in the primary auditory cortex (AI) of the cat. *Journal of Comparative Neurology* 268: 38–48.

McConnell, S. K. 1985. Migration and differentiation of cerebral cortical neurons after transplantation into the brains of ferrets. *Science* 229: 1268–71.

———. 1988*a*. Development and decision-making in the mammalian cerebral cortex. *Brain Research* 472: 1–23.

———. 1988*b*. Fates of visual cortical neurons in the ferret after isochronic and heterochronic transplantation. *Journal of Neuroscience* 8: 945–74.

———. 1989. The determination of neuronal fate in the cerebral cortex. *Trends in Neurosciences* 12: 342–49.

———. 1990. The specification of neuronal identity in the mammalian cerebral cortex. *Experientia* 46: 922–29.

McConnell, S. K.; Ghosh, A.; and Shatz, C. J. 1989. Subplate neurons pioneer the first axon pathway from the cerebral cortex. *Science* 245: 978–82.

McConnell, S. K., and Kaznowski, C. E. 1991. Cell cycle dependence of laminar determination in developing neocortex. *Science* 254: 282–85.

Meister, M.; Wong, R. O. L.; Baylor, D. A.; and Shatz, C. J. 1991. Synchronous bursts of action potentials in ganglion cells of the developing mammalian retina. *Science* 252: 939–43.

Mellus, E. L. 1912. Development of the cerebral cortex. *American Journal of Anatomy* 14: 107–17.

Merzenich, M. M., and Kaas, J. H. 1982. Reorganization of mammalian somatosensory cortex following peripheral nerve injury. *Trends in Neurosciences* 5: 434–36.

Miller, E. A.; Goldman, P. S.; and Rosvold, H. E. 1973. Delayed recovery of function following orbital prefrontal lesions in infant monkeys. *Science* 182: 304–6.

Mitani A.; Shimokouchi, M.; Itoh, K.; Nomura, S.; Kudo, M.; and Mizuno, N. 1985. Morphology and laminar organization of electrophysiologically identified neurons in the primary auditory cortex in the cat. *Journal of Comparative Neurology* 235: 430–47.

Mitrofanis, J. 1992. Patterns of antigenic expression in the thalamic reticular nucleus of developing rats. *Journal of Comparative Neurology* 320: 161–81.

Mitrofanis, J., and Guillery, R. W. 1993. New views of the thalamic reticular nucleus in the adult and the developing brain. *Trends in Neurosciences* 16: 240–45.

Molliver, M. E.; Kostović, I.; and Van der Loos, H. 1973. The development of synapses in cerebral cortex of the human fetus. *Brain Research* 50: 403–7.

Mountcastle, V. B. 1957. Modality and topographic properties of single neurons of cat's somatic sensory cortex. *Journal of Neurophysiology* 20: 408–34.

Mower, G. D. 1991. The effect of dark rearing on the time course of the critical period in cat visual cortex. *Developmental Brain Research* 58: 151–58.

Mrzljak, L.; Uylings, H. B. M.; Kostovic, I.; and van Eden, C. G. 1992. Prenatal development of neurons in the human prefrontal cortex: II. A quantitative Golgi study. *Journal of Comparative Neurology* 316: 485–96.

Neville, H. J.; Schmidt, A.; and Kutas, M. 1983. Altered visual-evoked potentials in congenitally deaf adults. *Brain Research* 266: 127–32.

Nguyen, C.; Mattei, M-G.; Mattei, J-F.; Santoni, M-J.; Goridis, C.; and Jordan, B. R. 1986. Localization of the human N CAM gene to band q23 of chromosome 11: The third gene coding for a cell interaction molecule mapped to the distal portion of the long arm of chromosome 11. *Journal of Cell Biology* 102: 711–15.

Nudo, R. J.; Jenkins, W. M.; and Merzenich, M. M. 1990. Repetitive microstimulation alters the cortical representation of movements in adult rats. *Somatosensory Motor Research* 7: 463–83.

Ogden, T. E., and Miller, R. F. 1966. Studies of the optic nerve of the rhesus monkey: Nerve fiber spectrum and physiological properties. *Vision Research* 6: 485–506.

Ogren, M. P., and Hendrickson, A. E. 1977. The distribution of pulvinar terminals in visual areas 17 and 18 of the monkey. *Brain Research* 137: 343–50.

Olavarria, J., and Van Sluyters, R. C. 1984. Callosal connections of the posterior neocortex in normal-eyed, congenitally anophthalmic, and neonatally enucleated mice. *Journal of Comparative Neurology* 230: 249–68.

O'Leary, D. D. M. 1989. Do cortical areas emerge from a protocortex? *Trends in Neurosciences* 12: 400–406.

O'Leary, D. D. M., and Stanfield, B. B. 1989. Selective elimination of axons extended by developing cortical neurons is dependent on regional locale: Experiments utilizing fetal cortical transplants. *Journal of Neuroscience* 9: 2230–46.

O'Leary, D. D. M.; Stanfield, B. B.; and Cowan, W. M. 1981. Evidence that the early postnatal restriction of the cells of origin of the callosal projection is due to the elimination of axonal collaterals rather than to the death of neurons. *Developmental Brain Research* 1: 607–17.

O'Rourke, N. A.; Dailey, M. E.; Smith, S. J.; and McConnell, S. K. 1992. Diverse migratory pathways in the developing cerebral cortex. *Science* 258: 299–302.

Pallas, S. L.; Gilmour, S. M.; and Finlay, B. L. 1988. Control of cell number in the developing neocortex: I. Effects of early tectal ablation. *Developmental Brain Research* 43: 1–11.

Pallas, S. L.; Roe, A. W.; and Sur, M. 1990. Visual projections induced into the auditory pathway of ferrets: I. Novel inputs to primary auditory cortex (AI) from the LP/pulvinar complex and the topography of the MGN-AI projection. *Journal of Comparative Neurology* 298: 50–68.

Pandya, D. N.; Karol, E. A.; and Heilbronn, D. 1971. The topographical distribution of interhemispheric projections in the corpus callosum of the rhesus monkey. *Brain Research* 32: 31–43.

Pini, A. 1993. Chemorepulsion of axons in the developing mammalian central nervous system. *Science* 261: 95–98.

Pons, T. P., and Kaas, J. H. 1985. Connections of area 2 of somatosensory cortex with the anterior pulvinar and subdivisions of the ventroposterior complex in macaque monkeys. *Journal of Comparative Neurology* 240: 16–36.

Posner, M. I.; Petersen, S. E.; Fox, P. T.; and Raichle, M. E. 1988. Localization of cognitive operations in the human brain. *Science* 240: 1627–31.

Rakic, P. 1971. Neuron-glia relationship during granule cell migration in developing cerebellar cortex: A Golgi and electronmicroscopic study in Macacus rhesus. *Journal of Comparative Neurology* 141: 283–312.

Rakic, P. 1972. Mode of cell migration to the superficial layers of fetal monkey neocortex. *Journal of Comparative Neurology* 145: 61–84.

———. 1974. Neurons in rhesus monkey visual cortex: Systematic relation between time of origin and eventual disposition. *Science* 183: 425–27.

———. 1975. Timing of major ontogenetic events in the visual cortex of the rhesus monkey. In N. A. Buchwald and M. A. Brazier (eds.), *Brain Mechanisms and Mental Retardation* (New York: Academic Press), pp. 3–40.

———. 1976a. Prenatal genesis of connections subserving ocular dominance in the rhesus monkey. *Nature* 261: 467–71.

———. 1976b. Local Circuit Neurons. Cambridge, Mass.: MIT Press.

———. 1977. Prenatal development of the visual system in rhesus monkey. *Philosophical Transactions of the Royal Society of London* 278: 245–60.

———. 1978. Neuronal migration and contact guidance in the primate telencephalon. *Postgraduate Medical Journal* 54: 25–40.

———. 1981a. Development of visual centers in the primate brain depends on binocular competition before birth. *Science* 214: 928–31.

———. 1981b. Neuronal-glial interaction during brain development. *Trends in Neurosciences* 4: 184–87.

———. 1985. Limits of neurogenesis in primates. *Science* 227: 1054–56.

———. 1988a. Defects of neuronal migration and the pathogenesis of cortical malformations. *Progress in Brain Research* 73: 15–37.

———. 1988b. Specification of cerebral cortical areas. *Science* 241: 170–76.

———. 1991. Development of the primate cerebral cortex. In M. Lewis (ed.), *Child and Adolescent Psychiatry: A Comprehensive Textbook* (Baltimore: Williams & Wilkins), pp. 11–28.

Rakic, P; Bourgeois, J.-P.; Eckenhoff, M. F.; Zecevic, N.; and Goldman-Rakic, P. S. 1986. Concurrent overproduction of synapses in diverse regions of the primate cerebral cortex. *Science* 232: 232–35.

Rakic, P., and Goldman-Rakic, P. S. 1984. Use of fetal neurosurgery for experimental studies of structural and functional brain development in nonhuman primates. In R. A. Thompson, J. R. Green, and S. D. Johnson (eds.), *Prenatal Neurology and Neurosurgery* (New York: Spectrum), pp. 1–15.

Rakic, P., and Nowakowski, R. S. 1981. The time of origin of neurons in the hippocampal region of the rhesus monkey. *Journal of Comparative Neurology* 196: 99–128.

Rakic, P., and Riley, K. P. 1983. Overproduction and elimination of retinal axons in the fetal rhesus monkey. *Science* 219: 1441–44.

Rakic, P., and Sidman, R. L. 1968. Supravital DNA synthesis in the developing human and mouse brain. *Journal of Neuropathology and Experimental Neurology,* 27: 246–76.

———. 1969. Telencephalic origin of pulvinar neurons in the fetal human brain. *Zeirschrift Anatomy Entwickl.-Gesch* 129: 53–82.

———. 1970. Histogenesis of cortical layers in human cerebellum particularly the lamina dissecans. *Journal of Comparative Neurology* 139: 473–500.

Richman, D. P.; Stewart, R. M.; and Caviness, V. S. 1973. Microgyria, lissencephaly, and neuron migration to the cerebral cortex: An architectonic approach. *Neurology* 23: 413.

Richter, E. 1912. Die Entwicklung des Globus Pallidus und das Corpus Subthalamicus. *Monographien aus dem Gesamtgebiete der Neurologie und Psychiatrie* (Berlin: Springer), pp. 1–131.

Ritvo, E. R.; Freeman, B. J.; Scheibel, A. B.; Duong, T.; Robinson, H.; Guthrie, D.; & Ritvo, A. 1986. Lower Purkinje cell counts in the cerebella of four autistic subjects: Initial findings of the UCLA–NSAC autopsy research project. *American Journal of Psychiatry* 143: 862–66.

Rockland, K. S., and Lund, J. S. 1982. Widespread periodic intrinsic connections in the tree shrew visual cortex. *Science* 215: 1532–34.

Roe, A. W.; Pallas, S. L.; Hahm, J.-O.; and Sur, M. 1990. A map of visual space induced in primary auditory cortex. *Science* 250: 818–20.

Santacana, M.; Heredia, M.; and Valverde, F. 1990. Transplant connectivity in the rat cerebral cortex: A carbocyanine study. *Developmental Brain Research* 56: 217–22.

Sarich, V. A. 1985. A molecular approach to the question of human origins. In R. L. Ciochon and J. G. Fleagle (eds.), *Primate Evolution and Human Origins* (Menlo Park, Calif.: Benjamin/Cummings), pp. 314–22.

Schaefer, G. B.; Bodensteiner, J. B.; Thompson, J. N., Jr.; and Wilson, D. A. 1991. Clinical and morphometric analysis of the hypoplastic corpus callosum. *Archives of Neurology* 48: 933–36.

Schambra, U. B.; Sulik, K. K.; Petrusz, P.; and Lauder, J. M. 1989. Ontogeny of cholinergic neurons in the mouse forebrain. *Journal of Comparative Neurology* 288: 101–22.

Schlaggar, B. L., and O'Leary, D. D. M. 1991. Potential of visual cortex to develop an array of functional units unique to somatosensory cortex. *Science* 252: 1556–60.

Schmahmann, J. D. 1991. An emerging concept: The cerebellar contribution to higher function. *Archives of Neurology* 48: 1178–87.

Schmechel, D. E., and Rakic, P. 1979a. A Golgi study of radial glial cells in developing monkey telencephalon: Morphogenesis and transformation into astrocytes. *Anatomy and Embryology* 156: 115–52.

———. 1979b. Arrested proliferation of radial glial cells during midgestation in rhesus monkey. *Nature* 277: 303–5.

Schneider, G. E. 1973. Early lesions of superior colliculus: Factors affecting the formation of abnormal retinal projections. *Brain, Behavior, and Evolution* 8: 73–109.

———. 1981. Early lesions and abnormal neuronal connections. *Trends in Neurosciences* 4: 187–92.

Schwartz, M. L., and Goldman-Rakic, P. S. 1982. Single cortical neurones have axon collaterals to ipsilateral and contralateral cortex in fetal and adult primates. *Nature* 299: 154–55.

———. 1991. Prenatal specification of callosal connections in rhesus monkey. *Journal of Comparative Neurology* 307: 144–62.

Schwartz, M. L.; Rakic, P.; and Goldman Rakic, P. S. 1991. Early phenotype expression of cortical neurons: Evidence that a subclass of migrating neurons have callosal axons. *Proceedings of National Academy of Science, USA* 88: 1354–58.

Selemon, L. D., and Goldman Rakic, P. S. 1985. Longitudinal topography and interdigitation of corticostriatal projections in the rhesus monkey. *Journal of Neuroscience* 5: 776–94.

———. 1988. Common cortical and subcortical target areas of the dorsolateral prefrontal and posterior parietal cortices in the rhesus monkey: Evidence for a distributed neural network subserving spatially guided behavior. *Journal of Neuroscience* 8: 4049–68.

Shatz, C. J.; Chun, J. J. M.; and Luskin, M. D. 1988. The role of the subplate in the development of mammalian telencephalon. In A. Peters and E. G. Jones (eds.),

Cerebral Cortex, vol. 7: *Development and Maturation of Cerebral Cortex* (New York: Plenum Press), pp. 35–58.

Shatz, C. J., and Luskin, M. B. 1986. The relationship between the geniculocortical afferents and their cortical target cells during development of the cat's primary visual cortex. *Journal of Neuroscience* 6: 3655–68.

Shatz, C. J., and Rakic, P. 1981. The genesis of efferent connections from the visual cortex of the fetal rhesus monkey. *Journal of Comparative Neurology* 196: 287–307.

Sherman, S. M., and Spear, P. D. 1982. Organization of visual pathways in normal and visually deprived cats. *Physiological Reviews* 62: 738–855.

Simonds, R. J., and Scheibel, A. B. 1989. The postnatal development of the motor speech area: A preliminary study. *Brain and Language* 37: 42–58.

Siwe, S. A. 1927. Das Gehirn: Die mikroskopische Entwicklung des Grosshirns nach der Geburt. In K. Peter, G. Wetzel, and F. Heindrich (eds.), *Handbuch der Anatomie des Kindes* (Munich: Bargman), pp. 609–32.

Smith, A., and Sugar, O. 1975. Development of above normal language and intelligence 21 years after left hemispherectomy. *Neurology* 25: 813–18.

Steindler, D. A.; Cooper, N. G. F.; Faissner, A.; and Schachner, M. 1989. Boundaries defined by adhesion molecules during development of the cerebral cortex: The J1/tenascin glycoprotein in the mouse somatosensory cortical barrel field. *Developmental Biology* 131: 243–60.

Stryker, M. P., and Harris, W. A. 1986. Binocular impulse blockade prevents the formation of ocular dominance columns in cat visual cortex. *Journal of Neuroscience* 6: 2117–33.

Sur, M.; Garraghty, P. E.; and Roe, A. W. 1988. Experimentally induced visual projections into auditory thalamus and cortex. *Science* 242: 1437–41.

Sur, M.; Pallas, S. L.; and Roe, A. W. 1990. Cross-modal plasticity in cortical development: Differentiation and specification of sensory neocortex. *Trends in Neurosciences* 13: 227–33.

Thompson, C. I.; Schwartzbaum, J. S.; and Harlow, H. F. 1969. Development of social fear after amygdalectomy in infant rhesus monkeys. *Physiology and Behavior* 4: 249–54.

Thong, I. G., and Dreher, B. 1986. The development of the corticotectal pathway in the albino rat. *Developmental Brain Research* 25: 227–38.

Udin, S. B., and Fawcett, J. W. 1988. Formation of topographic maps. *Annual Review of Neuroscience* 11: 289–327.

van der Kooy, D. 1984. Developmental relationships between opiate receptors and dopamine in the formation of caudate-putamen patches. *Developmental Brain Research* 14: 300–303.

Van der Loos, H., and Dörfl, J. 1978. Does the skin tell the somatosensory cortex how to construct a map of the periphery? *Neuroscience Letters* 7: 23–30.

Van der Loos, H., and Woolsey, T. A. 1973. Somatosensory cortex: Structural alterations following early injury to sense organs. *Science* 179: 395–98.

Verbitskaya, L. B. 1969. Some aspects of the ontophylogenesis of the cerebellum. In R. Llinas (ed.), *Neurobiology of Cerebellar Evolution and Development*, proceedings of the first international symposium of the Institute for Biomedical Research, American Medical Association, Education & Research Foundation (Chicago, Ill.: AMA), pp. 859–74.

von Economo, C. 1927. *Zellaufbau der Grosshirnrinde des Menschen*, Berlin: Springer.

Walsh, C., and Cepko, C. L. 1992. Widespread dispersion of neuronal clones across functional regions of cerebral cortex. *Science* 255: 434–40.

Webster, M. J.; Ungerleider, L. G.; and Bachevalier, J. 1990. Lesions of inferior temporal area TE in infant monkeys produce reorganization of cortico-amygdalar projections. *Social Neuroscience Abstract* 16: 618.

———. 1991. Connections of inferior temporal areas TE and TEO with medial temporal-lobe structures in infant and adult monkeys. *Journal of Neuroscience* 11: 1095–116.

Wiesel, T. N., and Hubel, D. H. 1963. Single-cell responses in striate cortex of kittens deprived of vision in one eye. *Journal of Neurophysiology* 26: 1003–17.

———. 1965a. Comparison of the effects of unilateral and bilateral closure on cortical unit responses in kittens. *Journal of Neurophysiology* 28: 1029–40.

———. 1965b. Extent of recovery from the effects of visual deprivation in kittens. *Journal of Neurophysiology* 28: 1060–72.

Williams, R. W., and Herrup, K. 1988. The control of neuron number. *Annual Review of Neuroscience* 11: 423–53.

Williams, R. W., and Rakic, P. 1985. Dispersion of growing axons within the optic nerve of the embryonic monkey. *Proceedings of National Academy of Science, USA* 82: 3906–10.

Wilson, A. C.; Carlson, S. S.; and White, T. J. 1977. Biochemical evolution. *Annual Review of Biochemistry* 46: 573–639.

Witelson, S. F, 1976. Sex and the single hemisphere: Specialization of the right hemisphere for spatial processing. *Science* 193: 425–27.

Withington-Wray, D. J.; Binns, K. E.; Dhanjal, S. S.; Brickley, S. G.; and Keating, M. J. 1990. The maturation of the superior collicular map of auditory space in the guinea pig is disrupted by developmental auditory deprivation. *European Journal of Neuroscience* 2: 693–703.

Woolscy, T. A. 1990. Peripheral alteration and somatosensory development. In J. R. Coleman (ed.), *Development of Sensory Systems in Mammals* (New York: Wiley), pp. 461–516.

Woolsey, T. A., and Wann, J. R. 1976. Areal changes in mouse cortical barrels following vibrissal damage at different postnatal ages. *Journal of Comparative Neurology* 170: 53–66.

Yakovlev, P. I. 1969. Development of the nuclei of the dorsal thalamus and of the cerebral cortex. In S. Locke (ed.), *Modern Neurology: Papers in Tribute to Derek Denny Brown* (Boston: Little, Brown), pp. 15–53.

Yakovlev, P. I., and Lecours, A.-R. 1967. The myelogenetic cycles of regional maturation of the brain. In A. Minkowski (ed.), *Regional Development of the Brain in Early Life* (Oxford: Blackwell), pp. 3–70.

Zecevic, N., and Kostovic, I. 1980. Synaptogenesis in developing neostriatum of the human fetus. *Neuroscience Letters Abstract Supplement* 5: 311.

3

Neurodevelopmental and Genetic Syndromes

The neurobiological processes involved in intrauterine and postnatal brain development were described in Chapter 2. This chapter will review common neuromigrational disorders and genetic syndromes, as well as acquired lesions that are associated with atypical patterns of cognitive development. Pediatric neuropsychologists are likely to encounter children with these problems, since they cover a spectrum of neuropsychological dysfunction ranging from subtle cognitive deficit and learning disabilities to more severe impairment and mental retardation.

NEUROMIGRATIONAL DISORDERS

Neuromigrational disorders (NMDs) range from those that involve a small, isolated area to those that involve large brain regions. Neuronal migration begins at around the 8th gestational week and is completed by week 16 (Sidman & Rakic 1982; Barth 1987). Disorders of neuronal migration may be associated with chromosomal anomalies, fetal infection (for example, cytomegalovirus), disturbance of the intrauterine environment, vascular insufficiency, and genetic or neurodegenerative processes. Neuromigrational disruptions have been reported in several rare disorders such as maple syrup urine disease—a disorder of branched-chain amino acids that presents shortly after birth (Kamei et al. 1992)—and Zellweger (hepato-cerebral-renal) syndrome—a peroxisomal disorder (Evrard et al. 1978).

Before the development of the computed tomograph (CT) scan, it was not possible to identify even gross brain anomalies in living children without invasive procedures. CT scans reveal anomalies such as clefts, porencephalies, and abnormally thickened gyri, but they do not pick up subtler migrational anomalies. However, high-resolution magnetic resonance imaging (MRI), using powerful magnets and thin-slice techniques, can detect NMDs (Byrd et al. 1989; Palmini, Andermann, Olivier et al. 1991). Positron emission tomography (PET) complements information obtained from MRI. These neuroimaging techniques have advanced our understanding of various anomalies and of regional brain development, and they enable us to relate specific brain anomalies to cognitive syndromes (Jernigan & Bellugi 1990; Sarnat 1987).

In the following subsections, a number of migrational abnormalities are described (see Table 3-1).

Lissencephaly (Agyria)

The cortical surface is smooth and fissureless in the developing fetus, but gyral and sulcal markings are readily seen by birth (Chi, Dooling, and Gilles, 1977). *Lissencephaly* is a brain malformation that results in a smooth cortical surface. This developmental anomaly reflects a profound disturbance in neuronal migration prior to 16 weeks of gestation (Dieker et al. 1969; Miller 1963; Norman 1980).

The cortex is markedly thickened and the normal six-layered cortex (see Chapter 2) is reduced, usually to four layers; layer II, which receives cortico-cortical input, and layer IV, which receives thalamocortical input, are absent (Stewart, Richman & Caviness 1975). Pachygyria (abnormal, broad gyri, with all six layers present) and agyria (absent gyri) are often observed. Normal gyral patterns may exist in certain regions, such as the orbito-frontal, basal temporal, and cingulate cortices. Hypoplasia in the corpus callosum and heteropia (neurons that are not in their expected locations) in the olivary nuclei often occur (Stewart, Richman & Caviness 1975). The brainstem and cerebellum appear grossly normal.

A number of etiological factors may lead to lissencephaly. Chromosomal abnormalities were noted. Miller-Dieker syndrome is the result of a deletion of the short arm of chromosome 17 (Schwartz et al. 1988). Norman-Roberts syndrome is an autosomal recessive form (Ianetti et al. 1992). Fukuyama muscular dystrophy (Fukuyama, Haruna & Kawaruza 1960) and "muscle-eye-brain" disease (Santavuori et al. 1989) are also associated with lissencephaly. Lissencephaly has also been reported as a secondary result of congenital cytomegalovirus infection (Hayward et al. 1991).

Children with lissencephaly have a characteristic facial appearance: a promi-

Table 3-1 Anomalies of the Developing Brain

Lissencephaly (agyria)
Megalencephaly
Unilateral megalencephaly (hemimegalencephaly)
Diffuse cortical dysplasia
Schizencephaly
Focal cortical migrational anomalies
Periventricular nodular or laminar heterotopia
Agenesis of the corpus callosum
Arhinencephaly
Holoprosencephaly
Macro cisterna magna
Anomalies of the cavum septum pellucidum

nent forehead, bitemporal hollowing, short nose with upturned nares, protuberant upper lip, and small jaw. Effects of the condition include severe growth and developmental retardation, decreased spontaneous activity, and hypotonia at birth, with later development of hypertonia. The child may have difficulty swallowing and eating, may respond minimally to visual or auditory stimulation, or may have abnormal ocular pursuit. Seizures, often severe, are associated with lissencephaly (Gastaut et al. 1987).

Megalencephaly

Megalencephaly refers to a large head (that is, macrocephaly—head circumference more than two standard deviations above the mean) and a large, heavy brain (for instance, a twofold weight increase). True megalencephaly involves increased numbers of neurons and glia, giant heterotopia, and disrupted neuronal migration (DeMyer 1972). Children with this abnormality are typically mentally retarded, although the retardation is sometimes relatively mild (as in cerebral gigantism or Soto's syndrome).

Unilateral Megalencephaly (Hemimegalencephaly)

Unilateral megalencephaly is a rare malformation. Children with this anomaly present with mental retardation; seizures; severe EEG abnormalities; macrocephaly; overgrowth (hemihypertrophy) of the face, head, body, and/or limbs ipsilateral to the enlarged hemisphere; and neurological deficits. Seizures are often intractable, and hemispherectomy of the abnormal hemisphere is performed, but the outcome is often not as good as in other clinical situations. Unilateral megalencephaly can be associated with neurocutaneous syndromes such as linear nevus sebaceous syndrome of Jadassohn (Hager et al. 1991) and hypomelanosis of Ito.

Hemimegalencephalic brains have an array of migrational anomalies (polymicrogyria, pachygyria, ectopic neurons), increased numbers of glial cells, and markedly increased neuronal size, resembling the giant cells seen in tuberous sclerosis. The cortex is thickened, and white–gray matter demarcation is poor. Normal cytoarchitecture in selected areas is reported, such as the hippocampal formation and the calcarine area (Manz et al. 1979). Basal ganglia and cerebellar abnormalities are common. Remarkably, the uninvolved hemisphere reportedly has a normal cytoarchitectonic arrangement. However, Rintahaka et al. (1993) conducted a PET scan study of eight megalencephalic children and noted that half had patchy hypometabolic areas on the nonhemimegalencephalic side (as well as some hypermetabolic areas) that correlated with a poorer prognosis following surgery.

Diffuse Cortical Dysplasia

Diffuse cortical dysplasia refers to a generalized NMD (also called *band heterotopia, double cortex,* and *generalized cortical dysplasia*) involving a symmetrical, subcortical layer of neurons that have failed in their migration to the cortical surface. The cortex may have a normal gyral pattern and six layers; or it may have anomalous broad gyri and four layers; or it may have a decrease in number and depth of sulci without true macrogyria, as well as poor white–gray matter demarcation and dilated ventricles. Development is normal until close to 1 year of age, when seizures start to occur and development slows (Palmini, Andermann, Olivier et al. 1991). The seizure disorder may involve infantile spasms, Lennox-Gastaut (Ricci et al. 1992), or other multifocal epilepsy. Older children are almost always retarded and have seizures and EEGs consistent with Lennox-Gastaut syndrome. Some children experience only slight intellectual impairment and late onset of epilepsy; their seizures are often easily controlled with anticonvulsants (Livingston & Aicardi 1990).

Schizencephaly

Schizencephaly is characterized by clefts in the parasylvian region and in the precentral and postcentral gyri of one or both hemispheres. There are two types: schizencephalies with fused lips (type 1) (Yakovlev & Wadsworth 1946*a*); and those with separated lips, often accompanied by hydrocephalus (type 2) (Yakovlev & Wadsworth 1946*b*). Bilateral clefts are not necessarily symmetrical. Migrational abnormalities are not restricted to the region of the cleft, and they may involve other cortical areas. Schizencephaly is easily detected on CT and MRI scans (Barth 1992) and can be picked up by ultrasound in neonates, but MRI provides much more detail (Chamberlain, Press & Bejar 1990).

Children with schizencephaly may have seizures, hydrocephalus, microcephaly, mental retardation, and significant motor handicap. Some affected children, however, have normal-range IQs, with only focal neuropsychological deficits congruent with cleft location. For example, three subjects with clefts predominantly involving the left hemisphere manifested evidence of greater left- than right-hemisphere impairment (speech and language deficits, impaired finger and tactile form recognition) as well as pathological left-handedness and right-limb hypoplasia (Aniskiewicz et al. 1990). Familial cases of schizencephaly were reported (Tilton et al. 1988; Hosley, Abroms & Ragland 1992; Hilburger et al. 1993).

Focal Cortical Migrational Anomalies

Neuromigrational disorders may be restricted to small cortical areas. Seizures and/or specific neuropsychological and neurological deficits are the usual presenting signs. Depending on the cortical area affected, the seizure manifestations and the neuropsychological profile can be quite different. Focal cortical dysplasia has been reported in numerous areas: both rolandic areas (Andermann et al. 1987); the occipital lobe, associated with congenital hemianopsia (Tychsen & Hoyt 1985); a single dysplastic microgyrus in the left insular cortex, with severe developmental dysphasia and oromotor apraxia (Cohen, Campbell &

Yaghmai 1989); and bilateral perisylvian dysplasia (developmental Foix-Chavany-Marie syndrome) associated with facial-lingual diplegia, sucking and swallowing problems in infancy, and a severe expressive speech deficit (Becker, Dixon & Troncoso 1989).

Several case reports indicate that other family members are affected, suggesting a genetic etiology. For example, in the case reported by Cohen, Campbell & Yaghmai (1989), the patient's brother had dyslexia. Bilateral perisylvian dysplasia was reported in twins (Graff-Radford et al. 1986) and in siblings (Palmini, Andermann, Aicardi et al. 1991). In a description of the *open opercular sign,* Tatum et al. (1989) described four children who presented failure of normal development of the sylvian fissure coupled with serious developmental deficits.

Periventricular Nodular or Laminar Heterotopia

Periventricular nodular heterotopia refers to clumps of neurons that did not migrate properly and instead became small nodules on the walls of the lateral ventricles. They resemble the heterotopia observed in tuberous sclerosis. Heterotopia may also be found in the white matter overlying the ventricles, where it has the same signal characteristics on MRI as the cortical mantle. These displaced clumps of neurons may show metabolic patterns resembling cortex on PET scans (Lee et al. 1994). Three females in one family had periventricular nodular heterotopia, and two of the patients had normal intelligence (Kamuro & Tenokuchi 1993).

Abnormalities of the Corpus Callosum

The corpus callosum appears between the 8th and the 12th gestational weeks (see Chapter 2). As early as the 6th gestational week, cortical fibers cross the lamina reuniens and the anterior commissure. By the 12th week, callosal fibers cross between the anterior commissure and the hippocampal commissure (the dorsal lamina reuniens). By the 17th gestational week, the fetal corpus callosum resembles a minature version of the adult corpus callosum. Although partial or complete agenesis of the corpus callosum is quite obvious on MRI scans, careful measurement of callosal area (relative to age- and sex-matched norms) may reveal more subtle abnormalities. Normative data on the ratio of corpus callosum area to total intracranial vault area are available. These data suggest that the development of the corpus callosum continues well into adulthood, and that it occurs at different rates at different times. For example, Schaefer et al. (1990) reported that no significant changes in callosal size occurred between preschool (up to 5 years old) and elementary school children (6 to 10 years old), but a large increase occurred between elementary school children and adolescents (11 to 15 years old). Corpus callosum area measured longitudinally with MRI for 11- to 61-year-old subjects revealed continued growth through age 20 to 29, with a subsequent plateau in rate of change (Pujol et al. 1993).

Agenesis of the Corpus Callosum

Agenesis of the corpus callosum has a prevalence of 1 to 3 per 1000 (Myrianthropoulos 1974). Schaefer, Bodensteiner et al. (1991) reported that 1% of 307 neurogenetics clinic patients had complete or partial corpus callosum agenesis. Jeret et al. (1987) reviewed a large group of agenesis cases and reported that total or partial callosal agenesis is characteristic of certain neurological syndromes, including *Aicardi's syndrome* (infantile spasms, chorioretinal lacunae, mental retardation, and presumed X-linked dominance, with lethality in males); *Andermann's syndrome* (an autosomal recessive syndrome characterized by retardation, areflexia, paraparesis due to a progressive sensorimotor neuropathy, and sometimes associated with psychosis [Filteau et al. 1991]); *Shapiro's syndrome* (excessive sweating, with reduction of body temperature to hypothermic levels); and *Acrocallosal syndrome* (polydactyly and severe retardation, possibly an autosomal dominant mutation).

Agenesis of the corpus callosum is also associated with some cases of *Apert's syndrome* (de León et al. 1987), occurs at increased incidence in schizophrenics (Swayze et al. 1990), can follow intrauterine exposure to toxins (as in fetal alcohol syndrome) (Wisniewski et al. 1983), and is seen in neural tube developmental defects such as spina bifida, aqueductal stenosis, and Dandy-Walker syndrome (see Chapter 7). It is also seen in association with a number of inborn errors of metabolism, such as hyperglycinemia (Dobyns 1989), Hurler's syndrome (Jellinger et al. 1981) and Leigh's syndrome (Carleton, Colins & Schimpff, 1976), probably reflecting exposure of the fetus to toxic metabolites that affect neuronogenesis (Kolodny 1989). In addition, agenesis is associated with other neuronal migrational anomalies such as polymicrogyria, hydrocephalus, and arhinencephaly.

A number of physical anomalies were described with partial or complete agenesis of the corpus callosum. These include hypertelorism (wide-set eyes), low-set and posteriorly rotated ears, high-arched palate, and cardiovascular defects. Clinically, children may be microcephalic, have seizures, and be mentally retarded. However, agenesis may also be an incidental finding in apparently normal children. Commonly, partial agenesis involves the posterior rather than anterior region. *Partial agenesis of the corpus callosum* typically involves the splenium; but cases of anterior agenesis of the corpus callosum, associated with other significant brain anomalies, were reported (Schaefer, Shuman et al. 1991). Anterior involvement has been detected principally in children with myelomeningocele (Fletcher et al. 1992).

Careful assessment of patients with agenesis of the corpus callosum reveals specific but different patterns of neuropsychological deficit. Some investigators suggest that these result from competition for neuronal resources (Gazzaniga 1970). Specific deficits reported include visuospatial deficits (Dennis 1977); impaired syntactic abilities (comprehending, producing, or repeating syntactically complex sentences; and deficient metalinguistic and pragmatic knowledge, but phonological and lexical-semantic strengths coupled with intact memory (Dennis 1981; Sanders 1989). Intact perceptual and cognitive perspective-taking was reported in two siblings with callosal agenesis (Temple & Vilarroya 1990). Persisting synkinesia (difficulty making isolated finger movements) was reported (Dennis 1976).

OTHER DEVELOPMENTAL BRAIN ANOMALIES

The following subsections describe developmental brain anomalies that affect structural development, occur in cortical and/or noncortical regions, and may involve NMDs. In general, these anomalies are associated with a significant degree of cognitive dysfunction.

Arhinencephaly and Holoprosencephaly

Arhinencephaly refers to congenital absence of the olfactory bulb and tracts associated with fusion of the cerebral hemispheres (olfactory aplasia). Cortical NMDs, optic pathway and long-tract abnormalities, fusion of the basal ganglia or thalami, cerebellar hypoplasia and heterotopia, dentato-olivary dysplasia, and agenesis or hypoplasia of the corpus callosum are associated with this condition. The term *holoprosencephaly* applies to associated cerebral and facial malformations (DeMyer, Zeman & Palmer 1964). Midface hypoplasia (secondary to maldevelopment of the frontonasal process) leads to a variety of lip, nose, palate, and eye anomalies. Eye position ranges from hypotelorism (closeset) to a single midline eye. Children with this malformation are severely retarded. Holoprosencephaly is associated with anomalies of chromosomes 7, 13, and 18 and undefined autosomal recessive forms (Kobori, Herrick & Urich 1987).

Macro Cisterna Magna

The cisterna magna (cerebellomedullary cistern) is a posterior fossa space that receives cerebrospinal fluid flowing out of the foraminae of Magendie and Luschka (see Chapter 7). Until recently, macro cisterna magna was considered a normal variant. However, of 14 children with an enlarged cisterna magna, a substantial number were boys with neurodevelopmental problems and other CNS anomalies (Bodensteiner et al. 1988), suggesting that this structural deviation may be a marker for neuronal and brain maldevelopment.

Anomalies of the Cavum Septum Pellucidum

The septum pellucidum is an anterior midline structure with two leaves (lateral processes) located just below the genu of the corpus callosum and between the anterior horns of the lateral ventricles. The cavum refers to the separation of these two leaves—a normal finding in the fetus. It has been found as late as 34 gestational weeks in normal prematures, and it can be seen in about 80% of newborns (Larroche & Baudley 1961). However, it constituted a rare finding (2.2%) in a CT study of older children (Nakanno et al. 1981). Size is a consideration; that is, it is small when present. Although its presence has been considered to be a normal variant, it seems likely that, with improved neuroradiological imaging, the presence of a large cavum septum pellucidum (over 1 cm) will become a marker for neurodevelopmental problems associated with anterior structures and the corpus callosum. Bodensteiner and Schaefer (1990) identified nine children with wide cavum septi pellucidi who had growth failure, optic nerve hypoplasia, and anomalies of the corpus callosum, in association with a variety of seizures and developmental retardation. Absence of a septum pellucidum has been reported to be associated with bilateral polymicrogyria (Siejka, Strefling & Urich 1989).

GENETIC AND CHROMOSOMAL ANOMALIES—BASIC CONCEPTS AND TERMS

Within the last decade, advances in molecular biology and increased knowledge about the human genome have led to an appreciation of the neuropsychological diversity of common genetic and chromosomal syndromes. It remains unclear how gene defects result in anomalous brain development and give rise to the characteristic neuropsychological profiles. Eventual understanding of the effects of these abnormalities on development depends on three different sources of information: the neuropsychological profiles of the various syndromes; the precise structural and functional anomalies of the brain that are characteristic of each syndrome; and the specific ways in which genes affect brain development and structure, and thus alter normal cognition. The Human Genome Project will ultimately provide the genetic information base. Syndromes currently grouped together because of their superficial resemblances may then be reclassified in terms of their genetic relationships. Details of current understanding of the neuropsychological profiles of children with some common syndromes are presented in the following subsections.

Each cell in the body (somatic cell) is *diploid:* it contains 23 pairs (for a total of 46) of identical, or almost identical chromosomes, with one chromosome in each pair coming from each parent. Twenty-two of these chromosome pairs are *autosomes,* and one is a *sex chromosome* pair. Females have two X chromosomes: a maternally derived X chromosome (X^m), and a paternally derived X chromosome (X^p) in each cell. Males have a maternally derived X chromosome and a paternally derived Y chromosome. *Mitosis* is the process that occurs when somatic cells divide and the pairs of chromosomes in each dividing cell are copied so that each daughter cell receives a duplicate of the genetic information complement.

Eggs and sperm *(gametes)* are *haploid:* they contain only one of each pair of the 22 autosomes, and 1 sex chromosome. *Meiosis* refers to the two-stage process in which gametes are produced that contain only one instead of two copies of each chromosome, thus maintaining a constant amount of DNA per cell from one generation to the next. Eggs contain X chromosomes; sperm may have either X or Y chromosomes. Therefore, an egg (containing an X chromosome) fertilized with a Y-chromosome sperm will develop into a male (XY); and an egg fertilized by an X-chromosome sperm will develop into a female (XX). The egg (but not the sperm) also supplies cytoplasm that contains mitochondria and other genetic information. Thus, the offspring (zygote) contains the standard genetic complement of diploid somatic cells—22 pairs of autosomal chromosomes (one from each parent) and 1 pair of sex chromosomes. Each chromosome contains long sequences of unique genetic code (genes), each at a specific locus. Genetic materials may be on the same chromosome (syntenic). *Linkage* refers to the proximity of genes to each other on the same chromosome. *Allele* is a term applied to the different forms that the genes at a specific locus can take. There can be many alleles, not just two. The Human Genome Project is systematically mapping these bits of genetic code, so at some point it will be possible to identify specific genes with specific disorders.

There is a standardized nomenclature for describing a chromosome (see Figure 3-1). Homologous pairs of chromosomes consist of two "arms" attached by a spindle fiber in a central region or *centromere,* and terminal portions or *telomeres.* A chromosome has a short arm (designated as "p") and a long arm (designated as "q"). In the late 1960s and early 1970s, special staining techniques were developed that differentially stained certain chromosomal regions, called *bands.* The banding patterns made systematic identification of *regions* possible. A region is the area of a chromosome that lies between two adjacent banding landmarks. The region or band nearest to the centromere (the proximal region) is numbered 1, and regions and bands are numbered consecutively outward (the segments near the tip are distal). Specific loci can be precisely identified by specifying the chromosome, the arm, the region, and the band in that sequence. Thus, 21q22, translates to chromosome 21, long arm, region 2, band 2, which identifies the area as being close to the centromere on the long arm.

A *karyotype* is the chromosomal complement of a given individual. Cells are cultured, stained, and photographed, and the chromosomes are arrayed on a page and then reviewed by the geneticist. A normal female karyotype is 46,XX; a normal male karyotype is 46,XY. The karyotype of a girl with typical Turner syndrome is 45,X. Deletions of genes or short regions are not evident on a karyotype (and thus, for example, the karyotype of Huntington disease is quite normal), but they are visible with molecular genetic analysis.

Chromosomal aberrations may arise during meiosis. *Nondisjunction* refers to the failure of the pairs of chromosomes to separate completely during meiosis, with resulting *trisomy;* that is, the somatic cells contain three sets of DNA rather than two. Trisomy can involve an entire chromosome (complete trisomy) or only a part of a chromosome (for instance trisomy 13, 18, or 21, Down syndrome). A gamete may be produced with only one copy of a chromosome *(monosomy).* For example, Turner syndrome (45,X) results in only one X chromosome. *Polyploidy* refers to having more than the standard complement of X or Y chromosomes (as is the case with XXXY or XYY individuals). *Complete monosomy* refers to the absence of an entire chromosome (45,X or Turner syndrome). Like partial trisomies, partial monosomies also exist, in which only a portion of a chromosome has been deleted. Recent molecular biological techniques have made it possible to identify deletion of very small areas of the

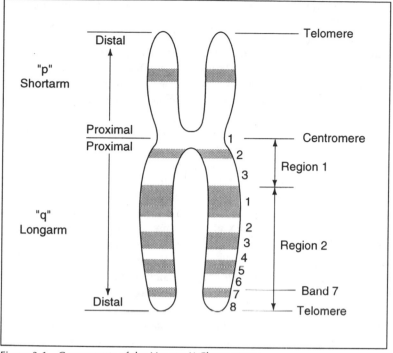

Figure 3-1 Components of the Human X Chromosome

human chromosome. *Balanced reciprocal translocation* refers to the exchange of chromosomal material between two chromosomes of different pairs.

Most normal organisms are made up of one cell line (cells having the same genetic information). *Mosaicism* refers to the intermingling of two different cell lines in one individual. For example, the karyotype of a girl with Turner syndrome who had two cell lines would be designated as 45,X/46,XX. Mosaicism can arise from nondisjunction or chromosome loss. Thus, some individuals may have both trisomic and normal cell lines. Parental mosaicism may give rise to offspring who are trisomic.

Expression of a gene depends on interaction with other genes and nongenetic factors. A distinction is made between the *genotype* (the specific complement of genetic material) and the *phenotype* (the external manifestation of the genetic anomaly, whether it be physical [as in albinism] or behavioral [as with the abnormal cognition and movements of Huntington's chorea]). *Penetrance* reflects the probability that a gene will be manifested in the bearer. If a gene is 60% penetrant, then 60% of all individuals carrying that gene will manifest the trait. Lack of penetrance refers to the absence of discernable effects of a gene; that is, the phenotype appears normal. *Expressivity* of a gene is the particular way a gene expresses itself. A gene may produce varying degrees of expression in different individuals. For example, some children with Down syndrome are severely retarded, with multiple cardiac and gut anomalies, while others are only mildly affected. Sex differences may affect expression of a gene, too.

Thus, boys are typically more severely affected in Tourette syndrome than are girls.

Classical genetic terminology classifies gene disorders as autosomal dominant, autosomal recessive, X-linked dominant, and X-linked recessive. *Autosomal dominant* traits result from vertical transmission of a single gene from an affected parent. Generally, males and females are affected equally, although expressivity may be sex-influenced. *Autosomal recessive* traits are expressed when the affected individual receives matching genes from each parent. Thus, children with Tay-Sach's disease must inherit the abnormal gene from each parent. Autosomal recessive traits are more common in children of consanguineous matings (that is, matings between closely related individuals such as father and daughter), or in genetically inbred populations, since these individuals have a much higher chance of carrying the same recessive gene.

In some cases, when a gene is X-linked (that is located on the X chromosome), the absence of a second X chromosome will result in the appearance of the disease. For example, Duchenne muscular dystrophy (DMD), transmitted by an X-linked gene, is rarely clinically apparent in females; but a girl with Turner syndrome who also has the DMD mutation may present with classical symptoms, since she lacks the second X chromosome.

X-linked inheritance refers to inheritance of a genetic defect that is present on the X chromosome. X-linked recessive traits are expressed only in the absence of the normal allele and are, therefore, seen in males who inherit the affected X chromosome, since they have only one X chromosome—the affected one. Since females with the affected X chromosome have an additional, normal X chromosome, they are phenotypically normal and generally do not manifest the trait. Consequently, they become unaffected carriers.

X-linked dominant traits are expressed in both males and females. If male offspring inherit the X-linked trait, it may result in fetal death. In these families, the offspring consist of unaffected males and 50% of unaffected and 50% of affected females, and there is a high rate of spontaneous abortion. For example, incontinentia pigmentosa (a disorder characterized by whorls of pigment on the skin and neural migrational anomalies) has a marked female preponderance and appears to be an embryonic genetic trait that is lethal in males.

In certain X-linked diseases, the expected pattern of inheritance does not occur. In fragile-X, for example, 20% or more of males with a documented fragile-X premutation are asymptomatic. Female offspring of these males are also asymptomatic, because they have a second, normal X chromosome. However, both male and female offspring of these carrier females may express the syndrome.

Females have a maternally derived X chromosome (X^m) and a paternally derived X chromosome (X^p) in each somatic cell. Thus, they potentially have twice the normal complement of X chromosome gene products. However, *X-inactivation* ("transcriptional silencing") prevents this from happening (Lyon 1991). This process occurs when methyl groups are added to deoxyribonucleic acid (DNA), randomly inactivating one set of X-chromosome genes; the result is a decrease of the XX chromosome products in females. As a result, the "dose" of X-chromosome gene products becomes the same in males and females (that is, dosage compensation). The signal for inactivation emanates from an area called the *X-inactivation center* on X_q. Thus, in normal females, tissue consists of two populations of cells—one derived from the paternal X and the other from the maternal X. Even when supernumerary X chromosomes exist (polyploidy—XXX or XXXXY), only a single X chromosome remains active. Certain specific genes escape X inactivation and are active on both X chromosomes (Fisher et al. 1990). To designate an X chromosome as inactive or active, the subscripts *i* and *a* are used: X_i or X_a.

Molecular genetics has identified several new important types of genetic processes and shed new light on the pathophysiology of inherited disorders. *Genomic imprinting* refers to the differential effect of a gene, a chromosome, or a chromosome set, depending on whether it was inherited from the mother or the father (Hall 1990). Thus, some genes inherited from the parent of one sex act differently from those inherited from the other parent. This is a result of an epigenetic modification (such as DNA methylation) of the imprinted genes (methylation) that occur in the two parents, and it yields different phenotypic manifestations. *Uniparental disomy* occurs when two copies of a gene, chromosome, or chromosome set are inherited solely from one parent, without the usual contribution from the other. Examples of imprinting and uniparental disomy are Prader-Willi syndrome and Angelman syndrome, which are described later in this chapter. Moore and Haig (1991) suggest that imprinted genes have persisted in evolution because this is a process that confers an advantage to some offspring at the expense of others. For example, offspring that have genetic information resulting in atypical placental growth, suckling, appetite control, and hypothalamic function would be at a disadvantage compared to other litter mates. The current human examples of imprinting (Prader-Willi, Angelman, and Beckwith-Wiederman syndromes) all have impairments in this area.

Another recently discovered type of genetic disorder, *trinucleotide repeats,* explains some puzzling patterns of inheritance and is of particular interest to neuropsychologists, because of its association with neuropsychiatric disorders (Ross et al. 1993). Examples of such conditions include fragile-X, myotonic dystrophy, Huntington disease, spinal and bulbar muscular atrophy, and spinocerebellar ataxia. Numerous examples of trinucleotide repeats were identified in normally occurring genes (Ross et al. 1993).

Nucleotides are the discrete chemical components of deoxyribonucleic acid (DNA) and ribonucleic acid (RNA). DNA consists of combinations of any of four organic molecules (bases)—thymine (designated T), adenine (A), cytosine (C), and guanine (G)—attached to a sugar (deoxyribose) and a phosphate molecule. DNA directs its own replication during cell division and directs the transcription to complementary molecules of RNA. RNA also consists of four bases, but thymine is replaced by uracil, and a different sugar molecule (ribose) is involved. Messenger RNA (mRNA) directs the synthesis of amino acids, which are the building blocks of proteins. Trinucleotide repeats are present in genomic DNA and consist of repeated units of three nucleotides. When they occur in the coding regions of genes, they direct the synthesis of repeating single amino acids.

In the neuropsychiatric diseases listed earlier, specific trinucleotide repeats occur. For example, the gene responsible for myotonic dystrophy (DM-1 or myotonin protein kinase) contains a CTG repeat; and the gene responsible for fragile-X is called FMR-1, which contains multiple repeats of the triplet CGG. The length of a trinucleotide repeat varies from one normal individual to another; thus, for instance, the length of the trinucleotide repeats that are associated with fragile-X range in normal individuals from 6 to 42 triplets. Some individuals, however, have a *premutation*—an allele with a slightly longer repeat (50 to 200 in fragile-X) that may persist unchanged for many generations. Persons with these premutations appear entirely phenotypically normal, but the premutations make the DNA sequence unstable. At some point, an increase in length occurs that continues to increase dramatically from one generation to the next (in fragile-X, this may involve as many as several thousand repeats). Increasing severity of the clinical manifestations accompany the increase in trinucleotide repeats. The process stops when the defects become so severe that reproduction of the repeated sequences is no longer possible. In rare cases (described in myotonic dystrophy), the long trinucleotide repeat may shrink back to normal size, with a resulting normal phenotype (Shelbourne et al. 1992; Brunner 1993). Rather than being *fixed* mutations, diseases resulting from trinucleotide repeats are *dynamic* mutations (Richards & Sutherland 1992) that can change from one generation to the next. Trinucleotide repeats explain the phenomenon of *anticipation* in these disorders: the clinical manifestations are manifested earlier and become much more severe with each successive generation. The amino acids coded by these sequences are widely expressed in the brain, with the specific form of expression depending on the particular amino acids and proteins involved. The precise way that the triplet repeats cause neuropsychiatric disease is not yet known. Fischbeck (1994) points out that some of these diseases may involve an increase in amount of gene product that is in some way neurotoxic. Further, there may be differences in the molecular expression of the triplet repeats, depending on the tissue examined. For example, white cells may have a different profile of repeats than saliva cells or brain cells (Taylor et al. 1994).

DISORDERS ASSOCIATED WITH DEFINED CHROMOSOMAL ANOMALIES

In the subsections that follow, several common chromosomal and genetic syndromes of interest to the neuropsychologist are reviewed. Included are Down syndrome, fragile-X syndrome, Turner syndrome, XYY syndrome, Prader-Willi syndrome, Angelman syndrome, neurofibromatosis, myotonic dystrophy, and Williams syndrome (see Table 3-2). Issues of interest include whether specific patterns of cognitive deficit are associated with these syndromes and, if so, in what ways chromosomal and genetic disorders affect the central nervous

Table 3-2 Disorders Due to
Chromosomal Abnormalities

Down syndrome
Fragile-X syndrome
Turner syndrome
XYY syndrome
Prader-Willi syndrome
Angelman syndrome
Neurofibromatosis
Myotonic dystrophy
Williams syndrome

system, leading to these cognitive profiles. The mechanisms appear to be quite variable and specific to the type of chromosomal defect. For example, trisomic states that have increased gene dosage may have different pathophysiologic features than do mosaic or monosmic states that have decreased gene dosage. Genetic deletions may result in specific deficits and characteristic neuropsychological profiles. Such studies are only now being conducted, aided by molecular biological techniques. Early results have found abnormalities of the dendritic tree or of synaptic organization in some trisomic states (Marin-Padilla 1972; Jay, Chan & Becker 1990; Huttenlocher 1991). Genetic syndromes may influence neuronal migration by affecting cell adhesion molecules or neurotransmitter systems (which have both a general growth-controlling feature and a specific neural transmission feature).

Down Syndrome

Down syndrome (DS) is the most common and extensively studied of the mental retardation syndromes associated with a defined chromosomal anomaly. Seguin first described the syndrome in 1846. In 1866, J. H. Langdon Down described the child's physical features and contributed to a confusing nomenclature by attributing epicanthic folds to Mongolian origin. In 1959, two groups of researchers (Lejeune, Gautier & Turpin and Jacobs, et al.) reported finding an extra chromosome 21 in DS patients. There are three cytogenetic types of DS: trisomy 21 (meiotic nondisjunction, accounting for 95% of all cases), translocation (accounting for 4% of cases); and mosaicism with a 21-trisomic clone and a normal disomic clone (accounting for 1 to 2% of cases). Trisomy of the entire chromosome 21 is not required. Down syndrome can result from trisomy of the distal portion of the long arm of chromosome 21 (21q22) (Hagemeijer & Smit 1977; Summit 1981). Only 95% of DS patients have complete trisomy, perhaps accounting for the observed clinical variation in this neurodevelopmental syndrome.

Down syndrome occurs with a frequency of 1 in 800 to 1 in 1000 live births. There is no particular ethnic predilection. The risk of having a DS child increases markedly with increasing maternal age. The risk is 0.71 per 1000 live births at ages 15 to 19 years, increasing to over 50 per 1000 live births at ages 45 to 49 years.

Characteristic dysmorphic features include a brachycephalic (short) head, upward-slanting palpebral fissures, epicanthic folds, Brushfield spots, a protruding tongue, and transverse palmar creases. Neonatal hypotonia is common. Many organ systems are affected. There is increased risk for congenital heart defect, congenital duodenal atresia and stenosis, and immunologic deficiency. Antibody response to vaccines is altered, and thyroid autoantibodies are increased. There is an increased risk for otitis media (Dahle & McCollister 1986).

Down syndrome patients have a 15- to 20-fold greater incidence of leukemia, compared to normal populations (Smith & Berg 1976) and a much higher risk of hematopoietic (blood-cell formation) dysfunction. There is also increased risk of seizures (50% in some series) in this population (Wisniewski et al. 1978). Alzheimer's disease (AD) is invariably found in persons with DS who are over the age of 40 years (Scott, Becker & Petit 1983). Neurofibrillary tangles and neuritic plaques (hallmarks of non-DS adults with AD) are not seen in brains of children under 10 years of age, but are seen in 15% of those 10 to 20 years of age, in 36% of those 21 to 30 years of age, and in 100% of those over 30 years of age (Wisniewski, Wisniewski & Wen 1985). DS patients over 50 years of age were found to have an array of neurocognitive impairments and "release" signs (for instance snout and grasp reflexes) (Thase et al. 1984). Young DS adults were identified as memory-impaired on the basis of their short delay savings scores on the Children's Version of the California Verbal Learning Test (Brugge et al. 1994). Subtle evidence of memory dysfunction might be seen in pediatric patients.

Methodological problems complicate the study of cognition in DS children, particularly in controlling for genotype, otitis media (which may adversely affect language competence), and the insidious emergence of AD. Most investigations of cognitive functioning have included only measures of general intelligence, with further neuropsychological investigation rarely conducted. The intelligence of DS children is quite variable, ranging from normal to severely deficient. Connolly (1978) reported on 180 children and adolescents with DS. The mean IQ (mostly Stanford-Binet) of this group was 44.3, with 40% of the sample having IQs over 40, and 1.6% having IQs over 50. This study was performed before modern molecular techniques were available, so characterization of the genotype was not performed. Fishler, Koch, and Donnell (1976) studied groups of mosaic and trisomic DS children. Mosaics had a significantly higher mean IQ than did trisomics (67 ± 13.8 vs. 52 ± 14.6). No significant correlation between percentage of normal cells and severity of cognitive deficit was found.

Typically, visuospatial abilities are relatively preserved, and language is impaired. In one series of 50 DS patients, all had learned to walk at between 2 and 6 years of age, but 10% had never spoken (Wisniewski et al. 1978). As a group, DS children are sociable, tractable, and lovable. The social behaviors of preschool-age DS children were studied in a play situation. The DS children displayed strength in nonverbal social interaction, with higher frequencies of social interactions and fewer requests for objects or assistance (perhaps attributable to a passive interaction style) and no deficit in symbolic play (Mundy et al. 1988).

Language deficits have consistently been identified in DS children and adults. Compared to Williams syndrome adolescents, DS subjects had difficulty with salient features of WISC-R vocabulary words, had Peabody Picture Vocabulary Test scores below their mental age equivalent, and had difficulty accessing exemplars of a semantic category on a fluency task. They also repeated words and strayed from the semantic category, and resorted to guesswork on tasks tapping syntactic comprehension (Bellugi et al. 1990). DS children matched for nonverbal mental age and mother's education had better vocabulary comprehension (Peabody Picture Vocabulary Test—Revised) than syntax comprehension. PPVT-R performance, but not syntax comprehension, improved with age. Difficulty processing sequential information was observed (possibly due to auditory short-term memory deficit or test artifact), and improvement with increasing age was not always noted. DS subjects also had difficulty with the Stanford-Binet Bead Memory subtest, but performed nonsignificantly better than controls on a Stanford-Binet Pattern Analysis subtest (Chapman, Schwartz & Kay-Raining Bird 1991).

Some investigators have suggested that there is right-hemisphere specialization for language in DS, based on dichotic listening task paradigms (Giencke & Lewandowski 1989; Pipe 1988). Tannock, Kershner, and Oliver (1984), however, suggested that the experimental paradigm may have involved right-hemisphere strategies. Piccirilli et al. (1991) used a dual task technique (naming pictures, right- or left-hand tapping task, and naming plus tapping with right hand and left hand). Three groups were included: DS retarded subjects, non-DS retarded subjects, and controls (matched for mental age). Both the DS and non-DS retarded subjects showed the same pattern of performance as controls, although the retarded groups performed less well on both tasks, and had a greater decrement in performance when concurrent tasks were carried out.

Brain weight of DS children has been measured as 76% of that of controls, and weights of brainstem and cerebellum were 66% of normal (Crome, Cowie & Slater 1966; Wisniewski, Wisniewski & Wen 1985). Brain configuration is abnormally round, with a short anterior–posterior diameter and a wide lateral diameter, narrowing of the superior temporal gyrus, and reduction of secondary sulci. Total intracranial volume in DS individuals was significantly less than in age-matched controls (Schapiro et al., 1990). The frontal lobes, operculum, and superior temporal gyrus were often small, with altered sulcal/gyral patterns. The ratio of cerebellar/brainstem weight to the cerebrum was also lessened. Studies of neocortex and hippocampus revealed decreased neuronal density (Ross, Galaburda & Kemper 1984; Wisniewski et al. 1986), abnormal dendritic spines (Marin-Padilla 1976), and atypical dendritic branching patterns (Becker, Armstrong & Chan 1986).

Schapiro et al. (1990) were unable to demonstrate any regional differences in cerebral metabolic rates for glucose between DS subjects and controls in the resting state. On the other hand, in a PET study comparing DS to age/sex-matched controls, Azari et al. (1994) noted no regional difference in the pattern of correlations. However, a discriminant function analysis using a left inferior premotor region (approximating Broca's area) and a left superior temporal region (approximating Wernicke's area) successfully classified all of the DS and and most of the control subjects.

Despite accumulated information about clinical and genetic aspects of DS, there is still little understanding of how the trisomic genetic defect produces anomalous brain structure and impaired cognition (see the review by Coyle, Oster-Granite, and Gearhart [1986]). Several investigations are underway to explore the underlying causes of brain anomalies in this disorder. First, several gene loci were identified on the crucial segment of the long arm of chromosome 21. In the trisomic condition, there is an increased gene dosage effect. How increased activity of certain enzymes reported in DS relates to alterations in brain development is unclear. Second, there is a mouse model of trisomy (mouse chromosome 16) that permits systematic study of the effect of the trisomic condition. Certain gene sequences are retained in the course of evolution, and a chromosome in one species may be homologous to a chromosome in another. The mouse model has many of the physical anomalies reported in DS (cardiac defect, atypical facies, immunologic defects, and reduced brain weight) but individuals with this condition do not survive the fetal period (Epstein, Lee, and Epstein 1980). Third, comparisons of brain structure (at both microscopic and anatomic levels) and neurochemical components of brain can be made between normal controls and DS patients.

Fragile-X Syndrome

Fragile-X syndrome is the second most common genetic form of mental retardation, after Down syndrome, and the most common inherited form. The estimated population prevalence is in the range of 0.73 to 0.92 per 1,000 males (Herbst 1980; Webb et al. 1986). In mentally retarded populations, 2 to 7% of males and 0.3 to 1% of females had the fragile-X chromosome (Jacobs, Mayer & Abruzzo 1986; Webb et al. 1986). Until recently, diagnosis required examining the tip of the long arm of the X chromosome for the presence of a slender thread. This "fragile site" was demonstrated in a culture medium lacking thymidine and folate. Now diagnosis is confirmed through a molecular diagnostic technique (Yu et al. 1991).

As described earlier, the trinucleotide repeat (CGG) is enormously increased in individuals with phenotypically apparent fragile-X, but only when the mutation is passed through the female to her offspring. This may be the result of genetic imprinting. Increased abnormal cytosine methylation occurs at or near the fragile-X site and inactivates the FMR-1 gene in the fragile-X region. The mutated allele is unmethylated in normal transmitting males, methylated only on the inactive X chromosome in their daughters, and totally methylated in most fragile-X males, although some are mosaic (Oberle et al. 1991). These inactivated genes are then passed on to the asymptomatic mother's children.

However, considerable difference exists in the size of the inherited fragments even in affected sibships (Oberle et al. 1991; Yu et al. 1991). The messenger RNA of the FMR-1 gene is highly expressed in brain and testes (the organs affected in fragile-X). The highest levels in the brain occur in the cerebellar granule cell layer, hippocampus, and neurons in the cerebral cortex (Hinds et al. 1993).

Fragile-X Males

The head circumference, height, and weight of fragile-X boys exceed those of normal peers (Sutherland & Hecht, 1985). By adulthood, however, only the head remains large. Boys have an elongated face, high forehead, prominent supraorbital ridges, midface hypoplasia, a broad nasal root, a prominent mandible, and large, underdeveloped ears (Nielsen, Tommerup & Mikkelsen, 1983). Hyperextensible joints, high-arched palate, pes planus, and velvety hyperelastic skin are frequently noted. Enlarged testicles (macroorchidism) are noted in 84% of fragile-X males, even prepubertal males (Bregman et al. 1987; Zachman et al. 1974).

Compared to developmentally disabled males and normal subjects, fragile-X males were found to have decreased size of the posterior vermis and increased size of the fourth ventricle (due to hypoplasia rather than atrophy)—an anomaly also reported in autistic patients (Reiss et al. 1991). This may reflect an embryonic effect on the timing of the migration of various neuronal populations into the cerebellum (Altman & Bayer 1985). Precisely how this anatomical finding relates to the behavioral anomalies of fragile-X males is not clear, but the cerebellum is increasingly implicated in attentional, sensory, motor, and language-processing functions. One possible explanation is that two genes related to cerebellar neural function were identified close to the fragile-X locus, although the relationship is still unclear. The $GABA_A$ receptor subunit gene (GABRA 3) has been mapped to the DXS374 locus in Xq28. GABA is the most common neurotransmitter in the cerebellum (Bell et al. 1989).

The IQ of males with fragile-X syndrome ranges from normal to profoundly mentally retarded (Chudley 1984; de la Cruz 1985). Several studies have suggested that IQ declines between childhood and adulthood. Young fragile-X boys tested in the mildly retarded range, whereas adult males were moderately to severely retarded (Hagerman, Kemper & Hudson 1985). Out of 21 fragile-X males who were tested twice between 5 and 19 years of age, 13 had a significant decline in IQ (Lachiewicz et al. 1987). Decline may coincide with the onset of puberty (Dykens et al. 1989) or the increased demand for abstract reasoning (Hagerman et al. 1989).

A recent multicenter study investigated whether the observed decline in IQ was a true finding or an artifact of the use of different test instruments at different ages (Hodapp et al. 1990). The study included 66 fragile-X males between the ages of 3 and 18 years (mean age: 9.21 years) at first testing and between 5 and 20 years at second testing. The mean interval between tests was $4\frac{1}{2}$ years. Average full-scale IQs declined from around 53 at first testing to 47 at follow-up; 77% of the subjects showed a decline in IQ score, with the most striking decline occurring between 11 and 15 years of age. Fragile-X males appear to reach a plateau with regard to their ability to learn more complex and abstract information, typically during early puberty. In addition, the largest decrements were noted in brighter children whose IQs had been above 60. The authors attributed this effect to reaching a "task-related wall"; in their view, chronological age is less important than the specific intellectual task.

Dysfluent, apraxic speech and echolalia, palilalia, and cluttering characterize the language of fragile-X boys with normal intelligence (Herbst 1980; Paul et al. 1987), but receptive language is relatively preserved. There is lack of consensus about social behavior. Some fragile-X males do not have social deficits disproportionate to their intellectual level and interact cooperatively and pleasantly (Chudley, de von Flindt & Hagerman 1987; de la Cruz 1985).

Fragile-X syndrome may be co-morbid with other disorders. For example, the incidence of fragile-X in autistic groups has varied from 8.4% (Bregman et al. 1987) to 16% (Wahlstrom et al. 1986). Conversely, between 17 and 60% of fragile-X males were reported to meet criteria for autism as well (Brown et al. 1986). Hyperactivity and attention deficit were reported in a large proportion of fragile-X males (Finelli et al. 1985). These symptoms were reported to respond to treatment with folic acid (Froster-Iskenius et al. 1986).

Fragile-X Females

Less information is available on specific characteristics of females with fragile-X syndrome. Fragile-X females often lack the dysmorphic features noted in males (Turner et al. 1980), although characteristic facial features were reported in some studies (Fryns 1986). The incidence of co-morbid psychiatric disorder is unclear; however, female carriers may be at risk for psychiatric disorder. Of 134 carriers, psychiatric disorder was present in 20% of the 46 intellectually impaired subjects and in 10% of 88 subjects of normal intelligence (Fryns 1986).

Specific frontal lobe deficits were found among women with the fragile-X gene (Mazzocco et al. 1992). No evidence of right-hemisphere impairment, dyslexia, or short-term verbal memory deficit was found. Rather, a consistent weakness in attentional functions, distractibility, shyness, impaired organizational skills, and difficulty with transitions was related to prefrontal deficits (Hagerman & Sobesky 1989). In another study, length of the CGG repeat, percentage of methylation of the mutation, and cytogenetic expression were compared to IQ in female carriers of the fragile-X gene. Those with a permutation (50 to 200 CGG repeats) had a mean IQ of 107 (none of these individuals had an IQ below 85). Among those with full mutation (over 200 CGG repeats), the mean IQ was 80.4. Three subjects (mosaics) had IQs of 100, 99, and 74. No significant relationship was found between percentage methylation of the mutant allele and IQ. Differences in the molecular characteristics of the mutation were seen in different tissues, suggesting that the molecular findings in white blood cells may not necessarily reflect the pattern of molecular expression in brain tissue (Taylor et al. 1994).

Turner Syndrome

Turner syndrome (TS) occurs in about 1 out of every 5000 live female births, but it is associated with high intrauterine lethality, so only about 1% of affected fetuses survive to term (Hook & Warburton 1983). Various genetic defects result in the TS phenotype. In about half, an X chromosome is absent (that is, XO). Another 10 to 15% are XO/XX mosaics, and the remaining cases involved one of a variety of structural anomalies, such as duplication of one arm of the X chromosome with loss of the other arm $(45Xi(X_q))$; 2 to 3% have a partial deletion of one X (Massa, Vanderschueren-Lodeweyckx & Fryns, 1992) or a ring chromosome. Some cases involve XY females with a TS extragonadal phenotype with deletions of the short arm of the Y chromosome (Y_p) (Magenis et al. 1984), suggesting that TS is the result of there being only one copy of a gene or genes common to the X and Y chromosomes. The TS phenotype may be the result of decreased production of a protein (RPF4) essential for cellular functioning that is coded by genes on both the Y and X chromosomes, such that the gene on the X chromosome is one of the few that escapes inactivation (Fisher et al. 1990).

Certain dysmorphic features and anomalies characterize TS children (Lippe 1990). At birth, babies often have edema, and oral-motor dysfunction (Mathisen, Reilly & Skuse 1992). Characteristic dysmorphic features and anomalies include low-set hairline, low-set ears, ptosis, micrognathia, high-arched palate, and atypical facies. There may be webbing of the neck or multiple neck folds— a result of a lymphatic clearing system defect. An unusual carrying angle of the elbow, short fourth metacarpals, short neck, and spinal deformities were noted. TS girls often have multiple pigmented nevi, a higher prevalence of coarctation of the aorta, and an elevated incidence of otitis and secondary hearing loss. They are short and have ovarian failure (the result of a lack of oocytes in early development, resulting in dysgenetic ovaries).

Neuropathological studies revealed NMDs (Kolb & Heaton 1975) and posterior right cerebral hemisphere impairment (Reske-Nielsen, Christensen & Nielsen 1982). In a PET scan study, decreased activity in the parietal and occipital lobes was noted in five women with TS (Clark, Klonoff & Hayden 1990).

TS girls do not have a uniform neuropsychological profile. There is considerable heterogeneity in the profile and in the severity of dysfunction. Verbal strengths contrast with particular difficulties on a wide range of nonverbal, visuospatial tasks. For example, in a recent study (Temple & Carney 1993), the TS group with the 45,X karyotype had a mean verbal > performance discrepancy of 14.5 points. Impairments in directional sense (Alexander & Money 1966), spatial reasoning (Money & Alexander 1966), part–whole perception (Silbert, Wolff & Lilienthal 1977), spatial construction and organization (McGlone 1985), mental rotation (Rovet & Netley, 1980; Shucard et al. 1992), and figure-drawing (Rovet 1992) were reported. Difficulty in visualizing outcomes of projects may be evident (Downey et al. 1991). Performance IQ often falls below verbal IQ (Rovet 1990); but 10 to 20% had superior nonverbal (to verbal) abilities (Pennington et al. 1985), and verbal fluency is·impaired. A selective difficulty with math is common (Rovet 1993). These children have social deficits and impaired facial affect recognition (McCauley et al. 1987) and are at risk for nonverbal learning disability (Rourke 1988). Deficits in executive function (Pennington et al. 1985; Waber 1979) and motor speed and coordination (McGlone 1985) were reported. Deficits were also reported in short-term memory (Williams, Richman & Yarbrough 1991), long-term memory, and visual memory (Waber 1979). In a study of event-related potentials (ERP) and reaction time (RT) of TS girls in three age groups, the ERPs in the younger TS subjects did not differ from those of controls. The ERPs of the older group, however, did differ from those of the age-matched control group and more closely resembled the younger group's, suggesting a failure of normal maturation. RTs were longer in the TS subjects, compared to controls. This study suggested that dissociable processes that had different maturational trajectories were present in TS girls (Johnson, Rohrbaugh & Ross 1993).

Prepubertal monozygotic twins discordant for TS were described by Reiss et al. (1993). The karyotype of the TS twin was 45,XO, while that of the normal twin was 45,XX. Both had a superior WISC-R full-scale IQ. The TS twin had a V > P IQ discrepancy of 25 points. There was a 3-point difference between verbal IQs, in contrast to an 18-point difference between performance IQs. The verbal comprehension factor scores (Sattler 1988) did not differ, but the perceptual organization factor scores differed by 21 points. On neuropsychological testing, the TS twin demonstrated visuospatial, attentional, executive function deficits relative to her normal twin. There was evidence of increased hyperactivity and impulsivity. An analysis of the MRI scans revealed larger regional CSF-to-brain ratios in the TS twin, including posterior fossa structures.

It is likely that, as more subjects are studied by molecular genetic techniques, the neuropsychological phenotype will be shown to be closely tied to genotype. Although TS girls with the classical XO genotype had a verbal > performance difference, those with mosaicism, isochromosomes, or deletions did not have a V > P discrepancy, and there were even P > V discrepancies in one case of isochromosome and one case of 45 XO ring X mosaicism (Temple & Carney 1993).

XYY Syndrome

In initial descriptions of XYY syndrome, no behavioral or physical abnormalities aside from mental retardation were noted (Hauschka et al. 1962; Sandberg et al. 1961). The association of aggressive behavior in XYY men with mental retardation was only noted later (Balodimos et al. 1966; Jacobs, Brunton & Melville 1965). The sampling procedures in these early studies were questionable (Owen 1972), however, since some samples were drawn exclusively from mental hospitals or prisons, or consisted entirely of tall men (Theilgaard 1986). In subsequent research, disturbances of cerebral development were described, consisting of migrational abnormalities and maturational delays (Brun & Gustavson 1972; Austin & Sparkes 1980).

XYY boys are not necessarily at risk for mental retardation, although this conclusion is controversial (Balodimos et al. 1966; Price & Whatmore 1967; Salbenblatt et al. 1987). In a sample of 23 cases from several centers, Stewart, Netley & Park (1982) noted that verbal and performance IQs were not particularly lowered. Despite this, more than half of the sample had educational difficulties, and mild developmental delays and learning problems were evidently common. In another study (Theilgaard 1986) 12 XYY and 16 XXY subjects were identified in a birth cohort of 31,438 males. Compared to controls, the full-scale WAIS IQs of these men were significantly lower. There were no differences between XYY and XXY males on other neuropsychological measures. There was a higher proportion of right-handers in the XYY group. XXY males were more ambidextrous. Finger tapping was slower in both groups. No difference was noted in visual-spatial performance. A substantial incidence of educational difficulties (52.6% of the sample) has also been reported (Stewart, Netley & Park 1982). Mild developmental delays and learning problems were observed in XYY males (Bender et al. 1984). The XYYs had particular difficulties in word retrieval, auditory discrimination, speed of processing, and retention of verbal information (Bender et al. 1983). The extent to which these individuals are at risk for antisocial behavior remains to be elucidated (Stewart et al. 1982).

Behavior problems and criminal tendencies were prominent in early case reports. More recent studies, however, suggest that the incidence of behavioral problems (15.8%) in 47 XXY males did not differ from that of the controls (Stewart, Netley & Park 1982) or was presumed related to severe environmental disturbance (Valentine 1982). A tendency toward higher activity levels, more negative mood, and temper tantrums was noted. It is difficult to establish that the disturbed behavior in XYY boys is solely related to the chromosomal anomaly, since multiple environmental factors may give rise to psychiatric disturbance (Ratcliffe & Field 1982). Moreover, psychiatric intervention often improves the behavior of these children.

Prader-Willi Syndrome

The prevalence of Prader-Willi syndrome (PWS) (Prader et al. 1956) is in the range of from 1 in 10,000 (Holm 1981; Cassidy & Ledbetter 1989) to 1 in 25,000 to 30,000 (Zellweger, 1981). More than half of the PWS patients have a cytogenetically detectable deletion in the chromosome 15q11-q13 region (Butler 1989) with additional deletions being diagnosed by molecular techniques (Knoll et al. 1990). The deleted chromosome 15 in PWS is always paternal in origin (Butler, Meaney & Palmer 1986; Nicholls, Knoll, Glatt et al. 1989). Recently, Nicholls, Knoll, Butler et al. (1989) studied two PWS patients in whom no DNA deletion could be discerned; instead, maternal uniparental disomy (UPD) of chromosome 15 was found (that is, no paternal contribution was involved). This work has subsequently been extended to include 18 PWS patients, and it unambiguously demonstrates maternal uniparental disomy (Mascari et al. 1992).

Children and adults with PWS have several consistent behavioral manifestations: they are obese; they have voracious appetites; they manifest poorly controlled food-seeking behaviors; and they gain weight at an accelerated rate. They have outbursts of aggressive, angry behaviors. Many of them also engage in self-injurious behavior, in the form of repetitive, compulsive skin-picking.

At birth, PWS children are typically hypotonic and fit into the "failure-to-thrive" category. As very young children, they are not obese and have a pleasant temperament. Obesity and hyperphagia do not appear until the preschool years, and PWS is frequently not diagnosed until after age 2, when the children accelerate off their weight growth curve. As they age, their food-seeking behaviors become a major management issue, to the extent that food must be locked away. These children will steal food from classmates, seek food in trash, and attempt to break locks on the refrigerator. They often respond angrily to attempts to limit food-seeking.

Other characteristics of this syndrome include mental retardation, short stature, hypogonadism (and infertility), small hands and feet, a stubborn, obsessive–compulsive personality, and a characteristic face (narrow bifrontal diameter with almond shaped eyes) (Butler 1989). PWS patients often manifest dysregulation of temperature and decreased sensitivity to pain.

Children with PWS have major language production deficits, that adversely affect articulation. These include hypernasality, dysfluency, and flaccid dysarthria. Speech apraxia has been reported (Branson 1981; Munson-Davis 1988). A longitudinal study of the phonologic abilities of one child found a phonologic developmental sequence that was similar to normal peers, but delayed (Dyson & Lombardino 1989). Hyperlexia has also been reported (Burd & Kerbeshian 1989).

Angelman Syndrome

Angelman syndrome (AS) is a rare neurological syndrome, also described as "Happy Puppet" (Angelman, 1965). It is frequently the result of a cytogenetic/molecular deletion in chromosome 15q11-q13. In contrast to PWS, however, the deletion is always maternal in origin (Knoll et al. 1989). Lack of the maternal chromosome 15q11-q13 region leads to the Angelman syndrome phenotype. Nicholls et al. (1992) have published cases of paternal uniparental disomy in AS. A third type of AS is familial, and patients show biparental inheritance for the 15q11-q13 region (Knoll et al. 1991). The biparental AS patients are clinically indistinguishable from the deletion and UPD patients (Zori et al. 1992). It is unclear whether a class of PWS patients with biparental inheritance of the 15q11-q13 region exists.

AS is associated with motor and mental retardation. Children with AS appear to be normal at birth, but they rapidly drift off developmental course. They seem able to process certain types of visuospatial information; and although their speech is limited to a few words at best, they can master simple signs and communicate with gesture. They are quite hyperactive, need little sleep, feed poorly, and are thin and of short stature, with a characteristic cheerful countenance. Severe seizures occur in most patients, particularly in AS deletion patients. Like PWS patients, AS patients are often hypopigmented.

Molecular analyses indicate that there is a deletion of the gene encoding the GABA$_A$ receptor beta3 subunit (GABRB3) in AS patients. This deletion lies within the deletion-critical region of AS (but the genetic loci of AS and PWS are distinct) (Saitoh et al. 1992). GABA is the major inhibitory neurotransmitter. A defect in inhibitory neurotransmission mediated by the GABA$_A$ receptor may play a role in the pathogenesis of AS (Saitoh et al. 1992). Deletion of the receptor loci may explain the difference in severity of seizures between the AS UPD and AS deletion patients.

Neurofibromatosis

Neurofibromatosis is recognized as being at least two separate genetic disorders (NF-1 and NF-2) (Barker et al. 1987; Rouleau, Wertelecki & Haines 1987). Both are inherited in autosomal dominant fashion, with considerable clinical and genetic heterogeneity, a high mutation rate, variable expressivity, and a complex pattern of penetrance (Riccardi & Lewis 1988).

The gene for NF-1 (Von Recklinghausen's disease) is located on the proximal long arm of chromosome 17 and is characterized by skin pigmentation (café au lait spots) and tumor formation. Neurofibromas—tumors that are usually found on peripheral nerves—lead to subcutaneous lumps and bone deformities. NF-1 affects 1 in 4000 people and accounts for over 85% of NF cases. The gene for NF-2 is located on chromosome 22 and results in CNS tumors (for example, acoustic neuromas and meningiomas). NF-2 is rare, occurring with a frequency of 1 in 50,000. Atypical forms of NF have been defined that do not fit either the NF-1 or the NF-2 category (Riccardi & Eichner 1986).

The diagnosis of NF-1 is based on the presence of two or more of the following seven features (National Institutes of Health Consensus Development Conference 1988): six or more café au lait spots exceeding 5 mm in greatest diameter in the prepubertal child, or exceeding 15 mm in greatest diameter in the postpubertal child; two or more neurofibromas of any type or one plexiform neurofibroma; freckling in the axillary or inguinal regions; optic glioma; two or more Lisch nodules (hamartomatous nodules of the iris, which can be seen on slit-lamp examination and which may be its only manifestation (Riccardi & Lewis 1988); a distinctive osseous lesion, such as sphenoid dysplasia, or thinning of long-bone cortex with or without pseudoarthrosis; and a first-degree relative with NF-1.

The gene for NF-1 codes for a large, ubiquitously expressed protein (Gutmann & Collins 1992) that may be involved in regulating the proto-oncogene ras. This may lead to the diffuse neuromigrational disturbance seen in NF-1, characterized by a disorganized cortical laminar pattern, cortical and subcortical heterotopia, atypical glial cell nests, gliosis, micronodular capillary changes, and hamartomatous lesions (Rosman & Pearce 1967; Rubinstein 1986). MRI scans reveal multiple areas of increased signal ("Unidentified Bright Objects" or UBOs) in the basal ganglia, posterior visual pathways, brainstem (Hurst,

Newman & Cail 1988), and cerebellum (Duffner et al. 1989) that are virtually pathognomonic for NF-1 children. These abnormalities are at least as sensitive for diagnosis as are Lisch nodules, which occur in 90% of NF-1 patients over 6 years of age (Goldstein et al. 1989). The abnormal signals were not correlated with brainstem auditory evoked responses, EEG abnormalities, seizures, cognitive status, or clinical neurological evaluation (Duffner et al. 1989), suggesting that they were glial nodules and hamartomatous lesions rather than NMDs. Recently, however, a clear correlation between UBOs in the basal ganglia and neurocognitive deficits was noted (Hofman et al. 1994).

The developmental problems of NF-1 children appear early. Children under the age of 18 months may already manifest atypical development, with motor delay an early finding (Riccardi & Eichner 1986). NF-1 children are at risk for mild mental retardation (Dunn 1987), seizures, learning disabilities (Eldridge et al. 1989) such as visuoperceptual motor deficit (Eliason 1986), memory deficit (Chapman, Korf & Urion 1989), attention deficit hyperactivity disorder (Eliason 1986), and possibly other behavior disorders. Analysis of Wechsler Intelligence Scale for Children profiles revealed that children with NF-1 performed within normal ranges for verbal comprehension, and within low normal limits for perceptual organization and freedom from distractibility (Eliason 1986). More recently, a significant verbal deficit was found in children with NF-1 who were compared with unaffected siblings (Hofman et al. 1994). Studies of children with NF-2 are less common. One would expect, however, that focal cognitive deficits related to focal CNS tumors would be observed.

Myotonic Dystrophy

Myotonic dystrophy is an inherited (autosomal dominant) multisystem disease. It has been shown to fall into the class of inherited disorders that result from a trinucleotide repeat, CTG, on a gene on chromosome 19 that encodes for myotonin-protein kinase. Recently, several cases with all the phenotypic features of myotonic dystrophy were reported, with normal-range CTG repeats, suggesting genetic heterogeneity (Thornton, Griggs & Moxley 1994). When the disorder appears in adults, the manifestations primarily involve progressive muscle weakness and myotonia (with cataracts), as well as skeletal and cardiovascular findings. The disorder manifests *anticipation;* consequently, when it presents in the neonatal period, the infant is severely affected. Such infants have low Apgar scores and respiratory difficulty, and they may die in the neonatal period. In utero, they have diminished movement and polyhydramnios (excessive amniotic fluid). There is a high incidence of macrocephaly, with dilated ventricles (Garcia-Alix et al. 1991). Neuropathological studies report migrational anomalies (Rosman & Kakulas 1966) and thalamic inclusions (Wisniewski, Berry & Spiro 1975).

Intellectual impairment has been reported in 25% to 75% of persons with myotonic dystrophy. Myotonic dystrophy is often diagnosed when there is early developmental retardation. In a neuropsychological study of adults, significant differences between controls and myotonic dystrophy subjects were found on digit span, paired-associate learning (nonrelated, "hard" pairs), verbal fluency, the Raven's Progressive Matrices Test, and the Mini-Mental State Examination. Focal white-matter lesions, increased skull thickness, and temporal lobe lesions occurred proportionately to the degree of intellectual impairment (Huber et al. 1989).

Williams Syndrome

Williams syndrome (WS) was first described in 1961 (Williams, Barratt-Boyes & Lowe), and this description was expanded by Beuren, Apitz, and Harmjanz (1962). These authors emphasized the characteristic "elfin" facial appearance and the presence of supravalvular aortic stenosis. Black and Bonham-Carter (1963) noted similarities between the facial appearance of children with idiopathic infantile hypercalcemia and those with cardiac lesions (described earlier). Although these children may have been clinically hypercalcemic as infants (Garcia et al. 1964), overt hypercalcemia is only rarely apparent in most children with WS (Preus 1984).

Williams syndrome has not been linked consistently to a specific gene, nor has the pathophysiology of the syndrome been clearly elucidated, although there has been some speculation about impaired calcitonin secretion in WS (Culler, Jones & Deftos 1985; Tschopp, Tobler, & Fischer 1984). It has been proposed that WS and supravalvular aortic stenosis are part of a spectrum for an autosomal dominant gene defect of variable penetrance and expression, with a gene frequency of 1 in 10,000 (Grimm & Wesselhoeft 1980). The relationship between early hypercalcemia and the morphogenetic abnormalities has not been elucidated, either. Large doses of vitamin D produce aortic lesions, craniofacial anomalies, and dental anomalies in animals, reminiscent of WS (Friedman & Mill 1969).

Facial features become more prominent with age. They include a broad forehead, medial eyebrow flare, stellate pattern of the iris, depressed nasal bridge, upturned nasal tip, malar flattening, prominent lips and a wide mouth. Teeth erupt late, with microdontia and rhizomikry (small roots), invagination of the incisors, malocclusion, and pathological folding of the buccal mucosa (Jensen, Warburg & Dupont 1976). In addition to supravalvular aortic stenosis, peripheral pulmonary stenosis may occur. The head has a typical dolichocephalic (long-headed) shape that Trauner, Bellugi, and Chase (1989) attribute to relative preservation of size of the posterior fossa.

Williams syndrome children are generally mildly to moderately retarded, although instances of severe retardation and of borderline to low average IQ are reported (Cortada, Taysi & Hartmann 1980; Pagon et al. 1987). Verbal IQ scores, while often deficient, tend to exceed performance IQ scores; but large verbal–performance IQ discrepancies are not typical (Arnold, Yule & Martin 1985; Kataria, Goldstein & Kushnick 1984; Udwin & Yule, 1991). Visuospatial deficits are marked and persist into late childhood and adolescence (Bellugi, Sabo & Vaid 1988; Pagon et al. 1987). These children are characteristically loquacious, with longer utterances than one would expect on the basis of their mental age (Bellugi et al. 1990). However, Crisco, Dobbs, and Mulhern (1988), using the Illinois Test of Psycholinguistic Abilities—Revised (Kirk, McCarthy & Kirk 1968) did not find any particular superiority of language functions, although visuospatial deficits were prominent. Reading recognition and comprehension may be relatively strong (Pagon et al. 1987). Hyperacusis of such severity as to preclude exposure to noisy household items such as vacuum cleaners has been reported (Martin, Snodgrass & Cohen 1984). These children showed high rates of emotional and behavioral disturbance on questionnaires (Udwin, Yule & Martin 1987).

In one study, Williams syndrome children were compared to DS children (Bellugi et al. 1990). Those with WS had relatively preserved language-processing ability (expressive and receptive vocabularies exceeded overall intelligence level) but were severely impaired on such cognitive tasks as conservation, seriation, and multiple classification. They performed poorly on WISC-R block design, the Developmental Test of Visual-Motor Integration (Beery 1989), and the Judgment of Line Orientation test (Benton, Varney & Hamsher 1978). Qualitative differences in ability to process focal versus global features of visuospatial stimuli have also been reported in children with DS and WS, compared to normals (Bihrle et al. 1989). The DS children reproduced global forms but were unable to replicate local forms. The WS children were able to recall local forms, but not the overall gestalt. Normal children had no difficulty with either local or gestalt elements of the designs (such as an uppercase letter D constructed out of a series of lowercase Y's). Although there was a suggestion of right-hemisphere deficit, no hemispatial neglect was found. In other studies, WS children used affective prosody and had good pragmatic skills (Reilly, Klima & Bellugi 1991). However, WS children were significantly different from age-matched and IQ-matched controls in terms of hyperactivity and poor peer relationships (Arnold, Yule & Martin 1985).

Trauner, Bellugi, and Chase (1989) compared the neurologic characteristics of age- and IQ-matched WS and DS patients, noting that the WS group had impaired oromotor skills (early suckling difficulties, later difficulty managing solids, and early motor language difficulties), evidence of cerebellar dysfunction, and graphomotor deficits. WS subjects were small for gestational age and more likely to have failure-to-thrive. MRI scans have not revealed focal cortical damage. Comparisons of DS and WS patients found that WS subjects had no reduction of overall size of posterior fossa structures; but cerebellar vermal areas I through V were slightly smaller and vermal areas VI and VII were significantly larger in WS (Jernigan & Bellugi 1990). In another study, WS patients had preserved neocerebellar volumes despite decreased cerebral volumes compared to DS (and in contrast to previous reports regarding cerebellar size in autistic subjecst) and in some cases a Chiari type I malformation (Wang et al. 1992).

ACQUIRED INSULTS TO THE DEVELOPING BRAIN

In the subsections that follow some other insults to the brain of the fetus and newborn infant are reviewed. These disorders were selected because they are relatively common and are sure to be encountered by neuropsychologists. For example, neuropsychologists are often called on to evaluate ex-prematures. The information provided next should help the reader identify some important risk factors, since specific insults are likely to be associated with certain patterns of cognitive deficit.

Cerebral Palsy

Cerebral palsy (CP) refers generally to severe motor handicap due to a static injury to the brain of the fetus or young infant. Implicit in the term is the concept of a nonprogressive injury, since some progressive neurodegenerative diseases are similar in appearance. Because the lesion occurs early in development, however, the neurological manifestations may change with maturation. For example, newborns with severe unilateral brain injury do not appear hemiparetic until the pyramidal tracts mature a few months later; athetosis may not be apparent in the young infant.

CP has been estimated to occur in 2 of every 1000 births. A number of prenatal and intrapartum factors lead to CP. CP was first described by Little, in 1862. He described hypoxic-ischemic encephalopathy and clearly linked what he called *spastic rigidity* to problems in the intrapartum and perinatal periods. Sigmund Freud related different clinical manifestations of CP into a single syndrome and suggested that it was not simply a process related to birth: "the anomaly of the birth process, rather than being the causal etiologic factor, may itself be the consequence of the real prenatal etiology" (Freud 1897). This view has proved to be remarkably prescient in terms of recent, large epidemiologic studies. For example, the National Collaborative Perinatal Project (Freeman & Nelson 1988; Nelson & Ellenberg 1986) found unequivocal evidence of intrapartum hypoxic insult in only a few children with CP. Out of a total of 54,000 pregnancies, 189 children were identified as having CP. Of this group of 189, 40 (21%) had at least one of three clinical markers consistent with asphyxia. However, only 17 of these 40 children (9%) had no major congenital malformation or other intrinsic defect that might have contributed to the poor outcome. Thus, when all information was taken into consideration, intrapartum risk factors by themselves contributed only slightly to the risk of CP. Because neuromigrational disorders may clinically resemble CP, doctors may sometimes attribute CP to intrapartum factors, in the absence of information indicating the presence of brain anomalies.

Children destined to develop CP may appear normal or hypotonic at birth (Ingram 1964; Cohen & Duffner 1981). Newborns may have significant cortical insult at birth but not manifest outward signs in the newborn period. Between 5 and 6 months of age, affected children develop a strong unilateral hand preference, and tightly fist the affected (hemiplegic) hand. Spasticity or athetotic hand posturing soon becomes apparent over the next 12 to 18 months. Fine motor skills are delayed. Problems in attaining normal milestones such as sitting up or rolling over are noted.

Several different patterns of CP can be identified. *Spastic diplegia,* characterized by leg spasticity with relatively normal arm function, is a common motor deficit in CP and typically appears between 6 and 12 months of age. Spastic diplegia is closely associated with prematurity. Ingram (1964) noted that 44% of infants with a birthweight under 2500 grams had spastic diplegia. Clinical manifestations vary with the degree of prematurity (Veelken et al. 1983). Spastic diplegia was associated with asphyxia in 89% of premature infants but in only 31% of full-term infants. Intrauterine factors were involved in 41% as the sole cause, and in 24% as a contributing factor. Spastic diplegia often is the result of *periventricular leukomalacia* (injury to white matter around the lateral ventricles underlying the germinal matrix). Intellectual subnormality was more common in full-term children with spastic diplegia; 45% had IQs below 70, in contrast to 15% for the ex-premature group. Fedrizzi et al. (1993) reported a long-term follow-up study of high-risk infants (mean gestational age of 29 weeks), and low-risk preterm controls (mean gestational age ranging from <32 weeks to 36 weeks), excluding infants with intraventricular hemorrhage, CNS malformation, and hyperbilirubinemia. On the Griffith's Mental Scale, the scores of the high-risk group were low, particularly on the eye–hand coordination subscale. On the WPPSI, at age 6 years, there was a marked difference in performance subtests between the small prematures and the controls. Fedrizzi et al. (1993) suggested that this reflects an evolving perceptual organization deficit. Although the problem of the mismatch in ages between the experimental and control groups is a concern, the finding of severe performance deficits coupled with fine motor deficits is informative.

In the small group of children among whom CP resulted from obstetrical factors, prematurity and hypoxic-ischemic encephalopathy were common. A hemiparesis may result from a thromboembolic vascular event that occurs in the last third of the pregnancy or in the early postnatal period (Hagberg, Hagberg & Olow 1984). Seizures in the neonatal period also contribute to the morbidity and poor outcome, but they usually result from hypoxic-ischemic encephalopathy.

Hypoxic-Ischemic Injury in the Newborn

Among infants with asphyxia (hypoxic-ischemic injury) in the neonatal period, 20% to 30% have cerebral palsy, mental retardation, or epilepsy. Despite modern obstetric techniques, asphyxia continues to occur in 2 to 4 out of every 1000 live term newborns. Markers of perinatal asphyxia include fetal heart-rate deceleration, low cord blood pH, thick meconium, and low 5- to 10-minute Apgar scores, although Apgar scores in isolation are not good prognostic indicators (Nelson & Ellenberg 1981). Half of the infants with asphyxia have seizures in the immediate postpartum period.

There are a number of different reasons for the susceptibility of the neonatal brain to hypoxic-ischemic injury. First, newborns are susceptible to CNS hypoperfusion resulting from systemic hypotension. Second, the neonatal brain has up-regulated excitatory aminoacid (EAA) receptors that play an important role in early learning and brain growth. However, they also predispose the developing brain toward increased injury during hypoxia (Hattori & Wasterlain 1990). Regions rich in glutamate (an EAA)—including Sommer's sector of the hippocampus, the thalamus, the brainstem, the cerebellum, and anterior horn cells of the spinal cord—are particularly affected by asphyxia. Another factor predisposing the neonatal brain toward sensitivity to hypoxia is active myelination of the region at the time of the hypoxic event.

Two general patterns of hypoxic-ischemic injury are seen in newborns (Myers 1972). One type results from partial but prolonged asphyxia. This affects the cerebral cortex—particularly the parasagittal area that lies in the "watershed" between the anterior and middle cerebral arterial distributions, the cerebral white matter, and the basal ganglia (Brann & Myers 1975; Pasternak 1987)—and it may result in damage to prefrontal and parietal cortical association areas. The other type results from a relatively brief period of total asphyxia, and is characterized by infarction of the brainstem and thalamus (Myers 1972). This type has a profound effect on subsequent motor and cognitive development. CT scans in infants often reveal hypodensities corresponding to areas of infarction and densities corresponding to hemorrhage. Some asphyxiated infants, however—particularly those with the acute asphyxic pattern—have normal CT scans but clearly demonstrable lesions on MRI (Pasternak, Predey & Mikhael 1991).

Different patterns of injury also result in different outcomes as the child matures. Children with parasaggital injury often have hypotonia and weakness in the upper extremities as neonates, with relatively mild motor impairment later. Basal ganglia damage in newborns evolves into choreoathetotic cerebral palsy with mental retardation. Neuropathological studies reveal *status marmoratus* of the basal ganglia. One interesting experimental model of hypoxic-ischemic damage to the striatum demonstrated that acetylcholinergic neurons were selectively involved (Burke & Karanas 1990), perhaps explaining the high incidence of movement disorder (dystonia, choreoathetosis) in survivors of these events.

Intraventricular Hemorrhage

Intraventricular hemorrhage (IVH) results from damage to the vessels in the highly vascular germinal matrix that lies around the horns of the lateral ventricles (Volpe 1989). In 80% of infants, the hemorrhage spills into the ventricular cavity. In addition to destroying the germinal matrix, the hemorrhage destroys precursors of cerebral glial cells. When severe, IVH results in increased intracranial pressure (ICP), damage to the white matter overlying the ventricles, and damage to the adjacent caudate nucleus. Almost all IVH occurs in prematures: the younger the infant, the greater the risk for IVH. Among preterm infants with low birthweights (less than 1500 grams), 30% to 65% suffer IVH as well as hypoxic-ischemic injury (Papile et al. 1979). Minor IVH (grades I and II) is often undetected in the newborn period, unless specifically looked for. Severe IVH (grades III and IV) is clinically apparent and usually results in severe mental and motor handicaps. In the first 3 years of life, 40% to 60% of infants with IVH manifest neurodevelopmental abnormalities, most prominent in the motor sphere (Krishnamoorthy et al. 1979; Bozynski et al. 1984). Motor deficits are not surprising, considering hemorrhage location. Although a rough correlation exists between outcome and amount of intraventricular blood, the extent of damage to periventricular tissue is an important prognostic factor (Guzzetta et al. 1986). In the presence of extensive damage to periventricular tissue (involving fronto-parieto-occipital areas), the outcome is poor: 80% of the infants died, and all survivors had motor deficits. Moreover, only 1 of the 37 affected infants had an IQ score over 80. When more restricted damage to periventricular tissue was involved, the mortality rate was only 37%; 20% of the survivors were free of motor deficit; 47% had IQs over 80; and 10% had normal motor and normal cognitive function. The most favorable outcomes occurred in infants who had unilateral lesions.

About half of all children with IVH show evidence of cognitive deficits in later childhood (Hynd, Hartlage & Noonan 1984). Even full-term newborns (2000 grams or more) who experienced IVH may develop cognitive and motor deficits. Williams et al. (1987) evaluated 35 preterm infants (1500 grams or less), with and without IVH, at ages 8 months and 12 months, and again $4\frac{1}{2}$ to 5 years later. Only subtle neurological deficits were noted in children without IVH. In contrast, 23% of those with IVH had significant motor findings, ranging from hyperreflexia to spastic diplegic CP with mild mental retardation. The group with hemorrhage had worse cognitive, motor, and neuromotor functioning. A high proportion of the hemorrhage group also experienced school difficulties.

Periventricular Leukomalacia

Periventricular leukomalacia (PVL) is a generally symmetrical, nonhemorrhagic, apparently ischemic injury of brain white matter in the premature infant. Takashima, Mito, and Ando (1986) have suggested that periventricular hemorrhagic infarction is prominent anteriorly, whereas hemorrhagic periventricular leukomalacia arises in the periventricular arterial border zones. This border zone is quite susceptible to ischemia, and this may contribute to hemorrhage.

DISORDERS ASSOCIATED WITH EXPOSURE TO HORMONES AND TOXINS IN UTERO

One way that early brain development can be affected is through intrauterine exposure to excessive amounts of naturally occurring hormones (Goy & McEwan 1980) or to neurotoxic substances such as alcohol.

Congenital Adrenal Hyperplasia

Congenital adrenal hyperplasia (CAH) is an autosomal recessive disorder of the adrenal 21-hydroxylase gene that causes decreased glucocorticoid production. The adrenals then produce increased amounts of androgen, which results in virilization. Some patients have increased mineralcorticoid production, with resulting salt-wasting. As a result, male and female fetuses homozygous for this disorder are exposed to high levels of androgens. While these may not be excessive ranges in normal males, the female fetus is exposed to a much higher than normal level of androgen. Nass and Baker (1991) hypothesized that, if intrauterine exposure to androgen was an etiological factor for learning disabilities, girls with CAH ought to have a higher incidence of learning disabilities than girls who were not exposed to androgen in utero. Using a control group of unaffected siblings, they found that, although affected females had (as a group) above-average intelligence (see also Resnick et al. 1986), their verbal < performance split was significantly greater than that in the controls. There was also a bias toward left-handedness in affected females (Nass et al. 1987). Tirosh et al. (1993) reported on 25 patients with CAH and left- and right-handed controls. A comparison of hand preference indicated that, proportionately, twice as many sinistrals were in the CAH as in the normal population. Immunologic disease was more common in CAH patients (28%) than in right-handed controls (8%), but 32% of the left-handed controls gave a history of immunologic disease. Dichotic listening revealed an unexpected right-ear/left-hemisphere superiority. These studies underscore the complex effects of intrauterine androgen exposure.

Intrauterine exposure to testosterone has been proposed as the pathophysiological mechanism underlying dyslexia, with a possible association with autoimmune disease (Geschwind & Galaburda 1985). Dyslexic brains have evidence of numerous heterotopia, suggesting early disturbance in neuronogenesis (Galaburda & Kemper 1979; Galaburda et al. 1985). Schrott et al. (1992) reported on a possible animal model,—New Zealand black (NZB) and BXSB mice, characterized by autoimmune disease and cortical ectopia.

Fetal Alcohol Syndrome

The diagnosis of fetal alcohol syndrome is based on three findings: evidence of central nervous system dysfunction; growth retardation; and a characteristic facial appearance. Many children with fetal alcohol syndrome are microcephalic. The dysmorphic facial features include anomalies of the palpebral fissures, a short upturned nose, thinned upper vermilion border and retrognathia (receding jaw). Ocular anomalies (strabismus, ptosis, microphthalmia), a cleft lip and palate, and small teeth are reported. Cardiac and urogenital defects are noted rarely (Clarren & Smith 1978). Neuropathological studies have revealed a wide variety of abnormalities, including dendritic spine anomalies (Ferrer & Galofre 1987); NMDs (Jones 1975); and agenesis of the corpus callosum, with anterior fusion of the frontal lobes, fusion of the thalamus and caudate nucleus, absent olfactory bulbs and tracts, and hypoplastic optic nerves (Coulter et al. 1993). Animal studies have suggested that prenatal alcohol exposure affects neurono-genesis in the cerebellum (Volk 1984; Mohamed et al. 1987a, 1987b). In one study, over 70% of children with fetal alcohol syndrome had speech and language deficits and hyperactivity. Most were mildly to moderately retarded (Iosub et al. 1981). When IQs were assessed at age 8 years, and again at age 17 years, the scores were remarkably stable (Streissguth, Randels & Smith 1991). However, studies of children with fetal alcohol syndrome are complicated by many confounding variables (such as low socioeconomic status, maternal drug ingestion, and smoking) that may also contribute to cognitive developmental abnormalities. The effect of "binge" drinking versus continuous relatively low levels of alcohol exposure has been questioned. In a controlled study using nonhuman primates, Clarren et al. (1992) demonstrated convincingly that early binge drinking, even when replaced subsequently with abstinence, resulted in later cognitive and behavioral dysfunction.

CONCLUSION

This chapter has reviewed common migrational anomalies, genetic anomalies, specific clinical syndromes, and some acquired lesions to the developing brain that are associated with neurocognitive deficits and behavioral problems. These conditions serve as models for various genetic and biochemical processes. Although it is currently difficult to relate information about brain development to the specific clinical manifestations of these syndromes with precision, a very exciting time in the field of developmental neurobiology and cognition lies ahead.

REFERENCES

Alexander, D., and Money, J. 1966. Turner's syndrome and Gerstmann's syndrome: Neuropsychologic comparisons. *Neuropsychologia* 4: 265–73.

Altman, J., and Bayer, S. 1985. Embryonic development of the rat cerebellum: III. Regional differences in the time of origin, migration and settling of Purkinje cells. *Journal of Comparative Neurology* 231: 42–65.

Andermann, F.; Olivier, A.; Melanson, D.; and Robitaille, Y. 1987. Epilepsy due to focal cortical dysplasia with macrogyria and the forme fruste of tuberous sclerosis: A study of 15 patients. In P. Wolf, M. Dam, D. Janz, and F. E. Drcifuss (eds.), *Advances in Epileptology,* vol. 16: *16th Epilepsy International Symposium* (New York: Raven Press) pp. 35–38.

Angelman, H. 1965. "Puppet" children: A report on three cases. *Developmental Medicine and Child Neurology* 7: 681–88.

Aniskiewicz, A. S.; Frumkin, N. L.; Brady, D. E.; Moore, J. B.; and Pera, A. 1990. Magnetic resonance imaging and neurobehavioral correlates in schizencephaly. *Archives of Neurology* 47: 911–16.

Arnold, R.; Yule, W.; and Martin, N. 1985. The psychological characteristics of infantile hypercalcaemia: A preliminary investigation. *Developmental Medicine and Child Neurology* 27: 49–59.

Austin, G. E., and Sparkes, R. S. 1980. Abnormal cerebral cortical convolutions in an XYY fetus. *Human Genetics* 56: 173–75.

Azari, N. P.; Horwitz, B.; Pettigrew, K. D.; Grady, C. L.; Haxby, J. V.; Giacometti, K. R.; and Schapiro, M. B. 1994. Abnormal pattern of cerebral glucose metabolic rates involving language areas in young adults with Down syndrome. *Brain and Language* 46: 1–20.

Balodimos, M. C.; Lisco, H.; Irwin, I.; Merrill, W.; and Dingman, J. F. 1966. XYY karyotype in a case of familial hypogonadism. *Journal of Clinical Endocrinology and Metabolism* 26: 443–52.

Barker, D.; Wright, E.; Nguyen, K.; Cannon, L.; Fain, P.; Goldgar, D.; Bishop, D. T.; Carey, J.; Baty, B.; Kivlin, J.; Willard, H.; Waye, J. S.; Greig, G.; Leinwand, L.; Nakamura, Y.; O'Connell, P.; Leppert, M.; Lalouel, J. M.; White, R.; and Skolnick, M. 1987. Gene for von Recklinghausen neurofibromatosis is in the pericentromeric region of chromosome 17. *Science* 236: 1100–1102.

Barth, P. G. 1987. Disorders of neuronal migration. *Canadian Journal of Neurological Science* 14: 1–16.

———. Schizencephaly and nonlissencephalic cortical dysplasias. *American Journal of Neuroradiology* 13: 104–6.

Becker, L. E.; Armstrong, D. L.; and Chan, F. 1986. Dendritic atrophy in children with Down's syndrome. *Annals of Neurology* 20: 520–26.

Becker, P. S.; Dixon, A. M.; and Troncoso, J. C. 1989. Bilateral opercular polymicrogyria. *Annals of Neurology* 25: 90–92.

Beery, K. E. 1989. *Revised Administration, Scoring, and Teaching Manual for the Developmental Test of Visual-Motor Integration*. Cleveland: Modern Curriculum Press.

Bell, M. V.; Bloomfield, J.; McKinley, M.; Patterson, M. N.; Darlison, M. G.; Barnard, E. A.; and Davies, K. E. 1989. Physical linkage of a $GABA_A$ receptor subunit gene to the DXS374 locus in human Xq28. *American Journal of Human Genetics* 45: 883–88.

Bellugi, U.; Bihrle, A.; Jernigan, T.; Trauner, D.; and Doherty, S. 1990. Neuropsychological, neurological, and neuroanatomical profile of Williams syndrome. *American Journal of Medical Genetics* Suppl. 6: 115–25.

Bellugi, U.; Sabo, H.; and Vaid, J. 1988. Spatial deficits in children with Williams syndrome. In J. Stiles-Davis, U. Bellugi, and M. Kritchevsky (eds.), *Spatial Cognition: Brain Bases and Development* (Hillsdale, N.J.: L. Erlbaum), pp. 173–298.

Bender, B.; Fry, E.; Pennington, B.; Puck, M.; Salbenblatt, J.; and Robinson, A. 1983. Speech and language development in 41 children with sex chromosome anomalies. *Pediatrics* 71: 262–67.

Bender, B. G.; Puck, M. H.; Salbenblatt, J. A.; and Robinson, A. 1984. The development of four unselected 47,XYY boys. *Clinical Genetics* 25: 435–45.

Benton, A. L.; Varney, N. R.; and Hamsher, K. 1978. Visuospatial judgment: A clinical test. *Archives of Neurology* 35: 364–67.

Beuren A. J.; Apitz J.; and Harmjanz, D. 1962. Supravalvular aortic stenosis in association with mental retardation and a certain facial appearance. *Circulation* 26: 1235–40.

Bihrle A. M.; Bellugi, U.; Delis, D.; and Marks, S. 1989. Seeing either the forest or the trees: Dissociation in visuospatial processing. *Brain and Cognition* 11: 37–49.

Black, J. A., and Bonham Carter, R. E. 1963. Association between aortic stenosis and facies of severe infantile hypercalcaemia. *Lancet* 2: 745–49.

Bodensteiner, J. B.; Gay, C. T.; Marks, W. A.; Hamza, M.; and Schaefer, G. B. 1988. Macro cisterna magna: A marker for maldevelopment of the brain? *Pediatric Neurology* 4: 284–86.

Bodensteiner, J. B., and Schaefer, G. B. 1990. Wide cavum septum pellucidum: A marker of disturbed brain development. *Pediatric Neurology* 6: 391–94.

Bozynski, M. E. A.; Nelson, M. N.; Rosati-Skertich, C.; Genaze, D.; O'Donnell, K.; and Naughton, P. 1984. Two-year longitudinal follow-up of premature infants weighing less than or equal to 1200 g at birth: Sequelae of intracranial hemorrhage. *Journal of Developmental and Behavioral Pediatrics* 5: 346–52.

Brann, A. W., and Myers, R. E. 1975. Central nervous system findings in the newborn monkey following severe in utero partial asphyxia. *Neurology* 25: 327–38.

Branson, C. 1981. Speech and language characteristics of children with Prader-Willi syndrome. In V. Λ. Holm, S. Sulzbacher, and P. L. Pipes (eds.), *The Prader-Willi Syndrome* (Baltimore, Md.: University Park Press), pp. 179–83.

Bregman J. D.; Dykens E.; Watson, M.; Ort, S. I.; and Leckman J. F. 1987. Fragile-X syndrome: Variability of phenotypic expression. *Journal of the American Academy of Child and Adolescent Psychiatry* 26: 463–71.

Brown, W. T.; Jenkins, E. C.; Cohen, I. L.; Fisch, G. S.; Wolf-Schein, E. G.; Gross, A.; Waterhouse, L.; Fein, D.; Mason-Brothers, A.; Ritvo, E.; Ruttenberg, B. A.; Bentley, W.; and Castells, S. 1986 Fragile X and autism: A multicenter study. *American Journal of Medical Genetics* 23: 341–52.

Brugge, K. L.; Nichols, S. L.; Salmon, D. P.; Hill, L. R.; Delis, D. C.; Aaron, L.; and Trauner, D. A. 1994. Cognitive impairment in adults with Down's syndrome: Similarities to early cognitive changes in Alzheimer's disease. *Neurology* 44: 232–38.

Brun, A., and Gustavson, K. H. 1972. Cerebral malformations in the XYY syndrome. *Acta Pathologica et Microbiologica Scandinavica* [A] 80: 627–33.

Brunner, H. G.; Jansen, G.; Nillesen, W.; Nelen, M. R.; de Die, C. E. M.; Höweler, C. J.; van Oost, B. A.; Wieringa, B.; Ropers, H.-H.; and Smeets, H. J. M. 1993. Brief report: Reverse mutation in myotonic dystrophy. *New England Journal of Medicine* 328: 476–80.

Burd, L., and Kerbeshian, J. 1989. Hyperlexia in Prader-Willi syndrome. *Lancet* (October 21): 983–84.

Burke, R. E., and Karanas, A. L. 1990. Quantitative morphological analysis of striatal cholinergic neurons in perinatal asphyxia. *Annals of Neurology* 27: 81–88.

Butler, M. G. 1989. Hypopigmentation: A common feature of Prader-Labhart-Willi syndrome. *American Journal of Human Genetics* 45: 140–46.

Butler, M. G.; Meaney, F. J.; and Palmer, C. G. 1986. Clinical and cytogenetic survey of 39 individuals with Prader-Labhart-Willi syndrome. *American Journal of Medical Genetics* 23: 793–809.

Byrd, S. E.; Osborn, R. E.; Bohan, T. P.; and Naidich, T. P. 1989. The CT and MR evaluation of migrational disorders of the brain: II. Schizencephaly, heterotopia and polymicrogyria. *Pediatric Radiology* 19: 219–22.

Carleton, C. C.; Collins, G. H.; and Schimpff, R. D. 1976. Subacute necrotizing encephalopathy (Leigh's disease): Two unusual cases. *Southern Medical Journal* 69: 1301–5.

Cassidy, S. B., and Ledbetter, D. H. 1989. Prader-Willi syndrome. *Neurologic Clinics* 7: 37–54.

Chamberlain, M. C.; Press, G. A.; and Bejar, R. F. 1990. Neonatal schizencephaly: Comparison of brain imaging. *Pediatric Neurology* 6: 382–87.

Chapman, C. A.; Korf, B. R.; and Urion, D. K. 1989. A specific memory deficit in a group of children with neurofibromatosis and learning disability. *Annals of Neurology* 26: 483.

Chapman, R. S.; Schwartz, S. E.; and Kay-Raining Bird, E. 1991. Language skills of children and adolescents with Down syndrome: I. Comprehension. *Journal of Speech and Hearing Research* 34: 1106–20.

Chi, G. J.; Dooling, E. C.; and Gilles, F. H. 1977. Gyral development of the human brain. *Annals of Neurology* 1: 86–93.

Chudley, A. 1984. Behavior phenotype. [In A. Chudley & G. Sutherland (eds.) *Conference Report: International Workshop on the Fragile X Syndrome and X-Linked Mental Retardation.*] *American Journal of Medical Genetics* 17: 45–53.

Chudley, A. E.; de von Flindt, R.; and Hagerman, R. J. 1987. Cognitive variability in the fragile X syndrome. *American Journal of Medical Genetics* 28: 13–15.

Clark, C.; Klonoff, H.; and Hayden, M. 1990. Regional cerebral glucose metabolism in Turner syndrome. *Canadian Journal of Neurological Sciences* 17: 140–44.

Clarren, S. K.; Astley, S. J.; Gunderson, V. M.; and Spellman, D. 1992. Cognitive and behavioral deficits in nonhuman primates associated with very early embryonic binge exposures to ethanol. *Journal of Pediatrics* 121: 789–96.

Clarren, S. K., and Smith, D. W. 1978. The fetal alcohol syndrome. *New England Journal of Medicine* 298: 1063–67.

Cohen, M.; Campbell, R.; and Yaghmai, F. 1989. Neuropathological abnormalities in developmental dysphasia. *Annals of Neurology* 25: 567–70.

Cohen, M., and Duffner, P. K. 1981. Prognostic indicators in hemiparetic cerebral palsy. *Annals of Neurology* 9: 353–57.

Connolly, J. A. 1978. Intelligence levels of Down's syndrome children. *American Journal of Mental Deficiency* 83: 193–96.

Cortada, X.; Taysi, K.; and Hartmann, A. F. 1980. Familial Williams syndrome. *Clinical Genetics* 18: 173–76.

Coulter, C. L.; Leech, R. W.; Schaefer, G. B.; Scheithauer, B. W.; and Brumback, R. A. 1993. Midline cerebral dysgenesis, dysfunction of the hypothalamic-pituitary axis, and fetal alcohol effects. *Archives of Neurology* 50: 771–75.

Coyle, J. T.; Oster-Granite, M. L.; and Gearhart, J. D. 1986. The neurobiologic consequences of Down syndrome. *Brain Research Bulletin* 16: 773–87.

Crisco, J. J.; Dobbs, J. M.; and Mulhern, R. K. (1988) Cognitive processing of children with Williams syndrome. *Developmental Medicine and Child Neurology* 30: 650–656.

Crome, L.; Cowie, V.; and Slater, E. 1966. A statistical note on cerebellar and brainstem weight in Mongolism. *Journal of Mental Deficiency Research* 10: 69–72.

Culler, F. L.; Jones, K. L.; and Deftos, L. J. 1985. Impaired calcitonin secretion in patients with Williams syndrome. *Journal of Pediatrics* 107: 720–23.

Dahle, A. J., and McCollister, F. P. 1986. Hearing and otologic disorders in children with Down syndrome. *American Journal of Mental Deficiency* 90: 636–42.

de la Cruz, F. 1985. Fragile X syndrome. *American Journal of Mental Deficiency* 90: 119–23.

de León, G. A.; de León, G.; Grover, W. D.; Zaeri, N.; and Alburger, P. D. 1987. Agenesis of the corpus callosum and limbic malformation in Apert syndrome (type I acrocephalosyndactyly). *Archives of Neurology* 44: 979–82.

DeMyer, W. 1972. Megalencephaly in children. *Neurology* 22: 634–43.

DeMyer, W.; Zeman, W.; and Palmer, C. G. 1964. The face predicts the brain: Diagnostic significance of median facial anomalies for holoprosencephaly (arhinencephaly). *Pediatrics* 34: 256–63.

Dennis, M. D. 1976. Impaired sensory and motor differentiation with corpus callosum agenesis: A lack of callosal inhibition during ontogeny? *Neuropsychologia* 14: 455–69.

———. 1977. Cerebral dominance in three forms of early brain disorder. In M. E. Blaw, I. Rapin, and M. Kinsbourne (eds.), *Topics in Child Neurology* (New York: Spectrum), pp. 189–212.

———. 1981. Language in a congenitally acallosal brain. *Brain and Language* 12: 33–53.

Dieker, H.; Edwards, R. H.; ZuRhein, G.; Chous, S. M.; Hartman, H. A.; and Opitz, J. M. 1969. The lissencephaly syndrome. *Birth Defects: Original Article Series* 5: 53–64.

Dobyns, W. B. 1989. Agenesis of the corpus callosum and gyral malformations are frequent manifestations of nonketotic hyperglycinemia. *Neurology* 39: 817–20.

Down, J. L. H. 1866. Observation on an ethnic classification of idiots. *London Hospital Report* 3: 259–62.

Downey, J.; Elkin, E.; Ehrhardt, A.; Meyer-Bahlburg, H.; Bell, J.; and Morishima, A. 1991. Cognitive ability and everyday functioning in women with Turner syndrome. *Journal of Learning Disabilities* 24: 32–39.

Driscoll, D. J.; Waters, M. F.; Williams, C. A.; Zori, R. T.; Glenn, C. C.; Avidano, K. M.; and Nicholls, R. D. 1992. A DNA methylation imprint, determined by the sex of the parent, distinguishes the Angelman and Prader-Willi syndromes. *Genomics* 13: 917–24.

Duffner, P. K.; Cohen, M. E.; Seidel, F. G.; and Shucard, D. 1989. The significance of MRI abnormalities in children with neurofibromatosis. *Neurology* 39: 373–78.

Dunn, D. W. 1987. Neurofibromatosis in childhood. *Current Problems in Pediatrics* 17: 445–97.

Dykens, E. M.; Hodapp, R. M.; Ort, S.; Finucane, B.; Shapiro, L.; and Leckman, J. F. 1989. The trajectory of cognitive development in males with fragile X syndrome. *Journal of the American Academy of Child and Adolescent Psychiatry* 28: 422–26.

Dyson, A. T., and Lombardino, L. J. 1989. Phonological abilities of a preschool child with Prader-Willi syndrome. *Journal of Speech and Hearing Disorders* 54: 44–48.

Eldridge, R.; Denckla, M. B.; Bien, E.; Myers, S.; Kaiser-Kupfer, M. I.; Pikus, A.; Schlesinger, S. L.; Parry, D. M.; Dambrosia, J. M.; Zasloff, M. A.; and Mulvihill, J. J. 1989. Neurofibromatosis type 1 (Recklinghausen's disease): Neurologic and cognitive assessment with sibling controls. *American Journal of Diseases of Children* 143: 833–87.

Eliason, M. J. 1986. Neurofibromatosis: Implications for learning and behavior. *Journal of Developmental and Behavioral Pediatrics* 7: 175–79.

Epstein, L. B.; Lee, S. H. S.; and Epstein, C. J. 1980. Enhanced sensitivity of trisomy

21 monocytes to the maturation-inhibiting effect of interferon. *Cellular Immunology* 50: 191–94.

Evrard, P.; Caviness, V. S., Jr.; Prats-Vinas, J.; and Lyon, G. 1978. The mechanism of arrest of neuronal migration in the Zellweger malformation: An hypothesis based upon cytoarchitectonic analysis. *Acta Neuropathologica* 41: 109–17.

Fedrizzi, E.; Inverno, M.; Botteon, G.; Anderloni, A.; Filippini, G.; and Farinotti, M. 1993. The cognitive development of children born preterm and affected by spastic diplegia. *Brain and Development* 15: 428–32.

Ferrer, I., and Galofré, E. 1987. Dendritic spine anomalies in fetal alcohol syndrome. *Neuropediatrics* 18: 161–63.

Filteau, M.-J.; Pourcher, E.; Bouchard, R. H.; Baruch, P.; Mathieu, J.; Bédard, F.; Simard, N.; and Vincent, P. 1991. Corpus callosum agenesis and psychosis in Andermann syndrome. *Archives of Neurology* 48: 1275–80.

Finelli, P. F.; Pueschel, S. M.; Padre-Mendoza, T.; and O'Brien, M. M. 1985. Neurological findings in patients with the fragile-X syndrome. *Journal of Neurology, Neurosurgery and Psychiatry* 48: 150–53.

Fischbeck, K. H. 1994. The mechanism of myotonic dystrophy. *Annals of Neurology* 35: 255–56.

Fisher, E.; Beer-Romero, P.; Brown, L.; Ridley, A.; McNeil, J.; Lawrence, J.; Willard, H.; Bieber, F.; and Page, D. 1990. Homologous ribosomal protein genes on the human X and Y chromosomes: Escape from X inactivation and possible implications for Turner syndrome. *Cell* 63: 1205–18.

Fishler, K.; Koch, R.; and Donnell, G. N. 1976. Comparison of mental development in individuals with mosaic and trisomy 21 Down's syndrome. *Pediatrics* 58: 744–48.

Fletcher, J. M.; Bohan, T. P.; Brandt, M. E.; Brookshire, B. L.; Beaver, S. R.; Francis, D. J.; Davidson, K. C.; Thompson, N. M.; and Miner, M. E. 1992. Cerebral white matter and cognition in hydrocephalic children. *Archives of Neurology,* 49: 818–24.

Freeman, J. M., and Nelson, K. B. 1988. Intrapartum asphyxia and cerebral palsy. *Pediatrics* 82: 240–49.

Freud, S. 1897. Infantile cerebral paralysis. Coral Gables, Fla.: University of Miami Press [1968] (L. A. Russin, translator), p. 142.

Friedman, W. F., and Mill, L. F. 1969. The relationship between vitamin D and the craniofacial and dental anomalies of the supravalvular aortic stenosis syndrome. *Pediatrics* 43: 12–18.

Froster-Iskenius, U.; Bödeker, K.; Oepen, T.; Matthes, R.; Piper, U.; and Schwinger, E. 1986. Folic acid treatment in males and females with fragile-(X)-syndrome. *American Journal of Medical Genetics* 23: 273–89.

Fryns, J. P. 1986. The female and the fragile X: A study of 144 obligate female carriers. *American Journal of Medical Genetics* 23: 157–69.

Fryns, J. P.; Jacobs, J.; Kleczkowska, A.; and van den Berghe, H. 1984. The psychological profile of the fragile X syndrome. *Clinical Genetics* 25: 131–34.

Fukuyama, Y.; Haruna, T.; and Kawazura, M. 1960. A peculiar form of congenital progressive muscular dystrophy: Report of fifteen cases. *Paediatria, Universitatis Tokyo* 4: 5–8.

Galaburda, A. M., and Kemper, T. L. 1979. Cytoarchitectonic abnormalities in developmental dyslexia: A case study. *Annals of Neurology* 6: 94–100.

Galaburda, A.; Sherman, G.; Rosen, G.; Aboitiz, F.; and Geschwind, N. 1985. Developmental dyslexia: Four consecutive patients with cortical anomalies. *Annals of Neurology* 18: 222–33.

Garcia, R. E.; Friedman, W. F.; Kaback, M. M.; and Rowe, R. D. 1964. Idiopathic hypercalcemia and supravalvular aortic stenosis. Documentation of a new syndrome. *New England Journal of Medicine* 271: 117–20.

Garcia-Alix, A.; Cabañas, F.; Morales, C.; Pellicer, A.; Echevarria, J.; Paisan, L.; and Quero, J. 1991. Cerebral abnormalities in congenital myotonic dystophy. *Pediatric Neurology* 7: 28–32.

Gastaut, H.; Pinsard, N.; Raybaud, C.; Aicardi, J.; and Zifkin, B. 1987. Lissencephaly (agyria-pachygyria): Clinical findings and serial EEG studies. *Developmental Medicine and Child Neurology*, 29, 167–180.

Gazzaniga, M. S. 1970. *The Bisected Brain*. New York: Appleton-Century-Crofts.

Geschwind, N., and Galaburda, A. 1985. Cerebral lateralization: Biological mechanisms, associations and pathology. *Archives of Neurology* 42: 428–59; 521–52; 634–54.

Giencke, S., and Lewandowski, L. 1989. Anomalous dominance in Down syndrome young adults. *Cortex* 25: 93–102.

Goldstein, S. M.; Curless, R. G.; Post, M. J. D.; and Quencer, R. M. 1989. A new sign of neurofibromatosis on magnetic resonance imaging of children. *Archives of Neurology* 46: 1222–24.

Goy, R. W., and McEwan, B. W. 1980. *Sexual Differentiation of the Brain*. Cambridge, Mass.: MIT Press.

Graff-Radford, N. R.; Bosch, E. P.; Stears, J. C.; and Tranel, D. 1986. Developmental Foix-Chavany-Marie syndrome in identical twins. *Annals of Neurology* 20: 632–35.

Grimm, T., and Wesselhoeft, H. 1980. The genetic aspects of Williams-Beuren syndrome and the isolated form of the supravalvular aortic stenosis: Investigation of 128 families. *Zeitschrift fur Kardiologie* 69: 168–72.

Gutmann, D. H., and Collins, F. S. 1992. Recent progress toward understanding the molecular biology of von Recklinghausen neurofibromatosis. *Annals of Neurology* 31: 555–61.

Guzzetta, F.; Shackelford, G. D.; Volpe, S.; Perlman, J. M.; and Volpe, J. J. 1986. Periventricular intraparenchymal echodensities in the premature newborn: Critical determinant of neurological outcome. *Pediatrics* 78: 995–1006.

Hagberg, B.; Hagberg, G.; and Olow, I. 1984. The changing panorama of cerebral palsy in Sweden: IV. Epidemiological trends 1959–1978. *Acta Paediatric Scandinavica* 73: 433–40.

Hagemeijer, A., and Smit, E. M. E. 1977. Partial trisomy 21: Further evidence that trisomy of band 21q22 is essential for Down's phenotype. *Human Genetics* 38: 15–23.

Hager, B. C.; Dyme, I. Z.; Guertin, S. R.; Tyler, R. J.; Tryciecky, E. W.; and Fratkin, J. D. 1991. Linear nevus sebaceous syndrome: Megalencephaly and heterotopic gray matter. *Pediatric Neurology* 7: 45–49.

Hagerman, R.; Kemper, M.; and Hudson, M. 1985. Learning disabilities and attentional problems in boys with the fragile X syndrome. *American Journal of Disease of Children* 139: 674–78.

Hagerman, R.; Schreiner, R.; Kemper, M.; Wittenberger, M.; Zahn, B.; and Habicht, K. 1989. Longitudinal IQ changes in fragile X males. *American Journal of Medical Genetics* 33: 513–18.

Hagerman, R. J., and Sobesky, W. E. 1989. Psychopathology in fragile X syndrome. *American Journal of Orthopsychiatry* 59: 142–52.

Hall, J. G. 1990. Genomic imprinting: Review and relevance to human diseases. *American Journal of Human Genetics* 46: 857–73.

Hattori, H., and Wasterlain, C. G. 1990. Excitatory amino acids in the developing brain: Ontogeny, plasticity, and excitotoxicity. *Pediatric Neurology* 6: 219–28.

Hauschka, T. S.; Hasson, J. E.; Goldstein, M. N.; Koepf, G. F.; and Sandberg, A. A. 1962. An XYY man with progeny indicating familial tendency to nondisjunction. *American Journal of Human Genetics* 14: 22–30.

Hayward, J. C.; Titelbaum, D. S.; Clancy, R. R.; and Zimmerman, R. A. 1991. Lissencephaly-pachygyria associated with congenital cytomegalovirus infection. *Journal of Child Neurology* 6: 109–14.

Herbst, D. S. 1980. Nonspecific X-linked mental retardation: I. A review with information from 24 new families. *American Journal of Medical Genetics* 7: 443–60.

Hilburger, A. C.; Willis, J. K.; Bouldin, E.; and Henderson-Tilton, A. 1993. Familial schizencephaly. *Brain and Development* 15: 234–36.

Hinds, H. L.; Ashley, C. T.; Sutcliffe, J. S.; Nelson, D. L.; Warren, S. T.; Housman, D. E.; and Schalling, M. 1993. Tissue-specific expression of FMR-1 provides evidence for a functional role in fragile X syndrome. *Nature Genetics* 3: 36–43.

Hodapp, R. M.; Dykens, E. M.; Hagerman, R. J.; Schreiner, R.; Lachiewicz, A. M.; and Leckman, J. F. 1990. Developmental implications of changing trajectories of IQ in males with fragile X syndrome. *Journal of the American Acadamy of Child and Adolescent Psychiatry* 29: 214–19.

Hofman, K. J.; Harris, E. L.; Bryan, R. N.; and Denckla, M. B. 1994. Neurofibromatosis type 1: The cognitive phenotype. *Journal of Pediatrics* 124: 51–58.

Holm, V. 1981. The diagnosis of Prader-Willi syndrome. In V. Holm, S. Sulzbacher, and P. Pipers (eds.), *Prader-Willi Syndrome* (Baltimore: University Park Press), pp. 27–44.

Hook, E. B., and Warburton, D. 1983. The distribution of chromosomal genotypes associated with Turner's syndrome: Livebirth prevalence rates and evidence for diminished fetal mortality and severity in genotypes associated with structural X abnormalities or mosaicism. *Human Genetics* 64: 24–27.

Hosley, M. A.; Abroms, I. F.; and Ragland, R. L. 1992. Schizencephaly: Case report of familial incidence. *Pediatric Neurology* 8: 148–50.

Huber, S. J.; Kissel, J. T.; Shuttleworth, E. C.; Chakeres, D. W.; Clapp, L. E.; and Brogan, M. A. 1989. Magnetic resonance imaging and clinical correlates of intellectual impairment in myotonic dystrophy. *Archives of Neurology* 46: 536–40.

Hurst, R. W.; Newman, S. A.; and Cail, W. S. 1988. Multifocal intracranial MR abnormalities in neurofibromatosis. *American Journal of Neuroradiology* 9: 293–96.

Huttenlocher, P. R. 1991. Dendritic and synaptic pathology in mental retardation. *Pediatric Neurology* 7: 79–85.

Hynd, G. W.; Hartlage, L. C.; and Noonan, M. 1984. Intracranial hemorrhages in neonates: Data on cognitive development. *International Journal of Clinical Neuropsychology* 6: 111–14.

Iannetti, P.; Schwartz, C. E.; Dietz-Band, J.; Light, E.; Timmerman, J.; and Chessa, L. 1992. Norman-Roberts syndrome: Clinical and molecular genetics studies. *Pediatric Neurology* 8: 355.

Ingram, T. T. S. 1964. The clinical findings in 79 patients with diplegia. In T. T. S. Ingram (ed.) *Paediatric Aspects of Cerebral Palsy* (London: E. & S. Livingstone), pp. 209–44.

Iosub, S.; Fuchs, M.; Bingol, N.; and Gromisch, D. S. 1981. Fetal alcohol syndrome revisited. *Pediatrics* 68: 475–79.

Jacobs, P. A.; Brunton, M.; and Melville, M. M. 1965. Aggressive behavior, mental subnormality and the XYY male. *Nature* 208: 1351–52.

Jacobs, P. A.; Mayer, M.; and Abruzzo, M. A. 1986. Studies of the fragile (X) syndrome in populations of mentally retarded individuals in Hawaii. *American Journal of Medical Genetics* 23: 567–72.

Jacobs, P. A.; Baikie, A. G.; Court Brown, W. M.; and Strong, J. A. 1959. The somatic chromosomes in mongolism. *Lancet* 1: 710.

Jay, V.; Chan, F.-W.; and Becker, L. E. 1990. Dendritic arborization in the human fetus and infant with the trisomy 18 syndrome. *Developmental Brain Research* 54: 291–94.

Jellinger, K.; Gross, H.; Kaltenbäck, E.; and Grisold, W. 1981. Holoprosencephaly and agenesis of the corpus callosum: Frequency of associated malformations. *Acta Neuropathologica* 55: 1–10.

Jensen, O. A.; Warburg, M.; and Dupont, A. 1976. Ocular pathology in the elfin face syndrome (the Fanconi-Schlesinger type of idiopathic hypercalcemia of infancy). *Ophthalmologica* 172: 434–44.

Jeret, J. S.; Serur, D.; Wisniewski, K. E.; and Lubin, R. A. 1987. Clinicopathological findings associated with agenesis of the corpus callosum. *Brain and Development* 9: 255–64.

Jernigan, T. L., and Bellugi, U. 1990. Anomalous brain morphology on magnetic resonance images in Williams syndrome and Down syndrome. *Archives of Neurology* 47: 529–33.

Johnson, R., Jr.; Rohrbaugh, J. W.; and Ross, J. L. 1993. Altered brain development in Turner's syndrome: An event-related potential study. *Neurology* 43: 801–8.

Jones, K. L. 1975. Aberrant neuronal migration in the fetal alcohol syndrome. *Birth Defects* 11: 131–32.

Kamuro, K., and Tenokuchi, Y. 1993. Familial periventricular nodular heterotopia. *Brain and Development* 15: 237–41.

Kamei, A.; Takashima, S.; Chan, F.; and Becker, L. E. 1992. Abnormal dendritic development in maple syrup urine disease. *Pediatric Neurology* 8: 145–47.

Kataria, S.; Goldstein, D. J.; and Kushnick, T. 1984. Developmental delay in Williams' ("elfin facies") syndrome. *Applied Research in Mental Retardation* 5: 419–23.

Kirk, S. A.; McCarthy, J. J.; and Kirk, W. D. 1968. *Illinois Test of Psycholinguistic Abilities, Revised.* Urbana, Ill.: University of Illinois Press.

Knoll, J. H. M.; Glatt, K. A.; Nicholls, R. D.; Malcolm, S.; and Lalande, M. 1991. Chromosome 15 uniparental disomy is not frequent in Angelman syndrome. *American Journal of Human Genetics* 48: 16–21.

Knoll, J. H. M.; Nicholls, R. D.; Magenis, R. E.; Glatt, K.; Graham, J. M., Jr.; Kaplan, L.; and Lalande, M. 1990. Angelman syndrome: Three molecular classes identified with chromosome 15q11q13-specific DNA markers. *American Journal of Human Genetics* 47: 149–55.

Knoll, J. H.; Nicholls, R.; Magenis, R.; Graham, J.; Lalande, M.; and Latt, S. 1989. Angelman and Prader-Willi syndromes share a common chromosome 15 deletion but differ in parental origin of the deletion. *American Journal of Medical Genetics* 32: 285–90.

Kobori, J. A.; Herrick, M. K.; and Urich, H. 1987. Arhinencephaly: The spectrum of associated malformations. *Brain* 110: 237–60.

Kolb, J. E., and Heaton, R. K. 1975. Lateralized neurologic deficits and psychopathology in a Turner syndrome patient. *Archives of General Psychiatry* 32: 1198–1200.

Kolodny, E. H. 1989. Agenesis of the corpus callosum: A marker for inherited metabolic disease? *Neurology* 39: 847–48.

Krishnamoorthy, K. S.; Shannon, D. C.; DeLong, G. R.; Todres, I. D.; and Davis, K. R. 1979. Neurologic sequelae in the survivors of neonatal intraventricular hemorrhage. *Pediatrics* 64: 233–37.

Lachiewicz, A. M.; Gullion, C.; Spiridigliozzi, G.; and Aylsworth A. 1987. Declining IQs of young males with the fragile X syndrome. *American Journal of Mental Retardation* 92: 272–78.

Larroche, J. C., and Baudley, J. 1961. Cavum septi lucidi, cavum vergae, cavum veli interpositi: Cavities de la ligne mediane. *Biology of the Neonate* 3: 193–236.

Lee, N.; Radtke, R. A.; Gray, L.; Burger, P. C.; Montine, T. J.; DeLong, G. R.; Lewis, D. V.; Oakes, W. J.; Friedman, A. H.; and Hoffman, J. M. 1994. Neuronal migration disorders: Positron emission tomography correlations. *Annals of Neurology* 35: 290–97.

Lejeune, J.; Gautier, M.; and Turpin, R. 1959. Le mongolisme, premier exemple d'aberration autosomique humaine. *Comptes Rendus de l'Academie des Sciences de Paris* 248: 1721–22.

Lippe, B. 1990. Physical and anatomical abnormalities in Turner syndrome. In R. Rosenfeld and M. Grumbach (eds.), *Turner Syndrome* (New York: Marcel Dekker), pp. 183–86.

Little, W. J. 1862. On the influence of abnormal parturition, difficult labors, premature birth, and asphyxia neonatorum on the mental and physical condition of the child, especially in relation to deformities. *Transactions of the Obstetrical Society (London)* 2: 293–96.

Livingston, J. H., and Aicardi, J. 1990. Unusual MRI appearance of diffuse subcortical heterotopia or "double cortex" in two children. *Journal of Neurology, Neurosurgery and Psychiatry* 53: 617–20.

Lyon, M. F. 1991. The quest for the X-inactivation centre. *Trends in Genetics* 7: 69–70.

Magenis, R. E.; Tochen, M. L.; Holahan, K. P.; Carey, T.; Allen, L.; and Brown, M. G. 1984. Turner syndrome resulting from partial deletion of Y chromosome short arm: Localization of male determinants. *Journal of Pediatrics* 105: 916–19.

Manz, H. J.; Phillips, T. M.; Rowden, G.; and McCullough, D. C. 1979. Unilateral megalencephaly, cerebral cortical dysplasia, neuronal hypertrophy and heterotopia: Cytomorphometric, fluorometric, cytochemical, and biochemical analyses. *Acta Neuropathologica* 45: 97–103.

Marin-Padilla, M. 1972. Structural abnormalities of the cerebral cortex in human chromosomal aberrations: A Golgi study. *Brain Research* 44: 625–29.

———. 1976. Pyramidal cell abnormalities in the motor cortex of a child with Down's syndrome: A Golgi study. *Journal of Comparative Neurology* 167: 63–81.

Martin, N. D. T.; Snodgrass, G. J. A. I.; and Cohen, R. D. 1984. Ideopathic infantile hypercalcaemia—A continuing enigma. *Archives of Disease in Childhood* 59: 605–13.

Mascari, M. J.; Gottlieb, W.; Rogan, P. K.; Butler, M. G.; Waller, D. A.; Armour,

J. A.; Jeffreys, J. A.; Ladda, R. L.; and Nicholls, R. D. 1992. The frequency of uniparental disomy in Prader-Willi syndrome: Implications of molecular diagnosis. *New England Journal of Medicine* 326: 1599–1607.

Massa, G.; Vanderschueren-Lodeweyckx, M.; and Fryns, J.-P. 1992. Deletion of the short arm of the X chromosome: A hereditary form of Turner syndrome. *European Journal of Pediatrics* 151: 893–94.

Mathisen, B.; Reilly, S., and Skuse, D. 1992. Oral–motor dysfunction and feeding disorders of infants with Turner syndrome. *Developmental Medicine and Child Neurology* 34: 141–49.

Mazzocco, M. M. M.; Hagerman, R. J.; Cronister-Silverman, A.; and Pennington, B. F. 1992. Specific frontal lobe deficits among women with the fragile X gene. *Journal of the American Academy of Child and Adolescent Psychiatry* 31: 1141–48.

McCauley, E.; Kay, T.; Ito, J.; and Treder, R. 1987. The Turner syndrome: Cognitive deficits, affective discrimination and behavior problems. *Child Development* 58: 464–73.

McGlone, J. 1985. Can spatial deficits in Turner's syndrome be explained by focal CNS dysfunction or atypical speech lateralization? *Journal of Clinical and Experimental Neuropsychology* 7: 375–94.

Menkes, J. H. 1990. *Textbook of Child Neurology,* 4th ed. Philadelphia: Lea & Febiger.

Miller, J. Q. 1963. Lissencephaly in two siblings. *Neurology* 13:841–50.

Mohamed, S. A.; Nathaniel, E. J.; Nathaniel, D. R.; and Snell, L. 1987a. Altered Purkinje cell maturation in rats exposed prenatally to ethanol: I. Cytology. *Experimental Neurology* 97: 35–52.

———. 1987b. Altered Purkinje cell maturation in rats exposed prenatally to ethanol: II. Synaptology. *Experimental Neurology* 97: 53–69.

Money, J., and Alexander, D. 1966. Turner's syndrome: Further demonstration of the presence of specific cognitional deficiencies. *Journal of Medical Genetics* 3: 47–48.

Moore, T., and Haig D. 1991. Genomic imprinting in mammalian development: A parental tug-of-war. *Trends in Genetics* 7: 45–49.

Mundy, P.; Sigman, M.; Kasari, C.; and Yirmiya, N. 1988. Nonverbal communication skills in Down syndrome children. *Child Development* 59: 235–49.

Munson-Davis, J. A. 1988. Speech and language development in Prader-Willi syndrome. In L. R. Greenswag and R. C. Alexander (eds.), *Management of Prader-Willi syndrome* (New York: Springer-Verlag), pp. 124–33.

Myers, R. E. 1972. Two patterns of perinatal brain damage and their conditions of occurrence. *American Journal of Obstetrics and Gynecology* 112: 246–76.

Myrianthropoulos, N. C. 1974. Epidemiology of central nervous system malformations. In P. J. Vinken, G. W. Bruyn, and H. L. Klawans (eds.), *Handbook of Clinical Neurology,* vol. 30 (New York: Elsevier), pp. 139–71.

Nakano, S.; Hojo, H.; Kataoka, K.; and Yamasaki, S. 1981. Age related incidence of cavum septi pellucidi and cavum vergae on CT scans of pediatric patients. *Journal of Computer Assisted Tomography* 5: 348–49.

Nass, R., and Baker, S. 1991. Learning disabilities in children with congenital adrenal hyperplasia. *Journal of Child Neurology* 6: 306–12.

Nass, R.; Baker, S.; Speiser, P.; Virdis, R.; Balsamo, A.; Cacciari, E.; Loche, A.; Dumic, M.; and New, M. 1987. Hormones and handedness: Left-hand bias in female congenital adrenal hyperplasia patients. *Neurology* 37: 711–15.

National Institutes of Health Consensus Development Conference Statement: Neurofibromatosis. 1988. *Archives of Neurology* 45: 575–78.

Nelson, K. B., and Ellenberg, J. H. (1981) Apgar scores as predictors of chronic neurologic disability. *Pediatrics* 68: 36–44.

———. 1986. Antecedants of cerebral palsy. *New England Journal of Medicine* 315: 81–86.

Nicholls, R. D.; Knoll, J. H. M.; Butler, M. G.; Karam, S.; and Lalande, M. 1989. Genetic imprinting suggested by maternal heterodisomy in nondeletion Prader-Willi syndrome. *Nature* 342: 281–85.

Nicholls, R. D.; Knoll, J. H.; Glatt, K.; Hersh, J. H.; Brewster, T. D.; Graham, J. M.; Wurster-Hill, D.; Wharton, R.; and Latt, S. A. 1989. Restriction fragment length polymorphisms within proximal 15q and their use in molecular cytogenetics and the Prader-Willi syndrome. *American Journal of Medical Genetics* 33: 66–77.

Nicholls, R. D.; Pai, G. S.; Gottlieb, W.; and Cantú, E. S. 1992. Paternal uniparental disomy of chromosome 15 in a child with Angelman syndrome. *Annals of Neurology* 32: 512–18.

Nielsen, K. B.; Tommerup, N.; and Mikkelsen, M. 1983. Clinical and cytogenetic findings in 26 mentally retarded males with the fragile X. *Clinical Genetics* 23: 241.

Norman, M. G. 1980. Bilateral encephaloclastic lesions in a 26 week gestation fetus: Effect on neuroblast migration. *Canadian Journal of Neurological Science* 7: 191–94.

Oberle, I.; Rousseau, F.; Heitz, D.; Kretz, C.; Devys, D.; Hanauer, A.; Boue, J.; Bertheas, M. F.; and Mandel, J. L. 1991. Instability of a 550–base pair DNA segment and abnormal methylation in fragile X syndrome. *Science* 252: 1097–1102.

Owen, D. R. 1972. The 47,XYY male: A review. *Psychological Bulletin* 78: 209–33.

Pagon, R. A.; Bennett, F. C.; LaVeck, B.; Stewart, K. B.; and Johnson, J. 1987. Williams syndrome: Features in late childhood and adolescence. *Pediatrics* 80: 85–91.

Palmini, A.; Andermann, F.; Aicardi, J.; Dulac, O.; Chaves, F.; Ponsot, G.; Pinard, J. M.; Goutières, F.; Livingston, J.; Tampieri, D.; Andermann, E.; and Robitaille, Y. 1991. Diffuse cortical dysplasia, or the "double cortex" syndrome: The clinical and epileptic spectrum in 10 patients. *Neurology* 41: 1656–62.

Palmini, A.; Andermann, F.; Olivier, A.; Tampieri, D.; Robitaille, Y.; Melanson, D.; and Ethier, R. 1991. Neuronal migration disorders: A contribution of modern neuroimaging to the etiologic diagnosis of epilepsy. *Canadian Journal of Neurological Sciences* 18: 580–87.

Papile, L. A.; Munsick, G.; Weaver, N.; and Pecha, S. 1979. Cerebral intraventricular hemorrhage (CVH) in infants < 1500 grams: Developmental follow-up at one year. *Pediatric Research* 13: 528.

Pasternak, J. F. 1987. Parasagittal infarction in neonatal asphyxia. *Annals of Neurology* 21: 202–4.

Pasternak, J. F.; Predey, T. A.; and Mikhael, M. A. 1991. Neonatal asphyxia: Vulnerability of basal ganglia, thalamus, and brainstem. *Pediatric Neurology* 7: 147–79.

Paul, R.; Dykens, E.; Leckman, J. F.; Watson, M.; Breg, W. R.; and Cohen, D. J. 1987. A comparison of language characteristics of mentally retarded adults with fragile X syndrome and those with nonspecific mental retardation and autism. *Journal of Autism and Developmental Disorders* 17: 457–68.

Pennington, B.; Heaton, R.; Karzmark, P.; Pendleton, M.; Lehman, R.; and Shucard, D. 1985. The neuropsychological phenotype in Turner syndrome. *Cortex* 21: 391–404.

Piccirilli, M.; D'Alessandro, P.; Mazzi, P.; Sciarma, T.; and Testa, A. 1991. Cerebral organization for language in Down's syndrome patients. *Cortex* 27: 41–47.

Pipe, M. E. 1988. Atypical laterality and retardation. *Psychological Bulletin* 104: 343–47.

Prader, A.; Labhart, A.; and Willi, H. 1956. Ein Syndrom von Adipositas, Kleinwuchs, Kryptorchidismus und Oligophrenie nach myatonieartigem Zustand im Neugeborenenalter. *Schweizer Medicinishe Wochenschrift* 86: 1260–61.

Preus, M. 1984. The Williams syndrome: Objective definition and diagnosis. *Clinical Genetics* 25: 422–28.

Price, W. H., and Whatmore, P. B. 1967. Behaviour disorders and pattern of crime among XYY males identified at a maximum security hospital. *British Medical Journal* 1: 533–36.

Pujol, J.; Vendrell, P.; Junqué, C.; Martí-Vilalta, J. L.; and Capdevila, A. 1993. When does human brain development end? Evidence of corpus callosum growth up to adulthood. *Annals of Neurology* 34: 71–75.

Ratcliffe, S. G., and Field, M. A. S. 1982. Emotional disorder in XYY children: Four case reports. *Journal of Child Psychology and Psychiatry* 23: 401–6.

Reilly, J.; Klima, E.; and Bellugi, U. 1991. Once more with feeling: Affect and language in atypical populations. *Developmental Psychopathology* 2: 367–91.

Reiss, A. L.; Aylward, E.; Freund, L. S.; Joshi, P. K.; and Bryan, R. N. 1991. Neuroanatomy of fragile X syndrome: The posterior fossa. *Annals of Neurology* 29: 26–32.

Reiss, A. L.; Freund, L. S.; Plotnick, L.; Baumgardner, T.; Green, K.; Sozer, A. C.; Reader, M.; Boehm, C.; and Denckla, M. B. 1993. The effects of X monosomy on brain development: Monozygotic twins discordant for Turner's syndrome. *Annals of Neurology* 34: 95–107.

Reske-Nielsen, E.; Christensen, A. L.; and Nielsen, J. 1982. A neuropathological and neuropsychological study of Turner's syndrome. *Cortex* 18: 181–90.

Resnick, S.; Berenbaum, S.; Gottesman, I.; and Bouchard, T. 1986. Early hormonal influences on cognitive functioning in congenital adrenal hyperplasia. *Developmental Psychology* 22: 191–98.

Riccardi, V. M., and Eichner, J. E. 1986. *Neurofibromatosis: Phenotype, Natural History, and Pathogenesis*. Baltimore: Johns Hopkins University Press.

Riccardi, V. M., and Lewis, R. A. 1988. Penetrance of von Recklinghausen neurofibromatosis: A distinction between predecessors and descendants. *American Journal of Human Genetics* 42: 284–89.

Ricci, S.; Cusmai, R.; Fariello, G.; Fusco, L.; and Vigevano, F. 1992. Double cortex: A neuronal migration anomaly as a possible cause of Lennox-Gastaut syndrome. *Archives of Neurology* 49: 61–64.

Richards, R. I., and Sutherland, G. R. 1992. Dynamic mutations: A new class of mutations causing human disease. *Cell* 70: 709–12.

Rintahaka, P. J.; Chugani, H. T.; Messa, C.; and Phelps, M. E. 1993. Hemimegalencephaly: Evaluation with positron emission tomography. *Pediatric Neurology* 9: 21–28.

Rosman, N. P., and Kakulas, B. A. 1966. Mental deficiency associated with muscular dystrophy: A neuropathological study. *Brain* 89: 769–88.

Rosman, N. P., and Pearce, J. 1967. The brain in multiple neurofibromatosis (von

Recklinghausen's disease): A suggested neuropathological basis for the associated mental defect. *Brain* 90: 829–37.

Ross, C. A.; McInnis, M. G.; Margolis, R. L.; and Li, S.-H. 1993. Genes with triplet repeats: Candidate mediators of neuropsychiatric disorders. *Trends in Neuroscience* 16: 254–60.

Ross, M. H.; Galaburda, A. M.; and Kemper, T. L. 1984. Down's syndrome: Is there a decreased population of neurons? *Neurology* 34: 909–16.

Rouleau, G. A.; Wertelecki, W.; Haines, J.; Hobbs, W. J.; Trofatter, J.; Seizinger, B.; Martuza, R.; Superneau, D.; Conneally, P.; and Gusella, J. 1987. Genetic linkage of bilateral acoustic neurofibromatosis to a DNA marker on chromosome 22. *Nature* 329: 246–48.

Rourke, B. P. 1988. The syndrome of non-verbal learning disabilities: Developmental manifestations in neurological disease, disorder and dysfunction. *Clinical Neuropsychologist* 2: 293–330.

Rovet, J. 1990. The cognitive and neuropsychological characteristics of females with Turner syndrome. In D. Berch and B. Bender (eds.), *Sex Chromosome Abnormalities and Human Behavior* (Boulder, Colo.: Westview Press), pp. 38–77.

———. 1992. Psychological characteristics of children with Turner syndrome. *Contemporary Pediatrics* (March/April): 13–21.

———. 1993. The psychoeducational characteristics of children with Turner syndrome. *Journal of Learning Disabilities* 26: 333–41.

Rovet, J., and Netley, C. 1980. The mental rotation task performance of Turner syndrome subjects. *Behavior Genetics* 11: 437–44.

Rubinstein, L. J. 1986. The malformative central nervous system lesions in the central and peripheral forms of neurofibromatosis: A neuropathological study of 22 cases. *Annals of the New York Academy of Science* 486: 14–29.

Saitoh, S.; Kubota, T.; Ohta, T.; Jinno, Y.; Niikawa, N.; Sugimoto, T.; Wagstaff, J.; and Lalande, M. 1992. Familial Angelman syndrome caused by imprinted submicroscopic deletion encompassing GABA_A receptor β_3 subunit gene. *Lancet* 339: 366–67.

Salbenblatt, J. A.; Meyers, D. C.; Bender, B. C.; Linden, M. G.; and Robinson, A. 1987. Gross and fine motor development in 47,XXY and 47,XYY males. *Pediatrics* 80: 240–44.

Sandberg, A. A.; Koepf, G. F.; Ishihara, T.; and Hauschka, T. S. 1961. An XYY male. *Lancet* (August 26) 2: 488–89.

Sanders, R. J. 1989. Sentence comprehension following agenesis of the corpus callosum. *Brain and Language* 37: 59–72.

Santavuori, P.; Somer, H.; Sainio, K.; Rapola, J.; Kruus, S.; Nikitin, T.; Ketonen, L.; and Leisti, J. 1989. Muscle-eye-brain disease (MEB). *Brain and Development* 11: 147–53.

Sarnat, H. B. 1987. Disturbances of late neuronal migrations in the perinatal period. *American Journal of the Diseases of Children* 141: 969–80.

Sattler, J. M. 1988. *Assessment of Children*. 3d ed. San Diego: J. Sattler.

Schaefer, G. B.; Thompson, J. N.; Bodensteiner, J. B.; Hamza, M.; Tucker, R. R.; Marks, W.; Gay, C.; and Wilson, D. 1990. Quantitative morphometric analysis of brain growth using magnetic resonance imaging. *Journal of Child Neurology* 5: 127–30.

Schaefer, G. B.; Bodensteiner, J. B.; Thompson, J. N.; and Wilson, D. A. 1991. Clinical and morphometric analysis of the hypoplastic corpus callosum. *Archives of Neurology* 48: 933–36.

Schaefer, G. B.; Shuman, R. M.; Wilson, D. A.; Saleeb, S.; Domek, D. B.; Johnson, S. F.; and Bodensteiner, J. B. 1991. Partial agenesis of the anterior corpus callosum: Correlation between appearance, imaging, and neuropathology. *Pediatric Neurology* 7: 39–44.

Schapiro, M. B.; Grady, C. L.; Kumar, A.; Herscovitch, P.; Haxby, J. V.; Moore, A. M.; White, B.; Friedland, R. P.; and Rapoport, S. I. 1990. Regional cerebral glucose metabolism is normal in young adults with Down syndrome. *Journal of Cerebral Blood Flow and Metabolism* 10: 199–206.

Schrott, L. M.; Denenberg, V. H.; Sherman, G. F.; Waters, N. S.; Rosen, G. D.; and Galaburda, A. M. 1992. Environmental enrichment, neocortical ectopias, and behavior in the autoimmune NZB mouse. *Developmental Brain Research* 67: 85–93.

Schwartz, C. E.; Johnson, J. P.; Holycross, B.; Mandeville, T. M.; Sears, T. S.; Graul, E. A.; Carey, J. C.; Schroer, R. J.; Phelan, M. C.; Szollar, J.; Flannery, D. B.; and Stevenson, R. E. 1988. Detection of submicroscopic deletions in band 17p13 in patients with the Miller-Dieker syndrome. *American Journal of Human Genetics* 43: 597–604.

Scott, B. S.; Becker, L. E.; and Petit, T. L. 1983. Neurobiology of Down's syndrome. *Progress in Neurobiology* 21: 199–237.

Seguin, E. 1846. *Le Traitment Moral, l'Hygiene et l'Education des Idiots*. Paris: Baillier.

Shelbourne, P.; Winqvist, R.; Kunert, E.; Davies, J.; Leisti, J.; Thiele, H.; Bachmann, H.; Buxton, J.; Williamson, B.; and Johnson, K. 1992. Unstable DNA may be responsible for the incomplete penetrance of the myotonic dystrophy phenotype. *Human Molecular Genetics* 1: 467–73.

Shucard, D. W.; Shucard, J.-L.; Clopper, R. R.; and Schachter, M. 1992. Electrophysiological and neuropsychological indices of cognitive processing deficits in Turner syndrome. *Developmental Neuropsychology* 8: 299–323.

Sidman, R. L., and Rakic, P. 1982. Development of the human central nervous system. In R. D. Adams and W. Haymaker (eds.), *Histology and Histopathology of the Nervous System* (Springfield Ill.: Charles C. Thomas), pp. 3–145.

Siejka, S.; Strefling, A. M.; and Urich, H. 1989. Absence of septum pellucidum and polymicrogyria: A forme fruste of the porencephalic syndrome. *Clinical Neuropathology* 8: 174–78.

Silbert, A.; Wolff, P.; and Lilienthal, J. 1977. Spatial and temporal processing in patients with Turner's syndrome. *Behavior Genetics* 7: 11–21.

Smith, G. F., and Berg, J. M. 1976. *Down's Anomaly*, 2d ed. New York: Churchill Livingstone.

Stewart, D. A. 1982. *Children with sex chromosome aneupoloidy: Follow-up studies. Birth Defects: Original Article Series* 18.

Stewart, D. A.; Netley, C. T.; and Park, E. 1982. Summary of clinical findings of children with 47,XXY, 47,XYY, and 47,XXX karyotypes. *Birth Defects* 18: 1–5.

Stewart, R. M.; Richman, D. P.; and Caviness, V. S. 1975. Lissencephaly and pachygyria: An architectonic and topographical analysis. *Acta Neuropathologica (Berlin)* 31: 1–12.

Streissguth, A. P.; Randels, S. P.; and Smith, D. F. 1991. A test–retest study of intelligence in patients with fetal alcohol syndrome: Implications for care. *Journal of the American Academy of Child and Adolescent Psychiatry* 30: 584–87.

Summitt, R. L. 1981. Specific segments that cause the phenotype of Down syndrome.

In F. F. de la Cruz and P. S. Gerald (eds.), *Trisomy 21 (Down Syndrome): Research Perspectives* (Baltimore: University Park Press), pp. 225–35.

Sutherland, G. R., and Hecht, F. 1985. *Fragile Sites on Human Chromosomes*. New York: Oxford University Press.

Swayze, V. W.; Andreasen, N. C.; Ehrhardt, J. C.; Yuh, W. T. C.; Alliger, R. J.; and Cohen, G. A. 1990. Developmental abnormalities of the corpus callosum in schizophrenia. *Archives of Neurology* 47: 805–8.

Takashima, S.; Mito, T.; and Ando, Y. 1986. Pathogenesis of periventricular white matter hemorrhages in preterm infants. *Brain and Development* 8: 25–30.

Tannock, R.; Kershner, JR.; and Oliver, J. 1984. Do individuals with Down's syndrome possess right hemisphere language dominance? *Cortex* 20: 221–31.

Tatum, W. O.; Coker, S. B.; Ghobrial, M.; and Abd-Allah, S. 1989. The open opercular sign: Diagnosis and significance. *Annals of Neurology* 25: 196–99.

Taylor, A. K.; Safanda, J. F.; Fall, M. Z.; Quince, C.; Lang, K. A.; Hull, C. E.; Carpenter, I.; Staley, L. W.; and Hagerman, R. J. 1994. Molecular predictors of cognitive involvement in female carriers of fragile X syndrome. *Journal of the American Medical Association* 271: 507–14.

Temple, C. M., and Carney, R. A. 1993. Intellectual functioning of children with Turner syndrome: A comparison of behavioural phenotypes. *Developmental Medicine and Child Neurology* 35: 691–98.

Temple, C. M., and Vilarroya, O. 1990. Perceptual and cognitive perspective taking in two siblings with callosal agenesis. *British Journal of Developmental Psychology* 8: 3–8.

Thase, M. E.; Tigner, R.; Smeltzer, D. J.; and Liss, L. 1984. Age-related neuropsychological deficits in Down's syndrome. *Biological Psychiatry* 19: 571–85.

Theilgaard, A. 1986. Psychologic study of XYY and XXY men. *Birth Defects: Original Article Series* 22: 27–292.

Thornton, C. A.; Griggs, R. C.; and Moxley, R. T. 1994. Myotonic dystrophy with no trinucleotide repeat expansion. *Annals of Neurology* 35: 269–72.

Tilton, A. H.; Krywanio, M.; Greene, C.; Nadell, J. M.; and Posas, H. 1988. Schizencephaly: Familial occurrence. *Neurology* 38: 5398.

Tirosh, E.; Rod, R.; Cohen, A.; and Hochberg, Z. 1993. Congenital adrenal hyperplasia and cerebral lateralizations. *Pediatric Neurology* 9: 198–201.

Trauner, D. A.; Bellugi, U.; and Chase, C. 1989. Neurologic features of Williams and Down syndromes. *Pediatric Neurology* 5: 166–68.

Tschopp, F. A.; Tobler, P. H.; and Fischer, J. A. 1984. Calcitonin gene related peptide in the human thyroid, pituitary and brain. *Molecular and Cellular Endocrinology* 36: 53–57.

Turner, G.; Brookwell, R.; Daniel, A.; Selikowitz, M.; and Zilibowitz, M. 1980. Heterozygous expression of X-linked mental retardation and X-chromosome marker fra(X) (q27). *New England Journal of Medicine* 303: 662–64.

Tychsen, L.; and Hoyt, W. F. 1985. Occipital lobe dysplasia: Magnetic resonance findings in two cases of isolated, congenital hemianopsia. *Archives of Ophthalmology* 103: 680–82.

Udwin, O., and Yule, W. 1991. A cognitive and behavioral phenotype in Williams syndrome. *Journal of Clinical and Experimental Neuropsychology* 13: 232–44.

Udwin, O.; Yule, W.; and Martin, N. 1987. Cognitive abilities and behavioural characteristics of children with idiopathic infantile hypercalcaemia. *Journal of Child Psychology and Psychiatry* 28: 297–309.

Valentine, G. H. 1982. The growth and development of six XYY children: A continuative report. *Birth Defects* 18: 219–26.

Veelken, N.; Hagberg, B.; Hagberg, G.; and Olow, I. 1983. Diplegic cerebral palsy in Swedish term and preterm children. *Neuropediatrics* 14: 20–28.

Volk, B. 1984. Cerebellar histogenesis and synaptic maturation following pre- and postnatal alcohol administration. *Acta Neuropathologica* 63: 57–65.

Volpe, J. J. 1989. Intraventricular hemorrhage in the premature infant—Current concepts. Part I. *Annals of Neurology* 25: 3–11.

Waber, D. 1979. Neuropsychological aspects of Turner's syndrome. *Developmental Medicine and Child Neurology* 21: 58–70.

Wahlström, J.; Gillberg, C.; Gustavson, K.-H.; and Holmgren, G. 1986. Infantile autism and the Fragile-X: A Swedish multicenter study. *American Journal of Medical Genetics* 23: 403–8.

Wang, P. P.; Hesselink, J. R.; Jernigan, T. L.; Doherty, S.; and Bellugi, U. 1992. Specific neurobehavioral profile of Williams' syndrome is associated with neocerebellar hemispheric preservation. *Neurology* 42: 1999–2002.

Webb, T. P.; Bundey, S. E.; Thake, A. I.; and Todd, J. 1986. Population incidence and segregation ratios in the Martin-Bell syndrome. *American Journal of Medical Genetics* 23: 573–80.

Wisniewski, K.; Dambska, M.; Sher, J. H.; and Qazi, Q. 1983. A clinical neuropathological study of the fetal alcohol syndrome. *Neuropediatrics* 14: 197–201.

Wisniewski, K.; Howe, J.; Williams, D. G.; and Wisniewski, H. M. 1978. Precocious aging and dementia in patients with Down's syndrome. *Biological Psychiatry* 13: 619–27.

Wisniewski, K. E.; Laure-Kaminionowska, M.; Connell, F.; and Wen, G. Y. 1986. Neuronal density and synaptogenesis in the postnatal stage of brain maturation in Down syndrome. In C. J. Epstein (ed.), *The Neurobiology of Down Syndrome* (New York: Raven Press), pp. 29–44.

Wisniewski, K. E.; Wisniewski, H. M.; and Wen, G. Y. 1985. Occurrence of neuropathological changes and dementia of Alzheimer's disease in Down's syndrome. *Annals of Neurology* 17: 278–82.

Wisniewski, H. M.; Berry, K.; and Spiro, A. J. 1975. Ultrastructure of thalamic neuronal inclusions in myotonic dystrophy. *Journal of Neurological Science* 24: 321–29.

Williams, J.; Richman, L.; and Yarbrough, D. 1991. A comparison of memory and attention in Turner syndrome and learning disability. *Journal of Pediatric Psychology* 16: 585–93.

Williams, J. C. P.; Barratt-Boyes, B. G.; and Lowe, J. B. 1961. Supravalvular aortic stenosis. *Circulation* 24: 1311–18.

Williams, M. L.; Lewandowski, L. J.; Coplan, J.; and D'Eugenio, D. B. 1987. Neurodevelopmental outcome of preschool children born preterm with and without intracranial hemorrhage. *Developmental Medicine and Child Neurology* 29: 243–49.

Yakovlev, P. I., and Wadsworth, R. C. 1946a. Schizencephalies: A study of the congenital clefts in the cerebral mantle: I. Clefts with fused lips. *Journal of Neuropathology and Experimental Neurology* 5: 116–30.

———. 1946b. Schizencephalies: A study of the congenital clefts in the cerebral mantle: II. Clefts with hydrocephalus and lips separated. *Journal of Neuropathology and Experimental Neurology* 5: 169–206.

Yu, S.; Pritchard, M.; Kremer, E.; Lynch, M.; Nancarrow, J.; Baker, E.; Holman, K.;

Mulley, J. C.; Warren, S. T.; Schlessinger, D.; Sutherland, G. R.; and Richards, R. I. 1991. Fragile X genotype characterized by an unstable region of DNA. *Science* 252: 1179–81.

Zachmann, M.; Prader, A.; Kind, H. P.; Häfliger, H.; and Budliger, H. 1974. Testicular volume during adolescence: Cross-sectional and longitudinal studies. *Helvetica Paediatrica Acta* 29: 61–72.

Zellweger, H. 1981. Diagnosis and therapy in the first phase of Prader-Willi syndrome. In L. R. Greenswag and R. C. Alexander (eds.), *Management of Prader-Willi Syndrome* (New York: Springer-Verlag), pp. 15–22.

Zori, R. T.; Hendrickson, J.; Woolven, S.; Whidden, E. M.; Gray, B.; and Williams, C. A. 1992. Angelman syndrome: Clinical profile. *Journal of Child Neurology* 7: 270–80.

II

The Pediatric Neurological and Neuropsychological Evaluation

4

The Pediatric Neurological Examination

Neuropsychologists and neurologists share an interest in the relationship of brain and behavior. The training of a neurologist stresses lesion localization and pathology—*where* a lesion is located (that is, in the muscle, in the peripheral nerve, in the spinal cord, or in the brain), and *what* might have caused that lesion. Behavioral neurologists and neuropsychologists focus specifically on "where and what" aspects of brain systems that subserve cognition and behavior, rather than on all aspects of the nervous system. In particular, neuropsychologists must be familiar with the essentials of the neurological examination, so they can better interpret the data from these along with results of the physical examination.

Clinical examinations performed by the great neurologists of the nineteenth century (including Charcot, Dejerine, and Wernicke) defined the examination approach that remains in use today. Although specific clinical maneuvers used by neurologists have not changed much since that time, interpretations of abnormal findings have been modified substantially on the basis of information from experimental and clinical studies and of the enormous growth of knowledge about nervous system function.

The "neurological examination" is really a collection of many different examinations. Based on patient history, the neurologist formulates hypotheses about the specific areas of the nervous system that are likely to be involved, and then conducts a general neurological screening examination (essentially a global "circuit check"). The initial hypotheses are then retained or discarded, and additional ones are generated. New hypotheses are tested using more detailed and specific *subroutines*—specialized neurological assessments that represent extensions of the neurological examination. These may include electrophysiological, neuroradiological, biochemical, and neuropathological studies. For example, if Patient A complains of weakness and loss of sensation in the right foot, the hypothesized location is at the level of the peripheral nerve or spinal cord. If Patient B complains of word-finding problems and weakness of the right hand, the hypothesized site is the left perisylvian cortical region.

Screening (a brief sampling of relevant functions) provides initial information about whether these hypotheses are true; the more focused examination (the subroutine) allows for evaluation of that specific area. Thus, if Patient A's screening examination reveals weakness, atrophy, areflexia, and sensory loss of the right lower leg, subroutines will focus on the peripheral nerve, and may include electromyographic (EMG) and nerve conduction studies. If hyper-reflexia is present, however, the emphasis will shift to the spinal cord. Patient B's subroutine examination will emphasize language and other aspects of cognition, and it is likely to include additional neuropsychological and neuroradiological studies.

Often, considerable congruence exists between the information obtained from neurological examinations and that obtained from neuropsychological ones. A discrepancy between these results is of clinical interest and suggests that data reevaluation is needed. For example, a patient who has a right hemiparesis and language difficulty is scarcely surprising; but aphasia in the context of a florid cerebellar syndrome is worthy of further exploration. As more is learned about brain function, areas previously believed not to participate much in cognition have come under scrutiny. The cerebellum, for example, is no longer viewed as being exclusively a neuronal machine for controlling motor movements. Evidence of its important role in higher cognitive functions is accumulating (Schmahmann 1991).

The standard neurological examination was designed for adults. Techniques and interpretation must be modified for the very young and the very old. Some aspects of the standard examination cannot be performed by infants (for instance, they do not walk), and the Babinski sign and grasp reflexes (indicating pathology in the adult) are normal in infants. For their part, the aged normally manifest diminution of vibratory and position sense, negating "evidence" of sensory impairment. Moreover, features of the child's physical and neurological status not examined in a classical neurological evaluation provide information about the nervous system nonetheless. These include dysmorphic features (anomalous facial and somatic features) and "soft signs."

The neurological examination has two stages: assessment and interpretation. It is possible for two examiners to disagree about the presence or absence of specific signs (for instance, degree of hyperactivity of deep tendon reflexes, aspects of the sensory examination) but still agree about the differential diagnosis. Multiple factors affect the level of agreement (Koran 1975). These reflect the nature of the judgment to be made. Dichotomous (yes/no) judgments tend to invite greater levels of agreement than Rikert scale–type measurements. There also tends to be higher levels of agreement among examiners with more training and experience. And agreement is higher in studies in which normal (rather than abnormal) persons are examined. Among neurological patients, repeated assessments may improve performance, but they may also result in fatigue effects and diminished performance. Finally, signs may fluctuate during the course of a day; for example, a patient may manifest greater disability and more florid signs in the evening than in the morning.

This chapter provides an overview of the general pediatric neurological examination, including history-taking and conducting an examination, with particular emphasis on aspects of the examination that are relevant to the pediatric neuropsychologist. Other subjects addressed include how to interpret information derived from the neurological examination, limitations of the examination, and its significance to neuropsychology. The reader may wish to refer to a comprehensive textbook of neuroanatomy or pediatric neurology for a more thorough presentation of anatomical and clinical features of the neurological conditions discussed (see the Preface).

THE NEUROLOGICAL HISTORY

The history is a review of events leading up to the current neurological problem. With pediatric patients, history must often be obtained from another person, such as a parent or other caretaker. However, even a young child can often provide lucid information about a problem. History-taking consists of two parts. The first part consists of a relatively unstructured description of the onset and course of the illness, supplemented by questions about the presence or absence of specific symptoms and their evolution. The second part consists of structured information obtained about the mother's obstetrical history, the delivery, the baby's status and behavior in the neonatal period, and developmental milestones. Medical history is reviewed. This includes a "review of systems"—questions related to specific body systems. For example, "Is there a history of bowel disturbance, nausea, vomiting, jaundice, abdominal pain . . . ?" elicits information about the gastrointestinal system. Family history and psychosocial information are also reviewed, including school history and the development of social behavior.

GENERAL PHYSICAL EXAMINATION

The child's height, weight, and head circumference are measured and compared to normative standards. For example, a height of 43½″ falls at the 50th percentile for a 5-year-old male, but is far above the 95th percentile for a 3-year-old and is below the 3rd percentile for a 7-year-old. Similarly, head circumference is compared to age and sex norms. Vital signs—blood pressure, temperature, pulse, and respiration—are measured. The child's general appearance is observed. Does the child look pale or sick? Are there signs of weight loss or of an unkempt appearance? Is the child obese or too thin? The general physical includes examination of the head, eyes, ears, nose, throat, heart, lungs, abdomen, skin, and genitalia. Specific features of the hair, skin, teeth, nails, facial appearance, and body are examined carefully.

MENTAL STATUS EXAMINATION

The mental status examination is familiar terrain for the neuropsychologist. First, level of consciousness is assessed. Is the child alert and relating to his or her environment (both physical and social aspects)? Is there evidence of self-awareness? Is the child irritable, inattentive, or distractible? Second, motor activity is observed. Is there restlessness or a marked paucity of spontaneous movement? Are movements stereotypic or random? Third, affect is checked. Does the child seem withdrawn and sad, furiously angry, or remarkably happy? Fourth, language is observed. Is spontaneous language grammatical, uttered with a normal prosodic contour, and fluent? Is verbal communication limited to a few sparse words or phrases? Is there evidence of reciprocal social give and take? Fifth, how the child relates to parents and strangers is noted. How a young child plays with toys may also have important diagnostic implications. Does the child merely bang or finger a toy, or is there evidence of imaginative, symbolic play? Spontaneous behavior is extremely important, as well (see Chapter 5). Formal assessment of mental status, orientation (person, place, and time), memory, backward digits, and a brief academic screen can be carried out with older children, but this effort often overlaps the neuropsychological assessment.

CRANIAL NERVE EXAMINATION

There are twelve cranial nerves. Each is located in the brainstem and receives innervation from various cortical areas (see Table 4-1). Each is considered separately in the subsections that follow.

Cranial Nerve I: Olfactory Nerve

Although humans are notably poor smellers compared to other mammals, examination of the olfactory system often proves helpful in neuropsychological

Table 4-1 Cranial Nerves and Their Major Functions

Cranial Nerve	Function
I. Olfactory	Smell
II. Optic	Vision
III. Oculomotor	Eye movement
IV. Trochlear	Eye movement
V. Trigeminal	Mastication movements; facial sensation; corneal reflex
VI. Abducens	Eye movement
VII. Facial	Facial sensation and movement; taste
VIII. Acoustic (cochlear, vestibular)	Hearing; balance; coordination; orientation in space
IX. Glossopharyngeal	Mouth sensation and movement; taste; autonomic visceral responses
X. Vagus	Mouth sensation and movement; autonomic visceral responses
XI. Spinal accessory	Neck and shoulder muscles
XII. Hypoglossal	Tongue movement

analyses. The distal processes of the olfactory nerve are ciliated processes that penetrate the mucous membrane of the upper portion of the nasal cavity. Molecules of odor dissolve in the mucus and come in contact with a specific receptor that triggers neuron firing. The neuron carries the signal, via unmyelinated nerves, through the cribriform plate to synapses in the olfactory bulbs. These neurons run posteriorly in the olfactory tract and divide at the olfactory trigone into medial and lateral olfactory striae. The medial olfactory striae end on the paraolfactory area, subcallosal gyrus, and inferior cingulate gyrus. The lateral olfactory striae pass under the temporal lobe and terminate in the uncus, anterior hippocampal gyrus, and amygdaloid nucleus.

Smell is tested in each nostril separately by presenting a vial of a readily identifiable fragrance (such as oil of lemon, coffee, or vanilla). Substances such as camphor, menthol, and ammonia also stimulate nasal sensory nerve endings and should not be used. Disorders of smell, although not often tested in children, may provide clues to underlying pathology. For example, unilateral anosmia may be the first sign of a sphenoidal ridge meningioma. One expects a child with agenesis of the olfactory bulbs to be anosmic. However, local infections (sinusitis) and allergies may also diminish smell.

Cranial Nerve II: Optic Nerve

The optic system consists of a series of multisynaptic neuronal pathways that connect the retina and visual cortex. The visual receptors—the rods and cones—synapse with two layers of cells in the retina: bipolar cells and ganglion cells. For each eye, the axons of ganglion cells pass through the fibrillar layer of the retina and exit the eyeball at the optic disk (papilla) to form the *optic nerve*. The nasal fibers partially cross in the optic chiasm and join with uncrossed temporal fibers from each eye. After leaving the optic chiasm, these axons constitute the *optic tract* that synapses in the lateral geniculate body. The *optic radiation* consists of the axons of the cells of the lateral geniculate body that ends in the visual cortex (striate area, Brodmann's area 17). The axons are arranged in an exquisitely localized manner; they sweep around the anterior surface of the temporal horns of the lateral ventricles to form a broad tract that underlies the lateral and occipital horns on its way to the striate area (Meyer's loop).

Assessment of the visual system involves progressive steps. First, *visual acuity* is assessed, at both far and near distances. Pictures of objects or shapes are often used in testing children who do not yet read. If the child wears glasses, it is important to know whether vision is corrected to normal acuity. Second, *visual fields* are assessed in the cooperative child by the confrontation method. The child's field is compared to the examiner's visual field. The child, positioned 2 to 3 feet away from the examiner, fixates on the examiner's nose. The child and the examiner each cover one eye (for instance, the examiner's right and the child's left). The examiner then brings a test object (a white- or red-topped pin, a pencil or a finger) into the field of vision, and the patient is asked to report when the object is first seen. Variants of this technique involve flicking a finger in the visual field or asking the patient to count one or two fingers. Young children, or those who cannot cooperate with confrontation testing, can be tested by drawing the child's attention to an object and then swinging it into the visual field and noting when the child turns to look at the object. Confused patients can also be tested by rapidly bringing a hand into the visual field ("threat") and observing a reflex blink.

When visual stimuli are presented in both fields simultaneously ("double simultaneous stimulation"), *visual neglect* can be assessed. Multiple single and double stimuli are presented randomly, and the child reports when and where the stimuli are seen. If the child perceives a single stimulus in a visual field but is seemingly unaware of it when it is accompanied by a simultaneous contralateral stimulus, neglect of the visual stimulus is noted.

A number of specialized instruments for visual field testing, such as perimeter and tangent screen methods, can be employed. However, these methods require full patient cooperation and attention.

Common visual field defects follow certain patterns. *Hemianopsia* (or *hemianopia*) refers to a loss of the left or right half of the visual field. A *homonymous* hemianopsia involves the loss of the temporal half of the field of one eye and the nasal half of the field of the other eye. This sign immediately identifies the lesion as being located behind the optic chiasm: the nasal field is affected in the eye ipsilateral to the lesion, and the temporal field is affected in the eye opposite to the lesion.

Another common field defect is a *bitemporal* hemianopsia, in which the temporal fields of both eyes are affected. This condition results from a lesion impinging on the optic chiasm (for instance, a pituitary tumor). *Binasal* hemianopsias are quite rare.

Quadrantanopsias or *quadrantic hemianopsias* involve only a quarter of the visual field (generally the temporal field). These result from lesions of the optic radiations. Temporal lobe lesions affecting Meyer's loop—the pathway that courses from the lateral geniculate through the temporal lobe (lateral to the ventricle) and terminates on the lower lip of the calcarine fissure—produce a superior quadrantanopsic field defect. Parietal lesions affecting the portion of the optic radiation that runs through the parietal lobe and terminates on the upper lip of the calcarine fissure produce inferior quadrantanopsic field defects.

Such altitudinal field cuts (involving the upper or lower halves of the visual field, or the superior or inferior quadrants) help the examiner locate lesions involving the posterior optic pathways and are of particular interest. There are two parallel processing systems: the ventral "what" system, involved with object recognition, that runs inferiorly from the occipital cortex through inferior parietal cortex into the temporal lobe; and the dorsal "where" system, involved in visuomotor performance and spatial perception, that is connected dorsally into the superior parietal area. These systems have been extensively studied in experimental animals (Ungerleider & Mishkin 1982), and dissociations between these two systems can be shown in humans. Patients with ventral pathway lesions, which are associated with superior field cuts, have impaired object perception and imagery. Patients with visual–spatial deficits, which are associated with inferior field cuts, cannot reach for objects, locate them accurately in space, or find their way around a given environment (Levine, Warach & Farah 1985). Rapcsak, Cimino & Heilman (1988) describe a woman with a superior parietal lesion who described her cows as "floating," because their feet were lost in an inferior field cut.

Defects of color vision, particularly when they affect one visual field *(hemiachromotopsia)* are of particular interest because of their association with alexia. Patients with achromotopsia are able to recognize shapes and dimensions of objects but have color vision loss, so the world appears gray in the affected field. One of the original alexic patients described by Dejerine (1891) had a hemiachromatopsia. Achromatopsia is observed with lesions of the fusiform and lingual gyri that spare the calcarine cortex and optic radiations (Damasio et al. 1980). Bedside testing for achromatopsia is conducted by presenting colored chips (those from the Token Test work well) following visual field testing procedures. We have observed a least one child who had achromatopsia in the context of an acquired alexia (Fennell & Voeller, personal communication). More complex color vision assessments involving multiple hues are available, such as the Farnsworth dichotomous test for color blindness (Farnsworth 1947).

Visual field defects that vary in size and shape, and may be restricted to only one eye, are called *scotomas*. Lesions affecting retinal neurons—for instance, toxoplasmosis or multiple sclerosis—can produce scotomas. Finally, scotomas can result from a widening of the blind spot (as in chronic papilledema), but these are often detected only with meticulous tangent screen testing.

The fundoscopic examination permits examination of the retina with special magnifying instruments. There are two different systems of ophthalmoscopy: direct and indirect. Direct ophthalmosocopy, which is preferred by ophthalmologists, involves using a hand-held lens and a light source mounted on the head. Indirect fundoscopy involves using an ophthalmoscope, which combines both of these components in one instrument. To inspect fundi adequately, it is often necessary to dilate the pupil. On occasion, an uncooperative child may need sedation. The optic disk or papilla (the point at which the optic nerve and the central artery and vein penetrate the globe), the fovea or macula (a small area lateral to the optic disk that contains the highest concentration of neurons), the general appearance of the retinal surface, and the blood vessels of the eye are all examined.

Fundoscopic examination permits detection of various ocular and central nervous system diseases. For example, it may reveal chorioretinitis, suggesting a congenital viral or protozoan disease such as cytomegalovirus, rubella, or toxoplasmosis. Certain genetic neurodegenerative diseases frequently present characteristic findings. For example, a "cherry red" spot is the result of abnormal accumulation of lipids in the ganglion cell layer of the retina and is characteristic of the retinal degeneration seen in Tay-Sachs disease (GM2 gangliosidosis), as well as in other metabolic storage diseases. Head trauma can often cause hemorrhage in the fundi. In the presence of increased intracranial pressure, elevation and reddening of the optic disk with engorgement of the retinal vessels is evidence of papilledema (swelling). Similar optic disk swelling (papillitis) is seen in optic neuritis. In optic atrophy, often due to optic nerve injury (for example, after a bout of increased intracranial pressure or as a result of an optic nerve glioma), the optic disk appears chalky white, with thinned blood vessels. In optic neuritis and optic atrophy, visual acuity is decreased.

Cranial Nerves III, IV, and VI: Oculomotor, Trochlear, and Abducens Nerves

Eye movements are controlled by an intricate system that involves retinal, vestibuloocular, and cortical inputs. Visual inputs trigger eye movements that bring visual stimuli detected at the periphery into the central visual field (foveal vision), and maintain foveal fixation on a moving target. Ascending inputs from vestibular nuclei provide information to the oculomotor system about the position of the body in space. The frontal eye fields (near Brodmann's area 8) and the supplementary eye fields are involved in generating goal-directed, voluntary eye movements (gaze) and in inhibiting these movements (Fuster 1981; Guitton, Buchtel & Douglas 1985; Verfaelli & Heilman 1987).

Normally, the eyes are yoked, with resulting conjugate eye movements; that is, as the right eye moves to the right, the left eye also moves to the right at the same rate and with the same deviation, so a visual target is maintained at the same point in the visual map. When eyes do not move in the same direction, they are said to be *dysconjugate*.

There are two types of conjugate eye movements: fast eye movements or saccades, and slow eye movements. Both types of movement are controlled by brainstem neural systems. Different firing patterns of the neuronal pools in the brainstem determine the specific type that occurs (Fuchs & Luschei 1970). Saccadic movements are present at birth, before the emergence of slow eye movements (Atkinson 1984; Roucous, Culee & Roucous 1983).

Fast eye movements are under both reflexive and voluntary control ("look to the left"). Reflex eye movements are triggered by the sudden appearance of a visual stimulus in the peripheral visual field, or by a sound. These movements are integrated at the level of the superior colliculus (Stein, Goldberg & Clamann 1976). Stimulation of the superior colliculus elicits conjugate eye movements, with a coordinated head and body turn toward a specific spot. This constellation of eye, head, and body movements is called the *orienting response, visual grasp reflex,* or *foveation reflex* and is involved in attention. The stimulus to fast eye movements is a retinal error induced by displacement of the visual stimulus. This results in a high-frequency burst of firing in the neural pulse generator, associated with a tonic spike frequency that triggers a fast, unalterable shift in eye position. The generator and integrator are in the pontine paramedian reticular formation (PPRF) close to the nuclei of the abducens nerve.

Slow (smooth pursuit) eye movements, on the other hand, are tracking movements that involve fixation on a moving target. The slow eye movement system is conjugate, smooth, and capable of continuous modification. It requires constant computation by the visual system of velocity mismatch signal between eye and target. The foveal area of the visual cortex, as well as of the cerebellum, plays an important role in slow eye movements.

A third type of eye movement, called *vergence movements,* are dysconjugate and also occur under the control of brainstem neural systems. The typical vergence movement occurs when a fixated object is brought close to the face and the eyes move inward to maintain fixation and avoid diplopia (double vision). Humans (and other primates) have an intricate system that links the degree of accommodation and pupillary constriction to the position of the fixated object. When a object is regarded close up, three events (called the "near reflex") take place to bring the object into sharp focus: widening of the lens of the eye (accommodation); convergence of the eyes; and constriction of the pupils.

Pupillary Reflexes

The diameter of the pupil is controlled by the relative balance of iris sphincter and dilator muscles. Pupils constrict in the presence of light and during accommodation. The motor pathway starts at the nucleus of Edinger-Westphal, close to the oculomotor complex in the brainstem; then it courses through parasympathetic fibers, traveling with the oculomotor (third) nerve to the ciliary ganglion and finally to the pupillary sphincter. Damage to the optic nerve (so that the incoming light stimulus cannot be transmitted) or lesions of the oculomotor (third) nerve disrupt pupillary constriction.

Opticokinetic Nystagmus

Opticokinetic nystagmus (OKN) is elicited by using a drum or black-and-white striped tape. When these are rotated in front of the child, either horizontally or vertically, nystagmoid movements of both eyes are normally elicited. These eye movements have a fast/slow phase. Although OKN is physiologically complex and neural mechanisms are not entirely elucidated, it is a valuable maneuver to use in assessing integrity of the visual and oculomotor systems. Cortical lesions (particularly parietal ones) or brainstem lesions will disrupt OKN. Asymmetrical OKN may be seen in a patient with a unilateral parietal lesions.

Eye Movements and Pupillary Reflexes

Eye movements are assessed by having the child follow a target in all directions of gaze. Their range is evaluated and abnormalities are noted (for instance, nystagmus or dysconjugate movements). Pupillary reflexes are tested by directing a light into each pupil and observing the light reflex in each eye. Pupillary constriction and accommodation are checked by having the patient focus on objects at near and distant points.

The child is also asked to look to the right or to the left, to demonstrate voluntary control of eye movements. If the child cannot look to the right or to the left, but follows a target or looks reflexively at an object that suddenly intrudes into the visual field, the condition is called *ocular apraxia.*

Normally, organisms do not respond to every stimulus that impinges on them. When a child is unable to inhibit gaze at nonrelevant stimuli, the child is said to be *distractible*. Distractible eye movements are reported in adults with prefrontal lesions or dysfunction in the prefrontal–subcortical pathways (Guitton, Buchtel & Douglas 1985). In children, lesions involving the cranial nerve nuclei or cortical control centers can cause distractible eye movements— for instance, brainstem gliomas. An interesting case of a young man who sustained extensive bilateral occipital lesions at birth was reported. Although he could make voluntary saccades, smooth pursuit movements were impaired (Rizzo & Hurtig 1989). Occasionally, a child will have a congenital fourth-nerve palsy, a marker for other brainstem and cranium anomalies (Bale et al. 1988).

Cranial Nerve V: Trigeminal Nerve

The fifth cranial nerve consists of a large sensory component that subserves sensation over the face, conjunctivae, and mucous membranes of the nasal and oral cavities, and a motor portion that innervates the muscles of mastication (the masseter, temporal, and internal and external pterygoid muscles).

Facial sensation is tested by applying light touch and pin to the face, testing all three divisions of the trigeminal nerve. The corneal reflex is tested by applying a small filament of a cotton swab to the cornea, eliciting a prompt blink (subserved by the facial nerve). Movements of the jaw—closing and opening the mouth and moving it from side to side—are controlled by the motor division of the trigeminal nerve.

Cranial Nerve VII: Facial Nerve

The seventh nerve is a complex mixed nerve, with both motor and sensory components. The motor segment controls facial movements, which play an extremely important role in human social signaling. Facial nerve nuclei are the largest motor nerve nuclei in the brainstem (Tomasch 1963). Approximately 7000 to 10,500 nerve cells are subdivided into highly differentiated cellular groups, with each neuron controlling relatively few muscle fibers, permitting discrete, finely fractionated face movements. The forehead receives innervation from both hemispheres, whereas the rest of the facial muscles are innervated by the contralateral hemisphere. A small motor component innervates the inner ear and the base of the tongue. A small component of the facial nerve carries parasympathetic fibers to the lacrimal gland (tears) and other glands of the nasal and oral cavity (saliva and mucus). A sensory component conveys taste information from the anterior two-thirds of the tongue. The seventh nerve also conveys sensory information from a small area around the ear.

Two types of lesions involving the seventh nerve can be distinguished on the basis of neural supply to the forehead. A peripheral facial nerve lesion (damage to the seventh cranial nerve nucleus or to the nerve at any point after it leaves the brainstem) results in inability to move either the forehead or the lower face on the same side as the lesion. The patient has a smooth, unwrinkled face, flattening of the nasolabial fold, widening of the palpebral fissure and inability to raise the eyebrows, wrinkle the forehead, frown, or smile on the side of the lesion. If severe enough, the patient cannot close the eye and saliva runs down the lip on the affected side. The neurologist can determine the precise point in the nerve at which the lesion occurs by examining the other functions of the nerve that leave the pathway at variable points. A central facial nerve lesion involves descending pathways before they reach the facial nucleus. This lesion results in weakness of the lower face only—sparing the forehead, which receives innervation from both hemispheres.

Central weakness can be further divided into two types: emotional facial paresis (the face is symmetrical when the patient smiles volitionally, but emotional smiling results in asymmetry of the central type); and volitional facial paresis (asymmetrical smiling of the central type during voluntary smiling, with symmetrical facial expression on emotional smiling) (Monrad-Krohn 1924). Emotional facial paresis results from interruption of connections between the thalamus and the frontal or mesial temporal lobes, implicating the anterior limb of the internal capsule rather than an anterolateral thalamus (Hopf, Muller-Forell & Hopf 1992; Graff-Radford et al. 1984; Gelmers 1983). Lesions in the subthalamic region and dorsal midbrain also result in emotional facial paresis. Lesions producing voluntary facial paresis involve either motor cortex or the pyramidal tract, and imply sparing of the frontal and temporal lobes and of the basal ganglia (Hopf, Muller-Forell & Hopf 1992). It is also seen in the anterior operculum syndrome (Foix-Chavany-Marie syndrome) (Ferrari, Boninsegna & Beltramello 1979; Mao et al. 1989).

The nature and presence or absence of facial movement asymmetry may provide information regarding the "timing" of early lesions. Lenn and Freinkel (1989) noted that most children with prenatal unilateral lesions had bilaterally intact facial movements, whereas most children with postnatal unilateral lesions had impaired facial movements contralateral to the lesion. Children who had prenatal bilateral lesions had bilateral impairment of facial movements. Facial motor responses of children under $2\frac{1}{2}$ years are bilateral, rather than unilateral, suggesting that prior to this age both crossed and uncrossed corticobulbar pathways project to the seventh cranial nerve nucleus. At around age $2\frac{1}{2}$ years, this bilateral response gives way to a unilateral (adult-pattern) response, suggesting that the population of uncrossed neurons is markedly attenuated at this time (Duchowny & Jayakar 1993). Monrad-Krohn (1924) also reported a "facial contracture"—the persistence of a grimace—secondary to a contralateral corticalspinal tract injury incurred in early life, but presumably after $2\frac{1}{2}$ years.

Cranial Nerve VIII: Acoustic Nerve

The eighth cranial nerve has two components: the cochlear nerve (subserving hearing), and the vestibular nerve (subserving balance, coordination, and orientation in space).

The cochlear nerve transmits impulses from the hair cells in the organ of

Corti in the inner ear to the cochlear nuclei in the pons. The impulses are then transmitted by a series of relay centers to the primary auditory cortex. Simple screening tests can be performed in the office to check a child's hearing. The ability to hear the examiner's normal speaking voice or a whisper, although not precise, is still a good screening test. Being able to hear fingers rubbing together close to the ear or a watch ticking is another good bedside assessment. The Rinne test involves comparing bone and air conduction. A tuning fork is struck and then placed against the mastoid process and the child indicates when the sound can no longer be heard. It is then placed next to the external auditory meatus (without being restruck), and the child is asked if it can be heard. The child should be able to hear the tuning fork in the latter location, since air conduction is normally better than bone conduction. The Weber test involves striking the tuning fork and then placing it on the vertex of the skull. It should be heard equally well in either ear. In conduction deafness, the sound will be heard better in the involved ear; in sensorimotor deafness, it will be heard better in the normal ear.

The vestibular nerve conducts impulses from the semicircular canals, the utricle, and the saccule in the inner ear to the vestibular nuclei. The system is widely connected to the cerebellum, to the cranial nerves subserving eye movements (through the medial longitudinal fasciculus), to the thalamus, and to multiple cortical areas. Vestibular system dysfunction is likely when the child complains of dizziness, experiences nausea and vomiting, tilts to one side, or falls in one direction. Nystagmus (involuntary rapid horizontal or vertical eye movements) is often present.

Cranial Nerves IX and X: Glossopharyngeal and Vagus

These nerves arise from nuclei in the same area of the medulla and travel together along their route from the skull and along the neck. Except in the most specialized examination, they are examined simultaneously, because their functions are closely related. The sensory branches of the glossopharyngeal nerve innervate the pharynx, palate, and ear canal, and control taste sensation in the posterior third of the tongue. The vagus nerve controls the movements of the soft palate, pharynx, and larynx; it is involved in swallowing and gagging, and controls the parasympathetic autonomic nerves to the viscera (cardiac rhythm and function of the stomach and intestines). The gag reflex, which is subserved by both nerves, is triggered by applying a tongue blade or swab to the back of the pharynx. Paralysis of the vagus on one side results in weakness of the soft palate and pharynx, absence of gag reflex on the affected side, and loss of laryngeal sensation. Increased heart rate is another possible consequence.

Cranial Nerve XI: Spinal Accessory

The spinal accessory nerve arises out of the medulla. It is geographically close to—and overlaps functionally with—the vagus and glossopharyngeal nerves.

The spinal portion of cranial nerve XI controls two neck muscles: the sterno-cleidomastoid (head turning) and the trapezius (shoulder shrug).

Cranial Nerve XII: Hypoglossal Nerve

The hypoglossal nerve arises from nuclei in the medulla and controls the movements of the tongue. It supplies all the intrinsic and extrinsic muscles of the tongue (except for the palatoglossus). Clinical testing of tongue movements involves observing the tongue at rest. If there is a peripheral lesion (such as Werdnig-Hoffman disease), the tongue will be atrophic, and possibly fasciculating. The child is asked to protrude the tongue and move it in and out, side to side, and up and down. With unilateral weakness or paralysis, the protruded tongue deviates toward the lesioned side. In children with oral buccal apraxia or anterior operculum (Foix-Chavany-Marie) syndrome, tongue movements are poorly executed. Abnormal movements of the tongue can be seen in dyskinetic states (such as Sydenham's chorea).

SENSATION EXAMINATION

Sensory testing refers to assessing a child's ability to perceive information about the outside world through skin sensations. A variety of peripheral sensory receptors reside in skin, including free nerve endings and specialized, encapsulated nerve endings. The sensory examination involves assessing position and vibratory sensation. Sensory testing presupposes a reasonable level of cooperation, conciousness, attention, and communicative ability on the patient's part. Confused and semiconscious children, retarded or autistic children, children with whom one does not share a common language, and very young children cannot be tested reliably.

Assessment is performed by presenting the child with a stimulus and precisely observing the response. If a young child responds promptly to a stimulus on one side of the body but responds only some of the time to a stimulus on the other side, or withdraws only after a long delay, the response is clinically relevant and suggests sensation problems on the slow-to-respond side. Depending on the testing and observations of the child's movements and gait, the examiner may initially focus on different specific body areas for sensation testing. Essentially, five types of sensation are examined: pain, temperature, vibratory sense, position, and tactile perception.

The basic sensory examination can be conceptualized as having two levels: primary sensation, relevant to peripheral nerve and spinal cord; and cortical sensation, requiring processing at the level of the brain. A very detailed assessment of dermatomal or peripheral nerve maps may be necessary for some children. For others, such as those with lesions affecting the spinal cord, concern about lesion level predominates. Dissociations of sensory modalities are also of interest.

Primary Sensory Testing

To assess pain, the child is asked to identify where a pin touch is made and to describe the stimulus. A child with a sensory deficit may perceive a painful sharp stimulus as a dull touch. Alternatively, sensation may be perceived differently on one extremity than on the other. The ability to perceive temperature (hot and cold sensations) is carried along the same pathways as pain. Peripheral sensory deficit is defined in terms of dermatomal or peripheral nerve maps in spinal cord or peripheral nerve lesions. Vibratory sensation is tested by applying an oscillating tuning fork to a bony prominence, such as the toe joint, ankle, or wrist. The child's response indicates that vibration (as opposed to touch) is elicited. Some children have difficulty perceiving vibratory sensation distally, but have no difficulty at more proximal joints. The neurologist compares the ankle to the knee, or the wrist to the elbow. In children with posterior column disease, vibratory sensation in the upper extremities may be intact, whereas there is a marked loss of vibratory sensation in the lower extremities. Position sense is tested by grasping a digit (finger or toe) and moving it either up or down over a short distance (perhaps 1 millimeter). The child indicates the direction of movement. Tactile sensation is tested by brushing the skin with a wisp of cotton. The patient indicates whether a touch is felt, and where. Testing two-point discrimination lends itself to quantification, but this has rarely been extensively examined in children. Cope and Antony (1992) reported normal values for children aged 2 to 13 years. Children 6 and older responded reliably, compared to only 20% of those aged $3\frac{1}{2}$ to 4 years.

Cortical Sensory Testing

To neurologists, cortical sensory testing measures complex, associational sensory information processing. There are five distinct somatosensory association cortices in the human: the primary somatosensory (SI); the ventrolateral association cortices (SII, SIII, and SIV); and the dorsomedial association cortex (supplementary sensory area). Each area has a characteristic cytoarchitecture and specific patterns of thalamocortical and corticocortical connectivity. Damage to ventrolateral somatosensory cortex produces tactile agnosia (impaired object recognition), with impairment of size, shape, and texture discrimination. This is reminiscent of the visual ventral pathway (the "what" system). Lesions of dorsomedial association cortex are typically associated with apraxia and deficits in sensorimotor integration, possibly analogous to the visual "where" system (Caselli 1993).

A complex sensory examination designed for adults has been described that includes extinction, barognosis discrimination (sorting identical objects of different weights, according to weight), texture (four grades of sandpaper), dimension (four wooden rectangular blocks), shapes, substance (such as wood), and tactile object recognition (Caselli 1991*a*, 1991*b*). A similar complex sensory examination for children does not exist, although there is a standardized bimanual test of tactile object recognition (Ayres 1972).

Tactile extinction refers to whether a child who can respond to a single, isolated stimulus extinguishes (or neglects) that same stimulus when it is presented simultaneously with another stimulus. The other stimulus is generally presented on a contralateral homologous body area, but it is also possible to demonstrate ipsilateral extinction—for example, with the face extinguishing the hand. The Quality Extinction Test presents a variety of tactile materials (carpet, velvet, metal, wire grating) mounted on a board and requires verbal responses (Schwartz, Marchok & Flynn 1977; Schwartz, Marchok, Kreinick & Flynn 1979). When the test was given to hemiplegic children and young adults, 23 of 39 patients (58%) manifested extinction (Lenti et al. 1991), and 19 extinguished the hand contralateral to the damaged hemisphere. Extinction was noted on the right hand in 4 patients with a right hemiparesis, 3 of whom had localized left frontal lesions. They did not find significantly more subjects with right-hemisphere lesions manifesting left-side neglect.

Finger localization refers to testing for two things: awareness of body schema, involving knowing where fingers are in space; and ability to identify or name touched fingers. A 50-item evaluation of finger localization was developed (Benton 1959). The subject must name a touched finger while watching, and then name the touched finger and identify pairs of touched fingers without visual input. A modification decreased the number of items to 20 (Levine 1980), and this test was administered to children between 6 and 12 years of age. An exponential increase in scores between 6 and 8 years of age was found, parallel to Benton's data. At around 9 years of age, rate of improvement slowed and reached an asymptote at around age 12. Naming with visual input was better than naming without visual input: 6-year-olds were able to name 88.4% of fingers under visual monitoring, but only 67.4% without; in contrast, 9-year-olds scored 99.3% and and 92.3%, respectively. The two-finger task was considerably more difficult (18.7% and 31.3% success rates at ages 6 and 9, respectively), in part because it involved more complex sensory and attentional components. The outside fingers of the hand were more accurately identified than those at the center. There was also a hierarchy of finger awareness: the thumb was more accurately localized than the little finger, followed by the index, middle, and the ring fingers. No substantial right–left differences were noted, except in a few 6-year-olds.

Gerstmann syndrome in the adult results from a dominant parietal lobe lesion and involves finger agnosia, dyscalculia, dysgraphia, and right–left confusion (Geschwind & Strub 1975). Constructional apraxia (difficulty in two- and three-dimensional constructional tasks) is frequently associated with Gerstmann syndrome (Critchley 1966). Gerstmann syndrome has been reported in children (Benson & Geschwind 1970; Spellacy & Peter 1978) and has sometimes been associated with disturbed oculomotor control and scanning (Pirozzolo & Payner 1978).

MOTOR EXAMINATION

The motor system subserves body movements through space and requires complex coordination across the whole neuraxis. The motor system examination involves simultaneous assessment of multiple, interdependent levels of the neuraxis, the brain (cortex, corticalspinal tracts, extrapyramidal system, and cerebellum), the spinal cord, and peripheral nerves and muscles. The central aspects of movement consist of the intention to move, motor planning, initiation, releasing the planned movement, and having that movement executed in smooth, organized fashion in space and real time by nerves, synapses, and muscles. The neurologist makes a determination of functional capacity only for the lowest part of the system involved. For instance, in the presence of severe muscle disease or peripheral nerve injury, a stroke affecting motor performance might be silent.

Gait

Walking involves two components: the capacity to maintain balance and an upright posture; and the ability to initiate and maintain rhythmic stepping. Standing and walking require complex interactions among visual, vestibular, and proprioceptive inputs. Arm movements or a shift in the center of gravity result in prompt compensatory shifts of the trunk (and sometimes of the legs and arms) to maintain balance. Starting to walk requires a shift in center of gravity, and stepping requires continuous, alternating, coordinated movements of legs, trunk, and arms.

The neurologist observes many different aspects of walking, including stride length, feet position (normally, close together for a narrow-based gait, or farther apart for a wide-based gait for stability), and symmetry in both the flow of movements and the position of the leg and foot in space. Upper extremity (associated) movements or arm swing are observed. For example, a child with a lateralized lesion may show decreased arm swing contralateral to the lesion. The child is also asked to perform a specific set of maneuvers: walking on heels, on toes, in tandem (one foot directly in front of the other, the heel of one foot against the toe of the other), walking on the sides of the feet, and hopping on either foot. In young children or those who cannot follow such requests, information is obtained by observing movement. Simply playing ball may provide a great deal of information about postural reflexes and gait, as the child runs, jumps, hops, turns, squats, and often assumes a quadrupedal position.

Muscle Tone

Muscle tone refers to the normal state of muscle tension. Tone can be increased (hypertonia) or decreased (hypotonia), and there are patterns of alterations in tone. For example, spasticity is assessed by passive limb movement and is manifested by increased tone in (for example) flexors of the upper extremity, when the arm is flexed at the elbow and the hand and fingers tend to be fisted. In the lower extremities, spasticity is manifested by increased tone in the extensors—for example, tightness of the heel cord resulting in toe-walking. There may also be tightness of the hamstrings and the adductors of the thighs (that is, the child walks with bent knees that are pressed together). This results in a typical hemiparetic posture (flexion of the upper extremity and extension of the lower). Rigidity implies that both extensors and flexors have increased tension.

Tone is also tested by palpating the muscle at rest and by making passive movements through a range of motion. Tone is affected by several factors: ability to relax, inherent mechanical properties of the muscle and surrounding tissue, and alterations in neurons controlling motor tone. In some pathological conditions, muscle tone is affected independently of the nervous system. Patterns of hypertonia include cogwheel rigidity (characteristic of a basal ganglia disorder) and spasticity (implying corticalspinal tract damage). Hypotonia may be due to central impairment or to peripheral nerve and muscle disease.

While moving muscles and joints, the neurologist will suddenly passively stretch certain joints to check for *clonus*—a series of rhythmic involuntary muscle contractions. Clonus can also occur spontaneously in the context of severe spasticity. It occurs most frequently at the ankle, knee, and wrist. Thus, sudden dorsiflexion of the foot is likely to elicit clonus in a child with corticalspinal tract damage involving the lower extremities.

Muscle Strength and Mass

Muscle strength is assessed by asking the child to perform certain movements against gravity and against the resistance provided by the examiner. Muscle mass is assessed by feeling the muscle bulk at rest and in response to strength testing. Weakness reflects a range of dysfunction in brain, peripheral nerve, and muscle. For example, a child may appear weak because of inability to initiate or maintain a motor movement, because of cerebellar dysfunction affecting the ability to synergize motor outputs, or due to corticalspinal tract damage or peripheral nerve, muscle, or neuromuscular junction lesions.

Muscle Stretch Reflexes ("Deep Tendon Reflexes")

Deep tendon reflexes provides considerable information about nervous system function. In assessing deep tendon reflexes, one examines the integrity of a reflex arc, which consists of muscle length receptors, afferent nerve (transmitting the impulse to the spinal cord or cranial nerve ganglion), a spinal or brainstem reflex center controlled by downstream impulses from the cortex, and other upper motor neuron structures, efferent nerve (from spinal cord to muscle), and muscle. Deep tendon reflexes are elicited by stretching a muscle. This is accomplished by applying a rubber percussion hammer (reflex hammer) to a tendon (or related structure). This produces a rapid stretch of the muscle group involved and normally elicits rapid muscle contraction. For example, tapping the patellar tendon (the "knee jerk") stretches the muscles and the organs monitoring muscle length (extrafusal fibers and muscle spindles) of the quadriceps, the large anterior thigh muscle, that is anchored to the tibia by the patellar tendon. The patellar tendon stretch results in a rapid stretch of the quadriceps and elicits a rapid reflex contraction of the quadriceps that causes the lower leg to jerk upward.

Deep tendon reflexes can be elicited at a number of points on the upper extremities (for instance, biceps, triceps, and brachioradialis), legs (for instance, knee, ankle, adductors of the thigh, and hamstring), and body. A jaw jerk can be elicited. De Jong (1979) lists over 30 different stretch reflexes, but many would be elicited only in a specific clinical context. Reflexes are compared on the two sides of the body. It is important to position the limbs similarly and to use the same force to elicit a reflex. The speed, amplitude, and recruitment of other muscle groups is noted. Reflexes are typically graded as 0 (= absent), 1 (present, but hypoactive), 2 (normal), 3 (increased but still within the normal range), and 4 (pathologically brisk, with associated clonus). In the presence of corticalspinal tract damage, deep tendon reflexes are typically hyperactive (not only brisk but of increased amplitude, with spread to other muscle groups). With peripheral nerve damage, deep tendon reflexes are typically hypoactive or absent. In the presence of cerebellar damage, deep tendon reflexes may be pendular; that is, the leg swings back and forth for several oscillations. Brisk reflexes are evidence of spasticity.

The Babinski sign is elicited by stroking the lateral aspect of the foot, from heel to toe, with a sharp object capable of inducing a painful stimulus. The patient should be positioned so that the knee is extended and the ankle flexed. The reflex is mediated by spinal roots L5, S1 (in particular), and S2, and consists of plantar flexion of the toes. Although a particularly strong stimulus will recruit other muscle groups, only in persons with hyperactivity of the S1 spinal segment will the extensor hallucis longus be recruited, resulting in extension of the great toe. The Babinski sign is observed when the integrity of the corticalspinal tract is interupted (a lesion) or is otherwise physiologically dysfunctional (for instance, in deep sleep, in the presence of drug intoxication, or in other encephalopathic states). Although 93% to 94% of normal newborns will have a flexor response if the stimulus is not particularly painful (such as a thumbnail) (Rich, Marshall & Volpe 1973), a painful stimulus will elicit an extensor response in 95% (Ross, Velez-Borras & Rosman 1976), reflecting the immaturity of the corticalspinal tracts. After about 12 months of age, however, the response becomes flexor, and the Babinski sign assumes a pathologic significance (Bodensteiner 1992).

One might conclude that the Babinski sign would be abnormal in older children with evidence of upper motor neuron injury, but this is not necessarily so. Marcus (1992) described 57 children who suffered brain injury in early childhood (53 before the age of 1 year). All had evidence of upper motor neuron lesions (such as quadriplegia, diplegia, or hemiplegia). The vast majority (80.8%) had flexor plantar responses; in only 11.5% were the reflexes extensor. Plantar flexor responses were observed even in children whose lesions occurred at age $2\frac{1}{2}$ years.

PRAXIS EXAMINATION

Praxis refers to the ability to perform *learned* skilled movements. Apraxia, described early in the twentieth century (Liepmann, 1908), has been elaborated in studies of adults with precisely localized acquired neurological lesions (Rothi et al. 1988). *Apraxia* refers to an inability to perform movements that is not explained by weakness, incoordination, sensory loss, or inability to understand instructions (Geschwind 1975). Apraxia thus consists of inability or loss of ability to access or evoke movement representations of skilled actions (that involve three-dimensional motor sequences in time). These movement representations (praxicons) are stored in the inferior parietal lobe—usually, but not always, in the dominant hemisphere. Thus, praxis involves association cortex and is firmly linked to the dorsal pathway (the "where" system).

Apraxic deficits occur at two different levels: a production level, and a conceptual level. Although apraxia and aphasia often coexist, they appear to be dissociable. Four different types of apraxia are identified: ideomotor apraxia (impaired pantomime and imitation); dissociation apraxia (such as callosal apraxia) (Watson & Heilman 1983); ideational apraxia (impaired use of common objects, with preserved pantomime and imitation); and conceptual apraxia (for example, difficulty with tool-object knowledge) (Ochipa, Rothi & Heilman 1989, 1992).

Praxis is tested in adults by asking for pantomime of a series of skilled acts—both transitive acts (using a tool or instrument) and intransitive acts (a gesture such as a wave goodbye). Both limbs are tested. If errors are made in pantomime, the examiner models the gesture (for imitiation). Finally, the actual tool may be used. In addition, the ability to *comprehend* pantomimes and to associate tools with specific tasks and functions is tested. An apraxic adult who used a toothbrush as an eating utensil and appeared to lose the ability to associate a task with a tool has been described (Ochipa, Rothi & Heilman 1989).

A child who cannot perform a simple learned movement such as brushing teeth, combing hair, or waving goodbye, is considered *apraxic*. This inability occurs despite an otherwise normal neurological and motor examination. The apraxic child is distinguished from the child with motor problems, the dyspraxic or clumsy child. Frequently, studies of dyspraxia in childhood do not distinguish between motor system deficit and apraxic deficit. It may be that a functioning motor system is required to learn appropriate movement sequences. Studies of developmental dyspraxia have come mostly from motor learning theorists (Schmidt 1988) and occupational therapists (Ayres 1972). Only recently have attempts been made to integrate the brain-behavior model of apraxia and dyspraxic children (Goodgold-Edwards & Cermak 1990). These authors identified six impairment patterns in dyspraxic children: difficulty learning general rules or schemata about classes of motor actions; difficulty using perceptual cues, e.g. spatial location or object speed/trajectory; difficulty organizing somatosensory/vestibular information; trouble with problem-solving or adapting to a new situation; difficulty analyzing task requirements and components, using knowledge in an effective fashion; and difficulty preparing for upcoming actions. These deficits involve both praxis and *meta*-knowledge about the properties and execution of motor movements—that is, prefrontal cognition.

A standardized dyspraxia battery identified 24 dyspraxic children ranging in age from 5 to 12 years (Deuel & Doar 1992). They were further divided into subgroups of ideomotor dyspraxia and ideational apraxia. There was no correlation between full-scale IQ and test battery performance, suggesting that dyspraxia is dissociable from intellectual deficit. Katz, Curtiss, and Tallal (1992) administered rapid automatized naming and gesture tasks to language-impaired children at ages 4, 6, and 8 years, who were matched by age and IQ to normal controls. Members of the language-impaired group were impaired on both tasks, suggesting the presence of a generalized disability in processing rapid, sequential information, as well as a close relationship between language and praxis in childhood.

Handedness

Handedness is an important component of cerebral lateralization in humans. Two approaches are used to define handedness in individuals: manual skill, and manual preference for a specific task (Bishop 1989; Chapman & Chapman 1987; Raczkowski & Kalat 1974). Handedness is often defined by hand preference on a specific task. A number of approaches have been proposed (see review by Fennell 1986). Commonly, a standardized hand preference questionnaire is used. A second approach, which asks for self-report of hand preference, has the disadvantage of not identifying intensity of preference and may not correlate well with manual dexterity performance (Benton, Meyers & Polder 1962; Satz, Achenbach & Fennell 1967).

In infants and children, hand preference must also be defined within the context of a specific task. It is likely that neural networks subserving attention, vision, head position, praxis, corticospinal motor control, and language are somehow integrated into handedness. Long before birth, there is evidence of right thumb-sucking in most fetuses, starting around the 15th gestational week (Hepper, Shahidullah & White 1990). In infants, reaching movements are noted earlier than prehension. The hand preferred for unimanual use at age 7 months corresponds to the dominant hand in bimanual activities at 13 months (Ramsay 1980). By around 9 months, most babies have settled on the right hand (Harris 1982). A unilateral hand preference may be interspersed with ambidexterity until the baby is close to 24 months, however, and these fluctuations may be related to specific events in language development (see review by Butterworth & Hopkins 1993).

Anomalously early or late hand preference suggests neuromotor dysfunction. A striking preference for one hand before 1 year of age may be a marker of lateralized cerebral damage. An early sign of a hemiparesis is a consistent lateralized hand preference at around age 6 months for all tasks (without the fluctuations seen in normal children). Prolonged ambidexterity—that is, no sign of hand preference by age 3—is another marker of a possible neurodevelopmental problem. Since determining hand preference by relying on either parental observation or self-report may be misleading, it is valuable to ask the child to perform a series of actions and directly observe hand use and praxis.

MOTOR MOVEMENTS EXAMINATION

Neuromotor control may be a useful independent measure of developmental age, distinct from chronological age, and may serve as a marker for central nervous system dysfunction. Motor movements fall into four categories: motor sequences programmed into memory; movements that require visual monitoring; movements involving a single extremity; and movements involving the integration of both upper extremities. In each case, different brain areas are involved. Dissociations between internally generated movements that must be organized within a temporal framework versus movements that are paced by external stimuli have been demonstrated (Halsband et al. 1993). Premotor cortex on the lateral aspect of the hemispheres and the supplementary motor area in the mesial aspect of the hemispheres both send projections to primary motor cortex and receive separate thalamic inputs. Premotor cortex is involved in the integration of visual information into motor performance, and depends on sensory feedback. The supplementary motor area is involved when learned sequential movements using internalized pre-programmed movements are required (Goldberg 1985).

Normal children show rapidly increasing motor ability between the ages of 5 and 7 years (Denckla 1974; Neuhauser 1975; Wolff, Gunnoe & Cohen 1985). Denckla's tasks (repetitive toe-tapping, hand-patting, index finger–thumb taps, alternating heel–toe tapping, alternating hand–arm supination and sequential finger–thumb opposition) quantitatively assess motor system integrity in children.

Observations of motor overflow or associated movements are also noted. Defining the developmental range during which overflow movements are seen helps to define patterns of developmental pathology (Wolff, Gunnoe & Cohen 1983, 1985). These authors recommend identifying sensitive periods—developmental points at which more than 20% but less than 80% of children show definite associated movements. They described synkinesias induced by "stress gaits" (movements of heterologous muscles of the upper limbs on both sides of the body, induced by walking on heels, toes, and sides of the feet) and mirror movements, resulting from coactivation of homologous muscles on opposite sides of the body in school-age younger children. Stress-gait-induced synkinesias involving the upper extremities are in the sensitive range for first-graders. Mirror movements were noted in the kindergarteners on a finger-spreading task, and the number of mirror movements increased as one moved from the radial to ulnar aspect of the hand. Mirror movements may be sensitive indicators of developmental dysfunction, if they persist beyond age 10 years (Denckla & Rudel 1978; Wolff, Gunnoe & Cohen 1985; Woods & Eby 1980).

Young children have particular difficulty integrating movements of the two hands. During early stages of bimanual skill acquisition, unintended manual coactivation occurs at multiple levels of motor organization. As subjects learned a motor skill involving uncoupled hand movements, systematic errors were noted. The anterior callosum plays an important role in suppressing bimanual overflow (Jeeves, Silver & Milner 1988; Preilowski 1972).

Patterns of deficit recur on the neurological examination. For example, cortical spinal tract disease results in a *hemiparesis,* with decreased arm swing or possibly fisting of the hand, and a tendency to swing the foot and leg on one side *(circumduction).* Several maneuvers bring out subtle abnormalities. Walking on toes or on the sides of the feet tends to produce fisting and posturing of an upper extremity and is impaired in patients with muscle/nerve weakness. Heel-walking exaggerates mild corticospinal tract impairment, because the patient cannot dorsiflex the foot well. In the presence of basal ganglia disease, patients may move more slowly, have a short stride length, and demonstrate loss of upper-extremity-associated movements.

Another aspect of motor programming is movement in extracorporeal hemispace. Little is known about the unfolding of the neural representations of hemispace in the young child. However, young children often do not cross the midline, suggesting that they do not have a fully developed map of contralateral hemispace. By age 7 to 8 years, children begin to bisect lines like adults, with both hands erring to the left. Younger subjects tended to err to the left with the left hand and to the right with right the right hand. Placing the hand in contralateral hemispace did not affect performance (Bradshaw et al. 1988).

CEREBELLAR EXAMINATION

The cerebellum plays a crucial role in the programming of motor movements (Thach, Goodkin & Keating 1992). It is involved in starting, accelerating, maintaining, decelerating, and terminating movements. It affects the quality of the ongoing movement—for example, force, smoothness, and timing. Cerebellar dysfunction results in prolonged reaction time, prolonged initial movement, and impaired stopping. The child cannot maintain a constant force, and the normal smooth flow of movements is disrupted by a tremor. Impaired programming is manifested by disrupted timing between movement components.

Recent studies of cerebellar anatomy and physiology indicate that multiple representations of the body map exist within the deep cerebellar nuclei. Each map controls a specific aspect of body movement, and the maps operate in parallel. The Purkinje cells of the cerebellar cortex are linked together and project onto the deep nuclei. The nuclei are organized so that subgroupings are task specific. Learning a new movement sequence is possible because the parallel fiber links to Purkinje cells are adjustable and modulable.

Cerebellar dysfunction is manifested by loss of normal postural control. For example, being unable to adjust posture to compensate for sudden tilts, the child overcompensates and consequently the body sways. Children with cerebellar dysfunction typically have a *broad-based gait* and often are markedly unsteady or *ataxic*. If the gait disturbance is subtle, *tandem walking* is performed poorly.

Impaired movement termination of the extremities is called *dysmetria*. When a child performs fast movements, *hypermetria* (that is, moving beyond a target) may be manifested. This is due to delayed onset of activity in the antagonist muscles that serve to brake the movement (Hore, Wild & Diener 1991). When performing slow movements, the child may demonstrate *hypometria* (that is, falling short of the target). This is likely due to disturbance in the relationship between agonist and antagonist muscle groups, resulting in abnormal braking (Hallett, Shahani & Young 1975). *Rebound,* another manifestation of the loss of reflexive braking, is tested by having the child flex each arm at the elbow against resistance provided by the examiner. The examiner then lets go suddenly. Children with cerebellar disease may not be able to initiate braking of the flexion movement, and the arm will fly up and hit the child's nose or chest unless blocked. Cerebellar lesions interfere with a child's ability to maintain a constant force, but not to exert a maximal force. For example, writing requires co-contraction of virtually all arm and hand muscles (Smith, Wetts & Kalaska 1985).

Several other bedside tests of cerebellar function are routinely administered. *Rapid alternating movements* are tested by rapidly alternating between supination and pronation of the hand (rapid patting with the palms up and down). Failure to perform this movement smoothly is called *dysdiadochokinesia*. Patients with cerebellar lesions perform these movements slowly and lack the smooth rhythmicity seen in the normal performance. *Dyssynergia* or *assynergia* refers to the inability to perform movements in three-dimensional space using multiple sets of agonist and antagonist muscles. This is tested by the *finger-to-nose* test, by the *heel-to-shin test* (running the heel down the shin), or by the *toe-to-object test* (touching the toe to the examiner's finger). Florid dyssynergia is termed *decomposition of movement*. In the course of the finger-to-nose or toe-to-object maneuvers, *intention tremor* (also known as kinetic or terminal tremor) may be seen—another manifestation of cerebellar dysfunction. This oscillating tremor increases in amplitude as the moving limb approaches its target.

Hypotonia, hyporeflexia, and asthenia have been described as typical symptoms following acute cerebellar damage. However, these symptoms also occur after other lesions and only within a brief time period following damage. *Pendular reflexes* are another manifestation of cerebellar disease. For example, when the patellar tendon is tapped, the lower leg oscillates back and forth several times, rather than manifesting one jerk.

Cerebellar disease also affects motor control of the cranial nerves. One often sees *nystagmus* when the patient attempts to move the eyes toward a target. A characteristic *scanning, dysarthric* speech pattern may be observed, as well.

Evidence of the cerebellum's contribution to higher cognitive functions has also accumulated (Bracke-Tolkmitt et al. 1989; Leiner, Leiner & Dow 1986).

In a review article, Schmahmann (1991) noted that, although the pathways that reciprocally link cortical regions to the cerebellum (the cortico-ponto-cerebellar and cerebellar-dentate-thalamic projections) are incompletely understood, the cerebellum may correlate motor acts with mood states and with unconscious motivation, and thus may play a role in nonverbal communication. He suggested that a "dysmetria of thought" may produce a mismatch between reality and its perception, with a resulting erratic over- and undercorrection of thought and behavior.

OBSERVATIONS OF PHYSICAL CHARACTERISTICS

Head Size

The neurological examination of a child includes head circumference measurement, and normative comparison. A too large head (macrocephaly) or too small head (microcephaly) may indicate pathology. However, head size must be evaluated in relation to body size. For instance, is a prospectively microcephalic child also of short stature? When is head size pathological? A formula (Head circumference (cm^3)/Body weight (gm)) results in an almost constant average (10, with SD of 1), irrespective of sex and with only a slight decrease with age, enabling the examiner to judge objectively whether head size is larger or smaller than appropriate, and permitting early identification of pathology. This index is useful for ages up to 18 months (Nishi et al. 1992).

Extremity Measurements

Unilateral brain injury in a young child may result in asymmetrical extremity growth contralateral to the side of cerebral injury—for instance, a smaller leg on the hemiparetic side (Penfield & Robertson 1943). Are subtle growth asymmetries found in children with milder degrees of hemispheric injury or developmental disorders? Satz, Yanowitz, and Willmore (1984) reported that children in whom epilepsy appeared before 2 years of age had significantly shorter feet contralateral to the lesion. Aram, Ekelman, and Satz (1986) reported foot and hand measurements from children with CT-verified lateralized lesions and found significant right < left hand and foot length differences with left-hemisphere lesions and left < right hand and foot length differences for right-hemisphere lesions. The authors suggested a cut-off point of 0.2-cm difference—that is, an informal rule that the possibility of lateralized CNS lesion should be considered if the difference exceeded this amount. Similar results were found for children whose lesions occurred after age 2 years. No obvious relationship between lesion location and degree of foot asymmetry was found.

Changes in skull and face growth also reflect early lateralized injury. Children with unilateral cerebral atrophy may have a thicker skull, a more prominent sphenoid ridge, a steeper slope to the temporal ridge, and larger sinuses on the side of the atrophic brain. Observed on skull films, this is called the "Davidoff-Dyke-Masson" effect. Resulting midfacial region asymmetries, with a higher orbit on the side of the injury, may be seen.

Physical Anomalies and Dysmorphic Features

Certain physical anomalies serve as markers for chromosomal or neurodevelopmental problems. These are often associated with characteristic changes in facial appearance, hair distribution and type, or other body areas. For example, dysmorphic facial features may include malformations and anomalies of the configuration and set of the eyes (horizontal palpebral fissures versus up- or down-tilting of the lateral canthi), epicanthic folds, short nose with a large or depressed nasal root, and anomalies of the nares, philtrum, and columnella. Ears may be small or large, with variable shape. Examination of the hands may show the presence of transverse palmar creases, or atypical dermatoglyphic patterns. In some cases, the array of dysmorphic features is virtually pathognomonic of a syndrome. For example, upslanting palpebral fissures, prominent epicanthic folds, small ears, rounded head shape, and protruding tongue strongly suggest Down syndrome. A number of chromosomal syndromes and metabolic diseases that affect children are reviewed in Chapter 3.

Minor physical anomalies (MPAs) constitute a subset of dysmorphic features, such as head circumference outside the normal range; more than one hair whorl; fine electric hair; epicanthus; hypertelorism; malformed, low-set, asymmetrical, or soft and pliable ears; adherent ear lobes; high-arched palate; furrowed tongue; geographic tongue; curved fifth finger; single transverse palmar crease; wide gap between first and second toes; partial syndactyly of two middle toes; and third toe longer than second. The MPA approach has appeal because of the stability of the findings over time, the simplicity of administration, and good interobserver reliability. Although research on MPA has suggested a relationship between MPA scores at birth and activity levels (Quinn & Rapoport 1974; Waldrop et al. 1978), some studies failed to replicate these findings (Jacklin, Maccoby & Halverson 1980). In part, this may result from the fact that MPAs are basically a subset of physical features, and whether that subset represents the most important predictor to pathology is unknown.

From a developmental perspective, in embryogenesis the neural crest gives rise to cells that ultimately develop into sensory and autonomic ganglia, endocrine glands, components of the musculoskeletal system, the skin, the melanocytes of the skin, and its appendages. Teeth, nails, and hair are all derived from common embryologic structures. Thus, examination of these structures provides clues about events in embryogenesis that may, taken together, provide information about the nature of the problem. For example, a group of syndromes (Rieger syndrome, neurofibromatosis, incontinentia pigmenti, and hypomelanosis of Ito) involve disorders of pigmentation coupled with markedly disordered neuronal migration, and have been labeled *neurocristopathies* (Bolande 1974, 1981; Kissel Andre & Jacquier 1981).

Skin

The child's pigmentation relative to other family members may provide a clue to the presence of an underlying genetic or metabolic problem. For example, children with Angelman syndrome, Prader-Willi syndrome (anomalies involving deletion of chromosomal regions) (Hittner et al. 1982; Butler 1989), phenylketonuria, and homocystinuria (inborn errors of amino acid metabolism) are blond, fair-skinned, and blue-eyed, and often considerably less pigmented than other first-degree relatives. Severe malnutrition (kwashiorkor) will result in hypopigmentation. An increased incidence of blondeness has been reported in a large group of bright, but learning-disabled adults (Schachter, Ransil & Geschwind 1987).

Ocular albinism is characterized by normal skin and hair pigmentation but hypopigmentation of the optic fundus. There are several genetic variants, including an X-linked condition and an autosomal recessive type (Kinnear, Barrie & Witkop 1985). Ocular hypopigmentation is also seen in Prader-Willi, Chediak-Higashi, Waardenberg, and Apert syndromes (Drager 1986). Ocular albinism is associated with a spectrum of neuronal anomalies in the visual system: decreased number of uncrossed retinal ganglion fibers; disordered retinal ganglion cells and lateral geniculate; decreased foveal acuity; loss of binocular vision; congenital nystagmus; and night-blindness. The development of the optic cup occurs at around the end of the first month of gestation, and pigmented epithelium plays an important role in the development of these structures.

Small areas of focal depigmentation are observed in syndromes that involve disturbances of neuronal migration. For example, infants with tuberous sclerosis have characteristic hypopigmented spots, called *ashleaf macules*. Tuberous sclerosis is also associated with other skin lesions, such as adenoma sebaceum scattered over the nose, subunqual fibromas, and shagreen patches.

Café au lait spots—so-called because they are the color of coffee with cream—are prominent in neurofibromatosis and can also be seen in tuberous sclerosis. Pigmented nevi have been reported in association with arachnoid cysts and spinal cord anomalies, such as diastematomyelia and syringomyelia (Cilluffo et al. 1981). Abnormal pigmentation often reflects underlying abnormalities of neuronal migration. Thus, for example, swirls of abnormal pigmentation can be seen in incontinentia pigmentosa (a disorder that typically occurs in girls and is associated with mental retardation), Hypomelanosis of Ito, and linear nevus sebaceus syndrome.

Linear nevus sebaceus syndrome (epidermal nevus syndrome) is a neurocutaneous lesion in which the skin shows epidermal hypertrophy—typically keratinocytic, with some involvement of the dermis. The lesions do not cross the midline, but they may be bilateral. A high degree of association of epidermal nevus syndrome with nervous system involvement exists but exact incidence is difficult to determine. In four cases, none had severe retardation, 50% had seizures, and 75% had focal EEG abnormalities. Thickening of skull bones, facial asymmetry, and cerebral vasculature abnormalities were noted (Baker,

Ross & Baumann 1987). The skin lesion is typically ipsilateral to the brain lesion.

A number of rare mental retardation disorders are associated with ichthyosiform dermatoses. Rud syndrome (Rud 1927) involves ichthyosis, seizures, hypogonadism, and mental retardation, as well as polyneuropathy, short stature, neurosensory deafness, hypoplastic teeth and nails, retinitis pigmentosa, and nystagmus. Neuropathological findings include cerebral atrophy, hypomyelination, and unusual neuronal configurations (Stewart 1939).

Hair

Hair may be stubby, sparse, dull, or wooly in appearance. Abnormalities are defined under a light microscope or scanning electron microscope. For example, *trichorrhexis nodosa* refers to hair-shaft breakage with filaments protruding around the fracture site; *monilethrix* refers to a beaded appearance of the hair shaft; and *pili torti* refers to twisting of the hair shaft. Specific mental retardation disorders are associated with hair anomalies—for example, Menkes disease (Menkes et al. 1962), Pollitt syndrome (Pollitt, Jenner & Davies 1968), argininosuccinic aciduria (Brown 1971), and biotin deficiency (Coulter, Beals & Allen 1982). Trichothiodystrophy, a syndrome involving sparse, brittle, sulfur-deficient hair with trichorrhexis nodosa, is associated with mental retardation. In one case it was associated with partial agenesis of the corpus callosum, cortical atrophy, and unilateral optic atrophy (Rizzo et al. 1992) (see review by Itin & Pittelkow 1991). This is also called *BIDS syndrome* (brittle hair, impaired intelligence, decreased fertility, and short stature), *IBIDS* (includes ichthyosis), *PIBIDS* (all of the above, plus photosensitivity), *Sabinas syndrome,* or *Tay syndrome.*

Teeth and Nails

Dental anomalies include hypoplastic, unusually shaped or positioned teeth. Some dental anomalies are due to intrauterine disturbances, while others occur postnatally. Nail anomalies may be noted in association with skin and teeth abnormalities. For example, a case report noted dyschromic, dysplastic nails (Rizzo et al. 1992).

Odor

Certain syndromes are associated with characteristic odors, and the neurologist may assess olfactory cues. Neuropsychologists who work for several hours in close proximity to a child in a small, often poorly ventilated room may note a distinctive odor. For example, children with phenylketonuria have a musty odor; those with isovaleric acidemia have a "sweaty foot" odor; and a sweet odor is associated with maple syrup urine disease.

SOFT SIGNS

To render the adult neurological examination more suitable for examining children, since it is relatively insensitive to minor degrees of sensorimotor deficit, a "soft signs" adaptation was developed. Kennard (1960) defined *soft signs* as "equivocal" signs—signs that were subtle or inconsistently present. Many of these signs are found in children who have an array of developmental problems, but there is little agreement about their meaning. How one actually detects or measures the presence of these signs, their replicability, the question of interobserver reliability, and how well a particular sign or constellation of signs reflects the presence of cerebral dysfunction are important considerations.

One example of a standardized examination for soft signs is the Revised Neurological Examination for Subtle Signs (NESS) (Denckla 1985). Soft signs examined include stereognosis, graphesthesia, dysdiadochokinesis (hand pronation–supination), mirror movements, motor slowness, chorea and athetosis. This procedure for examining soft signs attempts to arrive at replicable standardized methods for expanding the examination of some components of a pediatric neurological examination, and some items overlap with the neurodevelopmental motor skills testing described earlier. The NESS test replaced the Physical and Neurological Examination for Soft Signs (PANESS). Studies conducted on the reliability of the PANESS (Mikkelsen et al. 1982; Stokman et al. 1986) found good interrater reliability, good test–retest reliability, reasonable interrater reliability for some items (such as for mirror but not involuntary movements) and some item unreliability (such as for stereognosis). Neurological assessments, whether they involve hard or soft signs, can be assessed reliably (Stokman et al. 1986; Vitiello et al. 1989).

What do soft signs mean? A significant deviation from the normal pattern of motor development, if it occurs at a sensitive period in childhood, may reflect neurodevelopmental disturbance that will remain stable into adulthood. Whether soft signs reflect particular *specificity* remains to be determined. If factors that result in soft signs (for example, overflow) are better understood in terms of developmental neuropathophysiology, their relevance to certain chronic developmental syndromes may be better understood.

Long-term follow-up studies of developmental outcome among children with soft signs (Hollander et al. 1991; Schonfeld, Shaffer & Barmack 1989) suggested that some of these indicators—for instance, dysgraphesthesia and dysdiadochokinesia—may present into adulthood, and that soft signs in childhood (in combination with childhood psychopathology) predict psychopathology in adulthood, as in the case of obsessive compulsive disorder (Hollander et al. 1990).

CONCLUSION

Neuropsychologists in a medical setting have a special need to understand fully the intent and methods of the neurological examination. In this chapter, the basics of the neurological examination, the information that can be derived from the assessment, and the significance of this information for the neuropsychologist have been discussed. An important aspect of the neurological assessment of the child consists of quantifying components of the examination so that they can reliably be compared to normative developmental standards by different examiners. It is important to individualize the neurological examination to generate the most valuable information, sampling the most appropriate behaviors out of the myriad possible developmental sequences.

REFERENCES

Aram, D. M.; Ekelman, B. L.; and Satz, P. 1986. Trophic changes following early unilateral injury to the brain. *Developmental Medicine and Child Neurology* 28: 165–70.

Atkinson, J. 1984. Human visual development in the first 6 months of life: A review and a hypothesis. *Human Neurobiology* 13: 144–79.

Ayres, A. J. 1972. *Sensory Integration and Learning Disorders.* Los Angeles: Western Psychological Services.

Baker, R. S.; Ross, P. A.; and Baumann, R. J. 1987. Neurologic complications of the epidermal nevus syndrome. *Archives of Neurology* 44: 227–32.

Bale, J. F., Jr.; Scott, W. E.; Yuh, W.; Sato, Y.; and Menezes, A. 1988. Congenital fourth nerve palsy and occult cranium bifidum. *Pediatric Neurology* 4: 320–21.

Benson, D. F., and Geschwind, N. 1970. Developmental Gerstmann syndrome. *Neurology* 20: 293–98.

Benton, A. 1959. *Right-Left Discrimination and finger localization; Development and Pathology.* New York: Hoeber Medical, Harper & Row.

Benton, A. L.; Meyers, R.; and Polder, G. J. 1962. Some aspects of handedness. *Psychiatry and Neurology* (Basel) 144: 321–37.

Bishop, D. V. 1989. Does hand proficiency determine hand preference? *British Journal of Psychology* 80: 191–99.

Bodensteiner, J. B. 1992. Plantar responses in infants. *Journal of Child Neurology* 7: 311–13.

Bolande, R. P. 1974. The neurocristopathies: A unifying concept of disease arising in neural crest maldevelopment. *Human Pathology* 5: 409–29.

———. 1981. Neurofibromatosis—The quintessential neurocristopathy: Pathogenetic concepts and relationships. *Advances in Neurology* 29: 67–75.

Bracke-Tolkmitt, R.; Linden, A.; Canavan, A. G. M.; Rockstroh, B.; Scholz, E.; Wessel, K.; and Diener, H.-C. 1989. The cerebellum contributes to mental skills. *Behavioral Neuroscience* 103: 442–46.

Bradshaw, J. L.; Spataro, J. A.; Harris, M.; Nettleton, N. C.; and Bradshaw, J. 1988. Crossing the midline by four to eight year old children. *Neuropsychologia* 26: 221–35.

Brown, A. C. 1971. Congenital hair defects. *Birth Defects* 7: 52–68.

Butler, M. G. 1989. Hypopigmentation: A common features of Prader-Labhart-Willi syndrome. *American Journal of Human Genetics* 45: 140–46.

Butterworth, G., and Hopkins, B. 1993. Origins of handedness in human infants. *Developmental Medicine and Child Neurology* 35: 177–84.

Caselli, R. J. 1993. Ventrolateral and dorsomedial somatosensory association cortex damage produces distinct somesthetic syndromes in humans. *Neurology* 43: 762–71.

Caselli, R. J. 1991*a*. Rediscovering tactile agnosia. *Mayo Clinic Proceedings* 66: 129–42.

———. 1991*b*. Bilateral impairment of somesthetically mediated object recognition in humans. *Mayo Clinic Proceedings* 66: 356–64.

Chapman, J. P., and Chapman, L. J. 1987. Handedness of hypothetically psychosis-prone subjects. *Journal of Abnormal Psychology* 96: 89–93.

Cilluffo, J. M.; Gomez, M. R.; Reese, D. F.; Onofrio B. M.; and Miller, R. H. 1981. Idiopathic ("congenital") spinal arachnoid diverticula. *Mayo Clinic Proceedings* 56: 93–101.

Cope, E. B., and Antony, J. H. 1992. Normal values for the two-point discrimination test. *Pediatric Neurology* 251–54.

Coulter D. L.; Beals, T. F.; and Allen R. J. 1982. Neurotrichosis: Hair-shaft abnormalities associated with neurological disease. *Developmental Medicine and Child Neurology* 24: 634–44.

Critchley, M. 1966. *The Parietal Lobes*. New York: Hafner.

Damasio, A. R.; Yamada, T.; Damasio, H.; Corbett, J.; and McKcc, J. 1980. Central achromatopsia: Behavioral, anatomic, and physiologic aspects. *Neurology* 30: 1064–71.

Dejerine J. 1891. Contribution à l'étude anatomo-pathologique et clinique des differences varietés de cècite verbale. *Memoires Societé Biologique* 4: 61–90.

DeJong, R. 1979. *The Neurologic Examination: Incorporating the Fundamentals of Neuroanatomy and Neurophysiology,* 4th ed. Hagerstown, Md.: Harper & Row.

Denckla, M. B. 1974. Development of motor coordination in normal children. *Developmental Medicine and Child Neurology* 16: 729–41.

———. 1985. Revised neurological examination for subtle signs. *Psychopharmacology Bulletin* 21: 773–800.

———. 1989. Neurological examination. In J. L. Rapoport (ed.), *Obsessive Compulsive Disorder in Children and Adolescents* (Washington, D.C.: American Psychiatric Press), pp. 107–18.

Denckla, M. B., and Rudel, R. G. 1978. Anomalies of motor development in hyperactive boys. *Annals of Neurology* 3: 231–33.

Deuel, M. K., and Doar, B. P. 1992. Developmental manual dyspraxia: A lesson in mind and brain. *Journal of Child Neurology* 7: 99–103.

Drager, U. C. 1986. Albinism and visual pathways. *New England Journal of Medicine* 314: 1636–38.

Duchowny, M., and Jayakar, P. 1993. Functional cortical mapping in children. *Advances in Neurology* 63: 149–54.

Farnsworth, D. 1947. *The Farnsworth Dichotomous Test for Color Blindness*. New York: Psychological Corporation.

Fennell, E. B. 1986. Handedness and its measurement. In H. J. Hannay (ed.), *Experimental Techniques in Human Neuropsychology* (New York: Oxford University Press), pp. 15–44.

Ferrari, G.; Boninsegna, C.; and Beltramello, A. 1979. Foix-Chavany syndrome: CT study and clinical report of three cases. *Neuroradiology* 18: 41–42.

Fuchs A. F., and Luschei, E. S. 1970. Firing patterns of abducens neurons of alert monkeys in relationship to horizontal eye movement. *Journal of Neurophysiology* 33: 382–92.

Fuster, J. M. 1981. Prefrontal cortex in motor control. In V. Brooks (ed.), *The Handbook of Physiology. Section 1: The Nervous System,* vol. 2: *Motor Control* (Bethesda, Md.: American Physiological Society), pp. 1149–78.

Gelmers, H. J. 1983. Nonparalytic motor disturbances and speech disorders: The role of the supplementary motor area. *Journal of Neurology, Neurosurgery and Psychiatry* 46: 1052–54.

Geschwind, N. 1975. The apraxias: Neural mechanisms of disorders of learned movement. *American Scientist* 63: 188–95.

Geschwind, N., and Strub, R. 1975. Gerstmann syndrome without aphasia: A reply to Poeck and Orgass. *Cortex* 11: 296–98.

Goldberg, G. 1985. Supplementary motor area structure and function: Review and hypotheses. *Behavioral and Brain Sciences* 8: 567–615.

Goodgold-Edwards, S. A., and Cermak, S. A. 1990. Integrating motor control and motor learning concepts with neuropsychological perspectives on apraxia and developmental dyspraxia. *American Journal of Occupational Therapy* 44: 431–39.

Graff-Radford, N. R.; Eslinger, P. J.; Damasio, A. R.; and Yamada, T. 1984. Nonhemorrhagic infarction of the thalamus: Behavioral, anatomic, and physiologic correlates. *Neurology* 34: 14–23.

Guitton, D.; Buchtel, H. A.; and Douglas, R. M. 1985. Frontal lobe lesions in man cause difficulties in suppressing reflexes glances and generating goal-directed saccades. *Experimental Brain Research* 58: 455–72.

Hallett, M.; Shahani, B. T.; and Young, R. R. 1975. EMG analysis of patients with cerebellar deficits. *Journal of Neurology, Neurosurgery and Psychiatry* 38: 1163–69.

Halsband U.; Ito, N.; Tanji, J.; and Freund, H.-J. 1993. The role of premotor cortex and the supplementary motor area in the temporal control of movement in man. *Brain* 116: 243–66.

Harris, L. J. 1982. Laterality of function in the infant: Historical and contemporary trends in theory and research. In G. Young, S. J. Segalowitz, C. Corter, and S. Trehub (eds.), *Manual Specialization and the Developing Brain* (New York: Academic Press), pp. 177–239.

Hepper, P. G.; Shahidullah, S.; and White, R. 1990. Origins of fetal handedness. *Nature:* 347: 431.

Hittner, H. M.; King, R. A.; Riccardi, V. M.; Ledbetter D. H.; Borda, R. P.; Ferrell, R. E.; and Kretzer, F. L. 1982. Oculocutaneous albinoidism as a manifestation of reduced neural crest derivatives in the Prader-Willi syndrome. *American Journal of Ophthalmology* 94: 328–37.

Hollander, E.; DeCaria, C. M.; Aronowitz, B.; Klein, D. F.; Liebowitz, M. R.; and Shaffer, D. 1991. A pilot follow-up study of childhood soft signs and the development of adult psychopathology. *Journal of Neuropsychiatry and Clinical Neurosciences* 3: 186–89.

Hollander, E.; Schiffman, E.; Cohen, B.; Rivera-Stein, M. A.; Rosen, W.; Gorman, J.; Fyer, A.; Papp, L.; and Liebowitz, M. 1990. Signs of central nervous system dysfunction in obsessive-compulsive disorder. *Archives of General Psychiatry* 47: 27–32.

Hopf, H. C.; Müller-Forell, W.; and Hopf, N. J. 1992. Localization of emotional and volitional facial paresis. *Neurology* 42: 1918–23.

Hore, J.; Wild, B.; and Diener, H. C. 1991. Cerebellar dysmetria at the elbow, wrist, and fingers. *Journal of Neurophysiology* 65: 563–71.

Itin, P. H., and Pittelkow, M. R. 1991. Trichothiodystrophy with chronic neutropenia and mild mental retardation. *Journal of American Academy of Dermatology* 24: 356–58.

Jacklin, C. N.; Maccoby, E. E.; and Halverson, C. F. 1980. Minor physical anomalies and preschool behavior. *Journal of Pediatric Psychology* 5: 199–205.

Jeeves, M. A.; Silver, P. H.; and Milne, A. B. 1988. Role of the corpus callosum in the development of a bimanual motor skill. *Developmental Neuropsychology* 4: 305–23.

Katz, W. F.; Curtiss, S.; and Tallal, P. 1992. Rapid automatized naming and gesture by normal and language-impaired children. *Brain and Language* 43: 623–41.

Kennard, M. 1960. Value of equivocal signs in neurologic diagnosis. *Neurology* 10: 753–64.

Kinnear, P. E.; Barrie, J.; and Witkop, C. J. 1985. Albinism. *Survey of Ophthalmology* 30: 75–101.

Kissel, P.; Andre, J. M.; and Jacquier, A. 1981. *The Neurocristopathies*. New York: Masson.

Koran, L. M. 1975. The reliability of clinical methods, data and judgments. *New England Journal of Medicine* 293: 695–701.

Leiner, H. C.; Leiner, A. L.; and Dow, R. S. 1986. Does the cerebellum contribute to mental skills? *Behavioral Neuroscience* 103: 998–1008.

Liepmann, H. (1908) *Drei Aufsatze aus dem Apraxiegebeit*. Berlin: Karger.

Lenn, N. J., and Freinkel, A. J. 1989. Facial sparing as a feature of prenatal-onset hemiparesis. *Pediatric Neurology* 5: 291–95.

Lenti, C.; Radice, L.; Cerioli, M.; and Musetti, L. 1991. Tactile extinction in childhood hemiplegia. *Developmental Medicine and Child Neurology* 33: 789–94.

Levine, D. N.; Warach, J.; and Farah, M. 1985. Two visual systems in mental imagery: Dissociation of "what" and where" in imagery disorders due to bilateral posterior cerebral lesions. *Neurology* 35: 1010–18.

Levine, M. D. 1980. Normative aspects of finger localization. In M. D. Levine (ed.), *A Pediatric Approach to Learning Disorders* (New York: Wiley), pp. 64–91.

Mao, C.-C.; Coull, B. M.; Golper, L. A.; and Rau, M. T. 1989. Anterior operculum syndrome. *Neurology* 39: 1169–72.

Marcus, J. C. 1992. Flexor plantar responses in children with upper motor neuron lesions. *Archives of Neurology* 49: 1198–99.

Menkes, J. H.; Alter, M.; Steigleder, G. K.; Weakley, D. R.; and Sung, J. H. 1962. A sex-linked recessive disorder with retardation of growth, peculiar hair and focal cerebral and cerebellar degeneration. *Pediatrics* 29: 764–79.

Mikkelsen, E. J.; Brown, G. L.; Minichiello, M. D.; Millican, F. K.; and Rapoport, J. L. 1982. Neurologic status in hyperactive, enuretic, encopretic, and normal boys. *Journal of the American Academy of Child Psychiatry* 21: 75–81.

Monrad-Krohn, G. H. 1924. On the dissociation of voluntary and emotional innervation in facial paresis of central origin. *Brain* 47: 22–35.

Neuhäuser, G. 1975. Methods of assessing and recording motor skills and movement patterns. *Developmental Medicine and Child Neurology* 17: 369–86.

Nishi, M.; Miyake, H.; Akashi, H.; Shimizu, H.; Tateyama, H.; Chaki, R.; Tuskuda, H.; Nomura, H.; Hatanaka, Y.; and Nishi, M. 1992. An index for proportion of head size to body mass during infancy. *Journal of Child Neurology* 7: 400–403.

Ochipa, C.; Rothi, L. J. G.; and Heilman, K. M. 1989. Ideational apraxia: A deficit in tool selection and use. *Annals of Neurology* 25: 190–93.

———. 1992. Conceptual apraxia in Alzheimer's disease. *Brain* 114: 2593–2603.

Penfield, W., and Robertson, J. 1943. Growth asymmetry due to lesions to the postcentral cerebral cortex. *Archives of Neurology* 50: 405–30.

Pirozzolo, F. J., and Payner, K. 1978. Disorders of oculomotor scanning and graphic orientation in developmental Gerstmann syndrome. *Brain and Language* 5: 119–26.

Pollitt, R. J.; Jenner, F. A.; and Davies, M. 1968. Sibs with mental and physical retardation and trichorrhexis nodosa with abnormal amino acid composition of the hair. *Archives of Disease in Childoood* 43: 211–16.

Preilowski, B. F. B. 1972. Possible contributions of the anterior forebrain commissures to bilateral motor coordination. *Neuropsychologia* 10: 267–77.

Quinn, P. O., and Rapoport, J. L. 1974. Minor physical anomalies and neurologic status. *Pediatrics* 53: 742–47.

Raczkowski, D., and Kalat, J. W. 1974. Reliability and validity of some handedness questionnaire items. *Neuropsychologia* 12: 43–47.

Ramsay, D. S. 1980. Onset of unimanual handedness in infants. *Infant Behaviour and Development* 3: 377–85.

Rapcsak, S. Z.; Cimino, C. R.; and Heilman, K. M. 1988. Altitudinal neglect. *Neurology* 38: 277–81.

Rich, E. C.; Marshall, R.; and Volpe, J. J. 1973. Plantar reflex flexor in normal neonates. *New England Journal of Medicine* 289: 1043.

Rizzo, M., and Hurtig, R. 1989. The effect of bilateral visual cortex lesions on the development of eye movements and perception. *Neurology* 39: 406–13.

Rizzo, R.; Pavone, L.; Micali, G.; Calveri, S.; and Di Gregorio, L. 1992. Trichothiodystrophy: Report of a new case with severe nervous system impairment. *Journal of Child Neurology* 7: 300–303.

Ross, E. D.; Velez-Borras, J.; and Rosman, N. P. 1976. The significance of the Babinski sign in the newborn: A reappraisal. *Pediatrics* 57: 13–15.

Rothi, L. J. G.; Mack, L.; Verfaellie, M.; Brown, P.; and Heilman, K. M. 1988. Ideomotor apraxia: Error pattern analysis. *Aphasiology* 2: 381–88.

Roucous, A.; Culee, C.; and Roucous, M. 1983. Development of fixation and pursuit eye movements in human infants. *Behavioural Brain Research* 10: 133–39.

Rud, E. 1927. Et tilfaelda af infantilisme med tetani, epilepsi, polyneuritis, ichthyosis of anaemi of pernicious type. *Hospitalstidende* 70: 525–38.

Satz, P., Achenbach, K. and Fennell, E. 1967. Correlations between assessed manual laterality and predicted speech laterality in a normal population. *Neuropsychologia* 5: 295–310.

Satz, P.; Yanowitz, J., and Willmore, J. (1984) Early brain damage and lateral development. In R. Bell, J. Elias, R. Green, and J. H. Harvey (eds.), *Developmental Psychobiology and Clinical Neuropsychology: Interfaces in Psychology* (Lubbock, Tex.: Texas Tech University Press), pp. 87–107.

Schachter S. C.; Ransil, B. J.; and Geschwind, N. 1987. Associations of handedness with hair color and learning disabilities. *Neuropsychologia* 25: 269–76.

Schmahmann, J. D. 1991. An emerging concept: The cerebellar contribution to higher function. *Archives of Neurology* 48: 1178–87.

Schmidt, R. A. 1988. *Motor Control and Learning*, 2d ed. Champaign, Ill.: Human Kinetic.

Schonfeld, I. S.; Shaffer, D.; and Barmack, J. E. 1989. Neurological soft signs and school achievement: The mediating effects of sustained attention. *Journal of Abnormal Child Psychology* 17: 575–96.

Schwartz, A. S.; Marchok, P. L.; and Flynn, R. E. 1977. A sensitive test for tactile extinction: Results in patients with parietal and frontal lobe disease. *Journal of Neurology, Neurosurgury and Psychiatry* 40: 228–33.

Schwartz, A.; Marchok, P.; Kreinick, C. J.; and Flynn, R. E. 1979. The asymmetric lateralization of tactile extinction in patients with unilateral cerebral dysfunction. *Brain* 102: 669–84.

Smith, A. M.; Wetts, R.; and Kalaska, J. F. 1985. Activity of dentate and interpositus neurons during maintained isometric prehension. In A. W. Goodwin and I. Darian-Smith (eds.), *Hand Function and the Neocortex* (Berlin/Heidelberg: Verlag), pp. 248–58.

Spellacy, F. and Peter, B. 1978. Dyscalculia and elements of the developmental Gerstmann syndrome in school children. *Cortex* 14: 197–206.

Stein, B. E.; Goldberg, S. J.; and Clamann, H. P. 1976. The control of eye movements by the superior colliculus in the alert cat. *Brain Research* 118: 469–74.

Stewart, R. M. 1939. Congenital ichthyosis, idiocy, infantilism and epilepsy: Syndrome of Rud. *Journal of Mental Science* 85: 256–65.

Stokman C. J.; Shafer, S. Q.; Shaffer, D.; Ng, S. K-C.; O'Connor, P. A.; and Wolff, R. 1986. Assessment of neurological "soft signs" in adolescents: Reliability studies. *Developmental Medicine and Child Neurology* 28: 428–39.

Thach, W. T.; Goodkin, H. P.; and Keating, J. G. 1992. The cerebellum and the adaptive coordination of movement. *Annual Review of Neuroscience* 15: 403–42.

Tomasch, J. 1963. Uber die Zahl und Grosse der Zellen in den motorischen Hirnervenkernen des Menschen. *Zeitschrift Mikropisch-Anatomische Forschung* 70: 298–314.

Ungerleider, L. G. and Mishkin, M. 1982. Two cortical visual systems. In D. J. Ingle, M. Goodale, and R. J. W. Mansfield (eds.), *Analysis of Visual Behavior* (Cambridge, Mass.: MIT Press), pp. 549–86.

Verfaelli, M., and Heilman, K. M. 1987. Response preparation and response inhibition after lesions of the medial frontal lobe. *Archives of Neurology* 44: 1265–71.

Vitiello, B.; Ricciuti, A. J.; Stoff, D. M.; Behar, D.; and Denckla, M. B. 1989. Reliability of subtle (soft) neurological signs in children. *Journal of the American Academy of Child and Adolescent Psychiatry* 28: 749–53.

Waldrop, M. F.; Bell, R. Q.; McLaughlin, B.; and Halverson, C. R., Jr. 1978. Newborn minor physical anomalies predict short attention span, peer aggression and impulsivity at age 3. *Science* 199: 563–65.

Watson, R. T., and Heilman, K. M. 1983. Callosal apraxia. *Brain* 106: 391–403.

Wolff, P. H.; Gunnoe, C.; and Cohen, C. 1983. Associated movements as a measure of developmental age. *Developmental Medicine and Child Neurology* 25: 417–29.

———. 1985. Neuromotor maturation and psychological performance: A developmental study. *Developmental Medicine and Child Neurology* 27: 344–54.

Woods, B. T., and Eby, M. D. 1982. Excessive mirror movements and aggression. *Biological Psychiatry* 17: 23–32.

5

Assessment of the Pediatric Patient

The delineation of brain–behavior relationships may be extremely important to the overall well-being and care of a child or adolescent. However, it is not always easy to obtain the needed behavioral sample in a testing situation. It may be especially hard to elicit cooperation under the stressful conditions associated with hospitalization, chronic illness, or a life-threatening condition. Yet it is possible to build skills, learn techniques, and develop abilities that ensure the greatest likelihood of success. Ideally, the examiner will possess the good judgment, empathy, and humor needed to work productively with a child in the relatively brief time usually allotted for investigating neuropsychological functioning in the clinical medical setting.

SCHEDULING THE EVALUATION

The reason for referral should be established when a parent calls to schedule an outpatient evaluation for a child. At this time, the examiner can explain the rationale for the evaluation and summarize how neuropsychological data may prove helpful. A description of the outpatient consultation process is useful to parents, so the examiner should provide information about the history-taking interview (which precedes testing), the review of available records, the expected duration of the direct evaluation, and the plan for scheduling an interpretive session. The interpretive session may be emphasized as a time for discussion of the practical implications of the data and of treatment recommendations. Since a comprehensive written report reinforces the interpretations and conclusions reached cooperatively in the interpretive session, the examiner may encourage parents to telephone if they have questions after reading the report. A follow-up phone call placed a few days after the report has been received may be a useful means to address final questions or concerns.

A similar course of contacts may be appropriate with inpatients and their parents. However, confinement makes the child more accessible for direct evaluation in several important ways. There is more opportunity to prepare the child for evaluation, more freedom to arrange a flexible schedule, and more chances for reevaluation after short time spans, which in turn makes it easier to document change between contacts.

REVIEW OF HISTORICAL INFORMATION

The evaluation process begins even before direct contact with a child begins. A thorough history review before the formal evaluation is advantageous. Traditionalists may argue that bias is introduced if information is obtained prior to data interpretation. But, there is greater value in clarifying a child's relevant medical and developmental history before test selection and administration than in waiting until after assessment to obtain such information.

The history may be obtained by personal interview with the parent or caregiver, by having the parent complete a questionnaire, by direct contact with the referring professional, and/or by chart or records review. Besides providing factual environmental, educational, and medical data, this review may permit preliminary judgments about family relationships and about the child's (and family's) coping strategies. It also supports preliminary judgments about the most appropriate test instruments to use.

The Questionnaire and Personal Interview

A combination of questionnaire and subsequent personal interview is particularly valuable. An accurate recapitulation of a child's developmental, medical, sociocultural, psychological, and academic background is desirable, together with a summary of the child's current circumstances. Unfortunately, obstacles may prevent successful elicitation of historical information through the interview or questionnaire format. While most parents respond favorably, some may be reluctant, unwilling, or unable to comply. For example, the parent of a child evaluated by court order may be unwilling to divulge information freely; an informant's lack of medical sophistication may diminish the accuracy of the historical data provided; a parent may possess an excellent fund of useful factual knowledge, but an inexperienced interviewer may omit relevant questions that would have elicited these data.

A questionnaire serves as a basic guideline. It elicits information that subsequently may be explored further in a pretesting interview. The interviewer must probe for omitted but important details, since parents do not always appreciate the extent of their knowledge about their child. Direct communication supplements the provisional outline obtained by questionnaire. The questionnaire varies from setting to setting, but the substance of most broad screening instruments remains similar. The questionnaire should elicit information about the pregnancy and delivery, early risk factors, progression of developmental milestones, deviations from normal growth and maturity, and any family history that has direct bearing on the patient's condition. It should also screen for associated medical or behavioral problems, identify past and current treatments and medication therapies, and inquire about preschool experiences and (for a school-age child) academic history. Inquiries about the child's personality; social relatedness to family members, other children, and other adults; and extracurricular interests are often included. A sample questionnaire is presented in Appendix A.

Sometimes a general questionnaire does not elicit sufficient information about a specific functional area. Consequently, more focused questions may be needed. Two examples of such questionnaires are presented as Appendices B and C. The first was developed by one of the authors (I. S. B.) to assist trainees in obtaining greater detail about a child's social and emotional functioning. For example, the likelihood of shared symptomatology with children diagnosed as having a learning disorder related to social or emotional factors may be tentatively explored with the questionnaire presented in Appendix B. Sometimes a specific patient population or research interest necessitates the development of additional focused questionnaires. Appendix C is an example of one developed for children with hydrocephalus.

Records Review

A preparatory review of outpatient or inpatient medical record data should be undertaken, including summaries of medical consultations, diagnostic procedures, and treatment regimens. Previous psychological or psychiatric reports may also allow for a more informed impression of the child. Observational notes about the child's (or family's) characteristic reactions may provide insight into the level of acceptance or recognition of a problem.

The inpatient setting may be a source of valuable observational data. Many individuals contribute behavioral data to the child's medical chart on a daily basis. The "nursing notes" and "progress notes" sections of a chart are especially useful. Medical staff often record observations that highlight their concerns; and these may be, in part, the basis for a neuropsychological referral. Information recorded about the child's adaptation to the hospital setting may then be compared and contrasted with the examiner's own direct experiences with the child. For example, a child may respond favorably to the play setting established by the neuropsychologist, whereas medical personnel in traditional white coats may only encounter withdrawal and hostility when the child associates their presence with previous invasive procedures. The circumstances under which differential behaviors are observed may be especially helpful in treatment and rehabilitative planning.

While medical records may contain valuable notations about behavior, the neuropsychological significance of the observations may not be recognized by the original observer. An opportunity exists to integrate these data, to educate staff about the significance of their observations, and to encourage recognition of the correlation between brain integrity and functional responses. However, a word of caution is in order: one should not assume that the conclusions expressed in the medical record are definitive. Neuropsychological data may alter or modify earlier presumptive diagnostic impressions. It is important to remain unswayed by previous suppositions, while seeking data to test or refute hypotheses about cognitive function.

For example, an intimidating pediatric neurologist examined a school-age child at bedside and concluded that failure to discriminate left from right, failure to perform simple arithmetic operations, inability to read simple words, and finger agnosia were diagnostic of a developmental Gerstmann syndrome (Benson & Geschwind 1970). The strongly stated note in the chart about the discrete left parietal lobe impairment had to be disregarded when the neuropsychologist succeeded in documenting the child's capacity to perform all of these tasks in a more relaxed setting.

Parents should be encouraged to bring household medical or school records for review. Family records may contain relevant information—for instance, baby books specifying precise dates of accomplished developmental milestones. School records are sometimes incomplete or inaccurately interpreted. For example, a child's report-card grades may seem to indicate acceptable progress; but a sympathetic teacher may have graded a chronically ill child leniently to offer encouragement. Thus, the grade may not accurately reflect level of achievement. Handwritten notes alongside the grade may clarify actual accomplishment or weakness.

PREPARATION FOR THE MECHANICS OF TESTING

Examiner preparedness is important to create an environment that fosters a child's active involvement in the diagnostic process. The examiner must anticipate diverse obstacles to test administration and make needed modifications. As the examiner becomes more experienced with different age levels and diagnostic groups, such individual adjustments become easier to carry out.

Administrative Planning

It is useful to prepare a checklist of tests that are to be administered and to attempt to estimate the order in which they will be given, prior to testing. This smoothes transition time between tests. It is generally best to allow for very little unstructured time, during which a child's attention may easily be diverted.

Prepared folders that contain score sheets for all tests suited to an age range are useful. There are often different forms for children of different ages, with appropriate adjustments made in advance. Available alternate forms for reevaluation may be substituted. A face sheet listing available tests by behavioral area is useful (a sample checklist is presented in Table 5-1). This sheet ensures that tests without accompanying forms are not forgotten during the encounter, (for instance, draw-a-person, alphabet writing, number sequencing, and incidental drawing tests). A second opportunity may not exist after testing concludes.

Equipment should be close at hand and functioning before testing begins. Belatedly realizing that needed materials are elsewhere, when a child cannot be left alone, presents an unnecessary problem that foresight solves. Plenty of extra paper, sharpened pencils, colored pens, batteries, light bulbs, and technical equipment should be kept handy. If multiple examiners are testing concurrently and sharing equipment, sessions should be coordinated so that instruments needed at different times are accessible to all.

Table 5-1   Test Face Sheet for Children

Name	DOB	DOT	Age

General Intelligence	*Executive*	*Achievement*
WISC-III	Wisconsin Card Sort	WRAT Reading
McCarthy Scales	Category Test	WRAT Spelling
Stanford-Binet	Ravens Matrices	WRAT Arith.
Bayley	Mazes	WIAT
Kaufman	Go No-Go	Woodcock-J
Other _____		

Language

Write name, address, phone number
Peabody Picture Vocabulary
Token Test
Verbal Fluency
Paragraph Production
WISC-III Vocabulary, Similarities
Boston Naming Test
ABCDEFGHIJKLMNOPQRSTUVWXYZ (oral and written) JFMAMJJASOND (months)
1,2,3,4,5,6,7,8,9,10 (count forward);
20-19-18-17-16-15-14-13-12-11-10-9-8-7-6-5-4-3-2-1 (count backward)

Aphasia Screening Test
Boston Diagnostic Aphasia Exam
parts: _____
_____
Name colors

Sensory/Motor/Tactual-Motor

Sensory Testing: tactile, auditory, visual
Finger Recognition
Number Writing/ Symbol Writing
Tactile Form Recognition
Left-Right-Personal/Extrapersonal
Luria Motor
Tactual Performance Test

Tapping
Grip
Pegs (grooved)
Purdue Pegboard
Lateral Dominance
Apraxia Exam

Nonverbal

Draw-a-Person;-Clock;-Bicycle;-Family
Rey-Osterrieth or Taylor Complex Figure
Beery or Bender-Gestalt
Line Orientation; Line Bisection

Vis-mot Impersistence
Ramparts Drawing
mnmnmnmnmn
Hooper Visual Organization

Learning & Memory

Selective Reminding Test & Delayed Recall; or California Verbal Learning Test
Verbal Paired Associates & Recall
Bender/Other_____ Design Recall
Hannay-Levin Continuous Recognition Memory
Children's Logical Memory Paragraphs & Delayed Recall
Rey-Osterrieth (or Taylor) Immediate & Delayed Recalls
Benton Visual Retention
Wide Range Assessment of Memory and Learning (WRAML)

Table 5-1 (continued)

Attention/Concentration/Orientation/Vigilance

Trail Making Test	Cancellation/Visual Search
Symbol Digit Modalities Test	Stroop
WISC-III-Coding	Money Road Map
WISC-III-Digit Span	Continuous Performance
Mazes	

Others

Baby Bird Story; Three Wishes
Projectives___ (list) _____

_____

Test Selection and Order of Administration

Tests are selected based on the child's age, the likelihood that questions formulated about the child will be answered, the ability of the child to master the test requirements, and the need to challenge the child sufficiently to reach valid conclusions about neurobehavioral functioning. Sometimes it is best to administer a test whose statistical properties make it technically invalid, since clinical value may outweigh test construction considerations. Tests for which age-appropriate normative data do not exist may prove critical in formulating a conclusion about neuropsychological functioning. For example, a decision was made to administer the Wechsler Intelligence Scale for Children-III to a bright 5-year-8-month-old with a history of intracerebral brain tumor, although the WISC-III normative data begin at 6 years of age. The child was deemed capable of responding to subtest items sufficiently well to establish a baseline level. In this instance, the child needed to be followed serially. Progression or stability of cognitive function as a consequence of surgery and subsequent treatment was a major concern. The decision to administer the measure early, relying on quantifying specific responses to the individual subtests as a baseline, served follow-up planning best. Administering another measure might not have yielded the most useful data for examining interval change.

Medical restrictions sometimes prevent standardized administration of tests, but including a test may still be sufficiently important to justify deviating from specified procedures. For example, an intravenous tube in the preferred upper extremity may invalidate all or some of the motor and manipulative tasks planned. Cautious interpretation of preferred extremity performance may still be made, ensuring a "minimal degree of accomplishment." Thorough evaluation of the nonpreferred upper extremity alone may also provide important data. This may be particularly appropriate when contralateral cerebral efficiency has not yet been documented. There is also a high likelihood that an inpatient's treatment may directly influence neuropsychological performance. Suspected effects of a current therapy should be noted. For example, the varieties of medications commonly prescribed by neurologists for seizure disorders are discussed in greater detail in Chapter 8.

Tests should be chosen that balance a child's strengths and weaknesses. Continuously experiencing failure may cause the child to terminate a test session prematurely. Interspersing hard and easy tasks encourages active cooperation and prolongs participation. Tests that tap known strengths may be administered after particularly hard tasks to counter feelings of failure. Even when a test seems too simple, its accomplishment may be a source of pride for a child, instilling greater confidence.

Test order may be dictated by a physical condition or personality characteristic. For example, a child with spina bifida—a congenital condition often associated with lack of bowel and bladder control—may require periodic breaks for urinary catheterization. Delayed retrieval tasks must not conflict with the child's planned break. Test order becomes significant for a potentially aggressive adolescent. In this instance, relatively nonthreatening tests are best administered early. Harder tasks, perceived as stressful, may stimulate an aggressive outburst and should be planned for later in the session. The likelihood of physical aggression is further diminished by positioning furniture to restrain a child and to enable quick evasion of any physical confrontation. For example, a child may be seated against a wall, with the table placed in front, essentially locking the child into a confined space. The examiner, sitting across the table, has convenient access to the door. Nearby staff may be alerted in advance that the testing may be perceived negatively, so a call for physical intervention will receive a quick response.

Notification of the Inpatient Unit

The examiner should consult the inpatient's unit staff to confirm that the child does not have a schedule conflict. The patient's assigned nurse usually can help arrange a time that will necessitate the least number of interruptions. It is helpful to carry a sign such as "Do Not Disturb, Testing in Progress" to attach to the child's door to minimize interruptions by hospital personnel whose need to enter the child's room is not immediate.

Once technical preparations are complete, contact with the child can be expected to proceed more smoothly. Additional steps that may be taken to facilitate assessment relate to the emotional responses inherent in the evaluative setting.

Building Rapport

Rapport is a prerequisite for a reliable and valid evaluation. This is especially crucial in tests of young children, but it is also essential for older children and adolescents. There are, of course, extreme differences between the young child and the maturing adolescent; and these differences influence how one controls the testing environment, how much latitude one gives a child during evaluation, and how involved the child becomes in the interpretive session that follows.

Regardless of the child's age, the techniques necessary to obtain the best sample of performance are similar. The specifics of their application, however, differ. For example, referral concerns may dictate the choice of measurement procedures that are perceived by a teenager as childish. To engage the reluctant teenager, one may offer a brief intellectualized rationale for employing a test, such as "Yes, I realize that this test seems kind of silly to you. I have to admit, it seemed kind of silly to me, too, the first time I gave it. However, I find it works extremely well in telling me important information about how well you remember what you hear. I need to give you this test to help me sort out how well you can do. So, let's try it now, and then we'll go on to something else I think you will like more."

A cooperative relationship is often established when a child and the family recognize the need to work together to sharpen the delineation of neuropsychological function. The examiner's introduction to the child and family offers the first opportunity to set a positive tone—one that (one hopes) will carry through the entire interactive process. The ease with which the child is introduced to the testing day will engender confidence in the parent as well as in the child.

It is often best to avoid addressing the child directly at first. This is especially true for young children. Rather, the examiner's first introduction (accompanied by a warm smile) should be to the parent; at this time, the examiner can say something about looking forward to working with the child. The parent's acceptance of the examiner is a positive sign for the child ("My mother isn't nervous meeting this person. She's going to trust me with this person."). The child also has a brief opportunity to study the examiner before becoming the focus of attention. Then, the parent introduces the examiner to the child; alternatively, the examiner may turn to face the child, make eye contact, and—speaking directly to the child—repeat the initial introduction. Often a very young child feels reassured if the examiner is open and smiling. The examiner should kneel down for very small children to reduce the disparity in size, and thereby appear less threatening. This approach generally lessens the strain of the initial meeting.

Dependence on the parent may be discerned, in part, through observations of the child's level of comfort at the introduction. Some children are quite confident and demonstrate their independence by easily separating from the parent. Others—particularly young children—may want their parents to accompany them to the testing room before they feel comfortable.

Chronological age influences the decision about parental involvement. Infants are best assessed with their parents present. Preschool-age children may require a parent to be present for a brief period of time and sometimes for an extended period. By 2 to 3 years of age, some children respond best with their parent nearby, but others confidently leave the parent. By 4 years of age, most children can be expected to separate successfully. A child who attends school often leaves the parent willingly and enters the testing session independently. An abnormal degree of dependence on the parent or signs of separation anxiety should be noted. Separation provides an opportunity to observe the child's self-confidence, ease around new adults, and degree of eagerness in approaching new situations.

It is important to prevent a traumatic break from the parent by allowing extra time for contact with the parent, if necessary, and by acknowledging concerns about leaving the safety of the parent's presence. The lure of what awaits in the testing room should be offered. The examiner should encourage exploration of the testing room or assembled boxes of toys, all the while assuring the child of the safe nature of the impending time together. An introductory explanation of the situation might proceed as follows: "I'm so glad we have a chance to be playing ['working'] together; I've planned a special day and brought special toys ['tests' for the older child] that I think will be fun." The examiner should clearly state the conditions for the child's return to the parent in attempting to wean the child slowly away from the parent: "We'll be out for lunch around 11:45, Mrs. Smith. Jason and I have a lot to do. Jason, your mother is going to wait right here for you while we go to my special room. Why don't you come take a look at all the special things I've brought to show you? I've been looking forward to our time together. What's your favorite kind of toy? Let's go see if I have anything close to that." Then, the examiner should slowly guide the child away.

When separation is possible, the examiner should let the child know that the parent cannot participate in the session. However, a parent may be allowed to accompany the child to the testing room. For example, the examiner may state in a firm but friendly way, "Andy, let's have your father walk with us to our room, so he will know where we are." Then, once the group has arrived, the examiner may go on to say "Mr. Smith, this is where we are going to play today while you wait in the waiting room. Andy, see all those colored boxes? They hold the games I brought to play with you today while your father waits outside. Andy and I will come and see you a little later, Mrs. Smith." At this point, the examiner encourages parent and child to part.

Selective Parent Involvement

There are two major exceptions regarding parent participation in the testing room. First, a parent's presence may be considered an asset when the examiner is assessing an infant. A greater degree of cooperation may then be possible. The parent should be instructed to carry out actions directly with the child, while the examiner observes these critically. In this setting, and with appropriate structure, the parent's presence will not interfere, and it may even ensure collection of more detailed relevant information than might otherwise have been obtainable for such a young child.

Second, it may be viable to introduce the parent to the testing session when it becomes clear that no further progress can be made, or when a young child shows no sign of separating from the parent initially. The parent's role in these cases is to help motivate the child to comply with the examiner's requests. This may be accomplished by having a young child sit in the parent's lap or (preferably) by having the parent sit out of the child's direct view. A previously reluctant child, aware of the parent's physical presence, often cooperates. The examiner should engage the parent actively only as necessary to achieve the testing objectives.

A parent does not play the role of silent observer easily. It is very difficult to watch one's child make a mistake and maintain restraint. Consequently, rules and expectations should be stated at the outset. The examiner must insist that the parent remain silent in the background, not respond for the child or provide clues or answers, and prompt the child only when motioned to do so by the examiner. Maintaining eye contact between examiner and parent and nodding "yes" or shaking head "no" are unobtrusive but effective means of keeping the channel of communication open between parent and examiner. The examiner should do this only for reinforcement of parental participation or non-participation—not in response to how well the child is actually doing.

Participating parents should be warned that they will likely observe their child failing tasks that they believe could be accomplished. The examiner must clarify the importance of these parental observations, which will be sought from the parent later since some infant tests allow reported accomplishments to be scored as "passing" although the behavior is not observed by the examiner. Meanwhile, however, the parent must be made to understand that interrupting or stating impressions aloud during the actual testing is counterproductive. The examiner can provide paper and pencil to allow for note taking; it is also helpful to encourage the parent to write down questions that may arise about the observed tests or the child's responses.

Lessening Anxiety

A long testing session under the supervision of an unfamiliar adult figure tends to produce anxiety. Children, even when well prepared, initially perceive testing as a potentially threatening situation. For example, young children may need reassurances that there will be no pain and that the examiner is simply a "play person." Older children often share the same worries, although they may hide their discomfort better. A tone of enjoyment and positive challenge should be set early to alleviate these concerns.

Children have many misconceptions about testing. A straightforward explanation of the purpose of the testing process may undo distortions engendered by limited parental explanation or fearful conjecture. Children commonly are concerned when they are told they must see a "doctor." Many children come to the testing session expecting blood tests or fearing other invasive procedures. For example, a mother pulled a crying 5-year-old boy into the office one morning, while he pleaded to the secretary "No shot! No shot!" The secretary quickly hugged him and assured him that no one was going to hurt him: the doctor was only going to play games with him. To prove her point, she gave him paper and crayons to draw with, let him roam the office, and showed him some of the toys. By the time the neuropsychologist was ready to see the child, he was relaxed and eager to proceed.

Other specific physical and verbal actions defuse preconceived notions of a threatening "doctor." A white coat and other accouterments of the medical staff should be avoided, except when testing must be done in a sterile environment. Otherwise, negative associations with a prior hospital or physician's office experience may arise. The examiner should assert clearly to a reluctant child, "I am not the usual kind of a doctor. I am a play person. Everything we will be doing today will be done across a table top (or on the rug)." The young child can be shown the colorful boxes of games immediately upon entering the room, to build confidence that the time to be spent with the examiner will be pleasant. The examiner should emphasize the enjoyable nature of the impending play (work) time and generate excitement about what is going to be a fun experience for both child and adult. With such assurances, the child's fears usually dissipate quickly.

While obviously important for younger children, the relaxed nature of a testing session also appeals to older children. They quickly realize that administration procedures are similar to school experiences. Like younger children, they are relieved that the tests will not hurt. All children need assurance that most of the tests will fall within their range of competency. They also need preparation for the eventuality that some of the tests will be difficult and that they may not be able to respond correctly to every question.

One way the neuropsychologist may further appreciate the child's perception of problems that have resulted in neuropsychological referral is by direct questioning—for example, "Why are you here today?" for the outpatient, or "Why do you think I've come to play with you in the hospital today?" for the inpatient. The answer offers insight about a child's perspective, and it provides an opportunity to correct any flaws or distortions.

A surprising number of children do not know why they are being tested. Since parents frequently do not give their children a clear explanation of the purpose, they may create their own. While perceptions may be accurate with good preparation, they are often distorted when preparation is insufficient. Confusion, fear, or ignorance of the true reason for evaluation makes the initial moments of an evaluation especially tense. The following examples of responses reflect some of the typical worries children express: "There is something broken in my head"; "I'm stupid and these tests will prove it"; "If I fail these tests I'll have to go back to the hospital"; "I'm here because I'm missing something inside my brain."

Such fears overwhelm children and make it difficult for them to relax and participate in the testing. Asking a child about the reasons for the visit helps to elicit these feelings and to understand the child's unique perspective on the medical problems that occasioned the evaluation. Testing may be perceived as a punishment for not doing well in school or for being ill. Some false impressions are never spoken aloud but may be expressed symbolically through drawing or play tasks. It is up to the examiner to judge what needs to be said to the child to increase comfort, to counter distortions, and to foster the best possible assessment process.

Once the child has communicated personal impressions about the reason for the evaluation, the examiner can provide an accurate but tactful explanation rectifying any misperception. For example, "In our time together today, I will have a chance to give you many tests [or 'games,' for the young child]. These will help me figure out what kinds of things you can do very well and where you might have some trouble. These are the same tests that are given to many other children your age. Some are easy and some are a little harder. There is no failing grade because sometimes children do better on certain tests than on others and that's perfectly OK. We all do some things very well and other things not quite as well. It is important for you to try your very best today because then I will be able to find out how we can help you."

Limiting uncertainties about what will occur in the testing room should ensure a child's optimal cooperation. Generally, a relaxed child will not express a need to seek parental support during the session. By initially briefing the child about how some items will seem very easy and others will seem very hard, the examiner encourages the child to understand that acceptance and approval can be obtained simply by trying one's best. Similarly, a strong statement that success on some items and difficulty with others is expected allows the child to encounter difficulty comfortably. A child may need to hear more than once that the examiner views failures on especially difficult items as perfectly normal. For example: "I know some of the questions are going to be harder than others, but this test is designed to make you stretch for answers. It's OK if you feel some are just too hard. You can let me know that you've done your best, and we'll go on to something else." Most children need to know that the examiner is an ally before they feel comfortable in a testing setting.

Finally, the examiner's introduction to the child may provide a sense of how the child reacts to new adult authority figures and novel settings. There are many aspects of the initial interaction to note, including motoric, verbal, and nonverbal. One useful step is to observe physical accommodations and how the child is positioned. For example, does the child retreat and cling to a parent or independently and willingly step forward? Does the child look the examiner in the eye or act shy and anxious? Another important point to observe is the child's response to play objects. For example, is the child secure reaching out to novel stimuli, or does the child seek parental or examiner approval first? A third significant element consists of the parent's verbal reactions to the child's actions. For example, does the parent express approval or disapproval? How appropriate are these responses, given the child's behavior? What is the child's reaction? Observations such as these provide a basis for initiating conversation meant to set the child at ease and to uncover clues about personality that may require further exploration.

INTRODUCTORY CONVERSATION

Informal conversation is one of the best ways to lay the groundwork for a productive evaluation. The inexperienced examiner may underestimate the value of engaging in casual conversation at the beginning of a test session. The experienced examiner, however, has learned the benefits of such discussion. Since it is informal, the conversation varies from child to child—for instance, discussion of a favorite game or activity, particular interests, friends, upcoming vacations, or parties. Such conversation is nonthreatening to most children.

While it enables both participants to become familiar with one another, it also provides an excellent opportunity for the examiner to formulate initial clinical impressions that may subsequently be supported through formal data acquisition.

Sensitivity to the child's perception of illness or cognitive change should temper the conversation's content. Greater understanding of how cognitive disruption affects the child's self-concept may be one outcome of the conversation. The neuropsychologist may learn about the child's coping strategies—how the child has struggled to overcome dysfunction, how frustrations resulting from unsuccessful efforts have been handled, how fear of failure impacts on performance, and/or what obstacles still impede recognition of the full spectrum of problems. Still, the initial conversation preceding testing is best used as a "warm-up". Later, more detailed exploration of these facets may be planned.

It is important to avoid the pitfall of asking questions that are too probing or are perceived as judgmental. A child may refuse to participate further if boundaries are not kept. Sensitive topics may be broached more easily once rapport is strengthened and the examiner is perceived as supportive. When a child is questioned about personal matters, it is helpful to notice which questions are directly answered, which questions are answered only indirectly, and which topics are avoided altogether. These may be explored further at a later time.

General, rather than specific, questions are perceived as less personally threatening and therefore are answered more easily. For example, a teenager may allude to illicit drug use but may find it awkward to respond to direct questions about personal involvement in drug or alcohol use. As an alternative to direct personal interrogation, the examiner may ask the teenager about drug use among friends or at school. The examiner must then gauge the likely nature and extent of patient involvement. Of course, many teenagers recognize the underlying purpose of such questions; but they may nonetheless respond, since they feel that personal revelations couched in these terms are protected. As the nonjudgmental discussion continues it may become possible to inquire more specifically about personal use.

Spontaneous informal conversation also provides an opportunity to note preliminarily any impairments of receptive or expressive aspects of speech and language formulation. Speech pattern, verbal fluency, articulation, tonal quality, vocabulary, and the general ability to communicate content effectively through verbal expression should be noted. Overt or subtle language difficulties, when detected, may become a focus during testing.

Observations made during the initial phase of testing highlight other behavioral areas that may require exploration during formal assessment. For instance, monotonic speech observed in the context of a clear failure to appreciate the social significance of nonverbal cues (such as gestures and facial expression) may stimulate exploration of the child's facility with other aspects of nonverbal information processing. Such characteristics may prove to be noncontributory, or they may serve as the first indicators of the presence of a nonverbal social/emotional learning disability (Wing 1981; Baron 1987). If the child fails to respond to verbal directions consistently, or repeated requests that instructions be repeated, the examiner should recognize the need for a formal hearing assessment prior to consideration of central nervous system involvement.

Introductions should be brief and should be sustained only until the child is comfortable enough to proceed with formal evaluation. On occasion, a child may attempt to extend the time allotted for chatting in an effort to avoid the real purpose of testing. In such a case, the examiner should not hesitate to direct the conversation to a close and focus instead on the formal tests. For example, the examiner might say, "That's very interesting, and I'd like to hear more later when we have time. But right now we need to take these tests ['play these games']," or "Let me write that down and we will come back to it later." These statements often successfully conclude attempts to avoid or postpone the evaluation. Rest breaks supply opportunities for promised further discussion.

INITIATING AND SUSTAINING TEST-TAKING BEHAVIOR

The start of testing provides an opportunity to offer unconditional praise. The examiner should ease the child into testing by first presenting a nonthreatening, familiar task that will result in successful performance. For example, young children frequently like to draw. Shape drawing or a draw-a-person are therefore good initial tests for children who do not have a delay in visuomotor integration. If graphomotor problems are known through history review, the examiner should choose a simple verbal task that can easily be accomplished, instead of a drawing test—for instance, stating the alphabet and the months of the year, counting backward, counting by serial 3's, or taking a picture vocabulary test. It is extremely important to provide positive reinforcement for all attempts to fulfill the testing demands.

Stress may certainly be expected to increase when a child must concentrate on a test that involves areas of real or perceived weakness. For example, a child may have auditory attention problems. If so, tests that depend on the child's capacity to sustain auditory attention should be interspersed throughout the testing day, not administered in close temporal sequence to one another. Paper-and-pencil tasks may be offered as a break. For example, after a particularly difficult verbal learning test, a shape-drawing task allows a young child to excel and regain confidence.

As testing progresses, the examiner should offer reinforcement for difficult tasks, remaining aware of the child's sensitivity to perceived failures. In particular, such reinforcement should include recognizing when a child expends great effort but anticipates failure, acknowledging this determination, and supporting continued effort. The form of reinforcement one chooses should be appropriate to the child's age. For example, the examiner may demonstrate overt physical responses such as clapping effusively and smiling broadly for a very young child. For older children and adolescents, the examiner may restate the importance of trying to do one's best. Verbal encouragement that acknowledges how hard a particular task seems and emphasizes the importance of making an effort is usually well received.

A child may be frustrated by an especially hard test. At such times, the examiner should acknowledge the attempt and the obstacles, saying, for example, "That was a very hard test for a child your age, but you made a very good effort. You did as well as any child your age should. However, the test is also meant to be given to much older children, and that's why it seems especially hard. It is important to try your best, but it's OK to find it hard and to let me know. Let's go on to something else now." Relief is usually immediately visible.

Fear of failing invariably arises during testing. Children manifest such fear in a variety of ways. Some children express their concern in a very obvious manner, while others adopt a more covert demeanor. For example, a child may ask, "Will I be held back if I fail these tests?" As the day progresses, remarks such as "How did I do?" and "Did I do better than other kids my age?" further reveal the child's insecurities. Sensitivity to the existence of such fears puts the examiner on guard for signs of performance anxiety, however subtle these may be.

It is helpful to make a statement at the outset of testing assuring the child that the tests are not of a pass/fail nature and indicating in advance that some of the required tasks will be very easy while others will be much more difficult. This prepares children for the experience of encountering questions they will not be able to answer. It remains for the examiner to determine the appropriateness of pushing a child to the limits on any given task. This determination, of course, depends on how frustrating the task is and on the child's emotional stability and/or level of resistance toward a task. In most instances, fear of failure inhibits children from venturing guesses and causes more resistance. Reassurance that the child cannot fail the test may encourage responses.

The examiner should leave unclear whether answers are right or wrong. It is important not to develop a pattern that the child can interpret, such as smiling every time a correct answer is given. Thus, indicating "good try" or "good guess" occasionally is fine, but it should not only be done for misses. If the child is not fooled by these attempts to bolster confidence, the examiner should again focus on the admirability of the effort: "I know this was hard for you, but I like the way you tried." In instances where the examiner feels compelled to acknowledge a child's poor performance, it is best to respond honestly but positively—acknowledging the weak performance but supporting the child. One approach would be to state "This task seemed more difficult for you than some of the others. Did you notice this too? I wonder why. Let's see if we can figure this out together."

In summary, reluctance to participate may be countered procedurally in a number of ways: *first*, by avoiding initial tasks that emphasize a known weakness (in particular, the one that precipitated the request for evaluation; *second*, by carefully determining the optimum order for administering of test items, avoiding giving one type of task in a short span of time when it clearly taps a weak area, and varying test order so that the child is not burdened with failure for an extended time; *third*, by providing only nonjudgmental, positive feedback; fourth, by anticipating behavioral changes over the course of a testing session (especially fatigue or frustration) and minimizing their impact by interrupting testing at logical rest points with brief conversations that lighten the mood and steer attention away from hard items the child has not mastered; and *fifth*, by attempting to elicit a more developed answer than "don't know" (DK) when this response is repeatedly offered. This last effort can be pursued in between tasks by encouraging the child to make a guess. The examiner can explain, "Guessing is much better than saying 'don't know.' You don't lose points for guessing, and a lot of times an answer you think you may know but aren't completely sure of is the right one. That's why sometimes guessing is just a way of trying your best." Encouragement to guess often eliminates the DK response in all but the specific instances when the child really is at a loss. It is also important that the child understand when time limits are not being imposed. Children need clear guidelines about what is expected during the session, updated as necessary. Even though a child was reassured earlier in the test session, additional supportive comments may be needed later.

SITUATIONAL FACTORS

Situational factors directly affect the success of the evaluative process. Advantages and limitations exist in both the outpatient and inpatient settings. Awareness of their existence and understanding of how they vary contribute to creating a setting that will ensure optimum behavioral sampling.

Outpatient Evaluations

Given the extended time a child must spend in testing, an environment conducive to examination must be created. The ideal environment enables the child to feel comfortable while offering little potential for distraction.

A positive initial impression is desirable. A pediatrician's waiting room often has toys and posters of cartoon characters or media personalities, as a way to alleviate tension associated with a doctor's visit. Although it is not always possible to decorate the office or waiting room in which the examiner will see a child, familiar, comfort-inducing details may be introduced, such as colorful toys that are easy to wash before the next child plays with them, teen magazines, and manipulative toys.

Decorating and furnishing the testing room creates an artificially engineered "warm" environment, rather than a sterile and intimidating clinical setting. Toys are calming and provide a means to engage the child in conversation and to redirect attention momentarily. For example, a shy child with a speech impediment may be reluctant to engage in spontaneous conversation but may open up and chatter un-self-consciously about an appealing doll. The opportunity to evaluate spontaneous conversation freely is often enhanced when attention is subtly redirected away from the child and toward an object.

One must carefully consider the content of decorations and their impact on the child and on testing process. Discriminating use of wall hangings, desktop objects, plants, and pictures is advantageous. For example, one neuropsychologist decorated her testing room with a tapestry containing a colorful array of animals. Although this seemed appropriate, she later observed children glancing over at the tapestry for clues when required to generate animal names on a verbal fluency test. This interference was nullified by substituting a colorful abstract print for the tapestry.

Appropriate furniture includes a smooth, level testing surface and stable chairs that do not swivel but do adjust for height. A small child who must try to reach a tall desk for a long period of time will tire easily. Given the high incidence of attentional deficits and hyperactivity among the pediatric population referred for neuropsychological testing, the relevance of chair type becomes evident. Active children frequently have trouble staying seated in their chairs, even for brief periods of time. Chairs that swivel or tip easily serve only as an added distraction that can impede the testing process. Seating rules need to be selectively applied, however. For instance, a child hanging upside down over a chair but nonetheless responding well to verbal questions should not be forced to sit upright. That request should be saved for a task where proper sitting position is essential for good performance.

For any number of reasons, it may be difficult for a child to sit in a chair. If so, the floor may be used as a testing surface instead. Given a choice between desk and floor, a young child will often choose the floor. For physically handicapped children, use of the floor may facilitate mobility. A small pad or area rug tucked away in a closet may be brought out if the room is uncarpeted. The examiner should keep in mind that using the floor as a testing surface is viable, effective, and—in some cases—a more desirable option.

Inpatient Evaluation

Several special issues are related to bedside evaluations. In general, the examiner wields less influence than when the interaction is one-to-one in a professional office. The immediacy of the child's medical problem determines a priority of care that supersedes the evaluative process. The neuropsychologist has reduced control over many factors affecting the inpatient evaluative process. There is diminished ability to establish rapport. Time constraints exist that increase the need for advance preparation. The testing session is more frequently interrupted by external activities that form a natural part of the hectic medical setting. The ill or disabled child may have serious misconceptions about the purpose of the evaluation, and the neuropsychologist must rely heavily on appropriate reinforcements to elicit desired behavior. Such inpatient testing situations place a burden on the neuropsychologist to be as flexible as possible in the face of complex circumstances. The ability to turn the action of the moment productively to one's own purpose becomes an important skill.

A rigid, "we must follow the rules" approach, which inherently discounts a child's shifting emotions, is likely to fail. For example, when faced with a child who has a limited attention span, the examiner must plan how best to use the allotted time, obtaining the needed data as quickly but as carefully as possible. Flexibility toward the order of test administration allows for more comprehensive screening of cognitive functions, whereas adherence to a strict order of test administration typically leads to failure to achieve the minimum goals of testing.

Limitations Related to Bedside Evaluation

External means of inducing comfort are not easily introduced in the inpatient setting. Inpatients most often are evaluated in their hospital beds, with all the unpleasant associations this setting raises for the children. Moreover, since the bed is the child's temporary "home," the child can simply turn over and go to sleep or refuse to continue, knowing that the examiner depends on the child's cooperation. In certain cases, permission to move the child to a testing room may be granted. Whenever possible it is advantageous to change the environment to one that is novel and pleasant for the child. Entering a room with games openly arrayed is a welcome break from hospital routine. When transport is not possible, enticing portable materials should be sterilized and introduced as a pleasant alternative. The examiner should bring along a large flat form to serve as a table top in case a bedside table cannot be adjusted to the correct height and comfort level. One or two objects of potential play interest will facilitate introductions and be useful during play breaks. For younger children, a puppet is particularly appealing, since it meets many of the criteria that support a productive testing session; it is portable and it is easily adapted to situations that may arise or that may be structured by the examiner for informational purposes. Any toy of intrinsic interest to the child will serve the same purpose.

Limited Chance to Develop Rapport

The inpatient child may be especially reticent and may initially view the examiner as an additional strange adult figure who might be the source of additional hurt or inconvenience. As a result, there is less time to establish a positive relationship and to obtain the desired degree of cooperation. Further, the child's focus may be distracted by other personnel who interrupt the testing process or by public address announcements. It is often helpful for the examiner to make an introductory visit to the child, explaining the visitor's role, identifying some of the tests (games) the visitor will be bringing along next time, and stating when the visitor will return. The initial visit allows the examiner to gauge the mental and physical capabilities of the child. On the return visit, the examiner can arrive with tests in hand, smiling and colorfully attired (to contrast with the white coats and hospital uniforms that often carry negative associations), and already known to the child. It is helpful, but not always possible, to have a parent or favorite nurse initially present at the bedside to diminish a young child's fears.

Time Constraints

Some time constraints prevail in the hospital room that are not present in the testing office. Work periods may be shortened or hampered by unforeseen scheduling patterns, medical procedures, consultations, visitation, and shared room assignments that result in a lack of privacy. For example, a nurse may arrive to take vital signs; physician rounds may reach the room while the examiner is in the midst of timing a test; a parent or relative may arrive for a visit; lunch may be served; linens may have to be changed; a therapist may arrive for a session; or a roommate may receive visitors.

The ill child likely requires more frequent rest breaks than does a healthy child. The inpatient testing is thus more likely to be completed in segments, even stretching across days. Different times of the day and different days of the week affect outcome, but they also provide a valuable index of behavioral sampling over time. The examiner must be succinct and move rapidly, but not as if rushed. The examiner's attitude influences the child's performance, so it is desirable to be perceived as relaxed and comfortable rather than harried, distressed, or irritated by uncontrolled interruptions. It is important to keep chronological notes about interruptions that may negatively affect test results.

Time limitations necessitate that the examiner use available time prudently. While the child works on a task that does not require ongoing instruction or intent observation, the examiner can discreetly score or evaluate some of the completed tasks. A quick estimate of weak areas will indicate which additional tests should be given and which may be unnecessary.

Distractions

Since children become distracted so easily, one should always attempt to minimize external stimuli. This becomes especially important in work with children who are very active or inherently subject to attentional variability. Of immediate notice to such children are tabletop objects. Fidgety children will grab at, pick up, or inquire about most things that are within view or reach. Simply removing interfering objects from the desktop may help restore the child's focus.

Noises may also be a distraction. Telephone interruptions are particularly intrusive, but the problem can easily be prevented by temporarily unplugging the phone. Loud noises from outside the room are harder to eliminate. However, a child who is sensitive to such distractions is likely to be just as sensitive in the classroom; and the practical conclusions reached during the analysis of the clinical data may lead to important recommendations about noise insulation for parents and teachers.

Busy halls may be problematic. Nurses should be alerted to the examiner's visit and a sign indicating that testing is in progress should be posted outside the door. The fewer the distractions, the more quickly the testing will progress. Rapid testing ensures greater interest of the child in more varied but shorter-lasting tasks. Pacing the presentation of items well, ignoring distractions (as a model for the child), and gaining the child's continuing interest in the variety of tests utilized are ways the examiner can help the child refocus and continue with the task at hand.

Examiner Response to Physical Disability

The examiner's actions give clear messages to the child being evaluated. The examiner must try to be aware of signals that convey negative messages unintentionally. Avoidance (such as looking away or failing to maintain eye contact), sighs in response to poor performance, slight shaking of the head when the answer is wrong, and/or a clearly legible "x" or "–" on the exposed answer sheet for wrong answers are all negative cues the child interprets to gain a sense of how the testing is progressing. These behaviors must be eliminated to support successful performances. If they become a pattern, they may well diminish the likelihood that a child will attempt to work up to capacity. It is difficult for any psychologist at any experience level to know and suppress every negative message that may be conveyed by a gesture or position. There is a natural sense of sadness and, for some, reluctance when encountering a child who is quite ill or incapacitated. It is immensely difficult to come face-to-face with a child sustained by life-support machines, distorted by disfigurement, or striving with serious unsightly physical deformities or injuries. Negative feelings may be elicited from an examiner even with regard to a physically able child who has cognitive impairment. Nonverbal facial and body language is easily detected and interpreted by children and adolescents. To combat these tendencies, awareness of one's own reaction to illness and disability is necessary, since this may allow an appropriate modulation of one's reactions. A colleague's objective observations of the testing process—through a one-way mirror or by silently observing the testing from afar—may aid in detecting cues that have become habitual or otherwise escape notice.

The examiner's nonpunitive, unconditional acceptance of the child or adolescent should be clearly communicated. It is essential to reach the child who may mask feelings about physical deformity but whose medical problems are overtly visible. A sad example of failure to appreciate a child's tenuous self-image follows. A psychology intern tested a wheelchair-bound boy who had multiple craniofacial abnormalities. She was clearly made uncomfortable by his unusual physical presence. Likely sensing her feelings, he found it difficult to respond to her. In frustration over his discomfort and lack of motivation, she soon raised her voice, telling him to try harder, that he "could do it, if he just paid attention and tried." This exhortation was an exact replication of the negative feedback he had been receiving from well-meaning but naïve parents and teachers. He completely rejected the intern and the examination process, just as he had the academic environment. A valid testing that might have provided valuable insight had to postponed. And because the examination process was unduly harsh, the child's next exposure was inevitably affected, at least in the initial stages.

Another example involves a teenager who arrived for evaluation surly, uncommunicative, and dressed outlandishly because he had been forced to come (and confront his weaknesses once again) and sit through another "boring" evaluation process. The examiner is obligated to attempt to reach this individual with the same care and sensitivity as would be accorded to young children (whose true feelings tend to be nearer the surface). The moments taken to establish a positive dyadic interaction are extremely valuable and set the tone for the entire session. If one cannot make positive social contact with an adolescent one will likely fail to sustain the individual's motivation and adherence to the test session requirements.

An ill and uncomfortable child will not be inclined to perform at full capacity. It is best to acknowledge this openly, so that at least a sample of behavior may be obtained. Physical limitations imposed by diagnostic or treatment procedures further complicate efforts; for example, the placement of an IV tube may interfere with fine motor skill assessment; a headache persisting days after a spinal tap procedure may interfere with concentration and/or the ability to adjust body position well enough to take tests; compromised sensory perception may be secondary to ophthalmological evaluation; and sedative effects may remain after a drug regimen. Allowances must be made for these extraordinary conditions. If evaluation must be conducted under adverse conditions, the examiner should administer the minimum valid test items and defer the rest until a fair sampling may be obtained under better circumstances. It is preferable to delay evaluation until conditions are more favorable.

Distorted Perceptions

The examiner should always be sensitive to the child's internalized distortions in a setting where medical problems are openly discussed but not well explained. An inadvertent message may create a fearful state. For example, a consultation was requested for a young girl who was mute after neurosurgery—a child familiar to the neuropsychologist through presurgical baseline evaluation. The child was to be reevaluated postsurgically but only after discharge from the intensive care unit. Days after awakening from surgery, however, she still had not spoken to family or medical staff. To cheer the patient, the neuropsychologist brought along a small gift—a girl's cosmetic set, which included a mirror. When offered the gift, the girl smiled and readily unwrapped it, reaching rapidly for the mirror. She held it up to her face, and the "mute" child *said,* sadly and pitifully "Is that what I look like?" She had had grave fears about what neurosurgery ("head surgery") really meant. She was not sufficiently prepared for the recovery room experience and thus was frightened and perplexed about what had actually been done to her, silently wondering about possible disfigurement. Until she viewed her reflection in the proffered mirror she had not realized that the bandages were only on her head, and that her face was still the same. Her anger and confusion had been overtly directed at the staff and her parents. The reassurance provided by viewing herself in the mirror allowed her to speak freely to everyone, and her concerns could then be dealt with openly and constructively.

Reluctance to be tested, fear of separation from a parent, and fear of the setting may all be invisible beneath a smile and a superficial appearance of cooperation. A brief time of "perfect behavior," however, soon gives way to the real scary thoughts that were not deeply submerged. A young child's eyes may well up with tears, or there may be a series of requests to leave the testing room: "I need to get a drink"; "I want to see my mother"; "I don't want any shots"; "I have to go to the bathroom". The child may become silent and withdrawn. These messages of discomfort need to be intercepted and allayed before they interfere with testing.

Items of intrinsic interest enable the examiner to engage the child in more difficult tasks. Ingenuity in the application of the equipment will extend the versatility of the instrument and allow assessment of a wider range of behaviors. Some children quickly let one know of their interest in an object. If the child finds colored blocks appealing, the examiner can extend their use—for instance, by examining math concepts, assessing color recognition and naming, building three-dimensional constructions, copying shapes made by the blocks, observing hand preference, and using them as a reinforcer. Colorful crayons and pencils encourage continued participation for visuomotor tasks, which the examiner may introduce as follows: "I know you don't like to draw, but why don't you try to draw the next shape with a different color pencil? Do you have a favorite color? Let's try to draw the picture with that color." They may thus stimulate a child to accept the challenge of a drawing test in spite of their earlier unsuccessful attempts using only an ordinary pencil. A pen that writes with two colors, or can produce a silver/gold outline with a single stroke, is often appealing even to a very resistant child.

Novelty is endearing, but the time span of the interest generated is often brief. Continued alertness to possible reinforcing items is helpful. The examiner should try to be aware of current trends and toys, and should attempt to learn more through initial conversations with the child. Asking about a favorite toy, TV show, or current fad enlightens the examiner and serves as an agreeable topic of conversation to most children. What the examiner learns from one child is applicable to the next.

THE DIFFICULT CHILD

Taking many tests in a short period of time is fun and stimulating for some children, but it evokes negative behaviors from others. These responses may parallel a teacher's complaints about the child's classroom behavior. In the one-to-one testing environment, however, a wider range of behaviors may be allowed, as long as these behaviors do not interfere with the assessment process. It is desirable to achieve a productive and pleasant relationship for the brief time that the examiner and the child are together, so that the child becomes positively involved in the evaluative process. No matter how long it takes to obtain full cooperation, the examiner must ensure that such cooperation is achieved. The creativity and empathy of the examiner will be put to work fully in the effort to obtain accord.

However, a child's mood and affect during testing vary. For example, a child may react one way during the early phase of the testing and then change as the testing progresses. Early shyness may give way to warmer interactions and positive involvement in the testing process; but conversely, early enthusiasm may wane with the stress of difficult items. The length of a thorough test session is often sufficient to permit the examiner to obtain valuable impressions about how a child reacts to success and failure. If the length is perceived as excessive by a child, however, negative behaviors will emerge.

As can be expected in any provoking situation, children employ a number of strategies intended to remove the source of stress. These maneuvers are more likely at times of fatigue or when a task taps an area of real weakness. Thus, it is important to note the temporal connection between a task and its associated negative behavior. For example, when a child's head is rested on the desk in response to a request for arithmetic calculation or repetition of number sequences, the reaction may be a silent retreat from the task. The requirement to manipulate numbers mentally may be the obstacle. Sometimes children make comments as they work that provide a glimpse of the cognitive process and strategies they prefer. For example, the way a child reasons and solves a complicated math problem may be clearer when the steps taken are spontaneously stated aloud. One may also overhear a child's uncensored vocal expression of feeling—for instance, their determination to succeed, or self-berating comments.

The pediatric neuropsychologist may utilize behavioral management principles and techniques when testing a difficult child. The systematic application of reinforcement contingencies are especially useful for the resistant young child, who needs greater support. For example, young children may work very hard for a small sticker, shiny star or token prize. Tokens may be collected along the way, with any number achieved sufficient to earn a final reinforcement. With some recalcitrant children who demonstrate a strong interest in the stopwatch, this object can be used effectively as a reinforcer. One may selectively improve on-task behavior by judicious sharing of the timepiece. A child may work longer when controlling the stopwatch; and the testing time may be extended with comments such as "Let's try three more questions and then you can time the fourth" or "After I time you on this visual search game, you can time how long it takes me to set up the next game."

Evaluation may be adapted in response to actual behaviors. For example, a child may request a drink of water to escape briefly from testing demands. The examiner might simultaneously explore the integrity of left–right discrimination and spatial orientation in association with the mundane aspect of the request rather than lose an opportunity to add to the clinical data base. This would involve directing the child to make the appropriate left and right turns—rather than simply escorting the child to a fountain—and follow behind to observe whether the turns are made correctly.

It may happen that a child's patience with the test session lessens until the child refrains from further cooperation and asks to see a parent. Instead of immediately acceding to the child's explicit request for a break, the examiner may propose one more short task before a brief break. This places control over the order of events firmly with the examiner and may help limit the frequency of interfering requests.

Inevitably, examiners occasionally encounter children who, for one reason or another, are difficult to evaluate. A discussion of commonly occurring behaviors that interfere with testing, as well as some helpful strategies for dealing with them, follows.

Withdrawal or Avoidance

Withdrawal or avoidance are commonly observed, especially in response to a growing sense of failure. Too many hard items in close temporal proximity may result in escape-oriented actions. For example, when a writing task is given, the child may give up trying, regress to more childish behavior, complain of somatic disturbances, or employ techniques such as asking for mother, for a drink, or for a trip to the bathroom. To engage the child actively again, it is helpful to identify which task demands elicited the avoidance behavior. The examiner should remind and reassure the child that the tests are deliberately designed to push the test taker to the limits, that no one gets everything correct or (as seems quite reassuring to many) that the item is actually intended for older children, and that a good effort is what really matters.

Repeated requests to leave the testing room typically arise only with a very young child. Observed in an older child, it becomes an issue of clinical significance, perhaps indicative of extreme frustration or overwhelming anxiety associated with demands that exceed capability. In general, withdrawal and avoidance behaviors may constitute a normal reaction to stressful conditions.

Manipulation and Testing of Limits

A child may actively try to determine the limits of permissible conduct in the one-to-one setting, often in order to be in a position to terminate administration of a particularly difficult task. A child may also attempt to determine the boundaries of acceptance and of punishment, similar to their experience of control issues at home. Maintaining control of the testing session becomes difficult when an uncooperative child is determined to direct the course of testing.

The ways in which children test limits vary considerably, ranging from subtle manipulation through direct confrontation. Whatever the child's tactic, the examiner must be prepared for such behaviors and must be able to regain control immediately when they occur. For example, an 8-year-old boy started to say "Don't know" when questioned—occasionally at first, and then in response to every question, despite encouragement to give his best guess. He presented quite a serious face, as if trying hard. After confirming impressions of deliberate intent by asking a few very simple questions (for instance, what letter comes after A?), the examiner clearly stated with a smile that it was obvious that the boy could answer many of the questions but that he had evidently decided to try to fool the examiner. The examiner said she appreciated how clever he was to fool her, but she reminded him of the purpose of the testing and warned that, in order for the examiner to help him, he must do his best; their time together would be useless, she said "if he didn't give it his best shot". Moreover, she explained *with a deep sigh,* they would have a very long day ahead of them and perhaps even need a *second* visit. Therefore, she concluded, she was going to ask the questions again, and this time the boy really needed to answer them the best he could. Addressing his bluff directly but positively elicited a big smile, and he was a perfect examinee for the rest of the testing.

It is necessary to set firm limits when manipulation is suspected. As in the preceding example, benignly informing the child that, if tests are not completed, a return visit will be necessary may give them sufficient motivation to cooperate. The examiner must be firm and consistent, no matter what tactic is chosen. If, for example, the examiner states that the next break will take place following completion of three more tasks, the stated contract must be maintained and a break must be given after three tasks. When terms of reward are clear and predictable, children are often better able to pace themselves and accept the limitations of the setting.

Somatic complaints are sometimes given. It is helpful if the examiner can distinguish the complaint's legitimacy. A child's behavior during a rest break is often a good indicator of how a child really feels. Healthy children often are active during these times, whereas children who are not feeling well may sit quietly or doze. For example, one child persistently complained of a stomachache when required to engage in puzzle assembly and block construction tasks. A short rest break was therefore offered, during which the child happily explored the testing room without complaint. The relief of symptoms was clearly contingent on the child's freedom to choose a task, and the stomachache complaint was simply a maneuver to stop testing. When a true illness is suspected, the examiner should notify the parent and postpone testing to a time when a valid performance may be obtained.

Lack of Motivation

An examiner is often confronted with a child who has a motivational problem that seriously impedes attempts to understand the child's true capacities, unless addressed directly. A reliable and valid assessment implies that a child has put forth appropriate effort in completing the tasks at hand. If an examiner suspects that a child is not trying his or her best, the recorded conclusions are in doubt, and the purpose of the evaluative process has not been met.

Motivation varies with a child's perception of task difficulty; that is, when confronted with tasks that they feel are too difficult, children may not exert as much effort as they would on a task where success is virtually guaranteed. The examiner should note specifically which tasks increase (and which reduce) motivation to perform. Sometimes the confidence gained through quick success fosters enough determination to enable the child to proceed with a difficult task. For example, a tapping test has great intrinsic interest and may be an ideal instrument when one wants to offer praise quickly. Children without obvious motor impairment cannot judge their level of success on this task and will be guided by the examiner's responses.

The younger the child, the better the chances are of obtaining a true estimate of function when the evaluation is scheduled early in the day. The influences of fatigue, hunger, and distress over preceding performances all gain momentum as the time period extends. It is best to establish rapport quickly, and to proceed with the most critical tests, while not initially pushing the child too much.

A child may not balance considerations of speed versus accuracy well. For example, some children will rush through a test seemingly unconcerned with performance but eager to terminate the task; their failure might trouble them very little. Others may rush to impress the examiner with their competence and find their failures disheartening. Still others may rush, accomplish the task well, but expend undue energy in the process. Clear directions that emphasize appropriate test-taking behavior should encourage optimal participation.

Children with psychiatric histories—for instance, conduct or behavioral problems, or reactive depression secondary to physical symptomatology—most frequently (but not exclusively) present with motivational problems at testing. However, any child might respond less than enthusiastically. A history of emotional problems alone is not fully predictive of what will ensue in testing. Any child is subject to moments of motivational loss or apprehension, and certain feelings (such as hunger or fatigue) or the tests themselves may elicit these more strongly.

Humor—but not sarcasm—may facilitate cooperation. For example, a shy 4-year-old girl refused to make eye contact or to respond verbally to direct questions. "How old are you?" was finally answered nonverbally, with four fingers held up. "You're 4!" said the examiner, "well, I'm 6½!". "No you're not!" exclaimed the child, laughing, and now ready to participate in the testing. Another reluctant young boy was amused when, after indicating his age (6) with fingers, he was asked "Are you married?" A 10-year-old diagnosed as an elective mute proved quite challenging. After 30 minutes of concerted attempts to obtain a vocal response failed, the child was asked his age. No response. He was then asked to indicate his age by holding up fingers. No response. Then, the examiner said softly, "If you're 10 years old, blink twice." He struggled not to blink but, of course, could not sustain staring. He laughed so hard that he relinquished control to the examiner and cooperated fully for the full test session.

Rest breaks may be utilized productively when a child produces minimal effort. It is inadvisable to allow a young child to see the parent during a break, the danger being that the child will not freely return to the testing room. A break as simple as standing up, exploring the testing room, or engaging in more active calisthenics diverts attention from structured tasks. Simultaneous assessment of coordination, gross motor control, and cooperative play is then possible. In instances where many breaks are necessary (as is often the case with very young children), informing the child that "after two more short tasks, we will take another break" may be sufficient stimulus to improve motivation.

A break is often helpful in reaffirming a child's willingness to proceed further. However, the child's experiences immediately preceding a break should be positive and warmly encouraging, allowing the child to reestablish confidence for the next portion. For example, the examiner should save and administer an easy task to the child just before a break, to ensure that the child leaves with good feelings about what has been accomplished.

A brief break for snack consumption may be useful, but food reinforcements should never be used unless prior approval from the physician or parent is obtained. Allergies and special diet restrictions make it difficult to rely on this type of reinforcement.

Hypoactivity, Overactivity, and Distractibility

It is expected that a child will decrease or increase activity during testing. The requirement for focused participation for an extended period of time in activities not of the child's choosing may result in overt physical indicators of discomfort—for instance, slumping in a chair, fidgeting, or out-of-seat behavior. These behaviors are best stopped only when they have the potential to exert a negative influence on the results.

A listless or lethargic child is particularly challenging. Periods of lethargy may be countered with requests for increased activity. For example, a young child who fails to respond to the usual verbal request to stand and stretch may respond to requests of Simple Simon: "Simple Simon says stand up . . . jump two times . . . show me your nose . . . elbow . . . left hand . . . my right elbow," and so on.

Distractibility is often inevitable. The child's capacity for self-monitored sustained performance will fluctuate. In most instances this should not be viewed as pathological but as a natural reaction to testing demands. A child's relative ability to focus and attend to information conveyed through the varying modalities is of clinical interest. For example, is the child reluctant or excited about tasks with a predominant auditory/oral presentation versus nonverbal/visual material? Do tactual manipulative tasks result in a changed level of interest? Environmental modifications can reduce distractibility. For example, test equipment may be selectively introduced, piece by piece, and extraneous objects may be removed from view.

Self-paced tasks frequently present problems for children, especially for those who are active or have attentional deficits. Thus, a child may skip certain questions (or a whole section) of a test. It is helpful to redirect the child, provided that standardized test procedures are not violated. Even violating standardized procedures should be considered, however, when this will provide important clinical information about true capabilities. For example, the examiner may wish to extend time limits to gauge how effectively a child performs a timed task. Knowing that the child can complete the task when given additional time alters conclusions based on the assumption that the task is beyond the child's grasp.

A child described as "spacey," "inconsistent," or "often daydreaming" may have underlying neurological dysfunction—for instance, a previously unrecognized seizure disorder. The timing and duration of blank staring spells or brief episodes of drifting or altered consciousness should be recorded. The examiner should also note whether the child can respond during the altered state and how easily the child returns to full responsiveness. Testing should be delayed or postponed when postictal confusion or lethargy occur. The examiner must confirm whether the parent or teacher is aware of these occurrences and must ensure follow-up with a physician in instances where a seizure disorder is suspected.

Resistance and Aggression

Some resistance is a natural part of testing and is acceptable as long as it does not interfere with the evaluative process. Extreme resistance needs to be dealt with directly. Hints of the level of a child's resistance are initially derived from waiting-room observations and separation behavior—for instance, a young child clinging to parents. Children who are resistant to all or part of the testing may complain about a headache or stomachache, or may ask to go to the bathroom or to get a drink of water in hopes of receiving a pardon from testing, as described earlier. The examiner must decide whether the child's complaint presents a justifiable basis for interrupting or concluding testing.

When the examiner anticipates that a child will not work for the full planned time, the most relevant tests should be administered early. Alternatively, if a weak area of functioning is known, other functions may be assessed first in anticipation of a failure to complete full testing. For example, an adolescent who was known to be abusing drugs was evaluated primarily to determine how severely compromised her conceptual reasoning skills were. Her resistance to testing was extreme, and a full testing was not expected. Early tests administered steered clear of conceptual demands, briefly assessing sensory and motor functioning, language, and vigilance. Finally a mental shifting task was given—the Wisconsin Card Sorting Test. This proved especially problematic. She tried briefly but could never make the important and necessary shift in ideas. The young lady then softly but adamantly stated "I will not do these tests," stood up, and left the testing environment. By anticipating such a response and sampling much that was overtly nonthreatening, the examiner successfully acquired a sufficient database prior to her departure to confirm the integrity of other functions. The confirmation of her impaired reasoning capabilities was clarified by her failure on the conceptual shifting task and by the extreme discomfort she exhibited when she found herself unable to meet the test's demands.

Aggression is occasionally observed and often is effectively handled by extreme but pleasant firmness. Sometimes, a change in the physical environment suffices. For example, a boy became physically assertive and prevented testing from continuing. A simple rearrangement of the furniture enabled the examiner to reestablish control and permitted the child to cooperate once again. The child was confined in an armchair with his back against the wall; and the examining table was then pushed up to him, essentially locking him into a small space. The examiner then sat across from the table, with nearest access to the door.

An examiner increases structure inversely to a child's level of cooperation, with the most stringent structure being imposed when a child's behavior becomes unmanageable. Although active children often require considerable structure, they are often cooperative and testing may proceed without the initiation of specific techniques to reduce activity level. In other instances, however, an uncooperative or aggressive child may prod the examiner to consider actions likely to shape appropriate test-taking behavior. For example, a decision to remove a child temporarily from testing may be effective. This was the case for a young boy who began throwing test equipment at an examiner. A 10-minute "time-out" procedure was instituted, during which the child spat and wildly kicked at the examiner. Nonetheless, sufficient calm was restored after 10 minutes to permit resumption of testing.

Judicious environmental management is also necessary. One does not wish to overstimulate a child who may not settle down easily. A child with a history of violence may be provoked to antagonism by excessive prompting for better performance, while another child without such a history may continue to work diligently. For example, when pushed too far, a 16-year-old retarded girl broke the wallboard by banging her head against it; a 13-year-old girl angrily broke a pencil holder; and a frustrated 8-year-old boy tipped over the examining table. One must be careful in determining the specific techniques that are needed and those that will be most appropriate under a given set of individual circumstances.

A child's failure to respond to subtle cues for good behavior is unusual. Children who respond negatively to testing are likely to have histories replete with details of similar negative actions in the academic setting. The child's range of responses to the examiner as authority figure will provide insight into reactions the child may have to parents, teachers, and other adults. They may also be useful in understanding interactions with peers. Thus, the child's experience with the examiner may well mirror quite accurately any maladaptation within the child's usual social milieu.

Cursing, physical aggression, or other instances of overt defiance in the presence of an authority figure are rare occurrences. These actions are "red flags" that signal the need for further exploration of relevant personality factors, parent effectiveness, school placement acceptability, neuropsychological integrity, and/or emotional etiologic factors.

Unusual Behaviors

Certain behaviors are more unusual and infrequently noted. Their presence should lead to consideration of coexisting or alternative etiologies. Examples from clinical practice include (but are not limited to) extreme affection, sullen avoidance, premature termination of a testing session by the child in spite of the presence of an authority figure, mutism, abusive verbalization or actions, rocking or head-banging, auditory or visual hallucinations, echolalia, bizarre or confabulatory speech, and obsessive attachment to an object.

In summary, children express discomfort in a multitude of ways. They experience a natural incidence of fatigue over time that may be counteracted in part by judicious selection of test instruments and by provision of short rest breaks. Testing cannot be reliably continued until interfering issues are resolved. Having initially established a positive interaction, provided unconditional acceptance, explained the day's events, formulated expectations for behavior, and structured the situation to include acceptance of a certain level of nonresponse, the examiner has set the framework for dealing effectively with any negative behavior when it occurs.

CONCLUSION OF TESTING

The risk of losing a child's cooperation becomes great if the examiner administers a difficult test early in the session. It is often best to save a hard task for last. For example, the Tactual Performance Test (TPT) is a highly threatening test that requires the child to remain blindfolded for an extended period of time. Since children often want to terminate testing once the TPT is concluded, the test is best administered only after all other data have been collected.

If a child permits one last task, a final brief and easy item may be given at the very end. For younger children, it is an opportunity to experience success before the session concludes. It is highly desirable for a child to leave an evaluation feeling good about the effort expended. The final success culminates the experience with a sense of accomplishment.

All children appreciate acknowledgment of their diligence and sustained effort, even when the tests were hard. Thus, the examiner may say, "I'm so proud of you. You did such a special job, even when my tests seemed difficult." The examiner should also express appreciation for the child's cooperation by offering praise in the parents' presence. This is also a good time to let the parents know how hard it is for a child to stay seated and concentrate for such a long period of time, and how it would therefore be natural if their child seems more active or needs to release feelings through physical activity right after the evaluation. The examiner should point out that spontaneous activity level might well increase, and that some exaggerated reactions are to be expected. Some form of special recognition by parents of their child's cooperation is appropriate. Often a parent of an outpatient volunteers that a trip to a fast-food restaurant or a visit to someplace special is planned. The examiner should indicate that the child is deserving. Offering a little toy or sticker to the young child is a friendly gesture that is often appreciated; this final token should not be contingent on performance, but should be offered to all children of an appreciative age.

If the parent has been told in advance that a meeting to review results will take place at a future date, the conclusion of the testing session is likely to focus on the child—and rightly so. The parent often follows the examiner's pattern, knowing that the future consultation will provide an appropriate opportunity for the examiner to answer any concerns that initiated the evaluation. On occasion, it may be important to talk to the parent privately at the conclusion of the testing. It is a delicate matter to accomplish this consultation without upsetting the child, who may feel that the adults have joined in a conspiracy. Excusing oneself and the parent for a brief time in order to "get paperwork done, like an address, phone numbers" presents a rationale for the child to feel less threatened by the ensuing private conversation. Alternatively, asking the child to "trade places" at the conclusion of testing also permits time to be spent with the parent: "Now that I have had some time with you, let me have a little time with your mom to explain what the tests were like. I'll explain a little now and you can explain some more on the way home."

The parent must also feel comfortable about the examiner's ability to obtain their child's best effort. Parents are bound to be anxious after waiting for the testing to conclude, and they will expect some statement from the examiner— even if only a confirmation that all proceeded well. This will allay most parental concerns until the interpretive session is held. If the child concludes the evaluation with a comment that seems to indicate that full cooperation was achieved ("This was more fun than I thought it would be" or "These games were fun; I could do more"), the stage is set for a valuable and productive follow-up interpretive session.

In the best of situations, the child will leave the testing room smiling or at least content with the knowledge that the challenges presented were met well. The neuropsychologist will have obtained a valuable data set that illuminates strengths and weaknesses. The parent will feel confident that a valuable assessment of the child was performed. The medical staff will have access to data about brain–behavior functioning that are valuable in subsequent efforts to provide high-quality care to the child and family.

The purpose of all of these strategies is to increase examiner efficiency. Examiner efficiency results in shorter testing sessions and generally happier children, surprised at how much fun testing can be.

CLINICAL OBSERVATIONS

Critically important information may be obtained by clinical observation. It is surprising how often this information does not receive the full attention it deserves. The most complete neuropsychological evaluation is one in which the diversity of the clinical experience is evaluated together with quantitative and qualitative data obtained from the administration of standardized test instruments. This approach provides the most sensitive assessment of an individual. The ability to recognize subtle behavioral abnormality is a skill that sharpens with time and broadens the efficacy of the neuropsychologist in the neurodiagnostic and treatment/rehabilitative roles.

Waiting-Room Observations

The opportunity for observation exists even before formal assessment is underway. For the outpatient and mobile inpatient, the waiting room is a more realistic setting than the testing environment, and it more closely approximates the natural environment. The child's spontaneous actions in the waiting room may vastly differ from those observed later in the structured, one-to-one encounter. These incidental observations, coupled with observations made during formal testing, extend the range of behavioral impressions.

A child in a waiting room is generally experiencing at least mild anxiety, feeling pressure to "be good," and perhaps recognizing that the appointment is important enough to permit a school absence. Concerns discussed at home between family members may have been overheard, leading to a distorted understanding of the reason for the professional visit. A child's reactions may therefore provide insight about how the visit is perceived, about self-image, and about the child's response to structure and authority.

For example, waiting-room play may reveal aggressive actions, with shooting and war themes predominating as emotional tension about the encounter reaches the surface. Anger about being brought to the office may be clear in the physical distance between parent and child or by negative behavior that embarrasses the parent, who wants to make a good impression. Passive play may indicate contentment or a need for parent approval. The child may sit close to the parent, with eyes cast down, and seem shy or fearful about separating for the actual testing. Healthy acceptance is revealed by a mutually positive parent–child interaction that is warm and caring.

Support Staff Observations

Office support staff may offer valuable input about relationships. An observant receptionist, familiar with the comparable behavior of many other children, should be able to discern distinctive differences in the way a particular child and family behave in the waiting room. The receptionist is often "invisible" to the family, and thus able to gain an unique perspective. Assistance in interpreting nuances of interaction between the child and parents, between the child and siblings, and between parents may be offered by the receptionist/observer. Clinically valuable anecdotes about waiting-room behavior may reveal dynamics not perceived from a sampling of behavior taken in the structured testing environment or brief interview, such as parental methods of behavioral control. Differences in behavior between occasions when the examiner is present and occasions when the examiner is absent are always of great interest. For example, before the examiner appears, a parent may snap at the child to do everything the examiner asks or expect punishment later; then, when the examiner is actually present, the parent may sweetly chide the child to be good. Similarly, parents who cannot support one another may visibly reveal such feelings in the waiting room (by sitting separately and in stony silence, for example, or disagreeing openly about the need for the visit), but may hide these feelings in the presence of the professional. Cold, distant, or hostile interactions before "the doctor" arrives may be a clue to the presence of marital strain, perhaps resulting from differing perceptions about the child. If the neuropsychologist is made aware of such observations, they may be beneficially factored into the overall formulation of results and addressed in the interpretive session.

Patient Interaction with Others

The interactive style of a child vis-a-vis siblings or other children in the waiting room is of interest—for instance, the child's ability to socialize or inability to maintain control. The visit of a young teenager, whose initial waiting-room behavior (when he was the only child in the room) and neuropsychological performance were appropriate, serves as an example. The testing was conducted one-to-one in a small uncluttered testing room. The child was focused and attentive to every aspect of the testing. Successfully concluding what appeared to be an uneventful test session, the child returned to the waiting room, which was now inhabited by another child. No longer able to contain himself, he lunged at the waiting child, and the two almost came to blows before the secretary and the examiner could forcibly separate them. Notably, his mother sat reading a magazine, seemingly oblivious to the commotion. She made no effort to separate the children nor to admonish her son. For her, it was just one more incident in a long line of negative actions taken by her son that characterized much of his waking day. Her effectiveness as a parent in control had severely diminished over time, and her silent call for help could not have been more clear. Coupled with test data (which did not reveal a focus of neuropsychological impairment), the behavioral observations proved central to further exploration of what later proved to be a diagnosis of Attention Deficit Disorder with Hyperactivity, and appropriate therapeutic recommendations were made.

Interaction of Patient and Parent

Useful clinical information may be derived from observation of parent–child interactions. How they relate to each other at the start of testing, at lunch time or on breaks, and at the conclusion of testing provide interesting clinical data. The first statement a parent makes when the child returns to the waiting room may be especially revealing. Is it directed to the examiner or the child? For example, immediately asking "Did you pay attention to everything the doctor asked?" implies that the child may have difficulties in this area that have concerned the parents and perhaps constitute a source of contention between parent and child. There is also the implication, however, that the parent trusts the child to respond truthfully. Addressing the same question to the examiner sets a different tone—omitting the child from the communication, just when the comfort of a reassuring hug or welcome upon emerging from the testing room would have been most desirable. As in any interpersonal interaction, the non-verbal signals between a parent and child also offer insight into the dynamics of the relationship. Facial expression and gesture should be noted.

How the child responds to the idea of returning to the parent is also significant. Does the child evince worry or eagerness? If the child seeks assurance that the examiner will only speak well of the time spent together, this suggests that parental reward or punishment may be contingent on what the examiner says. For example, some parents promise their children a special lunch or treat in exchange for cooperation. While this is a common (and often effective) technique it may also reveal important information about the family's typical child-rearing strategies. Such techniques may also be carried to an extreme. Using the reinforcer as a "bribe" or using threats to elicit good behavior can be poor behavioral control methods when applied frequently in a parent's repertoire. A potential complication is that these strategies draw the neuropsychologist into the parent–child contract when the parent requests verification that good behavior was maintained. These predetermined contracts to exact good behavior affect the child's perception of the testing day and alter the child's relationship with the examiner.

Observations During Testing

Children often find it hard to state their concerns and fears openly, but they quickly reveal important information indirectly, through less obvious channels. Drawings may provide explicit information that the child cannot verbalize; puppet play may reveal hidden feelings; and informal conversation may contain references to factual details not previously available in the history nor elicited from the parents with direct questioning. Children, who are likely to be tuned in to any family difficulties, are typically unwilling or unable to convey freely what they know. Sometimes the request to "draw a family doing something" or to state "three wishes" permits preliminary exploration of these attitudes.

For example, a child was referred because his grades had plummeted, from mostly A's and B's to all C's and D's. He was the only child of an unemployed single parent, and his allowance had been stopped because of financial constraints. Thus, a valued symbol of increasing responsibility had been removed, and the child had grave concerns about the future. Neuropsychological test data did not reveal the suspected learning disability nor a clear neuropsychological basis for the decline in grades. Consequently, the supposition was that the decline likely had a primary emotional basis. With this suspicion in mind, the child was asked "If you could have any three wishes granted, what would you ask for?" He only asked for two wishes—"world peace" and an "advanced computer chip within a computer chip." He could not be convinced to express a third wish. When asked specifically to "make a wish for himself and not for the world," he replied once again "an advanced computer chip," unable to personalize his wish. The economic stresses were occurring simultaneously with the emergence of his school problems, and it became clear that he could not respond at a personal level. The precipitous decline in performance was not the result of unrecognized neuropsychological influences, but represented a reaction to recent environmental factors. The need for supportive psychotherapeutic intervention for the family was obvious, and the subsequent intervention had a positive outcome.

Another revealing example of the ability of a child to communicate indirectly follows. A child was asked to "Draw a Family Doing Something." As it did for the child in the preceding example, the neuropsychological profile appeared to be completely intact. Referral stressed extreme learning difficulties. The family appeared to have no serious emotional issues, nor was concern ever expressed in the course of history taking or by any professional with whom they had consulted. But the resultant detailed drawing revealed a family at war. Each family member was drawn present at a picnic but engaged in a ferocious food fight. The father threw meatballs at the mother, who fought back. The siblings hurled food and dishes at each other, and an airplane let loose bombs of food on top of all family members and pets, with one exception. Only the patient was drawn untouched, although present in the scene. The dynamics revealed in the drawing were later explored and confirmed in the interpretive session. When the parents were informed about their son's perception of their family life, they readily acknowledged that serious marital problems existed and had been present for a long time, and they revealed that a separation was imminent. They had mistakenly thought that their children were unaware of these stresses.

Sometimes children will verbalize how much they like the examiner, or what fun they are having, or how glad they are that they are taking these tests. These comments typically occur when the task at hand is perceived as quite difficult. The children are seeking reassurance and acceptance from the only adult figure at hand, and attempting to ingratiate themselves with the person judging them. Whether naively or intentionally, such comments are spoken at times that may identify areas of concern or cumulative feelings of distress that need to be addressed. Such comments should always be viewed in the context in which they occurred, as a sign of potential need for extra support and reassurance.

Until one's knowledge and experience are sufficiently broad, fortuitous clinical observations of signs and symptoms of dysfunction are likely to be missed. For example, a novice examiner giving an aphasia screening test memorized the test instructions perfectly, administered the test flawlessly, and—in the absence of overt language errors—concluded that there was no indication of impaired language function. Yet the child's incidental conversation contained subtle errors, including incorrect word retrieval ("store" for "stool"), speech hesitations, the beginning sound of an incorrect word almost stated fully but quickly self-corrected, and circumlocutory speech revealing the effort inherent in searching for a word. These errors are more likely to pass unnoticed to unskilled ears. The examiner's carefully written documentation of such verbal output is important for later review and analysis of behavior. Such language errors reveal the effort inherent in language production and should be explored further.

A child is often well aware of a problem, while parents do not always fully appreciate such self-perception. Because a child may attempt to hide a weakness, it is important to observe when attempts to evade a task occur. Children naturally shy away from or refuse to engage in activities that require use of a weaker skill. An attempt to deflect the examiner by engaging in actions that have proved successful in other settings, such as the classroom, may be made. For example, a young girl with a visuomotor deficit would begin to chatter about all sorts of family events whenever a drawing task was presented. Another, who had a suspected auditory–verbal processing disorder, placed her head down on the desk and claimed to be too tired to continue when a verbal learning test was presented.

The examiner's impressions undergo modification throughout the evaluation in response to direct observations. These help guide the process of test selection and behavior sampling. The general categories listed in Table 5–2 have proved to be useful to trainees, encouraging them to focus on a range of behaviors that may be observed reliably for every child. Trainees are encouraged to make notes for each area listed and to summarize their overall impressions at the conclusion of the evaluation.

Physical Appearance

The examiner should record information regarding the child's general physical appearance to aid in personal recollection later. Specific physical attributes or mannerisms may be forgotten without written cues—particularly when the examiner must evaluate a number of other patients within a brief span of time. Relevant attributes include height, body type, clothing, color and cut of hair, blemishes, birthmarks, scars, and other distinctive physical features. For exam-

Table 5-2　General Behavioral Observations

Behavioral Area	Observations
Physical appearance	
Activity level	
Motivation	
Executive function	
Motor control	
Language	
Nonverbal behavior	
Attention	
Social interaction	
Emotional maturity	
Examiner's reaction	

ple, "Rebecca was small for her age, unkempt and in a ripped shirt; fingernails were dirty; she held her head tilted when she had to look at the printed page (has she had a vision examination?), had a wonderful laugh and was quick to follow instructions; anticipated requests well, but almost cried during hard tests."

Activity Level

The examiner should observe what changes stimulate more or less activity, since a child's activity level normally fluctuates throughout testing. As a task becomes harder, some children fidget, but others become still. The examiner should note the child's response to test rules and how a requirement for self-monitoring affects activity and production. Instances of overactivity (for instance, the child is out of seat in a nonproductive way, grabbing for items in the room, dropping things, hanging over the chair, or getting up and moving about in the middle of a task) or hypoactivity (for instance, the child is slumped over, lethargic, slow to respond, or yawning) should be noted, along with their temporal relationship to tasks.

Motivation

The examiner should note the conditions that enhance motivation, when poor compliance is rectified by the application of one or more successful "tricks" from a repertoire of actions that have previously improved the motivation of other children (several of these have been discussed elsewhere in this chapter), and when motivation is sustained well.

Executive Function

The examiner should observe the child's ability to reason and plan. This entails making preliminary determinations about how literal or stimulus-bound the child may be or how adept the child is at developing alternative strategies. Were generalities and abstraction comprehended sufficiently on an informal basis, or were step-by-step instructions needed? The examiner can confirm clinical impressions of a child's independence of thinking with parents in the interpretive session. These observations will facilitate later communication with parents about day-to-day functioning and validate (in their estimation) the examiner's ability to see their child accurately.

Motor Control

The examiner should note lateral dominance, left–right confusion, and any bilaterality. Other relevant observations relate to gross motor activity, developmental age, gait and balance, and gross motor skill efficiency. These observation can then be compared with the history—for instance, acquisition of motor developmental milestones such as crawling, sitting alone, walking, and riding a bicycle. In connection with written parts of the test, the examiner should observe fine motor control (such as pencil grip), note the placement of paper when the child is writing (whether it is normal or rotated and awkward), note any inordinate need to anchor the paper with one hand in order to write smoothly with the other, and inspect the resultant letter formation and line quality in written productions.

Compensatory movements may be observed. For example, the child may move closer to the examiner in order to hear more accurately, may reach for the wall while walking in order to maintain balance, or may turn the head to compensate for hemispatial neglect.

The examiner should also note unusual reactions to touch or sudden movement. For example, one child had an exaggerated startle to the examiner's routine touch for sensory testing—a seizure-like state induced repeatedly by touch. It was then necessary to evaluate whether this behavior had a neurological basis and/or whether psychiatric issues were relevant.

Associated body movements may reflect neurological dysfunction or may be a nervous mannerism or habit. The examiner should document all unusual motor movements such as tics, twitches, and involuntary actions. Have these been cited by teachers as disturbing in the classroom? Finger or hand movements may signal neurological disease—for instance, the hand-washing movements associated with Rett syndrome, a rare disorder of unknown etiology that exclusively affects females and is associated with developmental stagnation and subsequent decline, after normal development for approximately the first year of life (Reiss et al. 1993; Walton 1985). Mouth movements such as chewing or licking may precede a seizure. The examiner should note motor overflow activity—as, for instance, when one hand or finger is engaged in a task, and the contralateral side produces similar activity.

Language

The examiner should screen language development initially from spontaneous conversation and later with formal instrumentation (note intonation, inflection, volume, vocabulary, and grammar). It is important to be attuned to speech hesitations or impediments, a stammer or stutter, missed or misperceived verbal instructions for short or lengthy commands, words restated that differ slightly from what was actually said, incorrect word retrieval or naming deficit, letter or number reversals, and reversed order of writing (right to left instead of left to right). Further tasks for the examiner include noting whether instructions are understood, recording differential responses to verbal and nonverbal instructions, confirming that results of a hearing test fell within normal limits, and noting irrelevancies or confabulations as possible indicators of psychiatric disorder or aphasia.

Certain speech characteristics may trigger recognition of a specific neuropsychological deficit. For example, monosyllabic speech may indicate anxiety about the test situation, may mask speech dysfunction, or may represent a specific subset of learning disability characterized by social-emotional impairment—for instance, Asperger syndrome.

Nonverbal Behavior

Body position may indicate the child's comfort level. The examiner should maintain eye contact with the child to observe whether the child is participating with enthusiasm, whether distractions are interfering with full cooperation, and (more rarely) whether transient loss of consciousness is occurring, as will be observed when petit mal staring episodes occur. The examiner should also confirm that the results of a vision test fell within normal limits, and should note the child's use of visual space. For example, a 10-year-old child suspected of having an auditory/verbal learning disability made reading word recognition errors due to missing the initial (left-sided) letter sounds at a high rate, had a head positional posture that favored the right side of space for drawing tasks, and drew on the right side of the page. Further investigation revealed a hemispatial neglect correlated with early right-hemisphere hemorrhagic insult. Simple prompting sufficed to ensure that full scanning of the page was accomplished. The possibility of visual neglect had been overlooked in initial consideration of the reasons for poor school performance. Indeed, the data did not support diagnosis of a language-based learning disability.

Attention

The examiner should note duration of attention span; circumstances that enhance or impair attention, vigilance, or sustained focus; any preferential modality (for example, auditory, visual, tactual, or kinesthetic); and any differences between early and late testing (for example, before and after lunch).

Social Interaction

The examiner should note the child's comprehension of nonverbal social cues and gestures, observe whether the child engages in socially inappropriate actions or verbalizations, and note the appropriateness of the child's sense of humor. Bizarre behaviors should be recorded. Certain neuropsychological profiles are associated with deficient social skill acquisition and impoverished gestural learning and interpretation—for instance, nonverbal learning disabilities. Such observations may highlight specific deficits not commonly identified because of the relative rarity of connecting such behavior to the neurological substrate necessary for normal development.

Emotional Maturity

The examiner should note the ease of separation from parent. Does the child retreat emotionally? Is emotional ability prominent? How are failure experiences handled?

Examiner's Reactions

The examiner's own feelings about the child should be noted, in order to understand better the reaction of others in the natural setting. Was the child a delight—someone teachers would adore—or did the child's actions become irritating? Could the child make serious attempts to manipulate the situation effectively to his or her own advantage? How much examiner control was required to continue testing? How likely is it that such structure could be provided in a natural setting? Is the child submissive or intimidated by authority or defiant?

Observations in the testing environment do have a direct correlation with the natural setting. Parents are sometimes suspicious of a teacher's motivations and impressions of their child. Finding corroborating clinical observations during formal assessment may allow for a more open and honest appraisal of the child's strengths and weaknesses. Determining that misperceptions exist due to a previously unexplained medical or neuropsychological deficit will facilitate the process of unifying parents and teachers on the child's behalf. For example, one teacher complained about a child's reluctance to respond to requests for oral class participation. The parents, in contrast, reported no problem at home and felt the teacher was making unreasonable demands. In the course of history taking, it was learned that the child watched quite a lot of television and was not responsive to questions unless voices were raised. The child also sat very close to the set, although a vision test was normal. The possibility of a subtle hearing loss had not been entertained, and formal testing did reveal a hearing loss.

CONCLUSION

The opportunity to hone skills that enable one to obtain the best sample of behavior in the pediatric age group is present whenever the professional interacts with a child. In the clinical setting, the lessons learned are regularly applied to reach conclusions that affect the care and treatment of a child. Thus, informal experiences must meld with formal evaluation. The pediatric clinical neuropsychologist may then apply theoretical knowledge and understanding and generate hypotheses based on the richness and diversity of behavior sampled within the clinical setting.

REFERENCES

Baron, I. S. 1987. The childhood presentation of social emotional learning disabilities: On the continuum of Asperger's syndrome. Paper presented at the Fifteenth Annual International Neuropsychological Society Meeting, Washington, D.C.

Benson, D. F., and Geschwind, N. 1970. Developmental Gerstmann syndrome. *Neurology* 20: 293–98.

Reiss, A. L.; Faruque, F.; Naidu, S.; Abrams, M.; Beaty, T.; Bryan, R. N.; and Moser, H. 1993. Neuroanatomy of Rett syndrome: A volumetric imaging study. *Annals of Neurology* 34: 227–34.

Walton, J. 1985. *Brain's Diseases of the Nervous System*, 9th ed. New York: Oxford University Press.

Wing, L. 1981. Asperger's syndrome: A clinical account. *Psychological Medicine* 11: 115–29.

6

The Interpretive Session and the Report

After the neuropsychological evaluation of the hospitalized child has been completed, it is important to communicate the results and recommendations clearly. This chapter reviews the two most effective ways to communicate what has been learned: the interpretive session and the written report.

THE INTERPRETIVE SESSION

Purpose

The interpretive session serves three important functions. First, it is a time to meet with parents to review and clarify information that has already been obtained during the pretesting clinical history-taking, during interviews with third parties, and during testing. Second, it is a time to acquire new information by judicious questioning and observation. For example, additional insight about familial interpersonal relationships, the dynamic contributions of individual family members, or the suspected influence of emotional issues may be gained. Third, it is a time to educate parents about the relationship between a medical condition and their child's behavior. Data are translated into meaningful, clear, concise, and practical recommendations, and the family is prepared for anticipated residual effects of an illness and/or treatment. In certain circumstances, to facilitate coordinated care, other professionals may be included in the interpretive session—physician, teacher, social worker, or therapist. Results are therefore communicated directly to the individuals working most closely with the child and family.

Information Review and Acquisition

After the evaluation, but before the interpretive meeting, preliminary hypotheses about a child's neuropsychological integrity are generated. During the interpretive session, notes about the child's behavior during the structured testing session may be compared to personal observations made by parents. Through review and clarification of historical information and the addition of newly obtained, supplemental data, initial impressions may be confirmed.

For example, a 12-year-old girl, admitted to the hospital for observation following a closed head injury, experienced difficulty on tests of executive functioning that help determine how well a child can plan, organize, shift ideas, and develop novel solutions in problem situations (Passler, Isaac & Hynd 1985; Welsh & Pennington 1988; Welsh, Pennington & Grossier 1991). The Wisconsin Card Sort test—a measure that was originally developed for use with adults, but that now has demonstrated applicability to children—was one of the poorly performed tests. By 10 years of age, a normal child's performance on this measure is indistinguishable from that of normal adults (Chelune & Baer 1986). In this case, the results were preliminarily interpreted, in context with other data, as indicating deficit secondary to trauma. In the interpretive session, the parents reported that their daughter was a mature young lady who had no history of organizational difficulty or of decision-making weakness. She was described as creative, competent, and adaptable in a variety of practical situations. Had any preexisting deficits in executive capacity been identified by the parents, a conclusion of impairment secondary to the injury might have been altered.

The interpretive session may also be a time when parental reports invalidate presumptive formulations, necessitating modification of a hypothesis. For example, an 11-year-old boy who suffered a lightning-strike injury and serious cognitive deficit made a remarkable recovery over a 2-year course (Baron, Haney & Shelburne 1985). The final neuropsychological data revealed a persistent deficit in his ability to perform oral arithmetic, possibly suggesting a residual area of cerebral dysfunction. All other previously impaired functions had cleared entirely. In the interpretive session, the persistence of this one abnormality was mentioned. The parent shrugged, remarking that her son always had a problem with math; thus, this problem preceded the lightning strike.

Sometimes the interpretive session elicits previously omitted information that may be highly relevant to the presenting complaint. For example, a 13-year-old girl was evaluated because of complaints that poor memory and inattentiveness were affecting her school performance deleteriously. The medical history obtained by questionnaire and personal interview was noncontributory for any significant developmental problems, illness, or trauma. There was no family history of learning difficulty. The neuropsychological profile was perplexing. Rather than the anticipated profile of a specific learning disability, the data revealed a clear focus of dysfunction implicating posterior left cerebral regions maximally and a milder focus of dysfunction implicating a confined region of the right cerebral hemisphere. Analyses strongly suggested that these data represented residua of a closed head injury. On the questionnaire and in direct interview, however, the parents had asserted that the girl had never suffered a head injury. The data and their implication were nonetheless explained in the interpretive session. Only at that stage in the process did the parents finally recall an incident they had long suppressed, expressing amazement at their omission of this highly relevant accident. Their daughter had fallen down a flight of stairs 7 years earlier, suffered a closed head injury with loss of consciousness, and was hospitalized, but never required surgery. They neglected to mention this to their current pediatrician or to the referring pediatric neurologist. In this instance, a distinct neuropsychological profile led to further questioning about the history, which then stimulated recall of the relevant incident.

On occasion, a child's behavior or idiosyncrasy may appear clinically valuable but may lose significance once the interpretive session is held. Initially worrisome features of the child's behavior may be of less concern when also observed in a parent or reported in a sibling. For example, one may observe an unusual vocal quality or somewhat odd facial feature that, alone or in the context of other findings, raises concern about neurological abnormality. However, the voice pattern or physiognomic characteristic may be equally apparent in the child's parent. For instance, parent and child may exhibit similar difficulty making eye contact, raising questions about social-emotional skill development and the weight of genetic predisposition versus learned behavior. A parent may spell simple words incorrectly (perhaps noted on the intake questionnaire), stimulating questions about poor educational background or inherited learning disabilities. A parent may choose incorrect grammatical constructions that also characterized the child's seemingly poor verbal expression, perhaps indicating imitative style and not central nervous system dysfunction in the child. A parent and child may both speak in a monotone, with any neurological influence still to be decided. In fact, a child's individual characteristics may no longer appear singularly abnormal when considered in the context of immediate family members.

Parent Education

An educational framework may be established in the interpretive session. Data that clarify a child's adaptation to systemic or central nervous system disorder have been collected. These data may then enable constructive feedback, to introduce concepts of cognition, development, and brain–behavior relationships to the parents. It becomes a time to help parents make the intellectual and emotional adjustments necessary to enable them to take a positive sequence of steps for their child's benefit. To serve as effective advocates, parents must learn about the impact of a specific illness or injury on their child's behavior.

Beginning the Interpretive Session

At the beginning of the interpretive session, it is helpful to ask parents to explain why the neuropsychological evaluation was requested and what their expectations are. For example: "I have seen Cara's medical records, and I have spoken to your physician. However, it will be very helpful to me if you tell me in your own words why you think I have been asked to see your child and what you hope to learn from this evaluation." The response may clarify their understanding about the child's illness, how this illness or condition affects their child's brain function, and their perceptions of their child's strengths and weaknesses. The responses may also help define expectations for and (importantly) limitations of the information you are able to provide. For example, misguided impressions may be apparent when parents state that their primary interest is that the neuropsychologist assist in prescribing drugs, or when parents indicate a belief that these data will help determine whether their child will make a full recovery from an illness.

During the Interpretive Session

As the neuropsychologist guides and teaches parents in the interpretive session, parents begin to integrate information that will enable them to educate others who play an important role in their child's daily life—school personnel, therapists, other family members. Educating parents prepares them for the important role they will later assume as advocates. In this role, they must secure and enact modifications that ease the ill or injured child's adaptation to day-to-day demands and hasten adaptive reentry into the normal environment.

Parents frequently focus on their child's level of general intelligence, on the child's potential for success in a regular school curriculum, on what (if any) behavioral problems they should expect, and on whether there will be a full cognitive recovery. Without guidance, they are not likely to appreciate the specific but perhaps subtle symptoms of brain dysfunction that may be compromising their child's performances. For example, a child's hemispatial neglect may be overlooked, but such a deficit may seriously interfere with the acquisition of information from a classroom chalkboard. Or, a 10-year-old's continued bafflement about her left and right sides may become a family joke, without any realization that such behavior has a neurological explanation. The neuropsychologist may play an important role in helping parents recognize deficit or delay consequent to medical illness and in helping them place it in proper perspective.

Elaboration and provision of specific examples of strengths and weaknesses are helpful. However, the clinician must be careful not to overwhelm parents with unnecessary detail or complex vocabulary. For example, one need not explain the intricacies of IQ assessment and the statistical properties of test instruments to parents whose primary concern is the quality of their child's survival and ultimate cognitive prognosis. But such elements may be appropriately detailed for parents who are concerned about school placement or who must choose between available school-based intervention options.

It is always important to answer parents' specific questions honestly and directly. Some parents, however, may not freely ask direct questions about brain dysfunction. Fear or anxiety may make parents reluctant to ask relevant questions. Attempts should be made to address unstated concerns that seem appropriate to the circumstances. For example, parents may not raise questions about the late-appearing effects of combination chemotherapy and radiation therapy that their child received six years earlier for childhood leukemia. That such treatment is associated with late cognitive sequelae (see Chapter 10) may nonetheless need to be mentioned. A physiological explanation may reassure parents who suspect primary emotional causation or who feel guilty about their own contribution because they have been overprotective. Further, parents who have not freely asked questions before or have not communicated openly with each other may find it reassuring finally to be able to compare experiences. When steered in a correct direction, they may be able to arrange appropriate interventions. Teachers may also need to be familiarized with treatment effects associated with a particular medical therapy, in order to appreciate better how these may affect classroom performance. Parents who avoid relevant factors, or who have not had an opportunity to ask direct questions and to receive honest answers, cannot be expected to advocate effectively for their child.

Sometimes parents express unrealistic concerns or ask for immediate answers to unanswerable questions. For example, parents of a child in kindergarten asked for a professional opinion about their child's college potential. A parent of a very bright teenager who had just been discovered to have serious organizational difficulties requested an opinion about whether the child would succeed in medical school. One must place the current evaluation in perspective for parents. The risks of making erroneous statements about a child's future functioning are great. Childhood testing does not allow for firm predictions about adult success or failure. Correction of a parent's overemphasis on test results may be made and placed in context with considerations of experience, motivation, and opportunity.

An intense interpersonal interaction may develop during the interpretive session. Parental feelings that have not been previously disclosed may become apparent. When a neuropsychologist validates fears about brain injury, emotions previously well hidden in communications with other professionals—or even with other family members—may finally surface. Additionally, frustrations may build over time as numerous medical professionals are consulted, each conveying complex and sometimes contradictory messages. Because neuropsychological consultation is often obtained in middle or late stages of the process of dealing with an illness, one of the neuropsychologist's roles may be to sort out these mixed messages for parents and place them in appropriate context.

The emotional tone of a session inevitably dictates how much specific information may profitably be discussed and how that information may best be communicated to the parent. Some parents communicate their feelings well, and as a result an open dialogue may be maintained. Others can not express their feelings spontaneously, while they struggle to accept the reality of an illness and its implications for their child's future. The neuropsychologist's preliminary plans for presenting a careful outline of factual results must change to accommodate the parents' understanding and acceptance of the implications of an illness. For example, parents of a child with acquired profound brain dysfunction secondary to the effects of a high-grade intrinsic brain tumor and radiation therapy expressed unrealistic concern about the likelihood of their child's future enrollment in a highly competitive private college. They effectively diverted conversation away from more immediate issues related to diagnosis, treatment, and survival. By focusing on the idealistic future, they were able to postpone a more realistic exploration of immediate rehabilitative options and strategies that would, in turn, force them to face the harder realities.

Interpretation with Allied Professionals Present

The neuropsychologist, in consultation with the parents, must decide whether to include allied professionals in or to exclude them from the interpretive session. When parents consent, other professionals who work with the child may be included in the interpretive session. Factual data and practical considerations may then be communicated to all parties involved in treatment at one time, minimizing the potential for distortions that otherwise might occur in the absence of first-hand communication.

Because this session may become emotionally charged, however (as described earlier), it may sometimes be inappropriate to include others. If the neuropsychologist anticipates that the presence of other professionals may inhibit the expression of feelings and personal questions or concerns, a session should be restricted to the parents and neuropsychologist. A second interpretive session may then be considered if others directly involved in the child's care request consultation.

Techniques for the Interpretive Session

Gaining the Parents' Acceptance

Early in the interpretive session parents may be reserved and anxious about the results, perhaps questioning the validity of the process. Resistance, whether overt or covert, is not unusual. Parents may find it difficult to acknowledge that someone who has spent a relatively brief period of time with their child is able to impart reliable personal details and valid conclusions. They often visibly relax once they feel assured that the neuropsychologist has an accurate perspective about their child. Therefore, gaining the parents' acceptance is crucial.

The neuropsychologist may begin by discussing the child in a personal way. Parents will be relieved to know that the examiner took care to make the child feel at ease. For instance, "I really enjoyed meeting Bob the other day. I enjoyed being with him, but it was obvious he needed a little more time than others his age to warm up to strangers. I just took it easy, explained what we were going to do and let him guide me in conversation. He really became excited when he talked about his soccer team. I could tell that his role on the team means a lot to him. That conversation really helped him relax, and then he cooperated beautifully for the rest of our time together"; or "Alex has a very interesting way about him. He seems so shy at first, but then he opens up completely. He has a wonderful sense of humor. I noticed he uses that humor even when things are hard, to help him through some difficult times."

It is important for the parents to realize that the neuropsychologist may have valid insights about their child's personality style. For example, the neuropsy-chologist might confirm that "your child has a way of withholding information until he is sure he will be right," or "she has an endearing but sly way of trying to get away with the least effort," or "his approach to novel situations is hesi-tant but he has the capabilities to go forward with a little support," or "her behavior during tests, as well as the actual test results, suggests she will retreat in the face of too many stimuli" [an observation the neuropsychologist may then suggest that the parents have also made when they took the child to a new shopping mall or to visit new family friends]. As the parent recognizes that the specialist indeed has an accurate personal perspective, the groundwork is pre-pared for successful discussion of formal data.

These statements are made possible by reviewing clinical impressions, notes about the child's interactive style, and any idiosyncratic features that typify the child's performance. Parental acceptance of the validity of the evaluative pro-cess is more likely when the neuropsychologist is able to interpret clinical data and to predict the child's responses in real-life situations. The neuropsycholo-gist has the capacity to learn valuable information about a child in a brief time. When parents understands this, they are more likely to accept the process and (therefore) its results. Trust then develops, and the parents tend to listen to results with confidence in the professional.

Comparing Parents' Attitudes

It is simplistic (and incorrect) to assume that both parents have parallel impres-sions of their child and similar goals and expectations. When both parents are present in the interpretive session, differences in their attitudes toward their child's illness or injury may be discerned. For example, both parents may share a similar perspective about education but remain at odds over the best method to ensure academic attainment. Or one parent may deny the existence of any brain-related problems, while the other acknowledges the full implications of how a disease has affected the child's capabilities and self-image.

Verbal and nonverbal interactions between parents may be quite revealing. Verbal statements by each parent may be contradictory, may reveal overt dis-agreement, or may directly place blame on the partner rather than reflect a concordance of view. For example, one couple attributed the basis for their child's behavioral problem to quite different causes, and thus had disparate impressions about the role of praise and punishment. The nonworking parent spent more daily time with the child, had more occasion to observe the effects of the suspected deficit, and therefore rightly attributed greater emphasis to the problem's constitutional basis. The working parent, who spent relatively lim-ited time with the child, was unwilling or unable to acknowledge a true physio-logic basis for the problem and instead faulted the spouse's supposedly ineffec-tual child-rearing practices. A detailed presentation of factual information, together with examples of how the same deficit would affect personal perfor-mance in the work setting, enabled the working parent to better appreciate his son's struggle. It was then possible for the resistant parent to accept that the child was not merely willfully disobedient or in need of firmer punishment tactics. Once the existence of a neuropsychological basis for the behavior was finally acknowledged, the parents could begin to work together in their son's best interests. Recognition of the parents' difference in opinion enabled the neuropsychologist to correct false impressions and to elaborate on the actual situation to ensure complete understanding.

Nonverbal indications of discordant thinking may also exist. Tension may be reflected in actions rather than words, such as angry glances between the couple or physical distancing in their seating. Facial expressions and body language may assist the neuropsychologist in gauging a parent's comprehension, to determine when further elaboration is needed. Slight gestures of discomfort, tensing of muscles, or clouding or confusion expressed through eye contact may indicate that important information has been missed or that a line of reasoning has not been followed.

Practical examples ensure that parents understand an interpretation. For example, a 19-year-old girl experiencing serious learning problems several years after the rupture and repair of a right cerebral aneurysm was found to have problems in visuoperceptual organization, a significantly lowered performance IQ, and markedly impaired novel visual learning in the context of preserved verbal learning. The initial terminology used proved too complex, and the parents' discomfort was apparent as they looked away and shifted uncomfortably in their chairs. By shifting the conversation to examples of how such weaknesses would likely be expressed day-to-day in the academic setting, the neuropsychologist was able to reach the parents and to convey to them the practical implications of the data. The neuropsychologist suggested that their daughter might have difficulty interpreting graphs, charts, and figures, and might experience increased frustration in geography and geometry classes, but that she probably would enjoy history and literature more. All were confirmed as accurate statements. The neuropsychologist then explained the correlation between nonverbal processing and right cerebral regions and between verbal processing and left cerebral regions. The linking of test data, simple brain function lessons, and real-life experiences enabled the parents to understand their child's struggle better. Their daughter had indeed experienced such problems at school, but the reasons were now more clear and the parents were better able to assist her. Their body language was observed to change positively, along with their comprehension.

The interpretive session becomes a time to convey information about the child's brain functioning, to encourage open discourse, and to reinforce the lessons of brain–behavior functioning that parents must learn in order to assist the child. It quickly becomes obvious in parent consultations that couples are not always mutually supportive. However, patterns that have developed over time may be modified or set on a more positive course.

Communicating Results Simply

The neuropsychologist should communicate what is known in a well-integrated presentation. Much information needs to be communicated in a relatively brief time. Even when greater time is allotted for an interpretation, there is a limit to how much can be understood and retained during the first presentation. Too much information will confuse and overwhelm any parent. The specialist should plan on making sure that two or three main points are related and understood, with specific treatment recommendations and habilitative alternatives considered in detail.

Using Restatement

Having parents restate information in their own words is a valuable technique that allows the neuropsychologist to gauge their level of understanding, pinpoint information they may have missed, and identify differences in comprehension between them. For example, the mother of a boy with mildly impaired verbal learning appeared to understand the results well. When her husband was asked to restate the issues she had just described, however, he sought advice about appropriate punishment for failure to complete homework and for continuing low grades. His response highlighted a fundamental difference in understanding and attitude between the two parents. The father had remained silent but seemingly attentive while the neuropsychologist described the nature of his child's learning problems, while his spouse raised questions, and while the neuropsychologist outlined a sequenced series of remedial steps and educational options. But when his silence persisted and he was prodded for his opinions, his failure to appreciate fully the genuine reason for his child's school difficulties was revealed, as was the ongoing disagreement between the parents about how and when to impose disciplinary action.

Providing Examples of Strengths and Weaknesses

Focus on a deficit should never be permitted to overwhelm the balanced presentation of strength and weakness. The neuropsychologist generally has an opportunity to convey good news as well as to confirm deficiencies. The professional must not lose sight of the relative strengths that will carry the child through difficult times and serve as the means for recovery and rehabilitation. The endeavor to balance functions that are preserved against abilities that appear to be disrupted is commendable, but not easily accomplished. It is easy to forget the good points when one is concerned with presenting a deficit profile in a limited period of time. By emphasizing strengths, the neuropsychologist may enable the parent of a child with a neurological condition to experience relief that the child's performances are not as globally impaired as may have been feared. A presentation of strengths prior to a description of weaknesses bolsters the parents' ability to maintain perspective about which abilities are preserved and which require intervention.

The parent of a child who has a nonneurological medical problem may be especially unprepared for news of impaired brain function. A parent may have been unaware that brain dysfunction was a potential consequence of an illness and/or treatment. In such cases, the detection of any deficit at all may evoke subtle to extreme reactions that cannot be anticipated fully. By providing a balanced description of preserved and dysfunctional abilities, the neuropsychologist may help parents better comprehend the consequences of an illness and the impact it has had on their child.

One helpful strategy is to provide examples of daily activities at which the child may be predicted to possess competence or disability, as the formal results are discussed. For example, "I want to make these findings clear. We have talked about Barbara's difficulty in working with material that requires the mental manipulation of numbers, even though we know she can understand logical arithmetic concepts. You may have noticed this problem when she has taken courses at school that depended largely on oral arithmetic, when she has had to work without a paper and pencil, or when she has been shopping and has had to figure out whether she received the correct change. These situations all require her to respond in a way that she clearly has more trouble with than others her age. You may also have noticed that she finds math easier if she is allowed to use a calculator or if she writes her numbers down. She's probably right when she says that she just can't do math in her head and that studying doesn't help. There really is a good, neuropsychological reason why she has been experiencing so much trouble. And there are ways we can help her do better."

Parents may also be encouraged to relate actual anecdotal experiences that highlight their child's adaptation or that reflect the disruption consequent to a medical condition. The neuropsychologist may then relate the test data to these examples.

Encouraging Questions

To facilitate clear communication, the neuropsychologist should encourage interruptions and answer all questions which may arise during an interpretive session. Since the specialist can adjust emphasis in direct response to the level of the parents' comprehension, questions are a means of understanding how well the message has been communicated. Too often, parents feel that physicians involved in their child's care have given them too little time for asking questions. Parents may even look at their watch during an interpretive session and ask if they have to go now, since they are used to being rushed. It may be important to extend the length of an interpretive session, to allow parents extra time to comprehend the main points raised during it.

Defining Terminology

It may be necessary to introduce new terminology and unfamiliar concepts in the interpretive session. Common sense dictates that one should avoid technical jargon in favor of simple language to promote optimal understanding. Vocabulary that is too complex, or information that is presented too quickly, may leave parents bewildered. Yet parents may be reluctant to acknowledge their misunderstanding or misperception.

Definition and clarification with examples are especially useful. Concepts widely used in popularized form by the lay person may not be understood in their specialized form. For example, one cannot assume that college educated parents understand basic Intelligence Quotient concepts. Parents may assume that an IQ test allows for direct hypotheses about brain function and therefore provides a sufficient measure of the future success or failure their child will experience. Parents may believe that the IQ score represents a critical determinant of their child's future. It is then incumbent on the neuropsychologist to highlight the full range of clinical data obtained and to dispute the decisiveness of this one global score taken out of context.

It may also be important to emphasize to the parent that one score or one test does not generally define a deficit. It may be possible to explain how a profile emerges based on behavioral observations and results from many different tests. The neuropsychologist should reinforce, as necessary, the notion that any one test result often depends on a number of factors operating simultaneously. The profile helps determine which factors are most relevant to understanding a child's quality of response.

Encouraging Participation

As noted earlier, it is important to draw a silent parent into the discussion, to ensure that there is parallel comprehension. If one parent dominates the session, the neuropsychologist should actively prompt the silent parent for comments and should listen carefully to that parent's expressed understanding of the results and attitude toward the recommendations. This will permit the specialist to confirm that the parents' impressions are accurate, that the basis for a plan of action is shared, and that a positive foundation for further discussion between the parents exists.

Participation may also promote clearer interpretation. An implication about family dynamics may seem less threatening if the parent states the importance of the test result before the neuropsychologist does. For example, a 13-year-old boy was asked to "draw a family doing something"—a kinetic family drawing task that is a useful screening measure. The family was drawn at the beach. Mother, patient, and sister were drawn playing together in the sand. Father was drawn lying on his back, under a big umbrella, away from other family members. The umbrella shaded his face. The father was encouraged to interpret the picture. He nodded and said that his son perceived him as "not always available." He volunteered that his son might sense a need to be with him more, and that he knew he had not been as close to his son as his child obviously would have liked. Thus, the parent, and not the neuropsychologist, introduced a sensitive topic about family relationships and the interpretation was strengthened by the parent's involvement.

Parents often feel inadequately prepared to explain test results to their children. Since explanations are immensely helpful in strengthening channels of communication between parent and child, they are worth encouraging. Parents may be guided about appropriate terminology and examples that the child can comprehend; and through role playing, the child's flaws in comprehension may be amended. This technique encourages parents to be open and direct with their child about why the evaluation was undertaken and what was learned, and it may have a lasting influence after the parents have left the office.

Interpreting to the Child

In general, interpretations to the child are not routine, but they may be considered when the child is capable of understanding the results given. In some instances, an interpretive session with the child is important. Wheelchair-bound children with spina bifida who are approaching the years of sexual development may have questions about modesty that they do not want to discuss with a parent. A child with newly diagnosed partial complex seizure disorder may be teased by friends and need education about seizure disorders and guidance about how to handle peer relationships.

An interpretive session may be held with the child directly or it may be held with the child and parents together. Having the child attend an interpretive session has several advantages: the child is part of the interpretive process from the beginning and thus is unlikely to feel that secrets are being withheld from him or her; the child can ask questions directly, have misperceptions corrected, and have accurate perceptions verified; the child gets to hear an opinion from an objective party who is not burdened by parent–child conflicts or parental contradictions; and the neuropsychologist can stress good points directly to the child, rather than relying on the parents to communicate these strengths, when they are likely to be preoccupied with the child's problems.

In several situations, however, one may elect not to include a child in the interpretive session: the child may not be sufficiently emotionally mature to understand and integrate complex information without distortion; the child may not be intellectually capable of appreciating the results; there may be a risk of upsetting the child, even though parents may want the neuropsychologist to provide a direct interpretation to the child; the information may be sufficiently serious to warrant exclusion because the prognosis is dire; the child may have been an unwilling participant in this process all along, the additional visit necessitated by inclusion would probably be met with further resentment; the parents may need time to incorporate the information before deciding how to involve the child in the process; the presence of the child may hinder the parents' ability to raise questions freely and to expose their concerns and emotions; or the neuropsychologist may suspect abuse of the child and may wish to explore these suspicions further.

Obviously, it is possible to work out special compromise arrangements. The neuropsychologist may conduct two separate interpretive sessions—one for the parents, and one including the child. Or the parents may meet with the neuropsychologist at the beginning of the session, and the child may be called in later in the session. In the latter situation, it is often useful to ask the parents to communicate directly to their child what they have just learned. The information conveyed can be carefully monitored by the neuropsychologist. This approach allows the parent and child to communicate freely, as they would normally discuss important issues.

Summary

Parents may gain greater useful knowledge about their child as a result of the interpretive session. Concurrently, they learn more about how and why they have responded to their child as they have. The information gleaned from a neuropsychological evaluation may well alter parents' perceptions and broaden their understanding of their child so productively that the process constitutes a highly valuable intervention, independent of any other formal procedure.

REPORT PREPARATION

The written report is often the means by which the neuropsychologist communicates with others involved in caring for the child. It draws together all relevant observations into a useful clinical analysis of the child's neurobehavioral functioning. The report should be written soon after the interpretive session, while recommendations formulated in light of facts revealed in the conference are still fresh. The report remains a part of the child's permanent medical and psychological records and will influence decisions that affect the child's future. Conclusions must be well-documented. If not properly prepared, a neuropsychological report can lead to misperceptions and, at the extreme, to improper care and bad decision-making.

Clarity in Report Writing: Simplifying the Complex

In most situations, a single written report serves as a data summary for various readers who have different degrees of medical and psychological sophistication. Therefore, one must take care to present the data and their interpretation clearly. Because specialists in one discipline may find the terminology of another discipline puzzling, the language selected should be chosen with care. A neuropsychological report should succinctly but fully summarize what has been learned, and should do so in a comprehensible way. It is unfortunate when an interested reader dismisses a report as unhelpful. All too often, however, parents, school personnel, medical staff, or others involved in caring for the child characterize the written report as too confusing, too wordy, too full of jargon, or insufficiently detailed about recommendations. A number of actions may be taken to avoid these criticisms.

Defining Medical or Neuropsychological Terminology in Lay Terms

By the time a child is referred for neuropsychological evaluation, other psychological or medical evaluations have often been completed. Neuropsychological dysfunction may be known or suspected from these earlier data. For example, consultation may be requested because a child demonstrates behavioral deficits following a known head trauma. Or referral may be requested because all available clinical and neurodiagnostic data have not revealed any basis for a parent's observations of forgetfulness and attentional variability that purportedly began after the child suffered a mild head injury. In this latter case, the consultation is requested when a deficit is suspected but not confirmed. It is incumbent on the neuropsychologist to integrate these previous data with newly acquired neuropsychological results, and to present conclusions in a "reader-friendly" report in which technical language is minimized.

Using Standard Scores

One way to highlight strengths and weaknesses and to compare results of different tests is to use standard scores. Medical staff are generally knowledgeable about conversions of raw data into standard measurement units. Parents and school personnel may also have some familiarity with these concepts, since (for example) results of group tests administered through the schools are converted into standard scores. The reader of a report may therefore more easily understand the significance of a child's weakness when a conversion is employed. For example, one may write "Amy's verbal IQ falls at the 95th percentile, and her recall score for new verbal information falls at the 92nd percentile—essentially equal and excellent performances. However, her recall score for new visual information was considerably lower, falling only at the 25th percentile." The reader of the report can readily appreciate the differences in rank achieved by the child for tasks of different types—that is, verbal in contrast to visual modality, in this instance.

Not all data, however, may be interpreted by conversion into standard scores or into percentiles. The significance of specific errors or of individual scores that are untranslatable may require particular focus in a report to ensure that it is not overlooked. For example, one may write "David had a tendency to repeat words on a controlled word association test of one minute's duration—a measure of verbal fluency that tests the person's ability to rapidly retrieve on command single words that begin with the same letter. This tendency to repeat (or perseverate) is unusual for a 13-year-old. This behavior was observed in combination with difficulty in planning strategy on a maze task, impairment in a test of the ability to switch ideas, poor gross motor tapping speed with both right and left upper extremities, and poor ability in replicating a sequence of three hand movements. Such a pattern suggests that there may be impairment of the regions of the brain that are particularly involved in the planning and regulation of activity, and in the ability to initiate and inhibit action successfully. These results also correlate with clinical reports by David's parents that he often appears confused when he is asked to follow instructions and with reports by his teachers that he is often disorganized."

Including All Essential Points Discussed
in the Interpretive Session

Once the interpretive session is over, parents may forget some essential information, even if the neuropsychologist has succeeded in keeping information limited to a few central points. For parents, the report is their reminder. It summarizes the results of the neuropsychologist's time with child and the conclusions jointly reached by the neuropsychologist and the parents about appropriate courses of action to take in the child's best interest. It is extremely helpful to summarize these conclusions in writing in essentially the same terms that were used to formulate them orally.

The report conclusions should include six essential points:

1. Whether evidence of abnormality existed.
2. Which data appeared to be correlated with brain dysfunction.
3. Which functional systems of the brain these data implicate.
4. Which abilities appear to have been preserved as strengths.
5. How the child may demonstrate deficit in practical situations.
6. What options for enacting a therapeutic intervention may exist.

Parents tend to rely on this written record for additional information that eluded them once the interpretive session came to a close. Moreover (and importantly), they may require specific details in the future when interval change must be assessed.

Providing Real-life Examples That Reflect Brain Dysfunction

A written report may serve as a reminder of the relationship between the child's behavior in real-life situations and the effects of brain dysfunction. For instance, a child may show personality changes after a head injury, such as increased aggressiveness, irritability, and crying spells. Once the child is discharged from the hospital, episodes of anger in response to frustration with school demands may arise in the classroom. This frustration, and difficulties in regulating emotional responses as a direct consequence of the recent head injury, may jeopardize the child's classroom performance, even though no visible signs of the injury remain. Realistic examples in a report may be used as examples of what to expect in a natural environment once the child is no longer within the imposed structure of the medical setting.

Reaching a Variety of Readers

A report may be read by a disparate group of individuals, each with a different role in the care of the child. A physician, parent, or teacher may be drawn to different sections of a report, depending on their respective interests. Each may apply a different baseline of experience in understanding what they read. Variations in how one communicates the data are possible. For example, one may write an alternative report in the form of a letter to the parents. A child may also wish to read the report, but may have difficulty grasping the descriptions of strengths and weaknesses and understanding how they relate to personal situations. A separate letter may be written for this purpose. However, a single format is typically the most space- and time-efficient way to communicate data, neuropsychological conclusions, and recommendations. Consideration of the needs of various readers is possible even within a single report.

Writing for the Physician

In most cases, a physician has initiated the referral to answer specific questions that arose in the care of the child. The neuropsychological tests were selected with those questions in mind and were modified in the test session based on the child's responses. One focus of the written report is to address the reason for referral as stated by the person coordinating medical care.

It is often useful to include a paragraph in the summary of the report headed "Neurological Implications." This technical paragraph is written specifically for the physician, contains medical terminology, and summarizes assumptions about neuroanatomic correlations. The paragraph's significance and the substance of its contents may be clarified for parents in their conference time with the neuropsychologist.

Conclusions about the possibility of residual neurobehavioral impairment following a closed head injury, the likelihood of a slowly progressive deterioration in a child who has a mild degree of hydrocephalus secondary to a partially obstructive mass, the presence of cerebral impairment for the oncology patient who received central nervous system prophylactic chemotherapy several years ago, the correlation of neuropsychological data with the identification of abnormalities visualized with neurodiagnostic imaging techniques, and the issue of permanence versus transience of the symptoms for a wide variety of disorders may all be successfully discussed and summarized within this section of the report.

Some information may have to be communicated to a physician informally—for instance, when tentative conclusions are reached but confirmation has been insufficient to warrant its inclusion in a permanent record. An accompanying letter may serve this purpose nicely. For example, the clinician may have inferred that there is extreme tension in the parental home and may suspect that some of the patient's response to treatment may be related to problems in the home. A cover letter allows the neuropsychologist to communicate such impressions when some question still exists as to their validity.

Writing for the Parent

The interpretive session offers the specialist an opportunity to explain the neuropsychological process carefully and directly to the parents; the written report serves as the formal explanation of that discussion. As noted earlier, a child's strengths often receive less conference time than do the child's weaknesses. Parents naturally focus on deficits, wanting to understand them better and seeking advice about opportunities for remediation. The written report allows for an elaboration on the observed strengths, as well as for a clear restatement of the documented deficits.

Whereas the "Neurological Implications" section may be written primarily for the medical staff, a summary paragraph labeled "Neuropsychological Implications" may be written for all readers. This portion of the report usefully summarizes issues of brain–behavior relationships and specifies recommendations. It captures the focus of the interpretive session, highlights all main points, and elaborates them with recommendations for useful and practical steps to take in the child's best interest. Parents may be advised to refer to this paragraph when they wish to review the oral conference summary.

It may be desirable to follow up on one's recommendations, monitoring the success of an intervention program, recommending modifications of strategies that prove ineffective, and tracking progress and rate of maturation. This paragraph thus serves another reader, as well—the neuropsychologist reading the report sometime in the future.

Writing for the School

In the absence of school personnel at the interpretive session, a written report becomes central to bridging the gap between teacher and parent. Neuropsychological data are insufficient if they do not lead to useful interpretations of academic performance. An explanation or likely cause of a child's academic weaknesses may give a teacher a new perspective on a child. For example, even the best of teachers often tells a child "You could do better if you just tried harder." Sometimes, this is just not true. No matter how hard a child with a neurological deficit may try, the efforts may not be rewarded by greatly improved performance. In such a case, admonitions for more effort may only increase the child's emotional distress. A written explanation of why a child may not be succeeding may solve a teacher's dilemma of deciding how far to push a child. The report may also serve as a formal statement justifying the need for supplemental help. It may provide a stimulus for the school to provide modifications in the curriculum that will bolster weaker skills and reinforce stronger abilities. A more positive interactive relationship may be expected to develop between parent and teacher once these data are communicated to all parties.

The school may receive a copy of the report, with the parents' written permission. The neuropsychologist should offer to discuss the findings with school personnel directly, either by phone or in direct consultation. In some cases, a report may not appear to address a teacher's particular concerns or may receive less attention than it deserves because the teacher perceives it as complex and overwhelming. Parents should also take the opportunity to discuss the link between obtained test performance and observed academic performance directly with the school, using the report as a resource.

Recommendations may be included in the report to assist school personnel in identifying resources within their system that may benefit the child. When possible, the report should clearly specify a child's optimal learning style, caution against pressing a child in areas of identified weakness, and suggest compensatory actions that draw on the child's strengths.

Establishing and maintaining open channels of communication with the school may also be necessary to monitor the success of medical (for example, drug) or psychological (for example, behavioral modification) interventions, placement changes or deferments, alternate courses, remedial learning techniques, or tutorial or other resource services. Recommendations for the school are most helpful when they are specific, realistic, and neither already incorporated nor already tried and rejected. Be sure to specify which beneficial interventions the school has already implemented and which should be supported.

A written report should help parents initiate dialogue with the school about the consequences of neurological dysfunction. Parents may be encouraged to take the report directly to the school for a conference. More personalized attention to the child's situation may result from a direct meeting between parents and teachers. The teacher's questions may now be answered by parents who are more informed and better prepared to serve as the child's advocates.

Writing for the Child

Some children may respond well to their own special written note. One special touch that may be personally satisfying to a child is a personal letter that summarizes the test results in very simple language and highlights all the good capabilities observed. The letter should be written to the child's level of comprehension. If the child has been discharged from the hospital, it may be mailed directly to the child's home. A personal letter is often appreciated.

The letter may address the child's own special concerns, which may differ from those of the parents. For example, a child may express worry about suffering partial brain injury. A letter may provide a means to address such concerns and to offer the child comfort. A personal letter may also remind the child of the need to take personal responsibility for overcoming obstacles. It may also provide a way to reinforce messages that will come from the parents, lending credence to interpretations made by the parents that the child might not otherwise fully believe.

Special supportive messages may be conveyed. For example, a child may need encouragement to let teachers know more often when schoolwork becomes too difficult, when it is hard to follow along in class, or when the pressure of working within certain time limits becomes too great. It may also be an opportunity to thank the child for working so hard under difficult circumstances.

Inpatient Notes

Before writing a note into the medical chart—or a full report—it is very helpful to read the existing chart carefully to review the impressions of other personnel. The nursing notes section often contains detailed behavioral observations about the inpatient. Observations made by these and other staff members may offer clues to relevant diagnostic considerations, including observations whose neuropsychological significance was missed by the staff. For example, notes about "immature speech" in a head-injured adolescent may be recorded without recognition of the presence of aphasia. These data may also provide an opportunity to highlight the neuropsychological significance of a patient's behavior for the staff and to educate the staff further about the significance of neuropsychological data.

An inpatient note in the progress section of a child's medical record may precede the formal written report, or it may be the only report of the neuropsychologist's contact with the child. Members of the staff may offer better care for a child when they appreciate the range of capabilities that are preserved and the capabilities that are compromised. It may also be an opportunity to suggest practical guidelines for nursing personnel and others involved in the moment-to-moment care of a child. For example, suggestions about how to interact with the child may be made for a child with receptive language problems. Such a child may need to have directions presented in brief, clear, concrete phrases. A distressed child may not process information well about a procedure that must be performed; fearing pain, the child may require emotional support and calming before being able to listen to lengthy instructions. A child with a visual processing impairment may baffle some staff members who are unaware of the child's particular medical problems. In this case, suggestions may be made that personnel present themselves and visual material on the side of space to which the child is more attentive, that they encourage the child to monitor the full visual range, and that they use verbal and visual prompts to ensure full scanning to the neglected side of space—for instance, a colorful margin or bright stickers to which the child must refer when reading. One may suggest positioning the child so that the busy hall or TV is not placed on the neglected side.

Format of the Written Report

There is no definitive model for writing a report. Considering the preceding recommendations, however, a general format can be outlined as follows.

Sample Outline

The written report is clearer when divided into separate sections. A report constructed on the following format is likely to be 5 to 7 typed pages long.

Neuropsychological Evaluation

Identifying Information

- Name
- Date of birth
- Date of testing
- Chronological age

Reason for Referral

- Referral source
- Diagnosis (confirmed or presumptive)
- Specific clinical complaints that necessitated this referral

Relevant History

- Contributory birth and developmental history
- Family and social history
- Contributory medical history
- Educational background and current placement
- Previous psychological and psychiatric history

- Previous psychological or neuropsychological evaluations
- Other supportive help received in the past

Tests Administered

- Should include all measures employed, either by category of function (with names specified in the text of the report) or by specific itemized listing

Test Behavior and Results

- Physical characteristics and observed clinical behaviors, summarized succinctly, with specific examples of particularly useful clinical observations included
- Response to examiner's attempts to impose structure
- Ability to work for duration of the test session(s)
- Response to reinforcement strategies employed
- Circumstances that were sources of stress
- Examiner's judgment about whether the testing was reliable and valid
- Specific test results:
  - General Intelligence
  - Academic Achievement
  - Executive Functioning
  - Attention/Concentration/Orientation
  - Receptive and Expressive Language
  - Sensory–Perceptual Examination
  - Motor Examination
  - Visuomotor Integration and Visuoperceptive Skill
  - Memory
  - Others (such as personality inventories, projective drawings, and questionnaires)

Test Summary

- General summary statement of patient's reason for referral (for the reader who reviews conclusions first)
- Overall conclusions about neuropsychological integrity

Neurological Implications

- Written primarily for medical staff
- Summary statement of specific test results in support of each hypothesis proposed in this paragraph
- Applicable statements regarding:
  - Behavioral correlation with reason for referral
  - Behavioral correlation with other neurodiagnostic techniques
  - Likely etiology and differential diagnostic possibilities
  - Chronicity—that is, whether a longstanding or a recent problem
  - Diffuse or focal nature of noted deficits
  - Stability of profile or transient observations needing follow-up

Neuropsychological Implications

- Written for all, but medical terminology limited
- Intended to summarize findings at a less technical level
- All practical observations about the child's current behavior

- Implications for the child's future behavior
- Applicable statements about the child's learning profile and any presumed pre-existing learning disability
- Specific recommendations for the parents
- Specific recommendations for the school
- Modifications necessary as a result of compromised cerebral functioning
- Summary statement of the child's strengths and how to use them

Conclusion

A major focus of the neuropsychological process is to make meaningful recommendations that will positively affect the child's outcome. This is accomplished by collecting serial data to monitor the course of a medical therapy, by evaluating changes consequent to a specific remediation, and by making suitable recommendations for the inpatient stay, for school placement, and for academic interventions. These must be considered in light of documented neuropsychological strengths and weaknesses. The written report is a central vehicle for communicating knowledge gained about a child in the evaluative process. It should be thorough and specific in delineating practical steps to follow for treatment purposes. It must also be easily comprehended by various professional and lay readers.

CASE EXAMPLE

Following is an example of a completed written report. The child was referred for evaluation because of academic difficulties, but he also had a history of spina bifida, hydrocephalus, and attentional problems for which medication therapy had been attempted but was not noticeably successful. Comprehensive neuropsychological evaluation had never been obtained.

Neuropsychological Evaluation

NAME: R. F.

DOB: 1/1/87

DATE OF TESTING: 7/1/94

CHRONOLOGICAL AGE: 7 years 6 months

REASON FOR REFERRAL: Neuropsychological evaluation was requested by C. S., M.D., his pediatrician, to assist in determining R.'s level of neuropsychological function, since his persistent academic difficulties have been resistant to the usual helpful techniques. R. is diagnosed as having spina bifida and hydrocephalus.

RELEVANT HISTORY: R. was the product of a full term uncomplicated pregnancy. He was born by spontaneous, vaginal delivery and weighed 7 lbs., 11 ozs. There were no complications at birth but he had surgery at 12 hours of age to correct a meningomyelocele and to place a V-P shunt for hydrocephalus. He was discharged from the hospital at 10 days of age but was readmitted for shunt revision after a bout with meningitis at 5 weeks of age. There have been no other shunt revisions.

R. does not have bowel or bladder control. Reportedly, there have been no recent CT or MRI scans, and he has been presumed to be functioning well. Further medical history was nonsignificant. He has been in good health, with no subsequent hospitalizations. There have been no prior neuropsychological evaluations. A general cognitive assessment administered thirteen months ago found him functioning within average limits on the WISC-R. His verbal IQ was essentially equivalent to his Performance IQ. Weak visuomotor integrative skill, attentional problems, and a complex language retrieval problem were identified. All language art skills were judged impaired.

R. is currently taking Cylert, and the impression given by his parents was that there have been only "subtle changes." R. is presently in a fully mainstreamed second-grade class at Davidson Elementary School, which has an appropriate environment for wheelchair-bound children. He has made academic strides, but the pace has been slower than hoped for. His attitude about school has not always been positive.

TESTS ADMINISTERED: Neuropsychological evaluation was administered to assess the integrity of cerebral functions in the following areas: general intelligence, executive function, memory, receptive and expressive language, lateral dominance and motor function, sensory perceptual integrity, visual-motor integration and visuoperceptive skill, and attention and concentration.

TEST BEHAVIOR AND RESULTS: R. was a lively, blond-haired child with a ready grin and freckled face. He maneuvered his wheelchair with assurance. He participated willingly in the varying tasks at first, seemingly eager and in good spirits. He was quite talkative, perhaps demonstrating the "cocktail party chatter" so characteristic of children with hydrocephalus. His language appeared immature, both in content and with respect to his use of words. He appeared to have difficulty modulating vocal level, often speaking quite loudly. R. constantly remained sensitive to the examiner's responses, seeking to evaluate the effects of his actions. He interrupted testing frequently. Clinically, R.'s attention and concentration were poor. Distractibility was evident prominently throughout the testing day. He was quite sensitive to noises, and it was difficult to keep him on task, even with strong guidance and structure. Because his activity level and ability to focus were so variable, these results were judged to be of questionable reliability. Nonetheless, every effort was made to elicit optimal behavior, and clearly there were times when he cooperated fully.

General Intelligence:

Administration of the Wechsler Intelligence Scale for Children—Revised found R. to be functioning between borderline and low average limits. He earned a Verbal IQ of 81, a Performance IQ of 75, and a resultant Full Scale IQ of 77. These scores fell at the 10th, 5th, and 6th percentiles, respectively. In comparison to prior testing, these scores represented declines of 16 points, 20 points, and 19 points, respectively—a profound decrease, and thus of great concern.

Intrascale subtest score scatter existed. Within the Verbal Scale, his comprehension of appropriate social actions to take in varying situations fell within deficient limits. All other verbal subtests fell within low average to average limits. Within the

Performance Scale, serious impairment was noted on the coding subtest requiring eye–hand coordination; deficient performance was noted on the more complex visuoperceptual analytic and synthetic tasks of block design and object assembly; and average performance was noted on measures of attention to essential visual detail, picture sequencing, and motor planning.

Executive Functioning, Conceptual Reasoning, and Judgment:

A test was given that helped evaluate R.'s ability to switch mental set, while maintaining two sequences in mind simultaneously. This test, the Trail Making Test, required R. to draw a line in sequence between numbered circles on Part A and to alternate between numbered and lettered circles on Part B. Successfully performing this task depends on simple reasoning capacity, the ability to scan material visually for essential information, and/or the ability maintain vigilance for a visual search task. R. made a sequencing error on Part A, when connecting only numbers. On the mental shifting portion, he demonstrated slowed performance and an error when required to alternate between numbers and letters, resulting in an impaired performance.

The Raven's Progressive Matrices Test—a measure of nonverbal spatial reasoning—was also given. R. earned a score that fell between the 25th and 50th percentiles for a 7½-year-old. His score was average for a 7-year-old.

The Mazes subtest of the WISC-R—a measure of motor planning—was also given. R. earned a scaled score that fell within the average range.

Receptive and Expressive Language:

R.'s spontaneous conversation was fluent. He had no difficulty with oral automatic language sequences, stating the alphabet perfectly. When writing the letters, however, he produced a mirror image of the letter "J," and many letters were poorly formed. He counted aloud accurately and wrote numbers correctly. He did not state the months of the year in correct sequence.

The Peabody Picture Vocabulary Test—a measure of receptive language—was also given. R. earned a standard score of 88, which fell at the 22nd percentile. This score earned him an age equivalent of 6 years 7 months. This score was fairly compatible with expectations, given the WISC-R Verbal IQ results.

Verbal fluency was assessed with a test requiring R. to generate words that began with a specified phoneme, a controlled word-association task. On one occasion, he produced a word beginning with a different vowel. Otherwise, his performance was intact.

An Aphasia Screening Test was also given, and R. was able to read numbers, letters, simple words, and names; calculate simple problems; demonstrate appropriate action; and recognize body parts. He had great difficulty writing his name; and when copying the word "SQUARE," he omitted the horizontal line in the letter "A."

Lateral Dominance and Motor Function:

R. prefers his right upper extremity for writing tasks. He preferred his left upper extremity on most unimanual tasks. He was able to discriminate left from right accurately.

Comparisons of the functional efficiency of the two sides of the body were made. R. demonstrated superiority of the left upper extremity on a measure of motor speed, rather than the expected right-sided efficiency of function. Both sides tapped slightly slower than expected for age. On a measure of motor dexterity, R. was required to rapidly place pegs into holes of varying orientation. His left upper extremity performance was more adept than his right upper extremity performance, but both were impaired. Again, the expected right-sided efficiency was not documented. Unfortunately, prior data do not exist to make comparisons over time.

Tactual Motor Problem Solving:

The Tactual Performance Test—a measure of psychomotor problem solving—was given. This is a test with great utility for the population of hydrocephalic children. R. had great difficulty on this task, unable to place blocks into a formboard using either upper extremity alone, while blindfolded. For this task, he depends on tactile and kinesthetic cues exclusively. His total time for completion of the test was thus within impaired limits, and his incidental memory for the blocks was poor. He was unable to recall the spatial location of any of the blocks, using paper and pencil once the blindfold was removed.

Sensory–Perceptual Examination:

Tests of primary sensation were given, and R. had perfect performance on a test of bilateral tactile simultaneous stimulation. On a more integrative test of finger recognition, he had perfect performance; and on a test of fingertip symbol writing perception, he made minimal bilateral errors, with no clear pattern of lateralization evident.

Visuomotor Integration and Visuoperceptive Skill:

Problematic fine motor development was apparent whenever R. had to draw or write with a pencil. His handwriting was enlarged, irregular, and immature for his chronological age. He had great difficulty copying even simple geometric designs, with immaturity of visuomotor development apparent. His attempt to copy a complex figure revealed poor organization, and attempts to integrate elements in the design were not successful. He drew a poor replication of a figure in response to the request that he draw-a-person.

Learning and Memory:

A test of novel verbal learning and recall was given. R. demonstrated an acceptable immediate recall of words. He demonstrated the ability to learn a list over repeated trials, and he had an acceptable delayed recall of the word list. His pattern of performance suggested age-appropriate encoding, storage, and retrieval of novel auditory/verbal information.

Attention and Concentration:

R. was assessed with instruments that are particularly sensitive to attentional variability and fluctuation. Visual search tests were given. He was able to locate target stimuli amid a competing visual array adequately. However, he tended to omit stimuli on the right side of the page. The Stroop test of attention was also given, and his scores fell within average limits on each part. Digit Span, as noted above, fell within average limits. He was able to recall 5 digits forward and 3 digits backward. The coding subtest fell within deficient limits, as noted above.

TEST SUMMARY: R. was a 7-year-6-month-old right-handed boy with spina bifida and hydrocephalus for whom an evaluation was requested to obtain a current assessment of neuropsychological integrity. His general cognitive ability, as measured with the WISC-R, was now significantly lowered compared to prior testing—a worrisome result. Mental shifting between two automatic language sequences was not intact as it should be for a child of his chronological age and average level of intelligence. His attentional capacity was variable clinically, but on several tasks seeking to evaluate such functioning formally he had remarkably intact functioning for his age peer group. This would suggest that attention, vigilance, and concentration are not the only variables influencing these lowered results. Further, serious pure motor and fine motor dysfunction was evidenced on tests of handwriting, speed, dexterity, and tactual-motor problem solving. Visuoperceptual abilities appeared to be seriously impaired and less intact than previously documented. Aspects of receptive and expressive language appeared to be particularly problematic, especially written production. Motor and sensory examinations did not allow for hypotheses of strong lateralization but were not entirely intact either. A suggestion of right-sided neglect was obtained from a visual search task.

NEUROLOGICAL IMPLICATIONS: R. demonstrated a profile entirely compatible with hypothesizing diffuse cerebral dysfunction and moderate to severe learning inefficiency for both verbal and nonverbal stimuli. The error pattern and qualitative analyses of his responses are strongly reminiscent of a profile commonly seen for children with spina bifida and hydrocephalus. However, current functioning is markedly deficient in contrast to the profile that emerged on prior psychological testing. His profile would not be easily explained by hypothesizing only lack of interest in cooperating, attentional problems solely, or an emotional etiology.

It is of primary importance that R. receive an updated, thorough review of medical status, including neurodiagnostic studies as appropriate to evaluate his hydrocephalic condition. A possible interpretation of these results, given that no prior neuropsychological data exist for comparison, is that R. is no longer maintaining the desired physiological balance. These results may be a reflection of changes due to a slowly progressive condition. Should a treatable condition be determined to exist, the implications for the future are surely quite different than if it is determined that his hydrocephalus is well controlled. Mrs. F. has thus been strongly advised to contact Dr. S. (her pediatrician), and she volunteered that she will also be contacting Dr. M. (R.'s neurosurgeon when he was younger).

NEUROPSYCHOLOGICAL IMPLICATIONS: A detailed interpretive discussion was held with R.'s mother, and these results were carefully elaborated. The nature of R.'s learning difficulties were detailed and examples were provided. In addition to the above stated concerns about medical integrity, recommendations for school placement and supportive interventions were also discussed. Once medical stability has been determined to exist, these recommendations may require further elaboration. The following tentative recommendations are thus made:

1. R. will find himself at a distinct disadvantage when faced with requests to produce through the written channel. Lengthy written productions will therefore be particularly problematic. This problem will become increasingly evident as he progresses through school and greater written expressive functioning is expected of him. Accommodations that would be greatly helpful and should be considered as they become appropriate include (but are not limited to):

extended time limits for examinations
examinations with true/false formats, fill-in-the-blanks, or multiple-choice responses

oral presentation or dictation of material that may overcome the need for extensive written production

oral dictation by R. and transcription by another to demonstrate his acquisition of content

decreased emphasis on visuomotor function for math instruction (for instance, number stamps)

less demand that he copy from the chalkboard and increased provision of written handouts

decreased emphasis on writing, by grading content separately from neatness and form of written production

decreased repetitive writing

increased use of a typewriter or keyboard

2. Tutoring and individual help may be useful for specific academic weaknesses that have been identified by the school through classroom performance or achievement tests. R. should be maintained in a school placement where he will obtain considerable one-to-one teaching and support. Daily practice in writing skills and language arts must be maintained or increased. Defined rest periods should be interspersed with active learning periods.

3. The variability associated with neurological dysfunction is not always recognized, and the existence of this difficulty should be clarified for his teachers. R. may well experience good moments and bad moments, good days and bad days. This is characteristic of children with neurological illness or conditions. It is clear that R. demonstrates a profile of attentional weakness, for which he is currently receiving medication therapy. Since this was initiated in May, sufficient time has not elapsed to fully gauge the significance of the provision of such therapy. However, his behavior during this test session was not as well focused as desired. The evaluation of his medication trial is being coordinated through his pediatrician.

4. Given R.'s many learning difficulties, a multimodality learning strategy appears essential. Auditory/verbal cueing strategies should be paired with nonverbal tasks to elicit optimal performance, and visual cues should be provided for auditory/verbal information. Pairing of verbal information with visual imagery techniques may prove inherently interesting to this young child and should be attempted.

5. Emotional support may be required if R., aware of his problems and sensitive to his sometimes failed attempts to succeed, cannot cope successfully on his own. Continued sensitivity to his self-perception is warranted. Formal intervention may have to be considered in the future if current informal attempts to provide support do not suffice. Further, social perceptiveness may be reduced. R. may lack a proclivity for understanding nonverbal gestures, facial expressions, and clues, relying on his stronger verbal capabilities to discern the importance of a situation.

6. It is also recommended that R. obtain a diagnostic consultation with an occupational therapist to determine an appropriate intervention strategy and exercises to bolster his poor pure motor and visuomotor skills.

If I can answer any further questions, please do not hesitate to contact me at the above phone number.

Ida Sue Baron, Ph.D., ABPP
Diplomate in Clinical Neuropsychology
American Board of Professional Psychology

REFERENCES

Baron, I. S.; Haney, A.; and Shelburne, S. 1985. Lightning injury in a child: Case report. Poster presented at the Thirteenth Annual International Neuropsychological Society Meeting, February, 7, 1985, San Diego, California.

Chelune, G. J., and Baer, R. A. 1986. Developmental norms for the Wisconsin Card Sorting Test. *Journal of Clinical and Experimental Neuropsychology* 8(3): 219–28.

Passler, M. A.; Isaac, W.; and Hynd, G. W. 1985. Neuropsychological development of behavior attributed to frontal lobe functioning in children. *Developmental Neuropsychology* 1: 349–70.

Welsh, M. C., and Pennington, B. F. 1988. Assessing frontal lobe functioning in children: Views from developmental psychology. *Developmental Neuropsychology* 4: 199–230.

Welsh, M. C.; Pennington, B. F.; and Grossier, D. B. 1991. A normative-developmental study of executive function: A window on prefrontal function in children. *Developmental Neuropsychology* 7: 131–49.

III

Pediatric Medical Disorders and Their Neuropsychological Aspects

7

Hydrocephalus and Myelomeningocele

Hydrocephalus involves an imbalance in the production and absorption of cerebrospinal fluid (CSF)—a clear, alkaline fluid that circulates within and around the brain and spinal cord. CSF is isotonic with blood plasma but contains less protein. It is produced continuously within the cerebral ventricles, in part by the highly vascularized choroid plexus and in part by the cerebral capillaries of the ventricular system. When normal circulation pathways are interrupted or impaired, a progressive accumulation of fluid results. This abnormal condition enlarges the ventricular system, exerting pressure upward, downward, and outward on surrounding brain structures (Menkes 1990).

CEREBROSPINAL FLUID

Circulation Dynamics

The ventricular system is made up of paired lateral ventricles, each lying within one cerebral hemisphere, and the midline third and fourth ventricles (see Figure 7-1). The lateral ventricles connect via the foramina of Monro to the third ventricle. The choroid plexus is located within the lateral, third, and fourth ventricles. The fluid formed in the lateral ventricles flows out through the paired interventricular foramina of Monro to reach the third ventricle, through the cerebral aqueduct (aqueduct of Sylvius) to the fourth ventricle, and through the foramina of Luschka and the foramen of Magendie to enter the subarachnoid space surrounding the brain and spinal cord. It is reabsorbed into the venous circulation from the subarachnoid spaces by the arachnoid villi (Behrman, Vaughan and Nelson, 1987; Fishman 1980). The total volume of CSF within the central nervous system is about 50 ml in the newborn, and it increases to about 150 ml in the average adult (Cutler et al. 1968).

Functions

The CSF serves two principal functions: it acts as a buoyancy agent for the brain, cushioning it within the skull and absorbing effects of sudden blows; and

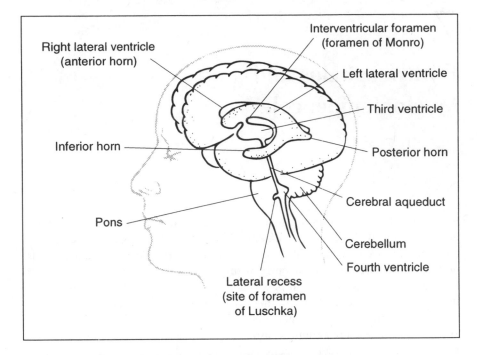

Figure 7-1   The Ventricular System: Lateral Projection

it provides a barrier between the brain and the blood (Menkes 1990). Suggestions that it has a role in the removal of waste products from central nervous system (CNS) metabolic processes, that it provides protection from certain bacteria, and that it serves in intracerebral transport have been advanced.

INCREASED INTRACRANIAL PRESSURE

When CSF pressures are elevated, the ventricular spaces within the brain begin to expand. Compensatory adjustments are made in response to increased fluid and pressure within the ventricular system. These may include transventricular absorption of the CSF, expansion of the skull when sutures have not yet closed, contraction of cerebrovascular volume, increase in ventricular surface area, and possibly a reduction in CSF fluid formation rate. Compensatory actions are not always sufficient, however. Ventricular enlargement may continue if complete obstruction of the CSF pathway exists and the pressure gradient persists. Continued expansion of the ventricles, unhalted by natural or mechanical means, may result in death by transtentorial herniation.

Increased intracranial pressure (IICP) can produce various neurological symptoms, depending on the rapidity with which the increase occurs (Fenichel 1988). In infants whose bony skull sutures have not fused, there may be tightening or bulging of the skin above the skull openings (fontanelles). Head size grows disproportionately fast for age. The infant may exhibit the so-called "sunset gaze" sign—so-called because the infant is unable to look up, and the pupils appear to be "setting" into the lower lid. Irritability and/or lethargy may result. The child's legs may be drawn up into a flexed position, or there may be diminished or absent deep tendon reflexes. The infant may also present with vomiting or may refuse feedings. In young children, urinary or bowel incontinence and headache complaints are more common. These symptoms may be accompanied by paralysis of the third and fourth cranial nerves. Occasionally, a child may appear to be healthy, but neuroimaging will reveal an enlarged ventricular system. A child without overt signs or symptoms of hydrocephalus may be at risk for developmental delay or other cognitive and behavioral symptoms (Barnett, Hahn & Palmer 1987; Fishman 1986), as is a child with overt manifestations of hydrocephalus.

PATHOPHYSIOLOGICAL CHANGES

Enlarging ventricles place the developing brain at risk along a number of dimensions. There may be stretching of axons, thinning of the calvarium (particularly over the cerebral gyri), atrophy of white matter, and compression of the cerebral mantle (brain tissue). Myelinization of the corpus callosum may be delayed (Gadsdon, Variend & Emery 1979). Subcortical pathways and structures may be compressed (Fletcher, Bohan et al. 1992). The olfactory tracts and optic nerves are often atrophic. There may even be selective thinning of the child's brain from the anterior regions to the occipital vertex (Dennis et al. 1981). The frontal lobes of the brain and their reciprocal connections to other brain regions may be at particular risk for vascular changes resulting from stretched anterior cerebral arteries (Mathew et al. 1975; Nauta 1971). As a result, neurobehavioral deficits may emerge (Eslinger et al. 1992). These pathophysiological changes may have particular impact on alertness, attention, memory, motor functioning, and language functions.

ETIOLOGY

Although childhood hydrocephalus can result from a number of diverse pathological brain processes (see Table 7-1), there are three main causes. First, hydrocephalus may result from obstructions within the ventricular cavities. Blockage may be due to malformations such as aqueductal stenosis. Alternatively, tumors arising from the lining of the ventricles or intruding into ventricular spaces from adjoining brain regions may also obstruct CSF dynamics (Menkes 1990; Leech & Brumbeck 1991). Blockage is also a common complication of a number of malformations involving the brain or the spinal cord (myelodysplasias) (Wills 1993). This type of childhood hydrocephalus accounts for about 60% of all cases. Second, hydrocephalus may be caused by blocked

Table 7-1   Possible Causes of
Hydrocephalus in Children

Congenital blockage
   Myelodysplasia
   Central nervous system malformation

Noncongenital blockage
   Hemorrhage
   Intracranial mass
   Inflammation
   Trauma

Cerebrospinal fluid overproduction
   Choroid plexus papilloma

absorption of the CSF within the cisterns or arachnoid villi over the cerebral cortex. This commonly results from thickening of the arachnoid or meninges following infections such as meningitis or from blockage of drainage secondary to hemorrhage—for instance, as a result of head trauma or prematurity (Menkes 1990). It is a common consequence of intraventricular hemorrhage in premature births (Fletcher, Francis et al. 1992; Volpe, Pasternak & Allan 1977). This type of hydrocephalus accounts for about 30% of all childhood cases. Third, excessive secretion of CSF may be occurring, due to overproduction by a choroid plexus papilloma. As a result, the arachnoid granulations on the cerebral hemispheres are unable to absorb the increased fluid volume (Milhorat 1975). About 1% to 4% of all cases of childhood hydrocephalus result from these benign papilloma growths, which may also block CSF circulation within the ventricles (Leech & Brumbeck 1991).

There is also a normotensive or "normal pressure" form of hydrocephalus—although this is a controversial entity. Children with this insidious condition present no overt signs or symptoms of active hydrocephalus, such as nausea, headache, or papilledema. Data suggest the existence of a group of asymptomatic children with clinically stable (that is, arrested) hydrocephalus, in whom abnormal neuropsychological test performances may indicate the need for CSF shunting and who will benefit from surgical intervention (Hammock, Milhorat & Baron 1976; Torkelson et al. 1985).

TYPOLOGY

Hydrocephalus is frequently described on the one hand as communicating or extraventricular, or on the other as noncommunicating, obstructive, or intraventricular, depending on the site of the abnormality or blockage that is impairing CSF circulation dynamics. The terms *communicating* and *extraventricular* refer to conditions in which the formation or absorption of the CSF is disturbed, although pathways within the ventricular system remain functional (Benson et al. 1970), or in which circulation in the subarachnoid space is obstructed. In such instances, the entire ventricular system becomes uniformly distended. For example, there may be a congenital failure of the subarachnoid spaces to develop, as in the Arnold-Chiari malformation. This malformation of the brainstem (elongated medulla oblongata) and cerebellum causes downward displacement of parts of the poorly developed cerebellum, fourth ventricle, and medulla into the cervical spinal canal, obstructing CSF flow around the brain stem in the subarachnoid space. Arachnoiditis, sagittal sinus obstruction, subdural collections, excessive CSF production, and connective tissue disorders may also lead to this type of hydrocephalus.

The terms *noncommunicating, obstructive,* and *intraventricular* refer to conditions that involve CSF circulatory abnormality directly within the ventricular system. Enlargement of the ventricular system occurs proximal to the site of obstruction. A common associated malformation is congenital *aqueductal stenosis,* which refers to a narrowing of the aqueduct of Sylvius (between the third and fourth ventricles). As a result of this narrowing, the aqueduct is unable to carry the full amount of CSF produced. Aqueductal stenosis may be a residual effect of an inflammation (for instance, viral), a result of compression by an external lesion (for instance, posterior fossa subdural hematoma), or (rarely) a sex-linked recessive trait. A Dandy-Walker malformation (cystlike formation) obstructs the fourth ventricle via cerebellar herniation (Menkes 1990). The Dandy-Walker syndrome may result from atresia of the foramen of Luschka and the foramen of Magendie or of cerebellar dysplasia. Neoplasm, a common cause of hydrocephalus in adults, may also cause childhood hydrocephalus. Neoplasms or tumors may be solid or cystic and may arise in any brain structure, although most childhood tumors develop in the cerebellum and brain stem regions (Menkes, 1990).

SYMPTOMATOLOGY

Clinical symptoms depend on the time of onset and on the severity of the imbalance between CSF production and resorptive capacity. When hydrocephalus develops before cranial sutures have fused, abnormal enlargement of the head circumference may result. Head circumference measurement is routine in pediatric examinations, and serial measurements of rapidly increasing head size should lead to further neurodiagnostic evaluation (such as by CT scan and/or MRI) to determine whether hydrocephalus is present. Other signs of infantile hydrocephalus—that is, increased intracranial pressure (IICP)—are a large, bulging anterior fontanelle (soft spot on top of the infant's head); separation of cranial sutures; downward deviation of the eyes; dilated scalp veins; and a high-pitched cry.

When the onset occurs later, the cranial sutures may already be closed. In such cases, there may be no obvious head enlargement to indicate the pathological state, and insidious deterioration may occur before the condition is detected. Instead, chronic papilledema seen on fundoscopic examination or recurring headache may first signal IICP. Headaches typically begin in early morning and intensify, often resulting in vomiting. Clumsiness, tremor, combined spasticity and ataxia (affecting lower limbs more than upper limbs), and urinary incontinence are associated symptoms.

ASSOCIATED MYELODYSPLASIA

Almost 70% of hydrocephalic conditions are associated with myelodysplasia (Shurtleff, Kronmal & Foltz 1975). The percentage of children with myelodysplasia who require shunting is between 65% and 90% (Smith & Smith 1973). *Myelodysplasia* refers to any of several malformations of the spinal cord and spinal meninges. Myelodysplasias can range from reasonably benign pilonidal cysts (Menkes 1990) to severe cases of spina bifida cystica—a group of congenital malformations involving failed neural tube closure early in embryogenesis. Several presumptive "causes" of spina bifida cystica have been identified, including maternal folic acid deficiency (Centers for Disease Control 1992), environmental teratogens, and genetic (hereditary) defects (Wills 1993).

MENINGOMYELOCELE

Meningomyelocele is one type of spina bifida cystica, in which the neural ectoderm developing into the spinal cord and nerve roots fails to separate from the epithelium, leading to an external sac containing CSF, incompletely formed meninges, and a malformed spinal cord. Meningomyelocele occurs with a frequency of from 1 to 5 per 1000 live births (Fishman 1986). The defect can be described according to the relative involvement of the spinal cord and meninges, as well as according to the vertebral level at which the defect occurred. The spinal cord has a segmental organization such that each segment is linked with musculature and organs of a particular body segment. The divisions, from top to bottom, are 8 cervical, 12 thoracic, 5 lumbar, and 5 sacral segments. Greater associated neurological deficits and cognitive deficits are described for higher spinal cord lesions. Approximately 75% of all myelodysplastic lesions, however, occur in lumbar or sacral spinal cord segments. As a result, there may be associated difficulties in the sensory or motor functions involved in ambulation, enervation of the bladder or bowels, spinal kurtosis or kyphosis, and (sometimes) lower limb wasting or hypertrophy (Fishman 1986). Hydrocephalus develops in approximately 90% of children who have meningomyelocele, as a result of aqueductal stenosis or the often associated Arnold-Chiari malformation.

Treatment of meningomyelocele is quite complex, due to associated neurological, orthopedic, bowel, and genitourinary difficulties (Fenichel 1988; Menkes 1990). Typically, the defect is apparent at birth, and the neonate has surgery to close the skin flap over the sac in order to prevent infection and to avoid further damage to the nerve roots caused by expansion of the sac. If there are associated deformities—for instance, an Arnold-Chiari malformation—or if the infant develops hydrocephalus, the child may shortly thereafter undergo a ventricular shunting procedure (discussed in a later section of this chapter). If left untreated, meningomyelocele can lead to life-threatening infections or death (Menkes 1990).

Once stabilized by surgery, the child begins a long treatment course for the associated neurological, orthopedic, and other medical problems resulting from the primary spinal cord lesion. For example, muscle contractures may occur that require surgical release. The child may develop chronic urinary tract infections, due to the presence of a neurogenic bladder. Physical therapy and occupational therapy help strengthen weakened muscle groups and assist in providing adaptive devices for eating and dressing. Special education services for the physically handicapped or learning disabled are often needed as the child enters the school system. Family residences may require adaptation for the handicapped, including wheelchair ramps, bathroom fixtures that accommodate a wheelchair, and special orthopedic devices to help in bed-to-chair transfers (such as a trapeze for lifting). Often the child's parents become both caregivers and advocates within the medical and educational community for their child's special needs.

As the child matures, additional orthopedic or neurosurgical procedures may be necessary to correct abnormal spine curvature, which can compromise respiratory function in the wheelchair-bound child. The family may require the services of a pediatric psychologist or child psychiatrist to help family members cope with the stresses of caring for a chronically disabled child (Varni & Wallander 1988). Financial or emotional stress may increase as parents and siblings adjust to the child's intensive care needs and as modifications in family lifestyle result. Behavioral problems consequent to having a brain disorder as well as to the child's response to the disease process may necessitate active intervention by health-care professionals who are specifically familiar with the multiply handicapped child with meningomyelocele.

OTHER MALFORMATIONS

Spina bifida occulta refers to the condition that results when neural closure fails but there is no involvement of spinal cord tissue and·thus no detectable neurologic deficit. If the spinal cord meninges herniate through the spinal column defect, but the spinal cord neural tissue is not involved, the anomaly is referred to as a *meningocele*. The presence of this type of spina bifida cystica has few associated neurologic consequences. An *encephalocele* refers to a lesion at the cranial level, involving a skull defect, and herniation of cerebral tissue through the defect. Associated sensory, motor, and cognitive deficits are expected.

DIAGNOSTIC PROCEDURES

A child with suspected or confirmed hydrocephalus undergoes a number of investigative procedures designed to confirm and define the hydrocephalic condition. The following may be included singly or in combination: *lumbar puncture* (often done serially), to measure CSF pressure; *constant-rate lumbar infusions*, to assess CSF absorptive capacity; short-term *continuous intracranial cerebral pressure monitoring*, to identify patients who will benefit from surgery (since their pressures rise intermittently but otherwise remain normal); *cerebral blood flow* studies; *electrophysiological* studies (for example, visual evoked responses and brainstem auditory evoked potentials); *electroencephalograms;* and *radiological* studies of the skull. *Computed tomogram* (CT) and/or *magnetic resonance image* (MRI) scans allow one to view, measure, and serially follow ventricular size and to detect periventricular hypodensity—a marker of pressure effects. Large ventricles but small sulci suggest hydrocephalus and not atrophy. *Radioactive iodinated serum cisternography* has been used to evaluate flow and dynamics, but it has poorer specificity and sensitivity. *Ventriculography* aids in revealing the site of an obstruction. Serial neuropsychological evaluation helps document a hydrocephalic profile, allows for assessment of interval change, and assists in evaluating the cognitive effects of treatment.

Measurement of the degree of hydrocephalus has varied among investigators. Some have measured cortical mantle thickness, brain mass, orbitofrontal circumference, or ventricle size. Dilatation of lateral ventricular size may be assessed by computing the ventricle–brain ratio (VBR), which is the area of lateral ventricles divided by the area of total intracranial contents times 100.

TREATMENT APPROACHES

If the hydrocephalus does not spontaneously arrest and if the condition is not temporary, intervention is required to prevent permanent CNS damage. When hydrocephalus is left untreated, a progressive decline can be expected, with herniation of the cerebellum a final, fatal result (Menkes 1990). The goal of treatment is to reestablish equilibrium between CSF production and reabsorption.

Various treatments have been attempted to reduce CSF formation and to bring about more effective drainage and absorption. In the past, attempts were made to reduce CSF formation by excising the choroid plexus or by using pharmacological agents (anti-secretory agents). Compressive head wrapping for milder cases was tried. Most effective treatments, however, have attempted to correct drainage and absorption directly. Procedures in this category include surgical removal of an obstructive lesion, bypass of an intraventricular blockage, and extracranial shunt diversions. An extracranial shunt procedure is a very common treatment. Prior to the use of modern shunting procedures, the mortality rate of untreated hydrocephalus was estimated to be about 50% with survivors at high risk for severe mental handicaps (Laurence & Coates 1962; Laurence 1969). Shunting has been accompanied by improved physical and mental outcome (Wills et al. 1990; Wills 1993).

Intracranial shunt procedures divert CSF away from an obstruction and into the subarachnoid space. These may be elected when the ventricular obstruction cannot be removed directly and when the subarachnoid space can meet demands for drainage and absorption.

Extracranial shunting procedures drain excess fluid from ventricular or lumbar subarachnoid spaces into an extracranial body compartment from which it can then be absorbed. If the procedure is successful, CSF pressure, volume, and flow decrease, and the ventricles regain normal pressure and diminish in size. Extracranial valve-regulated shunts to the peritoneum—such as the ventriculoperitoneal (VP) shunt—have become a standard surgical treatment for hydrocephalus. A plastic tube courses from a lateral ventricle down into the abdominal peritoneal cavity, where excess fluid is released for reabsorption and excretion. This procedure involves drilling a burr hole in the skull and placing a shunt (through which the CSF drains) under the scalp. There are several kinds of extracranial shunts and also several different shunt routes, including ventriculovascular, ventriculopleural, and lumboperitoneal, which are more common for adults (Leech & Brumbeck 1991).

Shunts have disadvantages, including the possibility of bacterial growth leading to ventriculitis, pulmonary emboli, and nephritis. Insertion of the shunt may be associated with hemorrhage. Shunt malfunction, infection and obstruction are common complications necessitating shunt removal, replacement surgery, and antibiotic therapy. These complications can be expected to affect cognitive outcome, quite apart from the hydrocephalus itself (Thompson, Eisenberg & Levin 1982; Wills 1993). Some evidence indicates that multiple shunt infections are associated with a higher incidence of cognitive impairment (Menkes 1990), although this finding is controversial. In part, this controversy relates to subject selection differences across studies (Donders, Canady & Rourke 1990; Wills 1993), to the use of different assessment measures, and to other potentially adverse confounding medical conditions that the child may have (Dennis et al. 1981). Even in the absence of such complications, elective shunt replacement may still be necessary to adjust for normal growth. Despite these problems, extracranial shunting remains the safest and most effective of the current therapies.

Shunt failures or infection are best detected early. Young children become acutely ill. In an older child, acute failure resulting in a rapidly progressive increase in intracranial pressure may present as headache, vomiting, stupor, and eventually coma. Children with chronic failure may exhibit school failure, lethargy, sleepiness, irritability, and gait deterioration.

NEUROPSYCHOLOGICAL STUDIES OF CHILDHOOD HYDROCEPHALUS WITH AND WITHOUT MENINGOMYELOCELE

As noted earlier, a number of factors affect the developmental outcome of the child with hydrocephalus and/or meningomyelocele. Among the factors that have been examined in research protocols to date are etiology of the hydrocephalus, duration, severity, timing of initiation of treatment, shunt complications,

Table 7-2 Neuropsychological
Problems Reported in Children
Shunted for Hydrocephalus

Lowered intelligence scores
Performance IQ lower than verbal IQ
Impaired oral discourse
Deficient nonverbal abilities
Variable executive function
Deficient motor/tactual abilities
Variable memory function
Variable attention and concentration
Deficient social maturity
Academic weaknesses

and associated neurological and CNS structural abnormalities (Baron & Gold-berger 1993; Dennis et al. 1981; Thompson, Eisenberg & Levin 1982; Donders, Canady & Rourke 1990; Fletcher, Bohan et al. 1992; Wills 1993; Wills et al. 1990). Each of these factors may have an impact, alone or in combination, on the presence of intellectual and neuropsychological disorder. The following subsections present an overview of research on the neuropsychological functioning of children with hydrocephalus, with and without associated CNS malformations (see Table 7-2). The review does not include studies of children who developed hydrocephalus secondary to head trauma or brain tumors (see Chapters 9 and 10).

Intellectual Functions

Early studies of untreated hydrocephalic children revealed that less than 40% of these children obtained IQ scores within the normal range (Laurence & Coates 1962; Laurence 1969; Yashon, Jane & Sugar 1965). However, IQ scores appeared to correlate with degree of physical disability. Lower scores were obtained by children who experienced symptoms of spasticity, ataxia, motor imbalance, or motor coordination problems. Subtest scatter on the Wechsler scales was more common in the more severe cases of hydrocephalus (Laurence 1969). Despite these associations, some children with very thin cortical mantles obtained scores within the normal range (Lorber 1980) and even had superior IQ scores after a corrective shunting procedure (Lorber 1968). Longer duration of untreated hydrocephalus was also found to be related to lower IQ scores (Foltz & Shurtleff 1963; Young et al. 1973).

More recently investigators have reported: a negative relationship between thickness of cortical mantle and IQ (Young et al. 1973; Thompson, Eisenberg & Levin 1982), an influence of the extent and configuration of cortical thinning on IQ (Dennis et al. 1981; Shurtleff, Foltz & Loesser 1973); differences in IQ abilities correlated with type of hydrocephalus (for instance, morbidity was expected to be lower in communicating versus noncommunicating hydrocephalus) (Raimondi & Soare 1974; McCullough & Balzer-Martin 1982); lower verbal skills associated with increased left lateral ventricle size (Bendarsky & Lewis 1990); and, a positive influence of shunt treatment on IQ (Dennis et al. 1981; Fletcher, Bohan et al. 1992).

In general, children with hydrocephalus—particularly if they have motor difficulties—may have lower performance IQs and, therefore, lower full-scale IQ scores on global intellectual measures such as the McCarthy (McCarthy 1972) and Wechsler (Wechsler 1974) scales. These data only reflect group mean scores, however, and (as noted earlier) the presence of hydrocephalus alone cannot predict an individual child's intellectual performance. Indeed, as the above studies suggest, there are few reliable predictors of impairments in intellectual function. Perinatal problems resulting in hydrocephalus compromise early cognitive development more than do comparable problems that do not result in hydrocephalus (Landry et al. 1984). A greater risk for adverse outcome seems to exist for children whose hydrocephalus is complicated by brain injury (Thompson, Eisenberg & Levin 1982), and for those with oculomotor or visual difficulties or with neuromotor deficits (McCullough & Balzer-Martin 1982). Within subgroups of hydrocephalic children, lower full-scale IQ (McCullough & Balzer-Martin 1982) and performance IQ scores were found for children with aqueductal, anterior third ventricle or foramen of Monro obstructions (Dennis 1985).

Perceptual–Motor Functions

Children with hydrocephalus often experience perceptual–motor problems. In addition to having problems with tasks found in the performance IQ section of general intelligence tests, these children may have particular difficulty with tasks involving visuomotor graphic skills such as copying geometric designs (Soare & Raimondi 1977) or on speeded tasks such as copying dots (Anderson & Plows 1977). Not surprisingly, there seems to be an association between global intellectual levels and perceptual–motor skills, with lower IQ scores associated with lower scores on visuomotor tasks (Tew & Laurence 1975; Spain 1974). Recent work suggests that children with hydrocephalus, with or without meningomyelocele, may be particularly adversely affected by speeded motor or visuomotor tasks (Donders, Rourke & Canady, 1991; Thompson et al. 1991), with many children evidencing dysgraphic problems. When time limits are not imposed and motor demands are limited, hydrocephalic children are more likely to exhibit average performance (Thompson et al. 1991). On more purely perceptual tasks, such as judgment of line orientation (Benton et al. 1983), the performance of groups of children with meningomyelocele, meningocele, or aqueductal stenosis was found to be related to right lateral ventricle size (Fletcher, Bohan et al. 1992). In the latter study, a positive correlation was found between verbal and nonverbal cognitive and neuropsychological measures, on the one hand, and size of the corpus callosum, on the other. Higher correlations were noted between nonverbal measures and corpus callosum size.

Memory

Relatively few studies have specifically assessed memory functioning of hydrocephalic children, despite the knowledge that an enlarging ventricular system may have direct negative effects on structures or pathways that are especially important for encoding and retrieval. Methodological weaknesses flawed many early attempts to address memory function in this population (Baron & Goldberger 1993).

The importance of controlling for IQ before one attributes poor performance to information-processing dysfunction or memory dysfunction has been emphasized (Cull & Wyke 1984; Prigatano & Zeiner 1985); and recent studies have attempted to control for intellectual level. Studies of two spontaneously remitted college-age hydrocephalic subjects reported impairments in verbal learning and memory (Richardson 1978). However, this has not been consistently observed in groups of children shunted for hydrocephalus (Donders, Rourke & Canady 1991; Fennell et al. 1987; Fletcher, Bohan et al. 1992; Spiegler 1984). Hydrocephalic children demonstrated age-appropriate performance on nonsense figure, face recognition, and short-story recall, but had deficient recall of unrelated words. However, no gross learning or memory deficiencies were noted when these children were compared to healthy children matched for IQ (Cull & Wyke 1984).

The absence of consistent evidence of problems in verbal and nonverbal memory and learning is somewhat surprising, given the presence of white matter pathway problems and the potential compression of hippocampal structures by ventricular dilatation (Dennis et al. 1981; Fletcher, Bohan et al. 1992). In part, this may be related to the choice of different measures across studies (Donders, Rourke & Canady 1991) or to the lack of sensitivity of the measures chosen to separate different groups of hydrocephalic children (Fletcher, Bohan et al. 1992). When deficits have been observed (Prigatano et al. 1983), they tend to reflect both initial learning difficulties and problems in long-term retrieval, which is aided by cueing. The pattern of performance deficits suggests that attentional dysfunction may lead to memory problems by disrupting initial encoding of new material to be learned. Problems in search may likewise impair long-term retrieval—a pattern sometimes described among patients with documented frontal–subcortical dysfunction.

Motor Functions

Fine and gross motor dysfunction is commonly reported in hydrocephalic children (Turner 1985). As noted earlier, gross motor difficulty involving gait, balance, or clumsiness may be seen (Shaffer et al. 1986; Sørenson, Jansen & Gjerris 1986). Among children with meningomyelocele, deficits in motor functions below the lesion level are ubiquitous, but impairments in fine motor skills of the upper limbs and impairments in hand–eye coordination are also common (Leech & Brumback 1991; Menkes 1990; Sand et al. 1974). Indeed, motor impairments are a uniform characteristic of the hydrocephalic child (Baron

1976; Baron & Goldberger 1993). Fine motor problems may be expressed as difficulties in copying designs or letters, as poor handwriting, as slowed writing speed, or as frank problems in fine motor coordination, speed, and dexterity (Fennell et al. 1987; Turner 1985). Among hydrocephalic children, the incidence of left-handedness is greater than expected, with estimates ranging from 20% to 40% of this population. The incidence of left-handedness appears to be higher in children with higher-level (thoracic-level) lesions; and consequently, a spinal rather than cortical basis has been proposed (Dennis et al. 1981). In addition, problems in finger-tapping speed (Fennell et al. 1987), in speeded dexterity measures (Thompson et al. 1991) and in coordination of the upper extremities (Woods 1979) have been reported. These deficits are compounded by the presence of oculomotor problems, as well as problems with gaze and accommodation (Clements & Kaushal 1970; Dennis 1985; Woods 1979; Zeiner et al. 1985). It is not surprising, therefore, that neuropsychological or cognitive measures that depend on visuomotor integrative skills (such as drawing) or on speed of motor response to visuoperceptual problems (such as block design construction) are frequently mildly to moderately impaired in hydrocephalic children (Baron 1976; Donders, Rourke & Canady 1991).

Language Functions

Frank language disorders are a relatively uncommon presentation in hydrocephalic children (Menkes 1990). While the literature contains references to clinical descriptions of the so-called "cocktail party" hyperverbality of the hydrocephalic child (Tew 1979) or "empty chatter" (Fleming 1968), this phenomenon of superficial and somewhat perseverative social speech patterns is more commonly seen in children with well below average intellectual abilities. One study of normal IQ hydrocephalic children did not support this syndrome, nor the view that deficits in syntax or pragmatics are a common feature of their expressive language (Byrne, Abbeduto & Brooks 1990). In another study, however, hydrocephalic children demonstrated deficits in understanding nonliteral and metaphoric discourse, suggesting that higher-order inferential language is more difficult (Dennis & Barnes 1993).

Some deficits in other aspects of language functioning have been reported among hydrocephalic children. For example, problems in receptive and expressive language development (Landry et al. 1988), in vocabulary definitions (Prigatano et al., 1983), in verbal fluency (Dennis et al. 1987; Donders, Rourke & Canady 1991; Fennell et al. 1987; Fletcher, Bohan et al. 1992), in understanding complex grammatical structures (Dennis et al. 1987), and in sentence repetition (Dennis et al. 1987; Fennell et al. 1987) have been reported among hydrocephalic children with and without meningomyelocele. Word-list recall deficiencies found in a group of 7- to 9-year-old children with hydrocephalus suggested that these children were unable to use appropriate semantic strategies when encoding was necessary (Cull & Wyke 1984).

Dennis and colleagues (1987) suggested that the behavior noted in earlier descriptions of the "cocktail party" syndrome may have been a product of the hydrocephalic child's struggles in word retrieval and word fluency. Their struggles may have led these children to rely on overlearned phrases and sayings in communicating with others. While fluency impairment has not yet been proved to be the critical factor, problems in word fluency and retrieval can have an obvious impact on measures of verbal memory for word lists (Cull & Wyke 1984). As a result, language problems may produce deviant scores on many verbal memory measures that are used to assess these children. Alternative explanations deserve further study—for instance, whether executive function impairment may exist that affects the child's ability to initiate and inhibit expressive verbal action or to organize verbal output, or whether a degradation of semantic information may occur (Baron & Goldberger 1993).

Attentional Functions

As noted earlier, descriptions of acute presentations of hydrocephalus describe arousal and alertness deficits in these patients (Menkes 1990). Parents of shunted children commonly report problems related to a shortened attention span, distractibility, and concentration (Fennell et al. 1987), suggesting elements of Attention Deficit Disorder without Hyperactivity. In the authors' experience, because these children often are not hyperactive, deficits in attention and verbal impulsivity may be the primary features of the ADD picture. Although parental reports and clinical descriptions of these children are available, few published studies have addressed the attentional abilities of hydrocephalic children (Horn et al. 1985; Zeiner & Prigatano 1982). Instead, deficits in attention have been inferred from performance on tests of digit span (digits backward), from difficulties in performing on embedded figures tasks (Willoughby & Hoffman 1979), and from poor initial learning on tests of verbal list learning (Donders, Rourke & Canady 1991; Thompson et al. 1991). When a formal computerized test of visual vigilance was administered to a small group of hydrocephalic children, increased errors of omission and commission were observed (Fennell et al. 1987). This same pattern of inattention and impulsive responding is comparable to the performance deficits observed in nonhydrocephalic children diagnosed with Attention Deficit Disorder (Barkley 1990).

As Wills (1993) recently observed, few published studies have directly addressed the types of attentional problems that these children manifest. In a recent review, Mirsky et al. (1991) propose that attention be viewed as consisting of four component behaviors: focus–execute; sustain; encode; and shift. By breaking down attention into component parts, each with a neuroanatomic substrate, clinicians may be able to study attentional disorders selectively in hydrocephalic children. Examples of clinical tests that could be employed to assess each of these domains include the following:

1. Focus–execute: letter cancellation tests and Trail Making Test (Reitan & Davison 1974).
2. Sustain: continuous performance tests.

3. Encode: arithmetic and digit span from the Wechsler scales.
4. Shift: Wisconsin Card Sorting Test (Grant & Berg 1948) and Stroop color word interference (Golden 1978).

Use of these measures might permit a more complete appreciation of the relationships between neuroanatomic compromise (due to lesion location) and attentional deficits among hydrocephalic children.

Psychosocial Functions

As noted earlier, children with hydrocephalus and/or spinal dysplastic syndromes may experience a number of physical, cognitive, and neurobehavioral problems that pose difficulties for the children and their families. School and learning problems, self-image and self-esteem problems, physical handicaps, and restrictions in vocational goals may be sources of stress and may negatively affect the child's adjustment. Family stresses—prevalent when a child is chronically handicapped—may produce marital discord, sibling adjustment and behavior problems, and role changes within the family structure (Dorner 1975; Donders, Rourke & Canady 1992). A recent review of quality-of-life issues for children undergoing intensive medical interventions in early life found that most families felt that the cost–benefit ratio in relation to outcome justified the associated strains of such aggressive interventions (Query, Reichelt & Christoferson 1990). However, more studies are certainly needed among hydrocephalic children and their families.

For example, few reports have examined specific affective disturbances among hydrocephalic children. In one study (Fennell et al. 1987), parent reports on standardized behavior checklists such as the Child Behavior Checklist (Achenbach 1991) suggested that many hydrocephalic children experience symptoms of depression and anxiety. However, this study failed to examine child self-report of these symptoms or to assess associated problems in self-esteem. Problems in self-monitoring and self-awareness have been reported among hydrocephalic children and may limit the utility of self-report measures to older and more high-functioning patients.

Finally, the clinician should be careful to obtain information regarding psychosocial adjustment and family functioning when examining the hydrocephalic child. In the authors' experience, greatest stress seems to occur when these children move from late childhood into adolescence. This period of development is normally beset with pressures and concerns regarding the child's developing independence from the family. Children with hydrocephalus and/or myelodysplasia (and their families) may experience even greater levels of stress during the adolescent years because of the additional burden resulting from this chronic condition (Baron 1976; Baron & Goldberger 1993). Adolescents and their families are often helped by supportive family therapy, which helps them develop ways of enhancing the child's independence while remaining aware of the limits imposed by their physical, neuropsychological, academic, and vocational needs.

CONCLUSION

Hydrocephalus, with or without associated myelodysplasias, can place a child at risk for a number of neuropsychological and behavioral problems. Besides the physical limitations (in ambulation, for instance) and medical problems that can accompany this condition, the child may experience problems in attention, intellectual functioning, language, fine motor skills, visuospatial skills, and visuoconstructional skills. There may also be difficulties in the modulation of emotional responses. Deficits in self-awareness and behavioral self-regulation may be present. School achievement is often problematic, and learning difficulties are not uncommon in these children. In addition, many stresses are associated with this chronic disability. These stresses include the limitations imposed by the child's physical disability, changes in family functioning required by the medical and academic needs of the child, and issues of self-esteem and self-worth with which the child must struggle. As the child matures, issues revolving around independence and separation from the family, dating, and future vocational goals become more prominent and (often) even more stressful for the child and the family.

Clinical neuropsychologists can play a key role in dealing with these problems by carefully describing the child's neurobehavioral deficits at each developmental stage, by communicating with the parents and the school to help them appreciate the child's particular strengths and weaknesses, by assisting in the development of appropriate strategies to enhance academic learning, and by suggesting and implementing therapeutic interventions for healthy social and emotional growth.

REFERENCES

Achenbach, T. M. 1991. *Manual for the Child Behavior Checklist/ 4–18 and the 1991 Profile*. Burlington, Vt.: University of Vermont, Department of Psychology.

Anderson, E. M., and Plows, I. 1977. Impairment of a motor skill in children with spina bifida cystica and hydrocephalus: An exploratory study. *British Journal of Psychology* 68: 61–70.

Barkley, R. A. 1990. *Attention Deficit Hyperactivity Disorder: A Handbook for Diagnosis and Treatment*. New York: Guilford Press.

Barnett, G. H.; Hahn, J. F.; and Palmer, J. 1987. Normal pressure hydrocephalus in children and young adults. *Neurosurgery* 20: 904–7.

Baron, I. S. 1976. Normal pressure hydrocephalus in children: Neuropsychological correlates. Unpublished doctoral dissertation, University of Maryland.

Baron, I. S., and Goldberger, E. 1993. Neuropsychological disturbances of hydrocephalic children with implications for special education and rehabilitation. *Neuropsychological Rehabilitation* 3: 389–410.

Behrman, R. E.; Vaughan, V. C. III; and Nelson, W. B. 1987. Nelson *Textbook of Pediatrics-13th Edition*. Philadelphia: W. B. Saunders, pp. 1304–6.

Bendarsky, M., and Lewis, M. 1990. Early language ability as a function of ventricular dilation associated with IVH. *Developmental Medicine and Child Neurology* 11: 17–21.

Benson, D. F.; LeMay, M.; Patten, D. H.; and Rubens, A. B. 1970. Diagnosis of normal pressure hydrocephalus. *New England Journal of Medicine* 283: 609–15.

Benton, A. L.; Hamsher, K.; Varney, N.; and Spreen, O. 1983. *Contributions to Neuropsychological Assessment: A Clinical Manual.* New York: Oxford University Press.

Byrne, K.; Abbeduto, l.; and Brooks, R. 1990. The language of children with spina bifida and hydrocephalus: Meeting task demands and mastering syntax. *Journal of Speech and Hearing Disorders* 55: 118–23.

Centers for Disease Control. 1992. Recommendations for the use of folic acid to reduce the number of cases of spina bifida and other neural tube defects. *Morbidity and Mortality Weekly Report* 41(RR-14): 1–7.

Clements, D. B., and Kaushal, K. 1970. A study of ocular complications of hydrocephalus and meningomyelocele. *Transactions of the Ophthalmology Society* 90: 383–90.

Cull, C., and Wyke, M. 1984. Memory function of children with spina bifida and shunted hydrocephalus. *Developmental Medicine and Child Neurology* 26: 177–83.

Cutler, R. W.; Page, L.; Galicich, J.; and Watters, G. V. 1968. Formation and absorption of cerebrospinal fluid in man. *Brain* 91: 707–20.

Dennis, M. 1985. Intelligence after early brain injury: II. IQ scores of subjects classified on the basis of medical variables. *Journal of Clinical and Experimental Neuropsychology* 7: 555–76.

Dennis, M., and Barnes, M. A. 1993. Oral discourse after early onset hydrocephalus: Linguistic ambiguity, figurative language, speech acts, and script-based inferences. *Journal of Pediatric Psychology* 18: 639–52.

Dennis, M. A.; Fitz, C. R.; Netley, C. T.; Sugar, J.; Harwood-Nash, D. C. F.; Hendrick, E. B.; Hoffman, H. J.; and Humphreys, R. P. 1981. The intelligence of hydrocephalic children. *Archives of Neurology* 38: 607–15.

Dennis, M.; Hendrick, E. B.; Hoffman, H. J.; and Humphreys, R. P. 1987. Language of hydrocephalic children and adolescents. *Journal of Clinical and Experimental Neuropsychology* 9: 593–621.

Donders, J.; Canady, A. I.; and Rourke, B. P. 1990. Psychometric intelligence after infantile hydrocephalus: A critical review and reinterpretation. *Child's Nervous System* 6: 148–54.

Donders, J.; Rourke, B. P.; and Canady, A. I. 1991. Neuropsychological functioning of hydrocephalic children. *Journal of Clinical and Experimental Neuropsychology* 13: 607–13.

———. 1992. Emotional adjustment of children with hydrocephalus and of their parents. *Journal of Child Neurology* 7: 375–80.

Dorner, S. 1975. The relationship of physical handicap to stress in families with an adolescent with spina bifida. *Developmental Medicine and Child Neurology* 17: 765–76.

Eslinger, P. J.; Grattan, L. M., Damasio, H.; and Damasio, A. R. 1992. Developmental consequences of childhood frontal lobe damage. *Archives of Neurology* 49: 764–69.

Fenichel, G. M. 1988. *Clinical Pediatric Neurology.* Philadelphia: W. B. Saunders.

Fennell, E. B.; Eisenstadt, T.; Bodiford, C.; Redeiss, S.; and Mickle, J. 1987. The assessment of neuropsychological dysfunction in children shunted for hydrocephalus. *Journal of Clinical and Experimental Neuropsychology* 9: 25–26 [abstract].

Fishman, R. A. (1980) *Cerebrospinal Fluid in Diseases of the Nervous System.* Philadelphia: W. B. Saunders.

Fishman, M. A., ed. 1986. *Pediatric Neurology*. Orlando, Fla.: Grune & Stratton.

Fleming, C. P 1968. The verbal behavior of hydrocephalic children. *Developmental Medicine and Child Neurology* Suppl. 16: 74–82.

Fletcher, J. M.; Bohan, T. P.; Brandt, M. E.; Brookshire, B. L.; Beaver, S. R.; Francis, D. J.; Davidson, K. C.; Thompson, N. M.; and Miner, M. E. 1992. Cerebral white matter and cognition in hydrocephalic children. *Archives of Neurology* 49: 818–24.

Fletcher, J. M.; Francis, D. J.; Thompson, N. M.; Brookshire, B. L.; Bohan, T. P.; Landry, S. H.; Davidson, K. C.; and Miner, M. E. 1992. Verbal and nonverbal skill discrepancies in hydrocephalic children. *Journal of Clinical and Experimental Neuropsychology* 14: 593–609.

Foltz, E. L., and Shurtleff, D. B. 1963. Five-year comparative study of hydrocephalus in children with and without operation (133 cases). *Journal of Neurosurgery* 20: 1064–78.

Gadsdon, D. R.; Variend, S.; and Emery, J. L. 1979. Myelination of the corpus callosum: II. The effect of relief of hydrocephalus upon the process of myelination. *Zeitschrift fur Kinderchirargie* 28: 314–21.

Golden, C. J. 1978. *Manual for the Stroop Color and Word Test*. Chicago: Stoetling.

Grant, D. A., and Berg, E. A. 1948. A behavioral analysis of degree of reinforcement and ease of shifting to new responses in a Weige-type card sorting problem. *Journal of Experimental Psychology* 38: 404–11.

Hammock, M. K.; Milhorat, T. H.; and Baron, I. S. 1976. Normal pressure hydrocephalus in patients with myelomeningocele. *Developmental Medicine and Child Neurology* 18: 55–68.

Horn, D.; Lorch, E.; Lorch, R.; and Culatta, B. 1985. Distractibility and vocabulary deficits in children with spina bifida and hydrocephalus. *Developmental Medicine and Child Neurology* 27: 713–20.

Landry, S. H.; Chapieski, L.; Fletcher, J. M.; and Denson, S. 1988. Three year outcomes for low birth weight infants: Differential effects of early medical complications. *Journal of Pediatric Psychology* 13: 317–27.

Landry, S. H.; Fletcher, J. M.; Zarling, C. L.; Chapieski, L.; Francis, D. J.; and Denson, S. 1984. Differential outcomes associated with early medical complications in premature infants. *Journal of Pediatric Psychology* 9: 385–401.

Laurence, K. M. 1969. Neurological and intellectual sequelae of hydrocephalus. *Archives of Neurology* 20: 73–81.

Laurence, K. M., and Coates, S. 1962. The natural history of hydrocephalus: Detailed analysis of 182 unoperated cases. *Archives of Diseases in Childhood* 37: 345–62.

Leech, R. W., and Brumbeck, R. A. 1991. *Hydrocephalus: Current Clinical Concepts*. St. Louis: Mosby Year Book.

Lorber, J. 1968. The results of early treatment of extreme hydrocephalus. *Developmental Medicine and Child Neurology* Suppl. 16: 21–30.

———. 1980. Is your brain really necessary? *Science* 210: 1232–34.

Mathew, N. T.; Meyer, J. S.; Hartmann, A.; and Ott, E. O. 1975. Abnormal cerebrospinal fluid–blood flow dynamics: Implications in diagnosis, treatment and prognosis in normal pressure hydrocephalus. *Archives of Neurology* 32: 657–64.

McCarthy, D. 1972. *McCarthy Scales of Children's Abilities*. New York: Psychological Corporation.

McCullough, D. C., and Balzer-Martin, L. A. 1982. Current prognosis in overt neonatal hydrocephalus. *Journal of Neurosurgery* 57: 378–83.

Menkes, J. H. 1990. *Textbook of Child Neurology,* 4th ed. Philadelphia: Lea & Febinger.

Milhorat, T. H. 1972. *Hydrocephalus and the Cerebrospinal Fluid.* Baltimore: Williams & Wilkins.

———. 1975. The third circulation revisited. *Journal of Neurosurgery* 42: 628–45.

Mirsky, A. F.; Anthony, B. J.; Duncan, C. G.; Ahearn, M. B.; and Kellam, S. G. 1991. Analysis of the elements of attention: A neuropsychological approach. *Neuropsychology Review* 2: 109–46.

Nauta, W. J. H. 1971. The problem of the frontal lobe: A reinterpretation. *Journal of Psychiatric Research* 8: 167–87.

Prigatano, G. P., and Zeiner, H. K. 1985. Information processing and reading competencies in hydrocephalic children. *Language Sciences* 7: 109–28.

Prigatano, G. P.; Zeiner, H. K.; Pollay, M.; and Kaplan, R. J. 1983. Neuropsychological functioning in children with shunted uncomplicated hydrocephalus. *Child's Brain* 10: 112–20.

Query, J. M.; Reichelt, C.; and Christoferson, L. A. 1990. Living with chronic illness: A retrospective study of patients shunted for hydrocephalus and their families. *Developmental Medicine and Child Neurology* 32: 119–28.

Raimondi, A. J., and Soare, P. 1974. Intellectual development in shunted hydrocephalic children. *American Journal of Diseases of Children* 127: 664–71.

Reitan, R. M., and Davison, L. A. 1974. *Clinical Neuropsychology: Current Status and Applications.* Washington, D.C.: V. H. Winston.

Richardson, R. T. E. 1978. Memory and intelligence following spontaneously arrested congenital hydrocephalus. *British Journal of Social and Clinical Psychology* 17: 261–67.

Sand, P. L.; Taylor, N.; Hill, M.; Kosky, N.; and Rawlings, M. 1974. Hand function in children with myelomeningocele. *American Journal of Occupational Therapy* 28: 87–91.

Shaffer, J.; Wolfe, L.; Friedrich, W.; Shurtleff, H.; Shurtleff, D.; and Fay, G. 1986. Developmental expectations: Intelligence and fine motor skills. In D. Shurtleff (ed.), *Myelodysplasias and exstrophies: Significance, prevention and treatment* (New York: Grune & Stratton), pp. 359–72.

Shurtleff, D. B.; Foltz, E. L.; and Loesser, J. D. 1973. Hydrocephalus: A definition of its progression and relationship to intellectual function, diagnosis, and complications. *American Journal of Diseases of Children* 125: 688–93.

Shurtleff, D. B.; Kronmal, R.; and Foltz, E. L. 1975. Following comparison of hydrocephalus with and without myelomeningocele. *Journal of Neurosurgery* 42: 61–68.

Smith, C. K., and Smith, E. D. 1973. Selection for treatment in spina bifida cystica. *British Medical Journal* 4: 178–87.

Soare, P., and Raimondi, J. 1977. Intellectual and perceptual–motor characteristics of treated myelomeningocele children. *American Journal of Diseases of Children* 131: 199–204.

Sørenson, P. S.; Jansen, F.; and Gjerris, F. 1986. Motor disturbances in normal pressure hydrocephalus. *Archives of Neurology* 43: 34–38.

Spain, B. 1974. Verbal and performance ability in preschool children with spina bifida. *Developmental Medicine and Child Neurology* 16: 773–80.

Spiegler, B. J. 1984. Verbal and spatial memory in children with hydrocephalus. Unpublished doctoral dissertation, University of Maryland.

Tew, B. 1979. The "cocktail party syndrome" in children with hydrocephalus and spina bifida. *British Journal of Disorders of Communication* 14: 89–101.

Tew, B., and Laurence, K. M. 1975. The effects of hydrocephalus on intelligence, visual perception and school attainment. *Developmental Medicine and Child Neurology* 17: 129–34.

Thompson, M. G.; Eisenberg, H. M.; and Levin, H. S. 1982. Hydrocephalic infants: Developmental assessment and computerized tomography. *Child's Brain* 9: 400–410.

Thompson, N. M.; Fletcher, J. M.; Chapieski, L.; Landry, S. H.; Miner, M. E.; and Bixby, J. 1991. Cognitive and motor abilities in preschool hydrocephalics. *Journal of Clinical and Experimental Neuropsychology* 13: 245–58.

Torkelson, R. D.; Leibrock, L. G.; Gustavson, J. L.; and Sundell, R. R. 1985. Neurological and neuropsychological effects of cerebral spinal fluid shunting in children with assumed arrested ("normal pressure") hydrocephalus. *Journal of Neurology, Neurosurgery, and Psychiatry* 48: 799–806.

Turner, A. 1985. Hand function in children with myelomeningocele. *Journal of Bone and Joint Surgery* 67: 268–72.

Varni, J. W., and Wallander, J. L. 1988. Pediatric chronic disabilities: Hemophilia and spina bifida as examples. In D. K. Routh (ed.), *Handbook of Pediatric Psychology* (New York: Guilford Press), pp. 190–221.

Volpe, J. J.; Pasternak, J. F.; and Allan, W. C. 1977. Ventricular dilation preceding rapid head growth following neonatal intracranial hemorrhage. *American Journal of Diseases in Children* 131: 1212–15.

Wechsler, D. 1974. *Manual for the Wechsler Intelligence Scale for Children—Revised.* New York: Psychological Corporation.

Wills, K. E. 1993. Neuropsychological functioning in children with spina bifida and/or hydrocephalus. *Journal of Child Clinical Psychology* 22: 247–65.

Wills, K. E.; Holmbeck, G. N.; Dillon, K.; and McLone, D. G. 1990. Intelligence and academic achievement in children with meningomyelocele. *Journal of Pediatric Psychology* 15: 161–76.

Willoughby, R., and Hoffman, R. 1979. Cognitive and perceptual impairments in children with spina bifida: A look at the evidence. *Spina Bifida Therapy* 2: 127–34.

Woods, G. E. 1979. Visual problems in the handicapped child. *Child Care, Health and Development* 5: 303–22.

Yashon, D.; Jane, J. A.; and Sugar, O. 1965. The course of severe untreated infantile hydrocephalus. *Journal of Neurosurgery* 23: 509–16.

Young, H. F.; Nulsen, F. E.; Weiss, M. H.; and Thomas, P. 1973. The relationship of intelligence and cerebral mantle in treated infantile hydrocephalus. *Pediatrics* 52: 54–60.

Zeiner, H. K., and Prigatano, G. P. 1982. Information processing deficits in hydrocephalic and letter reversal children. *Neuropsychologia* 20: 483–92.

Zeiner, H. K.; Prigatano, G. P.; Pollay, M.; Briscoe, C.; and Smith, R. 1985. Ocular motility, visual acuity and dysfunction of neuropsychological impairment in children with shunted uncomplicated hydrocephalus. *Child's Nervous System* 1: 115–22.

8

Epilepsy

This chapter reviews childhood epilepsy. In the first portion, prevalence, seizure classification, etiology, pathophysiology, and diagnostic techniques are reviewed. The next portion covers specific types of epilepsy, with special emphasis on those that first arise in childhood. Cognitive and neuropsychological functions in epilepsy are discussed in the third portion. And finally, the complex issue of the effect of antiepileptic drugs on cognition is addressed.

PREVALENCE

Epilepsy refers to recurrent convulsive or nonconvulsive seizures caused by local or generalized epileptogenic discharges in the brain. The prevalence of epilepsy in the pediatric population has been estimated as falling between 3.3 and 20.5 per 1000 (Cowan et al. 1989; Goodridge & Shorvon, 1983). The latter figure included all cases except those involving only febrile seizures. Prevalence dropped to 17.5 per 1000 when febrile and single seizures were excluded and to 10.5 per 1000 for active epilepsy and for persons receiving treatment. The prevalence rate was highest in children in the 1- to 4-year age range (Cowan et al. 1989).

SEIZURE CLASSIFICATION

In early nosologies, seizures were classified in terms of their clinical manifestations (for example, grand mal, petit mal, or psychomotor). External manifestations of seizures can be misleading, however, and they do not necessarily provide information about the specific brain areas involved, the underlying pathophysiology, or the appropriate treatment approach. New taxonomies are based on information from electroencephalographic studies, the natural history, and treatment response. The current nosology has been in use since 1989 (Classification of Epilepsies and Epileptic Syndromes—International League Against Epilepsy (ILAE). According to this system, epilepsy is divided into two groups: *localization-related* epilepsy (those that involve partial or focal seizures); and *generalized* epilepsy (those that involve seizures affecting diffuse brain areas bilaterally). These two groups are then subdivided into three types each: *idiopathic* (no clearly definable etiology, excluding genetic); *symptomatic* (seizures secondary to some definable factor or disease entity); and *cryptogenic* (epilepsies presumed to be symptomatic, but the precise etiology is occult) (see Table 8-1).

Localization-Related Epilepsy

Localization-related epilepsy (previously focal or partial) refers to seizure discharges that originate from a specific cortical area. These seizures may involve any of three types of symptoms: motor movements of a specific body part, if the seizure arises from motor cortex (for instance, hand twitching or leg jerking); sensory symptoms, if the seizure arises from cortex processing sensory information; or experiential symptoms, if neurons in association cortex are involved. Seizures involving complex cognitive or experiential phenomena (such as automatisms or altered mental state), with or without motor symptoms, are called *complex partial seizures (CPS)*. Focal seizures do not necessarily remain confined to their area of origin. They may spread to other areas within one hemisphere, or from one hemisphere to another, and become generalized.

A *Jacksonian march* refers to the spread of a focal seizure discharge from one area of cortex to another. For example, traveling upward from the lateral aspect of motor cortex along the rolandic fissure, a seizure might start with twitching at the angle of the mouth, followed by thumb and hand, lateral trunk, and leg movements. Similar "marches" may occur in other cortical areas. *Secondary generalization* refers to the spread of seizure activity from a specific focus to both hemispheres.

Generalized Epilepsy

Generalized epilepsy implies bilateral cerebral involvement. Generalized seizures have two forms: nonconvulsive and convulsive. *Generalized nonconvulsive epilepsy* involves a transient lapse of consciousness, sometimes associated with staring, blinking and minor motor automatisms. These seizures, previously called *petit mal* or *centrencephalic,* are now classified as *childhood absence epilepsy* or *juvenile myoclonic epilepsy. Generalized convulsive epilepsy* (previously grand mal) involves loss of consciousness with tonic–clonic motor movements. The *tonic phase* refers to rigid extension and stiffening of the trunk and limbs. This is followed by repetitive jerking or twitching of the head, trunk, and limbs—the *clonic phase*.

Atonic (astatic) seizures are characterized by a sudden loss of postural tone, with a drop of the head or trunk, that may be severe enough to result in a fall. *Myoclonic seizures* are marked by brief, lightning-like jerks of the extremities, head, or body.

Status Epilepticus

Status epilepticus refers to at least 30 minutes of continuous seizure activity or repetitive seizures that occur without the child regaining consciousness. Vari-

Table 8-1   Revised Classification of Epilepsies and Epileptic Syndromes

1. Localization-related (focal, local, partial) epilepsies and syndromes
     1.1 Idiopathic (with age-related onset)
         Benign childhood epilepsy with centro-temporal spike
         Childhood epilepsy with occipital paroxysms
         Primary reading epilepsy
     1.2 Symptomatic
         Chronic progressive epilepsia partialis continua of childhood (Rasmussen's syndrome)
         Syndromes characterized by seizures with specific modes of precipitation
         Temporal lobe epilepsies
             Amygdalo-hippocampal seizures
             Lateral temporal seizures
         Frontal lobe epilepsies
             Supplementary motor seizures
             Cingulate
             Anterior frontopolar
             Orbitofrontal
             Dorsolateral
             Opercular
             Motor cortex
             Kojewnikiow's syndrome (rolandic partial epilepsy)
         Parietal lobe epilepsies
         Occipital lobe epilepsies
     1.3 Cryptogenic
2. Generalized epilepsies and syndromes
     2.1 Idiopathic (with age-related onset, listed in order of age)
         Benign neonatal familial convulsions
         Benign neonatal convulsions
         Benign myoclonic epilepsy in infancy
         Childhood absence epilepsy
         Juvenile myoclonic epilepsy
         Epilepsy with grand mal (GTCS) seizures on awakening
         Other generalized idiopathic epilepsies not defined above
         Epilepsies with seizures precipitated by specific modes of activation
     2.2 Cryptogenic or symptomatic (in order of age)
         West syndrome (infantile spasms)
         Lennox-Gastaut syndrome
         Epilepsy with myoclonic-astatic seizures
         Epilepsy with myoclonic absences
     2.3 Symptomatic
         2.3.1 Nonspecific etiology
             Early myoclonic encephalopathy
             Early infantile epileptic encephalopathy with suppression burst
             Other symptomatic generalized epilepsies not defined above
         2.3.2 Specific syndromes
             Epileptic seizures related to specific disease states
3. Epilepsies and syndromes undetermined whether focal or generalized
     3.1 With both generalized and focal seizures
         Neonatal seizures
         Severe myoclonic epilepsy in infancy
         Epilepsy with continuous spike-waves during slow-wave sleep
         Acquired epileptic aphasia (Landau-Kleffner syndrome)
         Other undetermined epilepsies not defined above
     3.2 Without unequivocal generalized or focal features

Table 8-1 (*continued*)

---

4. Special syndromes
    4.1 Situation-related seizures
        Febrile convulsions
        Isolated seizures or isolated status epilepticus
        Seizures occurring only when there is an acute metabolic or toxic event (e.g., alcohol,
            drugs, eclampsia)

Source: Commission on Classification and Terminology of the International League Against Epilepsy (1989).

ous seizure types can occur during these long or repetitive seizures. Status epilepticus can be convulsive or nonconvulsive. Convulsive seizures can be generalized (primarily or secondarily) and can be tonic–clonic, tonic, clonic, or myoclonic. Convulsive status epilepticus is life-threatening. Nonconvulsive status epilepticus consists of continuous absence seizures or complex partial status epilepticus, and can be hard to distinguish without EEG monitoring (the child may appear "spacey"). *Epilepsia partialis continua* involves clonic activity of a small muscle group (for instance, finger or face twitching) due to involvement of a small cortical area and does not spread. The clonic activity may persist for days or months. Status epilepticus may be symptomatic, idiopathic, or cryptogenic. It may result from abrupt withdrawal of antiepileptic drugs (AEDs).

The Aura and Ictal, Interictal, and Postictal Periods

A series of defined time segments are associated with epilepsy. *Aura* refers to behaviors or experiential phenomena that occur at the seizure onset. The *ictus* is the actual seizure (the adjective *ictal* refers to behaviors associated with the ongoing seizure). *Postictal* refers to the period of time immediately after a seizure. *Interictal* is the period of time between epileptic events. Electroencephalograph (EEG) and positron emission tomography (PET) studies may produce dramatically different results at ictal and interictal periods.

ETIOLOGICAL FACTORS

Childhood epilepsy may result from focal cortical irritative lesions, such as those associated with brain tumors, arteriovenous malformations (AVMs), and cortical trauma. It may also be a consequence of hypoxia (for instance, hypoxic encephalopathy), infection (for instance, meningitis), or a neurodegenerative condition (such as the second stage of Tay-Sachs disease, during which seizures occur. The trigger may be a metabolic etiology such as hypoglycemia (low blood sugar), hyponatremia (low sodium), or biotinidase deficiency. Neonatal seizures are associated with hypocalcemia, hypomagnesemia, and hypoglycemia. Abrupt withdrawal from treatment with an AED can precipitate epilepsy. Seizures may also be a manifestation of a genetic neurodevelopmental syndrome. A genetic predisposition to epilepsy poses an additive risk for seizures from acquired factors.

Genetic Causes

Epilepsy may be familial. Generalized nonconvulsive epilepsy (petit mal) has a strong familial basis (Metrakos & Metrakos 1961), as does benign centrotemporal epilepsy—an idiopathic localization-related seizure disorder (Heijbel, Blom & Rasmuson 1975). Seizure types have been linked to specific chromosomes. For example, cases of juvenile myoclonic epilepsy were linked to chromosome 6, with evidence of genetic variability (Delgado-Escueta et al. 1994) and benign familial neonatal convulsions were linked to chromosome 20 (Ronen et al. 1993).

Twin studies indicate that age at seizure onset may be genetically determined. Segal, Chapman & Barlow (1991) described 11 pairs of monozygotic twins with idiopathic epilepsy, with a concordance rate of 91% for epilepsy and/or EEG abnormalities, and remarkable coincidence in the timing of seizure onset. Nine pairs were concordant for seizures. In one of the two discordant twin pairs, the asymptomatic twin had an abnormal EEG, and the epileptic twin did not.

Neuromigrational Disorders

Heterotopia and other focal NMDs (see Chapter 3) are now appreciated as important etiological factors in epilepsy. For example, severe neuronal ectopia was present in 42% of patients with epilepsy and in none of the normal controls. Resecting the focal lesions resulted in a good clinical outcome (Hardiman et al. 1988). In another study, 30 of 49 seizure patients had focal NMD (macrogyria, polymicrogyria and neuronal heterotopia) (Palmini et al. 1991a). Bilateral perisylvian dysplasia, diffuse cortical dysplasia ("double cortex"), hemimegalencephaly, megalencephaly, and nodular neuronal heterotopia were found in some patients (Palmini et al. 1991b). One report described four generations of females affected with nodular subependymal heterotopia associated with prolonged tonic–clonic seizures (Huttenlocher, Taravath & Mojtahedi 1994).

PATHOPHYSIOLOGY OF EPILEPSY

Seizures arise from a spontaneous discharge of a group of neurons that become progressively more active and *hypersynchronized,* and that *recruit* other neurons. The localized discharge spreads to involve more neurons firing synchronously, reflecting alterations in circuits of inhibitory neurons and neurotransmitter systems (McDonald et al. 1991; Wuarin et al. 1990). Viewing epilepsy as an imbalance between excitatory and inhibitory neuronal systems, however, may be an oversimplification. There is evidence that inhibition is actually increased in the epileptogenic regions of the hippocampus in individuals with CPS (Engel 1988). It is likely that several different mechanisms underlie epileptogenesis in different seizure syndromes.

In addition to cortical neuronal–level events, subcortical circuits play a prominent role in the initiation, propagation, and suppression of seizures, including thalamic nuclei (Velasco et al. 1989), basal ganglia, and substantia nigra (Gale 1988). Moreover, subcortical structures are involved in some of the seizure characteristics. Tonic motor seizures appear to have brainstem origin, and clonic seizures arise from forebrain (predominantly limbic) regions, with the substantia nigra playing an important role in motor behaviors. The substantia nigra is a critical site for the action of certain AEDs that involve the inhibitory neurotransmitter, gamma amino butyric acid (GABA) (Iadarola & Gale 1982).

Ongoing seizure activity may profoundly alter the structure and physiology of neuronal systems, and these alterations may contribute to the persistence of seizures. For example, dendritic spines and dendritic arborization may be reduced in the hippocampus of epileptic patients (Scheibel, Crandall & Scheibel 1974). When epileptogenesis was induced by kindling (discussed later in this section) structural changes consisting of axonal sprouting and synaptic reorganization in limbic pathways occurred before generalized seizures appeared. These structural changes were interpreted as increasing neuronal excitability and rendering the hippocampus more susceptible to epileptic events; they were not accounted for by neuronal loss (Sutula et al. 1988).

The age of the organism has an impact on the way excitatory and inhibitory systems affect neuronal activity and interact. For example, structural features (such as neuronal connections and synaptic systems) may be immature, or neurotransmitter systems (particularly inhibitory systems) may not be fully developed. Therefore, clinical features of childhood seizures, causal factors, and the seizure appearance may differ from the corresponding features in adults. Childhood seizures may also respond differently to AED than do adult seizures.

Experimental models exist for inducing seizures in the laboratory. Induction techniques do not necessarily produce the same seizure type, and the seizures often have specific patterns of response to AED. The models include maximal electroshock-induced seizures, induction by means of specific drugs (for example, pentylenetetrazol, picrotoxin, or bibuculline), and creation of a focal epileptic discharge by intracortical application of penicillin or alumina gel. There are also genetic animal epilepsy models (for instance, the baboon *Papio papio*, with photosensitive seizures; and inbred mice with susceptibility to audiogenic seizures (Neumann & Collins 1991). These models suggest that a primary effect of seizures is to disrupt learning, with greater impairment associated with greater seizure frequency (Holmes et al. 1990).

One experimental model, *kindling,* has relevance to developmental neuropsychiatric syndromes, such as panic and affective disorders (Post 1992). *Kindling* refers to repetitive induction of seizures in a restricted brain area of an animal (Goddard, McIntyre & Leech 1969). The brain is stimulated below the threshold required to produce seizures, so only afterdischarges are elicited in the early phase. Over time, however, the afterdischarges become progressively prolonged, and eventually actual seizures occur. These seizures ultimately become self-generating, at which point they begin to occur spontaneously, *without* the stimulation, and persist for the life of the animal. Limbic areas are particularly susceptible to kindling. Kindling induces generalized seizures more easily in young animals than in adults, indicating that the immature brain, because of poorly developed inhibitory systems, is less able than the adult brain to suppress seizure generalization (Haas, Sperber & Moshé 1990). Kindling produces no structural lesion but is a model for the physiological events surrounding epilepsy.

EVALUATING THE CHILD WITH EPILEPSY

A thorough personal and family history and clinical examination are essential for accurate seizure diagnosis. An adult patient's description of the events surrounding the seizure—the internal experiential phenomena—provides clues about the epileptic focus (for instance, a sense of fear, anxiety, or gastric discomfort; hallucinations; visual alterations in the size or shape of common objects). In children, this information can sometimes be elicited through careful questioning ("Some kids have a funny feeling in their stomachs; have you ever had this happen?"). Parental description of events surrounding the seizure episode is helpful, especially for a very young child. For example, a parent may observe autonomic changes, followed by fear, speech arrest, and right-side motor dysfunction. The neurological examination often permits differentiation between symptomatic and idiopathic epilepsy (see Chapter 4).

Seizures may consist of several sequential events. These experiential, sensory, and motor phenomena may be stereotyped or may vary. Different seizure types may be experienced by one patient. In one prospective study, experiential phenomena were reviewed, and characteristics of auras were related to the final diagnosis (Palmini & Gloor 1992). Auras were found in 93% of patients with temporal lobe onset, in 61% of the frontal lobe group, and in 100% of the parietal–occipital group. Auditory hallucinations occurred only in patients with temporal lobe foci. Somatosensory and visual/ocular auras were associated with parietal–occipital foci. Viscerosensory auras were more frequent in patients with temporal lobe (45%) than with frontal (6%) or parietal–occipital (9%) onset. In contrast, cephalic auras occurred in 24% of frontal patients, but in only 12% of temporal and 3% of parietal–occipital patients. Diffuse warm sensations were more frequent in frontal (18%) than in temporal lobe (2%) patients; they did not occur at all in parietal–occipital patients. Auras of vertigo and conscious confusion were rare and were not linked to a particular site. Experiential auras were more prevalent in patients with temporal lobe seizures (38%) than in those with frontal (4%) or parietal–occipital (6%) seizures. Viscerosensory and experiential auras were more predominant in right-side foci.

Head deviation contralateral or ipsilateral to the seizure focus is often an early seizure event. There is no consensus, however, about the correlation of head movements with a specific cortical focus (Ochs 1984; Wyllie et al. 1986; McLachlan 1987). Sustained ictal head deviation, when it occurs within a few seconds of an EEG seizure and without preceding automatisms, is a reliable sign of frontal lobe seizure origin (Jayakar et al. 1992).

Neurological function may remain altered for a variable period of time following a seizure. Todd (1855) described postictal hemiplegia lasting for a few hours to a few days following a seizure. Although it typically occurs after a focal seizure, a Todd's paralysis (or palsy) may occur on the more affected side after a generalized seizure. In adults, this is strongly correlated with a structural lesion in the contralateral hemisphere, but it is not so clearly localizing in children.

Specific cognitive sequelae of seizures may occur. For example, video and subdural EEG monitoring detected postictal behavioral changes related to the discharging temporal lobe; aphasic disturbances were common after left temporal onset, and emotional flattening and disorientation often followed right-side onset. Postictal automatisms occurred immediately after seizure, but these were rarely manifested with seizure spread (Devinsky et al. 1994). Apraxia may also occur postictally (Devinsky et al. 1993).

TREATMENT OF EPILEPSY

Regardless of epilepsy type, most seizures respond well to AED medication (discussed in a subsequent section of this chapter). Some seizures, however, are *intractable;* that is, no drug, combination of drugs (polytherapy), or dosage level can control the frequency of seizures and permit reasonable function. A child with intractable seizures may become a candidate for seizure surgery, in which the seizure focus site is excised or a segment of (or the entire) corpus callosum is sectioned to prevent seizure activity from spreading from one cerebral hemisphere to the other. A multidisciplinary team evaluates the risk–benefit ratio. The seizure focus site is identified, and the likelihood of cure by means of surgical excision is determined and weighed against potential side effects. For example, a left temporal lobe focus may overlap with a major language area. Wada testing (in which barbiturate is selectively injected into each hemisphere via the right and left internal carotids) is used to identify the hemisphere in which language exists and to assist the neurosurgeon in defining the region to be excised. Thus, for instance, left-side injection will make the patient with speech mediation under left hemispheric control unable to speak for a brief time. Presurgical assessment routinely involves simultaneous EEG and videotape recording, using a split-screen video technique. Patients are often withdrawn from AED. Sometimes, subdural electrodes are inserted to identify a focus clearly. Intraoperative recording and electrical stimulation may also be used.

DIAGNOSTIC TECHNIQUES

Electroencephalography

The electroencephalograph (EEG) machine, first developed in the 1930s, records brain electrical activity through scalp electrodes. This activity is then amplified and recorded on paper, video monitor, or computer. Since the 1930s, EEG technology has made considerable advances, including simultaneous multichannel recording (brain activity recorded simultaneously from different head areas) and computer generation of "paperless" recordings. The EEG frequency spectrum is divided into four different rhythms, each described in terms of units called hertz (Hz), with 1 hertz being equal to 1 cycle per second. The relevant frequency ranges are as follows: delta (less than 4 cycles per second); theta (4 to 8 cycles per second); alpha (8 to 13 cycles per second); and beta (over 13 cycles per second).

EEGs are typically recorded for at least 20 minutes, using scalp electrodes placed in a standardized array by the international 10–20 system (Jasper 1958). Technical adequacy depends on the EEG technician, who checks electrode application, recording, and the child's clinical state and level of consciousness. Baseline EEG activity varies with an individual's age and level of consciousness. The general level of EEG organization is noted—for example, the amount of alpha activity and slowing in various head areas. Typically, a preschool child's EEG alpha activity is less well developed and tends to be slower than an older child's. With maturation, well-developed occipital alpha activity is present during the resting, alert, eyes-closed state. Alpha disappears with eye-opening and drowsiness. Comparative EEG recording with the child awake and then with the child sleeping is common, because different EEG abnormalities emerge during different states.

Provocative techniques are routinely employed. *Hyperventilation* involves asking the patient to breathe rapidly and deeply for 3 minutes. This serves to "blow off" carbon dioxide and provoke latent EEG abnormalities. Children normally manifest EEG slowing in response to hyperventilation, but focal slowing or prolonged slowing after hyperventilation is abnormal. For example, hyperventilation in children with generalized nonconvulsive epilepsy (petit mal) may induce a typical episode of 3 per second spike-and-wave discharges. *Photic stimulation,* in which a strobe light flashes at different frequencies (or with different color frequencies) triggers photosensitive epilepsy. A *sleep deprivation* study may be helpful if a waking EEG is entirely normal; the patient is deprived of sleep prior to examination, to increase sleep time at the EEG laboratory. Certain EEG abnormalities are not usually observed in a waking record—for example, abnormal temporal lobe discharges. Sometimes a lengthy sleep recording is required, as in electrical status epilepticus induced by sleep (continuous spike-and-wave discharges occurring during slow-wave sleep, discussed later in this chapter).

While provocative techniques elicit abnormality in most patients, other approaches may be required in some cases. Standard EEG scalp electrodes only record activity over the convexity of the hemispheres—not from the mesial aspect of the temporal lobe, orbitofrontal cortex, or cortex deep in the sagittal sulcus. Special electrodes can be placed to record this activity. Thus, nasopharyngeal, sphenoidal, or supraorbital electrodes may be used.

Neuroimaging Studies

Neuroimaging studies are useful in the diagnostic evaluation of a child who has seizures. Computerized tomograph (CT) scans—particularly with contrast—may detect lesions such as small tumors, cysts, or an AVM, but they rarely visualize NMDs. Magnetic resonance imaging (MRI) scans are more useful in identifying NMD (Palmini et al. 1991a) or mesial temporal lobe asymmetries suggesting sclerosis. *Sclerosis* is a term used by pathologists to denote shrinkage and hardening of tissues. It implies gliosis and loss of nerve cells. In the hippocampus, the most vulnerable areas are CA4, CA1, and CA3. A higher incidence of abnormal MRI signals (indicating small tumors or gliotic/sclerotic areas) was found in the temporal lobes of epileptic patients (71%) than in controls (6.2%) (Kuzniecky et al. 1987). Volumetric measurements to identify hippocampal atrophy, combined with EEG localization, identified 18 of 20 (90%) patients referred for presurgical evaluation more reliably than did EEG localization (60%) or MRI localization (75%) alone (Murro et al. 1993).

Positron emission tomography (PET) or single-photon emission computed tomography (SPECT) scans have a role in seizure foci detection, although whether an ictal scan or an interictal scan is more reliable remains controversial. Ictal scans demonstrate regions of hyperperfusion, whereas interictal scans demonstrate "cold" spots (regions of hypoperfusion). Cerebral blood flow increases dramatically during seizures (Penfield, von Santha & Cipriani 1939). SPECT and PET scans may show involvement of large areas of brain in the course of CPS, making it possible to identify the hemisphere involved, but not to pinpoint the seizure focus specifically. Ictal SPECT is often able to localize foci in partial seizures not involving the temporal lobe (Marks et al. 1992). Henry, Mazziotta, and Engel (1993), using interictal PET scans in 27 subjects with refractory mesial TLE, found that 93% had areas of hypometabolism in the temporal lobe and in other areas. The ipsilateral thalamus was involved in 63% of these cases. A strong correlation between the degree of thalamic metabolic asymmetry and modality-specific memory dysfunction in patients with mesial TLE has been reported (Rausch et al. 1992). Theodore et al. (1992) reported that PET and quantitative measurements were helpful in identifying the affected temporal lobe when EEG was nonlocalizing, but concluded that these did not offer additional information when the surface EEG localized the focus.

SYNDROMES SPECIFIC TO CHILDREN OR OCCURRING FIRST IN CHILDHOOD

Certain epilepsies occur only in childhood or tend to appear first in childhood. These include juvenile myoclonic epilepsy, febrile convulsions, benign focal epilepsies of childhood, Landau-Kleffner syndrome, syndrome of epilepsy and continuous spike waves during slow-wave sleep, West syndrome, Lennox-Gastaut syndrome, and multifocal independent epileptiform discharges.

Juvenile Myoclonic Epilepsy

Juvenile myoclonic epilepsy represents approximately 7% to 8% of all epilepsies (Janz 1985). It is inherited, and asymptomatic parents and siblings have EEG abnormalities (Delgado-Escueta et al. 1990). Juvenile myoclonic epilepsy consists of absence seizures, myoclonic jerks, and generalized tonic–clonic (GTC) seizures (Grunewald & Panayiotopoulos 1993). The first manifestation is absence seizures, which appear between the ages of 5 and 16 years. These may present as fluctuating attention, because they are not associated with clear behavioral signs. They are followed in adolescence by myoclonic jerks that are typically worse in the morning. The patient may interpret these as "clumsiness" or "nervousness." The results of a neurological examination conducted at this stage typically fall within normal limits, although patients may have a tremor (Panayiotopoulos, Obeid & Tahan 1994). Generalized tonic–clonic seizures occur within months after myoclonic jerks appear. Juvenile myoclonic epilepsy continues into adulthood. These patients are sensitive to sleep deprivation and may be photosensitive; in addition, their seizures may be induced by alcohol consumption. The interictal EEG may show long, generalized 2.5- to 3.5-Hz spike/multiple-spike and slow-wave complexes, without alteration in level of consciousness or other clinical manifestations. Focal EEG abnormalities occur in over 50% of patients (Grunewald, Chroni & Panayiotopoulos 1992) and may lead to misdiagnosis as complex partial seizures. EEG abnormalities are often triggered by hyperventilation. Valproate is the preferred AED; and 90% of patients treated with it become seizure-free (Penry, Dean & Riela, 1989). Carbamazepine, however, is ineffective. Usually patients remain AED-dependent.

Febrile Convulsions

There are two types of febrile convulsions: benign febrile convulsions, and seizures triggered by fever. Benign febrile convulsions are familial, emerge in the second half of the first year of life, occur in the course of a fever exceeding 102°F, are generalized, are self-limited, and are not complex. Seizures triggered by fever are often symptomatic of underlying brain dysfunction and commonly evolve into nonfebrile seizures later in childhood.

Prolonged febrile seizures are associated with neuronal loss (counts below the lower limits of normal) in three hippocampal areas (H_1 zone, end folium, and dentate gyrus) (Sagar & Oxbury 1987). Cell loss was significantly greater when seizures occurred prior to age 3 years, and it was contralateral to the most involved seizure side. Some children subsequently have mesial temporal sclerosis and intractable epilepsy. In one study, 35% of TLE patients had a history of prolonged febrile convulsions. Volumetric measurements showed amygdala and hippocampal atrophy—the former more affected. Prognosis was good following seizure surgery (Cendes, Andermann, Dubeau et al. 1993).

Benign Focal Epilepsies of Childhood

Benign focal epilepsy of childhood occurs in otherwise neurologically normal children and has a good long-term prognosis. Seizures appear after age 2 years. They are typically brief and stereotyped, and they usually occur during sleep. There is familial incidence: 20% to 40% of patients had family members who also had these seizures in childhood (Dalla-Bernardina et al. 1992). Seizures typically disappear in adolescence (Lerman & Kivity 1991). EEG background is normal. Spikes have a characteristic configuration and localization that aids in diagnosis.

There are two main forms of benign childhood epilepsy: benign rolandic epilepsy, and benign occipital epilepsy.

Benign Rolandic Epilepsy

Benign rolandic epilepsy (BRE), also known as benign epilepsy with central-temporal spikes, is the more common type of benign childhood epilepsy, accounting for 16% of all epilepsies (Holmes 1993). Peak incidence of BRE occurs at between age 7 and age 8 years, and boys are more frequently affected than girls. About 98% to 99% of these children become seizure-free by age 16 years (Loiseau et al. 1988). Seizures arise from sensorimotor cortex lying along the rolandic (central) sulcus, which subserves oropharyngeal structures (throat, pharynx, tongue, and mouth) and hand and face areas. There is often a somatosensory aura (numbness or pins-and-needles), and consciousness is rarely impaired during daytime events. Seizure manifestations often switch from one body side to the other. Nocturnal seizures start with clonic mouth movements and difficulty controlling saliva, and they often secondarily generalize. Seizures may be focal or generalized, and they are infrequent or occur only once. EEG findings are distinctive and, with clinical manifestations, confirm diagnosis. The interictal EEG reveals high-amplitude diphasic spikes with prominent following slow waves at the midtemporal and central electrodes. EEG abnormalities may occur without overt clinical seizures or may reflect epileptic symptomatology. There is no increase in neurological examination abnormalities (van der Meij et al. 1992). It has been suggested that rolandic epilepsy is transmitted by an autosomal dominant gene with age-dependent penetrance (Blom & Heijbel 1989). Thus, rolandic spikes are found in 34% of siblings of children with rolandic epilepsy, but only 15% have symptomatic epilepsy.

Benign Occipital Epilepsy

The second form of benign childhood epilepsy is benign occipital epilepsy (BOE), also known as childhood epilepsy with occipital paroxysms. It is less common than BRE (Gastaut, 1982). Peak incidence of onset occurs at between age 5 and age 7 years, and most affected children no longer have seizures in adolescence. Visual symptoms include loss of vision, light flashes, complex-formed visual hallucinations, and changes in the shape and form of objects. Clinical motor seizures may involve GTC, CPS, or other seizure types. Some children experience headache and vomiting after BOE episodes, with a migraine-like profile. The interictal EEG reveals normal background activity with high-voltage diphasic occipital spikes, with characteristic morphology that occurs rhythmically and disappears promptly with eye opening. Darkness and loss of visual fixation increase the EEG abnormality (Panayiotopoulos 1989).

Other types of benign focal epilepsy have been reported. Children with benign complex partial seizures characterized by prominent affective symptoms (fearfulness) occurring briefly (for 1 or 2 minutes) followed by sleep have been reported (Dalla Bernardina et al. 1985). The interictal abnormality was a spike with a following slow wave or rhythmic sharp waves in frontotemporal or parietotemporal areas, either unilaterally or bilaterally. Benign frontal epilepsy was described in 11 children with focal seizures beginning between 4 and 8 years of age and disappearing by adolescence (Beaumanoir & Nahory 1983).

Landau-Kleffner Syndrome (Verbal Auditory Agnosia, Acquired Epileptiform Aphasia)

In Landau-Kleffner syndrome (LKS) (Landau and Kleffner 1957), a previously normal child develops progressive loss of expressive language in the context of paroxysmal EEG activity involving temporal lobe structures. LKS is one model of childhood brain dysfunction in which active seizure discharge in a specific area of developing cortex renders that area nonfunctional—although sometimes reversibly so.

More than 100 cases of LKS have been reported in the last 30 years, and evidence indicates that the language disorder is directly caused by epileptic discharges in critical language areas (Deonna 1991). Landau and Kleffner (1957) suggested that this persistent activity "in brain tissue largely concerned with linguistic communication results in the functional ablation of these areas for normal linguistic behavior." LKS may first appear as lack of responsiveness to verbal commands (Rapin et al. 1977) that becomes increasingly severe. Expressive language is not severely affected initially, but it deteriorates over time. The child may also become apraxic (Ansink et al. 1989). Ictal manifestations of hemiplegias with preservation of consciousness in children with LKS were distinguished from Todd's paralysis, which occurs after the seizure (Hanson & Chodos 1978).

Some children develop a dense auditory agnosia and cannot identify environmental noises, but others recover. Most, however, continue to have significant language-processing deficits (Deonna, Peter & Ziegler 1989). EEGs are abnormal, with several different patterns, including bilateral independent temporal or temporal–parietal spikes, generalized sharp waves or slow-wave discharges, and multifocal or unilateral spikes (Gomez & Klass 1983). Clinical seizures occur in about 80% of cases, with generalized motor seizures most common (Dugas et al. 1982). These seizures are often hard to control, but they improve over time. By age 10 years, only 10% to 20% have seizures, and these children are generally seizure-free by age 15 years (Beaumanoir 1985).

There is no evidence of CNS lesion in children with LKS. The clinical pattern is variable, with some children showing slow and continuous improvement after aphasia onset, and others experiencing a fluctuating course with progressive deficit (Paquier, Van Dongen & Loonen 1992). There is little correlation between the severity of the EEG abnormalities and the speech disorder, and they can fluctuate out of phase (Genton 1993). The older the child, the better the prognosis (Bishop, 1985). Children under age five years have an especially poor prognosis.

Children with LKS resemble deaf children in their inability to process syntax. They can use sign language and prefer the visual channel as a mode of communication (Bishop & Rosenbloom 1987). These childrens' strengths in social interaction suggest that they do not fall on the autistic spectrum. Coupled with the fact that there is no obvious brain lesion, the relationship between age of onset and outcome suggests that the seizure disorder produces these deficits by impairing language comprehension at a crucial stage.

The etiology of LKS is not clear. Brain biopsy was normal in two cases, but it revealed an inflammatory response consistent with a slow virus. A genetic etiology is a possibility, but few familial cases were described (Landau & Kleffner 1957; De Negri 1993). Monozygotic twins discordant for LKS were reported (Feekery, Parry-Fielder & Hopkins 1993). Gordon (1990) suggested that children with severe language deficits but preserved visuo-verbal functions may have an "unusual genetic or acquired pattern of cerebral organization" (p. 271) that makes them particularly sensitive to the impact of repetitive paroxysmal activity. Holmes, McKeever & Saunders (1981) viewed the epileptiform activity as being an epiphenomenon reflecting underlying abnormalities of speech areas rather than as being the direct cause of the aphasic disturbance, citing the fact that speech abnormalities in absence seizures were timed with the spike-wave discharge and consisted of speech arrest, decreased speed, and brief periods of receptive or expressive aphasia, whereas the speech impairment in LKS was not related to the aphasic disturbance.

Does treatment help, particularly in the absence of unequivocal clinical seizures? Nass and Petrucha (1990) described a 3-year-old boy with many features of pervasive developmental disorder who ceased to progress in language after initial speech acquisition. An EEG revealed generalized spike and polyspike activity. An MRI scan was normal. He was started on an AED, with rapid improvement in language output. Similar cases have been described (Deuel & Lenn 1977; Payton & Minshew 1987). In one report, the child had normal development until age 6 years (2 years after clinical seizure onset and an abnormal EEG). Within one week, the girl developed a severe expressive/receptive aphasia that responded to an AED. Subsequent aphasic episodes responded to manipulation of AEDs (Deuel & Lenn 1977).

The role of LKS in developmental dysphasia was explored in a study of 32 children with severe language impairment but without evidence of focal lesion or recurrent seizures (those with IQs below 70, hemiparesis, and recurrent seizures on AEDs were excluded). Two-thirds of the children had no clinical seizures. Repeated standard EEGs were consistently normal in 69% and were abnormal in 56% after sleep deprivation. However, overnight polygraphic EEGs were abnormal in all but 2 children (94%) (Echenne et al. 1992).

Syndrome of Epilepsy and Continuous Spike Waves During Slow-Wave Sleep (Electrical Status Epilepticus Induced by Sleep)

Epilepsy and continuous spike waves during slow-wave sleep (CSWS) resembles LKS to some extent. In both disorders, epileptiform discharges and substantial neuropsychological deficit occur in previously normal children. They differ in that language dysfunction is prominent and the seizure discharge is typically restricted to the temporal-parietal area in LKS, whereas CSWS involves frontal areas and associated cognitive deficits. Some clinicians stress the similarities between LKS and CSWS. For instance, Hirsch et al. (1990) view CSWS as the most severe form of LKS. Others believe that CSWS is distinct from LKS, citing the different cortical areas involved (Genton 1993). Adequate sleep studies need to be performed to make the diagnosis, since the waking EEG may be entirely normal, and since seizures (partial motor or generalized) may occur only at night or not at all. A case of LKS with pure acoustic agnosia, in which continuous spike wave discharges arising from temporal cortex occurred only during rapid-eye-movement (as opposed to slow-wave) sleep, was reported (Genton et al. 1992).

CSWS occurs in 0.5% of children with epilepsy (Morikawa et al. 1989). Previously normal children of preschool to early elementary school age develop profound behavioral and cognitive deficits in the context of a continuous spike-wave discharge during slow-wave sleep—that is, during at least 85% of slow-wave sleep (Jayakar & Seshia 1991; Patry, Lyagoubi & Tassinari 1971). This persistent abnormality usually lasts more than a year. Although cognitive deficits may persist, seizures usually disappear by adolescence. Perez et al. (1993) described five children aged 3 to 8 years with seizure onset occurring at between $2\frac{1}{2}$ and 5 years. Seizures consisted of focal motor activity with secondary generalization; and unilateral frontal foci spread to parietal regions in some children. All had uneventful perinatal histories, normal early development, and only subtle neurological motor signs. All waking EEGs were abnormal, with generalized discharges but normal background rhythms. Intense continuous spike-wave discharges occurred during at least 85% of slow-wave sleep periods. Treatment with ethosuximide and/or prednisone resulted in behavioral and cognitive improvement. The neuropsychological manifestations consisted of a declining IQ, perseveration, and impaired learning of new information. These children were inattentive, hyperactive, impulsive, aggressive, disinhibited, and prone to rapid mood changes. Language and naming were relatively preserved, but verbal fluency was impaired. Reasoning was impaired, and they could not understand "why" questions. Deterioration was rapid in two cases and slow and insidious in the others. With treatment there were rapid gains on intellectual measures (as much as 20 IQ points) and improved behavior. In another report, a child with CSWS was followed from initial seizure (age $3\frac{1}{2}$ years) into adolescence. Cognitive deterioration began shortly after the seizures started, and at age 18 years he functioned adequately only in a semi-supervised setting (Roulet et al. 1991).

West Syndrome (Infantile Spasms, Myoclonic Spasms of Infancy)

West syndrome refers to a triad of infantile spasms, hypsarrhythmic EEG, and mental retardation (Jeavons, Bower & Dimitrakoudi 1973). Over 150 years ago, West (1841) described the "bobbings of the head" of his young son. These movements occurred many times a day in clusters of "bowings and relaxings." Infantile spasms typically appear after the neonatal period, usually between 3 and 8 months of age. Babies can have flexor spasms (flexion of the neck, trunk, arms, and legs), extensor spasms (extension of neck, trunk, and extremities) or a mixed flexor–extensor pattern. As West noted, they occur in clusters and recur many times a day. Parents sometimes misinterpret crying episodes as colic. The EEG has a characteristic *hypsarrhythmic* pattern (Gibbs & Gibbs 1952), consisting of high-voltage slowing and multifocal spikes. The EEG is poorly organized, with asynchrony as well as focal abnormality and burst suppression (Hrachovy, Frost & Kellaway 1984). Frequency of spasms decreases by about 12 months, and they are rare after age 4 years. Infantile spasms are often a manifestation of serious underlying brain disease (for instance, tuberous sclerosis or pertussis encephalopathy). Over 40% of patients with a history of infantile spasms have a history of cortical NMD (Jellinger 1987). In 9% to 14% of cases, however, there is no obvious, definable etiology; that is, they are cryptogenic.

In one study, infants with infantile spasms and hypsarrhythmic EEGs had decreased total sleep time and marked reduction in rapid-eye-movement sleep that reverted to normal as infants responded to treatment (Hrachovy, Frost & Kellaway 1981). The authors suggested that the primary abnormality may occur at a pontine level and involve the serotonergic system. The preferred treatment is high-dose adrenocorticotropic hormone (ACTH), administered intramuscularly. A younger child has a better prognosis than an older (more than 12 months old) child. Steroids are another treatment option, but standard AEDs are often not helpful (Snead 1990). Why ACTH is effective is still unkown. Baram (1993) hypothesized that corticotropin-releasing hormone is a neuropeptide that has highly specific and potent convulsant properties, particularly in the immature brain, and that ACTH suppresses this endogenous convulsant.

There is a 10% to 20% mortality rate in West syndrome, and 75% to 90% of infants become mentally retarded, often in the moderate to severe range. Guzzetta, Crisafulli, and Isaya Crinó (1993) followed 31 infants diagnosed with myoclonic spasms for 28 to 60 months. They noted that, during the acute stage the infants had fluctuating arousal (were usually drowsy), irritability, and fluctuating task performance. They were able to reach and manipulate, but they could not engage in visually guided grasping or following. They also had marked impairment of social behavior and attention. Only 5 infants had developmental quotients over 60.

Children whose infantile spasms are cryptogenic have IQs closer to the normal range. In a prospective study, 38% of children without definable etiology had normal development or only mild retardation (Glaze et al. 1988). Ichiba (1990) reported on two children with West syndrome who were hyperlexic. They could fluently read Japanese and Chinese characters, numbers, Roman alphabet letters, and trademarks at age 3, but without comprehension. They had relative preservation of auditory memory, impaired visual retention and visual constructional abilities, and general impairment of associational abilities.

A review of CT and MRI scans on 98 children with infantile spasms found that 14 had posterior fossa abnormalities (including 6 Dandy-Walker cysts), 65 had supratentorial abnormalities, and 19 had normal scans (Schiffman et al. 1993). Infants with abnormal scans had lower developmental quotients than did those with normal scans. PET scanning may identify small focal lesions. Chugani et al. (1990) found that PET scans can effectively identify areas of cortical hypometabolism, representing focal NMD, in babies with cryptogenic infantile spasms. In a subsequent PET study of children with infantile spasms, Chugani et al. (1992) found an increase in local metabolic rates for glucose in the lenticular nuclei.

When the lesion is restricted to one hemisphere, it is sometimes possible to resect either a lobe or the entire hemisphere, with good results. Caplan et al. (1992) reported on a group of eight children with intractable infantile spasms who underwent surgery for focal structural lesions that either involved one lobe of a hemisphere or were restricted to one hemisphere, with clear improvement in the children's level of alertness and social behavior following surgery.

Lennox-Gastaut Syndrome

The Lennox-Gastaut syndrome (LGS) consists of intractable seizures associated with a generalized slow spike-and-wave discharge on EEG and mental retardation (Chevrie & Aicardi 1972). LGS emerges at around age 2 years (the overall range is from 1 to 7 years), and represents about 3% of childhood epilepsies. In some cases, infantile spasms precede LGS. Mental retardation is seen in about 80% of children. The younger the child is at onset, the greater is the child's risk of mental retardation. The risk increases further in the presence of an underlying neurological disorder. LGS often involves several different types of seizures—for example, classical and atypical absence, tonic, atonic, myoclonic, and complex partial. Seizures are often refractory to treatment. Other types of seizures—multifocal independent epileptiform discharges, electrical status epilepticus in sleep, LKS, partial complex seizures of frontal lobe origin, atypical benign partial epilepsy of childhood (Aicardi & Chevrie 1982), and occipital lobe epilepsy (Niedermeyer, Riggio & Santiago 1988), for instance— have an underlying similarity with LGS in that generalized slow spike-and-wave discharges occur during slow-wave sleep, although the waking EEG reveals a much more restricted discharge.

Multifocal Independent Epileptiform Discharges

The interictal EEGs of children with multifocal independent epileptiform discharges (MIED) show three or more foci of interictal epileptiform activity, with at least one focus present in each hemisphere. Clinically, these children have frequent, generalized, tonic–clonic seizures, often with intermixtures of several different seizure types that are hard to control (Noriega-Sanchez & Markand 1976; Blume 1978). The children are often mentally retarded. The seizures are resistant to AED treatment, but surgical treatment may be beneficial. In one report, four children had extensive scalp EEG recordings revealing MIED. However, each child had clinical seizures that appeared to be of focal origin, most with a "fencing posture." Three improved after surgery (Burnstine et al. 1991).

COMMON TYPES OF EPILEPSY ENCOUNTERED IN BOTH CHILDREN AND ADULTS

In this section, seizure disorders that begin in childhood and continue into adulthood or first emerge in adulthood are reviewed.

Complex Partial Epilepsy of Temporal Lobe Origin

Complex partial seizures (CPS) arise in temporal or prefrontal areas, often involve elaborate cognitive or experiential phenomena, and are associated with stereotypic behaviors (automatisms). Older nomenclature refers to these seizures as *psychomotor* or *temporal lobe epilepsy (TLE)*. These are sometimes called *petit mal* seizures by the lay public because their symptoms are not convulsive—that is, they do not involve tonic–clonic movements—but their EEG patterns and response to AED are quite different.

Seizures that arise from foci in the temporal lobe have been of particular interest to neurologists and neuropsychologists. Hughlings Jackson (1880–1881) described "elaborate mental states" associated with TLE. In 1933, Penfield (1975) was able to elicit a memory flashback with temporal lobe electrical stimulation. While these electrically elicited experiences seemed real, patients knew they were not.

Age may determine seizure characteristics. Duchowny (1987) described CPS in 14 infants under 2 years of age studied by video-EEG monitoring. Seizures consisted of a behavioral arrest and lateralized tonic posturing of one upper extremity with head and eye deviation (either adversive or contraversive), resembling a tonic neck response. Unilateral jerking of the eye or mouth and facial automatisms occurred in about half of the children. Although hard to assess, consciousness appeared to be impaired. Onset on the EEG was unilateral, but there were multifocal discharges. The infants were uniformly retarded. In contrast, a normal developmental outcome was reported for a group of children with a strong family history of seizures, normal neurological examination, onset during the first year of life, normal interictal EEG, and excellent response to treatment. The seizures occurred in clusters—as many as 10 episodes in one day—and were characterized by behavioral arrest, decreased responsiveness, staring, simple facial automatisms, and mild motor convulsive movements (head/eye deviation and clonic movements) (Watanabe et al. 1990).

The hippocampus, amygdala, and temporal lobe neocortex are often involved in these seizures and can contribute to both the characteristics of the epileptic event and the neuropsychological profile. Tumors, small AVMs, harmartomas, sclerosis, and NMDs represent major neuropathological etiologies of TLE. However, a substantial number of cases do not involve evident lesions, and therefore localization is not readily apparent. Moreover, many patients have evidence of bilateral TLE, since seizures tend to propagate to the other temporal lobe, despite there being only one focus. Surgery is an important treatment option.

Patterns of Seizure Spread in Temporal Lobe Epilepsy

As is the case with other epilepsies, those that arise in the temporal lobe may spread to involve other areas. Seizure spread may be associated with either an experiential phenomenon that the patient can describe or an observable behavior. In one study, 220 seizures from 53 patients with complex partial epilepsy of temporal lobe origin were analyzed (Gloor et al. 1993). Four main types of seizure spread were noted: Type 1, spread from mesial temporal structures to contralateral mesial temporal structures, before involvement of ipsilateral temporal isocortex; Type 2, spread from mesial temporal to ipsilateral temporal isocortex; Type 3, spread from mesial temporal to contralateral mesial temporal to contralateral isocortical temporal cortex, prior to extending into ipsilateral temporal isocortex; Type 4 (most common), spread from ipsilateral temporal isocortex to contralateral temporal regions. The authors suggested that seizures spread to the other hemisphere through the dorsal hippocampal commissural system.

Clinical Data Aiding Lateralization of the Focus.

Clinical observations may lead to lateralization of the focus. The role of speech phenomena in TLE was evaluated (Gabr et al. 1989). Analyses of 100 CPS videotaped in 35 patients during EEG monitoring found speech manifestations in 79 seizures. These consisted of vocalizations (not speech) in 48.5% of patients, identifiable speech occurring ictally in 34.2%, and abnormal speech (speech arrest, dysarthria, or unintelligible speech) in 51.4% (ictally or postictally). Among patients with *postictal* dysphasia, 92% had seizures originating from the dominant temporal lobe; and among those with *ictal* speech, 83% had seizure origin in the nondominant side.

Another localizing sign is lower-face weakness opposite the temporal lobe seizure focus (Cascino, et al. 1993). A detailed history of the experiential aspects of the seizure may be valuable in localizing CPS—for instance, the TLE patient's aura. The nature of the seizure may also provide information about which temporal lobe region is involved (Chee et al. 1993). Palmini, Gloor, and Jones-Gotman (1992) described a small group of TLE patients with pure amnestic episodes as one of their seizure manifestations—that is, episodes without alteration in consciousness, but with subsequent dense amnesia for the event. They observed that "impairment of consciousness" actually consisted of two separable phenomena: unresponsiveness and amnesia. They postulated that pure amnesic seizures occurred when mesial temporal structures were inactivated but temporal cortex was spared.

Gloor et al. (1982) suggested that experiential phenomena associated with TLE are the result of limbic structure activation rather than of temporal neocortex. In a depth electrode study of 35 patients with medically intractable seizures, 18 (52%) reported experiential phenomena that were either electrically elicited or part of the spontaneous seizure. Most of these experiences were described in terms of visualized images, rather than formed auditory perceptions. Some of the unusual experiential illusions involved time perception changes, such as "everything is slowing down."

Mesial Temporal Lobe Epilepsy

Mesial temporal lobe epilepsy (MTLE) accounts for the largest group of patients with medically intractable epilepsy who are successfully treated with neurosurgery (Dreifuss 1987). Although some patients have tumors, AVMs, or NMD, the most characteristic lesion is mesial temporal sclerosis (also called *Ammon's horn sclerosis* or *hippocampal sclerosis*). It was suggested that hippocampal (incisural) sclerosis was the result of a prolonged, traumatic birth (Earle, Baldwin & Penfield 1953), although this view was subsequently challenged (Babb & Brown 1987).

MTLE typically begins in mid-childhood. In one study, 67 patients without evidence of tumors, who ultimately had depth electrode EEG studies and mesial temporal lobectomy/ hippocampectomy, were described (French et al. 1993; Williamson et al. 1993). Mean age of onset was 9 years (with a full range of from 9 months to 32 years), with initial seizure occurring before age 17 years in 88%. Many had a history of febrile seizure (78%), and some had a history of head trauma (15%). Only 2 patients had a history of prolonged, difficult labor with forceps delivery, suggesting that incisural sclerosis is not a major factor. Of the study sample, 66 patients had CPS at initial episode, and 28% had GTC seizures, but these did not occur as the exclusive seizure type in any patient; 64 patients (96%) reported an aura preceding some or all seizures. The most common aura was abdominal visceral sensation—nausea, pressure, butterflies, or a rising epigastric sensation (these were not specific for MTLE). In 25 patients (39%), the aura did not include visceral sensations, but consisted most frequently of fear, smell, light-headedness, déjà vu, generalized somatosensory sensations, and "indescribable." About one-third had seizures that evolved over time, becoming progressively more elaborate. Neurological examination was normal in all but 3 patients. Neuropathological evaluation was possible for 59 of the 67 patients. Mesial temporal sclerosis was found in 48 (81%).

Mesial temporal sclerosis, if severe, can be seen on MRI scan. In the preceding studies (French et al. 1993; Williamson et al. 1993), CT scans were normal in all but 1 patient. In 23 of 28 patients, MRI found unilateral hippocampal atrophy. MRI evidence of MTL atrophy corresponding to neuropathological evidence of medial temporal sclerosis was generated in 91% of the cases, with one false negative and one false positive. Thus, a normal MRI does not rule out the diagnosis of mesial temporal sclerosis (Jackson, Kuzniecky & Cascino 1994).

When presurgical computerized volumetric measurements of the hippocampus and temporal lobe were correlated with neuropsychological findings, it was demonstrated that the left and right hippocampi were symmetrical in control subjects but that the hippocampus ipsilateral to the seizure focus was smaller in seizure patients (Lencz et al. 1992). Significant correlations with some verbal memory measures were observed for patients with left temporal lobe seizures.

Posterior Temporal Lobe Epilepsy

Clinical differences exist if epilepsy originates in anterior versus posterior temporal lobe regions. Automatisms often appear early in the seizure sequence and are pronounced with anterior temporal lobe seizures, while motor manifestations are not a major component. Seizures arising in posterior temporal cortex, common in the pediatric population, often start with behavioral arrest (Duchowny et al. 1994); speech disturbance is prominent (Lüders et al. 1991); and sometimes visual hallucinations occur. Motor seizures are followed by tonic stiffening of the contralateral arm, and then by clonic movements. Automatism occurs late in the sequence. The patients studied had interictal spike focus maximal in the posterior temporal scalp electrodes, or evidence of focal lesion. A case of seizures arising from the left fusiform gyrus, with adolescent onset and characterized by impaired spontaneous speech and language comprehension without loss of consciousness, was reported (Suzuki et al. 1992).

Amgydala Epilepsy

Consistent evidence of severe neuronal loss and gliosis in the amygdala of patients with intractable epilepsy who require surgery was reported (Hudson et al. 1993), whereas hippocampal sclerosis was found in only 65% to 73% of patients (Babb & Brown 1987; Bruton 1988). In one study (Hudson et al.

1993), hippocampal sclerosis patients exhibited significantly reduced performance relative to those without, and to controls, on a recognition memory test for words and on recall of simple geometric figures.

The role of the amygdala in epileptogenesis has only recently been appreciated. For example, when the amygdala was resected along with a small area of hippocampus, 63% of patients achieved seizure control (Feindel & Rasmussen 1991). In another study, 30 patients with intractable TLE and 7 patients with foci outside the temporal lobe had MRI volumetric studies of their amygdala, hippocampal formation, and anterior temporal lobe. Hippocampal formation measurements provided lateralization in 87% of subjects, whereas combined amygdala and hippocampus measurements provided lateralization congruent with the clinical data in 93% (Cendes, Andermann, Gloor et al. 1993).

Occipital Lobe Epilepsy

Only a small percentage of epilepsies involve the occipital lobe. In one series, seizures started between 1 and 26 years of age (with the mean age of onset 11 years). A circumscribed lesion (for instance, a low-grade neoplasm, cortical dysplasia, or hamartoma) was the etiological factor in 44% of cases. In most cases, the interictal EEG was localized to the posterior area. There were two types of seizure onset: elementary visual hallucinations (sparks or flashes), and loss of vision. A small percentage had complex visual hallucinations. Eye blinking often occurred. In 56%, visual field defects were the only abnormal neurological finding (Williamson et al. 1992). A case of acute cortical blindness in a 7-year-old boy in the context of bioccipital epileptogenic discharges was described. The seizure involved associated sensations of loud noises, abdominal pain, nausea, vomiting, ocular pain, and abrupt loss of vision, but the child preserved consciousness throughout the episode (Zung & Margalith 1993).

Parietal Lobe Epilepsy

Parietal lobe epilepsy consists of simple partial seizures with prominent sensory symptoms, including tingling sensations and a feeling of "electricity" that may remain in one area or may spread in a Jacksonian march. The body areas most involved are those with the largest cortical representation (hand, arm, and face). Seizures arising near the mesial aspect of the parietal lobe may give rise to genital sensations, and these often become secondarily generalized. A sensation of body part motion may be involved. There may be negative phenomena (for example, partial loss of a visual scene, loss of sensation, or numbness). Right parietal seizures may be associated with visual neglect (Heilman & Gregory 1980). Vertiginous sensations may be involved. Visual ictal phenomena may include *metamorphosia* (that is distortions of the shape of a common object). Parietal lobe seizures may spread into the adjacent temporal lobe, or those close to the midline may become generalized. Parietal lobe seizures affecting the dominant parietal lobe may also have ictal aphasic symptoms.

Frontal Lobe Epilepsy

Frontal lobe epilepsy (FLE) may be simple partial, complex partial, or secondarily generalized seizures, or a combination of these. It is associated with a wide range of atypical complex motor behaviors and automatisms. Although patients may be fully alert and in contact with the environment, they may experience emotionalized images that give a psychotic flavor to the event. Frontal lobe epilepsies are subdivided into supplementary motor seizures, cingulate seizures, anterior frontopolar region seizures, orbitofrontal, dorsolateral, opercular, motor cortex, and rolandic partial epilepsy (see Table 8-1).

FLE typically begins in childhood. In one series, mean age was 12 years (with a full range of from 5 to 21 years) (Williamson et al. 1985). Seizures may be frequent (25 to 100 per month), are often nocturnal, and may occur in clusters. FLE responds well to carbamazepine. Seizures may include axial, midline motor behaviors (vocal, respiratory, pelvic thrusting); symmetrical, bimanual activity (clapping, rubbing, snapping of fingers, hugging, manipulation of the genitals, cheerleader pose); or bipedal activity (bicycling leg movements or kicking). Vocalizations (humming, moaning) and cursing are often observed. The automatisms associated with these seizures are not stereotyped. Postictal confusion is minimal, if not absent.

A range of emotional/affective behaviors accompanies FLE—for example, laughter, sexual behaviors, screaming. One patient with a deep medial frontal lobe tumor had seizures associated with an aura of extreme embarrassment, followed by tonic movements of the left arm and other motor manifestations (Devinsky, Hafler & Victor 1982). Three patients experienced intrusive, horrific mental images (visions of murder, graveyards, or rats) in the context of deep orbital foci. There was no loss of consciousness; episodes lasted a few seconds to minutes; and the patients continued to interact and talk while the images occurred. They also reported anxiety, and aggressive behavior was prominent. Standard EEGs were normal, but enhancing techniques revealed discharges arising from deep orbitofrontal foci (Fornazzari et al. 1992). A 13-year-old girl was evaluated for inattention, for failing grades, for volatile, unpredictable, irritable, aggressive behavior, and for precocious sexual activity. During seizures, she briefly turned to the right, stared, and picked at her clothes (Boone et al. 1988).

Patients with FLE often have normal intelligence, but they may show deficits on "frontal" tasks. For example, the 13-year-old girl just mentioned was impaired on tasks involving motor speed, attention, response inhibition, and alternation, but had normal performance on the Wisconsin Card Sorting and verbal fluency tests. Her behavior and test performances improved dramatically with carbamazepine treatment, and she subsequently expressed remorse and shame for her behaviors.

Supplementary motor seizures (mesial frontal lobe epilepsy) often start in childhood. Waterman et al. (1987) described 12 such patients. Of these, 10 had had seizures starting prior to age 18 years and 1 had had them in infancy. Most had normal intelligence, and 9 had normal neurological examinations.

Seizures were frequent (25 to 100 per month) and consisted of vocal/respiratory affective behaviors (shouting, laughing, cursing, deep breathing, cursing, lip-smacking, swallowing, or chewing), bimanual and bipedal activity (clapping, hugging, bicycling movement), and axial movements (running, thrashing, shrugging shoulders). Seizures were often nocturnal and occurred in clusters. There was little or no postictal confusion. Awareness was variably preserved, and automatisms were typically unstereotyped.

Quesney et al. (1990) studied 40 FLE patients who had successful surgical removal of the parasaggital cortical (PSC) region ($n = 10$) or the anterolatero-dorsal frontal cortical region (ALDC) ($n = 30$). Nine of the 10 PSC patients had an aura, whereas 50% of the ALDC group had an aura. The aura of the PSC group was somatosensory, involving the contralateral aspect of the head, arm, or leg, and all had either partial or focal seizures with secondary generalization. The ALDC auras were more variable and complex, resembling those of TLE, and only half had partial motor seizures. Head turning occurred in about one-third of each group, but all PSC patients were aware of the head turn. Automatic behaviors occurred in 30% of the ALDC group, but these were absent in the PSC group.

Photosensitive Seizures

Photosensitive seizures are triggered by light flashes. Often encountered in children, video-game epilepsy is now well-recognized. Video games may be more effective triggers of electrocortical activation than standard laboratory maneuvers (De Marco & Ghersini 1985). In a literature review, seven children who experienced seizures, pounding headaches, and/or nausea while playing video games were found. Their EEGs revealed different patterns of abnormality, but all were generalized. Most had a photoconvulsive response. Treatment consisted of video-game avoidance or valproate, with good response (Maeda et al. 1990).

Reflex Epilepsy (Precipitated Seizures)

Reflex epilepsies (precipitated seizures) are consistently preceded by specific environmental or internal factors. Epilepsy may be triggered by a cognitive act (for instance, induced by thinking) (Wilkins et al. 1982), by use of a calculator (Yamamoto et al. 1991), or by writing and calculating with fingers (Hasegawa et al. 1981). *Familial rectal pain* is a form of reflex epilepsy (Schubert & Cracco 1992). Chronic rectal pain is unusual, since the reflex pain is both the trigger and the ictal manifestation. *Bathing-induced* seizures are unusual seizures that occur when young children are immersed in water (Lenoir et al. 1989).

Reading epilepsy is a form of reflex epilepsy (Bickford et al. 1956). The child has sensation of jaw and throat movements while reading; and these develop into actual myoclonic movements, become increasingly frequent if reading is continued, and culminate in a convulsion. Familial cases (with an autosomal dominant pattern of inheritance) and cases resulting from left hemisphere injury have been reported (Lee et al. 1980). In most cases, ictal discharges are localized to the left frontocentral area, but jaw jerks may be associated with a brief bilateral synchronous EEG discharge. A report of association with a left fronto-central lesion was described. Seizures occurred when the patient read aloud or silently (including simple and complex material, nonsense reading, and nonword reading). Humming did not trigger seizures. The least effective stimulus was single-word reading. It was suggested that seizures were specifically triggered by grapheme-phoneme transformations, that reflex epilepsy involves other aspects of language processing (such as writing), and that different reading epilepsy patterns may depend on the extent of epileptogenic cortex (Ritaccio et al. 1992).

Pseudoepileptic (Psychogenic) Seizures

Psychogenic seizures are not due to actual epileptogenic activity. They represent a difficult diagnostic problem and are often AED-resistant. Hospitalization and EEG video-monitoring may not result in a definitive diagnosis. Pseudoseizures differ from real seizures in that epileptiform EEG activity is not present during a seizure and postictal slowing does not occur. Diagnosis is easier when pseudoseizures involve motor behavior. When pseudoseizures involve psychic phenomena, however, the distinction is often complex. Careful history, direct observation, repeated EEG monitoring, and psychiatric evaluation help make the determination. An experimental paradigm was developed to evaluate the efficacy of inducing seizures by suggestion. The investigators contrasted 93 psychogenic epilepsy patients with 20 genuinely epileptic patients. Induction attempted with a standardized protocol was positive in 72 of the psychogenic cases, but in none of the epileptics. Sensitivity and specificity were high with a positive predictive value of 100% (Lancman et al. 1994).

COGNITIVE FUNCTIONING AND EPILEPSY

Cognitive impairment is correlated with epileptic activity in several ways: cognitive dysfunction occurring in the course of a clinical epileptic event; postictal cognitive dysfunction; transitory cognitive impairment occurring as a result of interictal epileptiform discharges; persisting cognitive dysfunction in children; cognitive deficits associated with atypical lateralization of function, secondary to reorganization of neuronal circuits; and nonspecific effects of epilepsy on cognition. A brief overview of these different types of cognitive impairment is presented in the following subsections. In addition, researchers have produced numerous descriptions of focal lesions that give rise to epilepsy and to specific cognitive and/or motor symptoms in adult patients. Review of this extensive literature, however, is beyond the scope of this chapter. For an overview, the reader is referred to Lishman (1987) and Bennett (1992).

Ictal Cognitive Dysfunction

The relationship between cognitive dysfunction and seizure activity is straight-forward. Ongoing behavior is disrupted during the spontaneous discharge of groups of neurons. The type of disruption and the resulting cognitive changes depend on the foci or brain regions involved in the seizure. In the preceding pages, examples of cognitive dysfunction occurring during ictal events were presented. These aphasic disturbances, impaired attentional capacity, and deficits in prefrontal functioning are frequent concomitants of ictal events. While tests selected for evaluation of the child with epilepsy do not differ substantially from tests normally selected for many other neurological conditions, the clinician may decide to administer tests selectively in order to evaluate these functional areas more thoroughly. Tests of attention/concentration/vigilance and mental shifting often provide evidence of the fluctuating behavior associated with epilepsy. A characteristic 'in-and-out' quality may be observed across test sessions and may be especially helpful when observed within a test session—for instance, unimpaired performance early in a session, followed by error on an identical task later in the same session (during the ictal event). The timing of the neuropsychological evaluation may also affect results. Clinical or subclinical seizures negatively influence behavior, although determination that there is an actual ictal event may be difficult. Once the event is confirmed, the examiner must decide whether testing can be reliably continued or is best postponed. For example, a brief focal discharge may not interfere with continued testing, but a generalized seizure with postictal confusion necessitates temporary discontinuation.

Postictal Cognitive Dysfunction

Since disruption in cognitive and motor processes may persist during the postictal period, clinical testing must be postponed when there is evidence of altered consciousness and/or resultant cognitive impairment. The type and the duration of these disruptions depend on the type and the focus of the seizure activity. Examples were also provided of specific dysfunction of local cortical circuits induced by clinically apparent epileptic activity (Devinsky et al. 1993; Devinsky et al. 1994), including postictal aphasic disturbances after left temporal onset, emotional flattening and disorientation after right temporal lobe onset, apraxia, and cognitive and behavioral deficits associated with FLE (Boone et al. 1988). Further, determining the relative effects of postictal disruption and AED therapy is difficult. Multiple test sessions may be helpful in making these distinctions.

Transitory Cognitive Impairment and Interictal Discharges

Subclinical seizures often escape clinical detection but can reliably be detected by EEG monitoring. The episodic disruption of normal neural activity resulting from interictal EEG discharges is called *transitory cognitive impairment (TCI)* (Aarts et al. 1984). When these interictal events are closely monitored with video and EEG, subtle, fleeting, behavioral changes are apparent. Cognitive deficits are clearly linked to the hemisphere in which the interictal discharge occurred. During continuous performance tasks, left-side discharges were associated with transient verbal impairment and right-side discharges with transient visuospatial deficit (Aarts et al. 1984; Shewmon & Erwin 1988). Shewmon and Erwin (1988) further demonstrated that the impairment was *timed* with the EEG discharge and that deficit fluctuated within an individual. When right- and left-hemisphere discharges occurred independently, the deficit was greater with the hand or visual field contralateral to the discharge, suggesting that the deficit was not due to chronic brain damage.

TCI is a spontaneous occurrence, but the effect is similar to what occurs with electrical stimulation of a small brain area. Stimulation disrupts the neuronal processing that occurs in an area (Ojemann 1983). Sometimes the effect is complex, involving both excitatory and inhibitory phenomena. For example, a patient with left limbic system discharges had impaired verbal task performance when interictal discharges were noted and had better performance when material was presented to the right hemisphere. There was little effect on visuospatial material. Conversely, right-hemisphere performance improved when the left hemisphere was adversely affected by discharges (Regard et al. 1985). Whether this reflects "rewiring," a selective inhibitory mechanism protecting the right hemisphere from effects of seizure activity, or elimination of tonic inhibition of the right hemisphere by the left side is unclear. It has been suggested that interictal discharges may impair important stages of learning in which newly learned information is "rehearsed, elaborated, and integrated with previously stored knowledge" (Binnie, Channon & Marston 1990, p. S4); that is, stages in processing higher order associations and consolidating memories may be disrupted.

Subclinical discharges may result in increased errors during neuropsychological testing. Seventy children (6 to 15 years of age) with either secondary generalized or partial epilepsy were tested with two continuous performance tests (a nonverbal, visuospatial task consisting of a computer-generated Corsi's Block Test and a visually presented word list). They showed a clear association between epileptiform discharges and errors. Right-side discharges impaired visuospatial performance, and left-side discharges affected verbal performance (Kasteleijn-Nolst Trenité et al. 1988; Kasteleijn-Nolst Trenité et al. 1990; Kasteleijn-Nolst Trenité, Siebelink & Berends 1990).

Persisting Cognitive Dysfunction

The impact of epilepsy on the immature brain may be long-lasting, as in the regression of language in LKS. Diverse cognitive functions may be affected. For example, enduring prefrontal deficits are seen in CSWS. Relatively subtle deficits may also be noted. For example, comprehension of emotional prosody in children with CPS of right temporal lobe onset fell below that of normal children but did not differ from that of the left-hemisphere onset group (Cohen et al. 1990).

Cognitive Deficits Associated with Cortical Reorganization in Childhood-Onset Epilepsy

Another complication in the neuropsychological evaluation of the epileptic child is the likelihood that there has been cortical reorganization of function. For example, although bilateral speech representation may be indicated, one hemisphere may actually dominate language function. Nass and Myerson (1985) described a left-handed boy with a left fronto-parietal vascular malformation who developed right focal seizures at age 18 months, with a Todd's palsy lasting several days. Seizures were intractable. Extensive neuropsychological testing at age 13 years revealed mild language deficit but normal intelligence. Preoperative Wada testing found no aphasia following either left or right amytal injection, and there was no speech arrest during left Sylvian fissure stimulation. Yet, global aphasia resulted after surgical removal of the lesion. Despite postoperative improvement, deficits associated with left hemisphere damage remained. Since the surgical site was not in the sylvian region, a more diffuse representation of language in the left hemisphere was suggested.

Kurthen et al. (1992) evaluated the interhemispheric dissociation of expressive and receptive language functions in patients with intractable childhood-onset epilepsy who had presurgical Wada evaluations. The majority (72.2%) were left-hemisphere dominant for language, 7.6% showed right-hemisphere dominance, and 20% had evidence of bilateral hemispheric language processing. Most had evidence of bilateral language representation—either predominantly lateralized to the left hemisphere, with minor representation of language on the right, or with clear double language function. Four patients (3.8%) had strong bilateral language representation, with evidence of interhemisphere dissociation of receptive and expressive functions. One patient had expressive language function represented in the right hemisphere and receptive function in the left; another had right receptive and left expressive function.

Nonspecific Effects of Epilepsy and Its Treatment on Cognitive Function

Less specific effects arise as the result of sleep disturbances associated with epilepsy that result in diurnal lethargy (Binnie, Channon & Marston 1990). In addition, epilepsy treatment (AED therapy) may affect cognition and learning, as reviewed in the following section.

LEARNING DISABILITY AND EPILEPSY

The literature suggests that children with epilepsy are at greater risk for learning disability (LD) (Rutter, Graham & Yule 1970; Stores 1978). An estimated

5% to 50% of epileptic children have learning problems (Thompson 1987). Aldenkamp et al. (1987) reported that approximately 30% of children with therapy-resistant epilepsy received special education, compared to 7% of matched controls. As epileptic children grew older, they tended to drop out of school; and by adolescence, only about 33% remained in school, compared to twice that many controls. In addition to complicating clinical assessment, these children's considerable test–retest variability poses methodological problems for cognitive studies (Farwell, Dodrill & Batzel 1985). One-time cognitive assessments were not prognostically reliable (Rodin, Schmaltz & Twitty 1986).

Risk factors for learning deficit include early epilepsy onset and prolonged (Dodrill 1986) or intractable (Kupke & Lewis 1985) seizures. Despite assumptions that an IQ decline with age and continuing seizures was to be expected, longitudinal study of 45 children failed to observe WISC-R verbal, performance, full-scale IQ, or subtest profile changes over a 4.2-year period, despite a high seizure frequency in most children (Aldenkamp et al. 1990). The authors noted that the first IQ test was conducted 5 years after epilepsy onset, and it was therefore possible that a decline had occurred early and was not reflected in later testing. Factor-analytical studies of intelligence test results indicated that the freedom from distractibility factor was most consistently lowered in patients with intractable epilepsy (Aldenkamp et al. 1990; Kupke & Lewis 1985; Rodin, Schmaltz & Twitty 1986). It is extremely difficult, however, to separate the effect of prolonged, poorly controlled seizures from the effect of chronic, high-dose AEDs.

Are specific types of seizures correlated with specific types of LD? Aldenkamp et al. (1990) noted that many studies were conducted before the concept of LD subtype was fully appreciated and did not fractionate LD into subtypes (Rourke 1985). Reading impairment and uncomplicated epilepsy were thought to be related in early studies (Rutter, Graham & Yule 1970; Stores 1978). Aldenkamp (1987) observed that arithmetic was often impaired in epileptic adolescents. In an attempt to relate type of epilepsy to type of LD, Aldenkamp et al. (1990) postulated four different LD typologies: a memory deficit type, with short-term and long-term memory disruption, possibly linked to temporal lobe onset seizures; an ADD type, linked to tonic–clonic seizures; a "speed-factor" type, characterized by slowing of information processing, associated with arithmetic LD, and correlated with polytherapy and long-term treatment with phenytoin; and a "problem-solving" type, associated with higher-order cognitive processing that was thought to be related directly to epilepsy.

PSYCHIATRIC DISORDERS IN CHILDREN WITH EPILEPSY

Children with epilepsy are at risk for psychiatric disorder (Rutter, Graham & Yule 1970; Hermann 1982; Hermann & Seidenberg 1989). It is unclear, however, whether seizures, associated neurocognitive deficits, medication, environmental factors, or chronic illness is most determinant.

Psychiatric Aspects of Temporal Lobe Epilepsy

A strong relationship exists between psychiatric disorders and CPS of temporal or frontal lobe origin. Ictal manifestations of seizures arising from these regions may have a distinctly psychotic tenor (Adebimpe 1977; Flor-Henry 1969). Engel, Ludwig, and Fetell (1978) described a girl diagnosed as catatonic schizophrenic, during a prolonged partial complex status epilepticus. Patients with frontal lobe partial complex seizures often experience complex hallucinatory phenomena while appearing quite alert, and this gives their condition a psychotic tone (Fornazzari et al. 1992). *Interictal psychosis*, in which patients have psychotic disturbances between bouts of seizures, has been reported. Caplan et al. (1991) described three children with left temporal lobe onset seizures and an interictal schizophrenia-like psychosis. These children met DSM-III criteria for schizophrenia, but they had intact affect and no "negative symptoms." They all demonstrated moderate to severe illogical thinking on the Kiddie Formal Thought Disorder Ratings (Caplan et al. 1989), and they resembled adults with interictal psychosis, although the symptoms emerged after a much shorter period of time than would be the case in adults.

Depression is also associated with TLE (Robertson 1985). Strauss, Wada & Moll (1992) reported that 40% of 85 patients with lateralized TLE were depressed. More men with left temporal lobe focus than with right temporal lobe focus were depressed; in contrast, no such right-left difference was noted in women. Whether children and adolescents with TLE are more prone to depressive disorder is not yet clear.

Fire-Setting

Fire-setting with associated photosensitive epilepsy may be a manifestation of temporal lobe seizures. Milrod and Urion (1992) described three boys with fire-setting, who had photoparoxysmal responses to intermittent photic stimulation and left temporal paroxysmal activity that remitted with AED treatment. A girl with fire-setting and other atypical behaviors exacerbated by watching TV was described by Meinhard, Oozeer & Cameron (1988). Interestingly, her father had visual prodromes followed by aggressive behavior and fire-setting.

Autism

Children who become increasingly "autistic" with epileptic discharges in limbic cortex have been reported (Rapin 1991). There is a higher incidence of epilepsy in children with autism than in the general population. Chronic seizures can also lead to behavioral regression, often with autistic features. Deonna et al. (1993) described two boys with tuberous sclerosis who had normal development and social behavior until the emergence of limbic system seizures. Thereafter, their social behavior and general development regressed, and they eventually met formal diagnostic criteria for autism. Treatment resulted in gradual diminution in autistic behaviors.

ANTIEPILEPTIC DRUGS

Antiepileptic drugs (AEDs) are a heterogeneous class of drugs that effectively control seizures with different physiological causes. AEDs control seizures through several different mechanisms. Currently, they are thought to modulate voltage-dependent neuronal ion channels, enhance activity of the major inhibitory neurotransmitter (GABA), or suppress excitatory amino acid (for instance, glutamate) neurotransmission.

The identity of AEDs can be a point of confusion because they have a generic (chemical) name, a trade name, and sometimes a unique American, British, or other European name (see Table 8-2). Each AED has an unique pharmacokinetic and metabolic pattern, its own specific therapeutic plasma-level range, specific dosing requirements (amount and time), a distinctive pattern of somatic and cognitive side effects, and specific symptoms of toxicity. Different AEDs are effective for specific seizure types.

AED metabolism is affected by other drugs (for instance, another AED or an antibiotic) that may affect plasma levels by altering the pharmacokinetics of detoxification. For example, drug–drug interactions may affect pharmacokinetics by competing for the same binding sites on plasma protein molecules or by inducing or inhibiting hepatic enzymes that metabolize AEDs. Whenever possible, neurologists avoid polypharmacy and maintain the patient on a single AED (monotherapy), using the lowest effective dose.

To interpret a patient's medication status correctly, the neuropsychologist needs to know the seizure type, the child's age and weight, the plasma level, and concurrent medications. Since young children tend to metabolize drugs more rapidly than do adolescents and adults, a child may need a larger dosage relative to weight than does an adult. Monitoring plasma AED levels is important because these guide dosage adjustments, confirm patient compliance, and provide precise information about a patient's tolerance of AEDs. It is also

Table 8-2 Common Antiepileptic Drugs

Generic Name	Trademark Name
phenobarbital	Luminal
primidone	Mysoline
diphenylhydantoin (phenytoin)	Dilantin
ethosuximide	Zarontin
carbamazepine	Tegretol
valproate (valproic acid)	Depakene
divalproex sodium	Depakote
diazepam	Valium
clonazepam	Klonopin
dicarbamate (felbamatol)	Felbamate
vigabatrin (gamma-vinyl GABA)	Sabril
gabapentin	Neurontin
lamotrigine (triazine)	Lamictal

important to discriminate between *dose-related effects* (responses that can be eliminated simply by decreasing the dose) and *side effects* (which are idiosyncratic and not necessarily dose-related) such as allergic reactions and hepatic or bone-marrow toxicity.

Another variable relates to generic versus brand-name drugs. Manufacturers must produce drugs whose content falls within certain specified ranges and a single-dose crossover bioavailability study in healthy male volunteers is mandated, but lot-to-lot variability is not studied (Oles & Gal 1993). Generic drugs may therefore vary in absorption characteristics and timing of the plasma-level peak, even though they are chemically identical. Further, drugs must be administered by an adult, or the child must remember to take them. Some AEDs require dosing two or three times per day. Patient compliance is an important problem, and as many as 30% to 50% of patients are noncompliant (Leppik 1988).

Commonly Used Antiepileptic Drugs

The following subsections briefly summarize salient information about common AEDs.

Phenobarbital (Luminal)

Barbiturates depress activity of all excitable tissues. The nervous system is extremely sensitive to this effect, which ranges from minimal sedation to general anesthesia, depending on dose. Barbiturates that are useful as AEDs exert a selective anticonvulsant action at a level below the level required to cause sedation. Phenobarbital (PB) has a long half-life (90 hours in adults, less in children). It is metabolized by liver microsomal enzymes, and 50% is excreted by the kidney, so phenobarbital levels may be elevated in patients with renal disease. Besides allergic reactions (such as rashes), major side effects of phenobarbital include sedation and depression. A 40% prevalence of major depressive disorder in children treated with phenobarbital, in contrast to 4% of those treated with carbamazepine, was reported (Brent et al. 1987). Phenobarbital may also cause paradoxical symptoms of inattention, hyperactivity, and disinhibition. Because of its undesirable behavioral side effects, phenobarbital is rarely prescribed as the first-line drug, but it remains an effective AED with a wide margin of saftey. The standard plasma level is from 10 to 25 (up to 40) μg/ml.

Primidone (Mysoline)

Primidone is closely related to phenobarbital. It is metabolized into two active drugs, phenobarbital and phenylethylmalonamide (PEMA). Both have long half-lives (for PEMA, 24 to 48 hours). There can be hematologic side effects and allergies (rashes). Toxic side effects include sedation, ataxia, diplopia, and nystagmus. Since these are often maximal when the drug is first started, low doses are prescribed initially, and larger doses are tolerated by accommodation.

Primidone is useful in the management of GTC, partial, and CPS of temporal lobe onset. Both phenobarbital and PEMA plasma levels are monitored.

Diphenylhydantoin or Phenytoin (Dilantin)

Phenytoin (PHT) is one of the most widely used AEDs. It suppresses electro-shock convulsions and is structurally similar to phenobarbital (Merritt & Putnam 1938). It is useful in managing a wide range of epilepsies, although not absence epilepsy. It is not sedative in ordinary doses. It has a half-life of about 24 hours, but the duration is dose-dependent. PHT is metabolized in the liver (hydroxylated by the microsomal enzyme system), and a number of drugs affect this enzyme system. PHT toxicity results in nystagmus, ataxia, diplopia, and other somatic symptoms. There were reports of a toxic effect on cerebellar Purkinje cells when PHT was administered over a prolonged period of time at high doses (Dam 1972). The therapeutic plasma level range for PHT is 10 to 20 μg/ml. PHT is heavily plasma-bound; for some purposes, "bound" and "unbound" forms of PHT are reported. For example, valproate interferes with plasma binding of PHT molecules.

Ethosuximide (Zarontin)

Ethosuximide was developed for treating generalized nonconvulsive epilepsy (petit mal, absence seizures). The plasma half-life is 30 hours. The drug is primarily metabolized by hepatic microsomal enzymes. Side effects are predominantly gastrointestinal (nausea, vomiting, and abdominal pain) and CNS (drowsiness, lethargy, photophobia, restlessness/agitation, and inattention). Systemic side effects include allergic reactions and bone-marrow depression. The therapeutic plasma level is in the range of from 40 to 100 μg/ml.

Carbamazepine (Tegretol)

Carbamazepine (CBZ) has been used since 1974. CBZ is highly effective in treating partial epilepsy—particularly TLE, frontal seizures, and benign rolandic epilepsy of childhood. Generic CBZ has been reported to yield underdosage (Koch & Allen 1987) or toxicity (Gilman, Alvarez & Duchowny 1993). CBZ is chemically related to tricyclic antidepressants. It has a short half-life and requires dosing two to three times per day. The drug is metabolized by hepatic microsomal enzymes. Side effects include lethargy, double vision, dizziness, nausea, and ataxia. There are rare but serious bone-marrow, liver, and allergic (Stevens-Johnson) side effects. The therapeutic plasma level ranges from 4 to 12 mcg/ml. CBZ also has psychiatric uses, and is helpful in the management of aggressive patients and in the treatment of atypical depression.

Valproate or Valproic Acid (Depakene), and Divalproex Sodium (Depakote)

Valproate (VPA) is a "modern" AED that consists of a simple branched-chain carboxylic acid. It may inhibit GABA transaminase or succinic semialdehyde dehydrogenase, increasing the amount of GABA available in the brain. It is rapidly absorbed orally, and peak concentration occurs in 1 to 4 hours. It is heavily (80% to 94%) bound to plasma proteins. Toxic CNS side effects are rare. Elevated levels of blood ammonia were reported in treated patients (Coulter & Allen 1981). Although the condition is obvious when florid (symptoms include stupor and increased seizures, subtler cases of hyperammonemia might result in subtle cognitive deficits. A major risk is fatal liver damage, occurring in 1 in 500 to 800 developmentally delayed children younger than 2 years of age who are on polytherapy (Dreifuss et al. 1989; Willmore, Triggs & Pellock 1991). In some cases, hepatic damage was related to underlying hepatocerebral degeneration rather than to VPA (Bicknese et al. 1992). VPA treatment is associated with carnitine deficiency (Ohtani, Endo & Matsuda 1982). VPA depletes carnitine, a nutrient found in meat and dairy products. Concurrent treatment with carnitine decreases the risk of liver damage (Coulter 1991). The therapeutic plasma range is 50 to 100 μg/ml; but because of rapid changes in plasma concentration, the dose per kilogram and the patient's clinical situation are also considered. VPA increases phenobarbital concentrations markedly and competes for plasma-binding sites with PHT. VPA is useful in treating generalized epilepsy, but it can also be effective in partial epilepsy. Photosensitive seizures are particularly responsive to VPA (Jeavons, Bishop & Harding 1986). VPA has been used to treat bipolar disorder in adults.

Benzodiazepines: Diazepam (Valium) and Clonazepam (Klonopin)

Benzodiazepines constitute a class of drugs widely used as sedatives and anti-anxiety drugs; they also have antiepileptic properties. Diazepam (valium) is used in treating status epilepticus. Clonazepam is used as a second-line AED in managing children with hard-to-control seizures. Their anticonvulsant effect is thought to be related to GABA-mediated neurotransmitter systems (Haefely et al. 1979).

Newer Antiepileptic Drugs

Four new AEDs will have been released by 1995. In phase II and phase III clinical trials, a double-blind, placebo-controlled, add-on trial is conducted on patients who are being treated with (and are unresponsive to) existing AEDs. These trials impose severe standards of safety and efficacy, overestimating toxicity and underestimating therapeutic benefit (Cereghino 1992). Only when extensive clinical experience has been accumulated does a clear picture of the side effects and the therapeutic efficacy of a new drug emerge.

Felbamatol or Dicarbamate (Felbamate)

Felbamate, released by the FDA in 1993, has a structure similar to that of meprobamate. In preclinical trials, it was effective in animal models and clinical populations for partial, complex partial, GTC, and absence seizures. It was targeted for use in children with Lennox-Gastaut syndrome. It appears to have a central alerting effect rather than being a sedative. Insomnia and anorexia with accompanying weight loss are prominent symptoms. Felbamate is metabolized in the liver and has a half-life of about 20 hours. It has a complex pattern in combination with other AEDs, increasing plasma levels of PHT, CBZ epoxide, and valproate, while decreasing CBZ plasma concentrations. PHT and CBZ increase the rate at which felbamate is metabolized, thus reducing the half-life to 11 to 16 hours. Valproate decreases the rate at which felbamate is metabolized.

Vigabatrin or Gamma-Vinyl GABA (Sabril)

Vigabatrin is a "tailor-made" molecule. It was developed to increase central levels of GABA (and therefore, to increase synaptic inhibition) by specifically and irreversibly inhibiting the enzymatic breakdown of GABA by the enzyme GABA-aminotransaminase. It is effective in partial—and to a lesser extent, in GTC—seizures. It may worsen absence and myoclonic seizures. There appears to be little dose–response relationship, suggesting an "all-or-nothing" effect. The recommended dose is in the range of from 40 to 80 mg/kg, although larger doses (up to 600 mg/kg/day) have been used. Interaction with other AEDs is minimal. Although the half-life of vigabatrin is relatively short (5 to 7 hours), the duration of action is longer than 24 hours because of its irreversible binding to the enzyme. It is not metabolized in the liver and has little impact on other AEDS, except for reducing PHT concentrations by an unknown mechanism. Therapeutic effects are not noted immediately, because it takes time to affect GABA levels. Side effects in adults have included rare reversible psychosis, drowsiness, fatigue, and dizziness. In children, agitation, somnolence, and ataxia were noted. Concerns that the drug might produce abnormalities in myelin have not been corroborated by any documentation in humans. McGuire, Duncan, and Trimble (1992) studied cognitive function (attention, mental speed, motor speed, central cognitive processing, and perceptuomotor performance) and made objective mood assessments in patients receiving 2 g/day of vigabatrin. They found a *decrease* in response time and no adverse effects.

Gabapentin (Neurontin)

Gabapentin was designed as a structural analog of GABA, the major inhibitory neurotransmitter. However, it does not appear to affect GABA or other neurotransmitter systems specifically. Gabapentin is effective in treating partial and secondarily generalized seizures. It has one unique pharmacokinetic property: its bioavailability decreases at high doses. It is primarily excreted by the kidney and has little effect on AED metabolism. It has low plasma-binding and virtually no defined toxicity.

Lamotrigine or Triazine (Lamictal)

Lamotrigine exerts antiepileptic action by inhibiting the presynaptic release of glutamate, an excitatory amino acid. It was effective in large, controlled add-on trials involving refractory partial seizures and in small-scale studies involving absence, myoclonic, and atypical absence seizures. Major adverse effects are dose-dependent dizziness, ataxia, diplopia, and allergy. Lamotrigine does not affect the pharmacokinetics of other AEDs.

Effect of Antiepileptic Drug Treatment on Cognition

Studies of the cognitive effects of AED treatment exist (Aldenkamp et al. 1987; Aman et al. 1990; Committee on Drugs 1985; Dodrill & Troupin 1977, 1991; Smith et al. 1987; Trimble 1990), but these often present conflicting results—due, in part, to complex methodological issues. The cognitive effects of AEDs may have been exaggerated because of methodological difficulties (Dodrill 1992). Experimental designs must control for a multiplicity of variables, and they benefit from inclusion of large, multisite populations. The following seven variables should be considered:

1. Epilepsy type, severity, age of onset, and etiology (whether symptomatic or idiopathic) vary, but all are important (Dam 1990). The site of the epileptic focus and the duration of the seizure may outweigh all other factors (Silvenius et al. 1984; Ojemann & Dodrill 1985).

2. AED choice may affect outcome. AEDs are chosen to control specific seizure types (for instance, CBZ is used for complex partial seizures). Certain diagnoses respond preferentially to a single AED, while others require polytherapy. Polytherapy increases study complexity, due to the impact of one AED on the pharmacokinetics of another.

3. AED toxicity may influence neuropsychological task performance. Since *how much* AED (that is, the drug's plasma level) appears to be more important than *which* AED, studies of the impact of AEDs on cognition must closely monitor plasma AED levels. In one report, PHT resulted in greater cognitive impairment than did CBZ. The differences disappeared, however, after subjects with PHT levels above a therapeutic range were excluded (Dodrill & Troupin 1991). Similarly, other studies reported that drug-induced cognitive impairment was strongly related to plasma AED levels, and that performance improved when these dropped into a therapeutic range (Aldenkamp 1987; O'Dougherty et al. 1987; Smith et al. 1987). Meador et al. (1990) experimentally controlled the relative amount of drugs, using plasma levels as percentages of the standard therapeutic range.

4. There is individual sensitivity to AED side effects; that is, some patients have idiosyncratic sensitivities to the cognitive effects of certain drugs at certain levels. Duration of drug therapy may be a factor; for example, side effects that arise early in treatment may differ from those that occur later (Kulig & Meinardi 1977).

5. Subject factors may have a significant impact on cognitive functions. For instance, a history of prior encephalopathy or of a focal lesion (not independent of seizure type) may be highly relevant to outcome.

6. Neuropsychological instruments need to be carefully selected. Several broad neuropsychological domains are usually evaluated in these studies,

including memory, attention, problem-solving strategies, and visuomotor speed and coordination (Gaillard 1980). The influence of motor speed alone may result in attributing adverse higher level intellectual or cognitive effects to an AED (Dodrill & Temkin 1989). Cognitive function deficits resulting from AEDs must be assessed on a test–retest basis (either off/on or on/off AEDs). Learning effects must be anticipated and controlled. The performances of epileptic children fluctuate markedly from test session to test session (Farwell, Dodrill & Batzel 1985), so test–retest reliabilities may be low and variance large.

7. Statistical analysis (power) problems increase as neuropsychological tasks increase in number. Assessing a multiplicity of tasks makes interpretations, comparisons, and meta-analysis from one study to another difficult. Longitudinal studies also implicate maturational effects that may require growth-curve designs.

Study conclusions vary as to which AEDs impair cognition, attention, or fine motor performance. Generally, phenobarbital and PHT are thought to impair cognitive and motor functioning, and VPA and CBZ are associated with fewer cognitive deficits; but these have not been consistent findings.

The immature nervous system may be more readily affected by AED treatment. Most studies have been relatively small and have been hampered by complications involving the preceding methodological issues. Aldenkamp et al. (1993) reported a multisite study involving 100 children, ranging in age from 7 to 18 years, who were seizure-free on a single AED (carbamazepine, phenytoin, or valproate), were paired with controls, and were withdrawn from medication over a three-month period, with individualized withdrawal schedules. Plasma levels were monitored, and EEGs were analyzed. Neuropsychological evaluation included computerized visual search, finger tapping, simple reaction time to auditory and visual stimuli, binary choice reaction time, and two short-term memory tests (involving serially and simultaneously presented words and figures). Both controls and experimental subjects showed a learning effect. Group differences were discerned in dominant-hand finger tapping of the epileptic subjects only in the baseline condition. Performance on the simultaneous memory task was significantly lower for the epileptics in both conditions; but performance on the serial memory task was lower only at baseline. In the absence seizure group, slower motor speed was noted (finger tapping and visual reaction time test at baseline; finger tapping after AED withdrawal). Impaired performance on binary choice reaction time and computerized visual search persisted in the absence seizure group, but not in other seizure types.

In another study, 63 epileptic children treated with VPA or CBZ for 12 months and 27 matched controls were evaluated; modest, transient effects on cognitive function were found that were attributed to subclinical seizures (Stores et al. 1992). Forsythe et al. (1991) randomly assigned 64 new cases of childhood epilepsy to one of three drug conditions and evaluated them three times within the year. CBZ in moderate dosage decreased performance on a memory task, but VPA and PHT did not.

A prospective, placebo-controlled discontinuation study compared polyphar-macy patients (PHT, CBZ, and VPA) to a control group that received one medication (Duncan, Shorvon & Trimble 1990). Tests of mental speech, atten-tion, performance of a learned skill, short-term memory, concentration, and simple coordinated hand movements were included. Simple motor skills were faster after discontinuation of PHT, CBZ, or VPA. Attention and concentration improved after discontinuation of PHT, but were unchanged after CBZ or VPA discontinuation. Vining et al. (1987) compared the effects of PB and VPA with a double-blind, counterbalanced crossover study of 21 children, using an extensive neuropsychological test battery. The AEDs did not differ in seizure control efficacy. Children on PB performed less well on four tests (WISC-R performance IQ, full-scale IQ, block design, and Berkley Paired Association Learning Test II). Behavioral changes (increased hyperactivity) were noted.

Farwell et al. (1990) compared intelligence quotients of young children who had at least one febrile seizure and were at increased risk for additional sei-zures. The children were randomly assigned to daily doses of PB or placebo. The authors found a depression of cognitive performance associated with PB administration, with indications of a disadvantage that outlasted AED adminis-tration by several months. PB administration did not benefit seizure prevention and the proportion of children remaining free of subsequent seizures did not differ between the two groups.

PSYCHOPATHOLOGY EMERGING IN THE COURSE OF AED TREATMENT

Landolt (1953) first described *forcierte Normaliserung* ("forced normaliza-tion")—development of a psychotic state by an epileptic patient when seizure control and EEG normalization are achieved. Pakalnis et al. (1987) described seven such patients, most of whom had CPS. They had no prior history of psychopathology, but each developed acute psychotic symptoms when AED treatment was instituted, good seizure control was attained, and EEGs were normalized.

Withdrawal of AEDs may result in increased clinically significant psychiat-ric symptoms (including anxiety, depression, hypomania, and bipolar or panic attacks). Savard et al. (1991) reported the occurrence of frank psychosis in patients with CPS, in the course of drug tapering. Ketter et al. (1994) noted that AED withdrawal–emergent psychopathology may be partly due to benefi-cial psychopharmacologic effects of AEDs, since reinstituting AEDs eliminated the psychopathologic symptoms.

SUMMARY

This chapter reviewed the major types of epilepsy, with special reference to those that have prominent effects in children. The various mechanisms by which epilepsy affects cognition and the impact of antiepileptic drug treatment on cognition and neuropsychological functioning were discussed.

REFERENCES

Aarts, J. H.; Binnie, C. D.; Smit, A. M.; and Wilkins, A. J. 1984. Selective cognitive impairment during focal and generalized epileptiform EEG activity. *Brain* 107: 293–308.

Adebimpe, V. R. 1977. Complex partial seizures simulating schizophrenia. *Journal of the American Medical Association* 237: 1339–41.

Aicardi, J. M., and Chevrie, J. J. 1982. Atypical benign partial epilepsy of childhood. *Developmental Medicine and Child Neurology* 24: 281–92.

Aldenkamp, A. P. 1987. Learning disabilities in epilepsy. In A. P. Aldenkamp, W. C. J. Alpherts, H. Meinardi, and G. Stores (eds.), *Education and Epilepsy, 1987* (Lisse/Berwyn: Swets & Zeitlinger), pp. 21–38.

Aldenkamp, A. P.; Alpherts, W. C.; Blennow, G.; Elmqvist, D.; Heijbel, J.; Nilsson, H. L.; Sandstedt, P.; Tonnby, B.; Wåhlander, L.; and Wosse, E. 1993. Withdrawal of antiepileptic medication in children—Effects on cognitive function: The multicenter Holmfrid study. *Neurology* 43: 41–50.

Aldenkamp, A. P.; Alpherts, W. C.; Dekker, M. J.; and Overweg, J. 1990. Neuropsychological aspects of learning disabilities in epilepsy. *Epilepsia* 31(suppl. 4): S9–S20.

Aldenkamp, A. P.; Alpherts, W. C. J.; Moerland, M. C.; Ottevanger, N.; and Van Parys, J. A. P. 1987. Controlled release carbamazepine: Cognitive side effects in patients with epilepsy. *Epilepsia* 28: 507–14.

Aman, M. G.; Werry, J. S.; Paxton, J. W.; Turbott, S. H.; and Stewart, A. W. 1990. Effects of carbamazepine on psychomotor performance in children as a function of drug concentration, seizure type and time of medication. *Epilepsia* 31: 51–60.

Ansink, B. J.; Sarphatie, H.; and Van Dongen, H. R. 1989. The Landau-Kleffner syndrome—Case report and theoretical considerations. *Neuropediatrics* 20: 170–72.

Babb, T. L., and Brown, W. J. 1987. Pathological findings in epilepsy. In J. Engel, Jr. (ed.), *Surgical Treatment of the Epilepsies* (New York: Raven Press), pp. 511–40.

Baram, T. Z. 1993. Pathophysiology of massive infantile spasms: Perspective on the putative role of the brain adrenal axis. *Annals of Neurology* 33: 231–36.

Beaumanoir, A. 1985. The Landau-Kleffner syndrome. In J. Roger, C. Dravet, M. Bureau, F. Dreifuss, and P. Wolf (eds.), *Epileptic Syndromes in Infancy, Childhood, and Adolescence* (London: John Libbey), pp. 181–91.

Beaumanoir, A., and Nahory, A. 1983. Les epilepsies bénignes partielles: 11 cas d'épilepsie partielle frontal a évolution favorable. *Revue de Electroencephalographie et de Neurophysiologie Clinique* 13: 207–11.

Bennett, T. L. 1992. *The Neuropsychology of Epilepsy.* New York: Raven Press.

Bickford, R. G.; Whelan, J. L.; Klass, D. W.; and Corbin, K. B. 1956. Reading epilepsy: Clinical and electroencephalographic studies of a new syndrome. *Transactions of the American Neurological Association* 81: 100–102.

Bicknese, A. R.; May, W.; Hickey, W. F.; and Dodson, W. E. 1992. Early childhood hepatocerebral degeneration misdiagnosed as valproate hepatotoxicity. *Annals of Neurology* 32: 767–75.

Binnie, C. D.; Channon, S.; and Marston, D. 1990. Learning disabilities in epilepsy: Neurophysiological aspects. *Epilepsia* 31(suppl. 4): S2–S8.

Bishop, D. 1985. Age of onset and outcome in "acquired aphasia with convulsive disorders" (Landau-Kleffner syndrome). *Developmental Medicine and Child Neurology* 27: 705–12.

Bishop, D., and Rosenbloom, L. 1987. Childhood language disorders: Classification and overview. In W. Yule and M. Rutter (eds.), *Language Development and Disorders: Clinics in Developmental Medicine,* Nos. 101/102. Oxford: Blackwood Scientific; Philadelphia: Lippincott, pp. 16–41.

Blom, S., and Heijbel, J. 1989. Benign epilepsy of childhood with centrotemporal spikes. In G. Beck-Mannagetta, V. E. Anderson, H. Doose, and D. Janz (eds.), *Genetics of the Epilepsies* (Berlin: Springer-Verlag), pp. 67–72.

Blume, W. T. 1978. Clinical and electroencephalographic correlates of the multiple independent spike foci pattern in children. *Annals of Neurology* 4: 541–47.

Boone, K. B.; Miller B. L.; Rosenberg, L.; Durazo, A.; McIntyre, H.; and Weil, M. 1988. Neuropsychological and behavior abnormalities in an adolescent with frontal lobe seizures. *Neurology* 38: 583–86.

Brent, D. A.; Crumrine, P. K.; Varma, R. R.; Allan, M.; and Allman, C. 1987. Phenobarbital treatment and major depressive disorder in children with epilepsy. *Pediatrics* 80: 909–17.

Bruton, C. 1988. *The Neuropathology of Temporal Lobe Epilepsy.* New York: Oxford University Press.

Burnstine, T. H.; Vining, E. P. G.; Uematsu, S.; and Lesser, R. P. 1991. Multifocal independent epileptiform discharges in children: Ictal correlates and surgical therapy. *Neurology* 41: 1223–28.

Caplan, R.; Foy, J. G.; Asarnow, R. F.; and Sherman, T. 1989. Information processing deficits of schizophrenic children with formal though disorder. *Psychiatry Research* 31: 169–77.

Caplan, R.; Guthrie, D.; Mundy, P.; Sigman M.; Shields, D.; Sherman T.; and Peacock, W. J. 1992. Nonverbal communication skills of surgically treated children with infantile spasms. *Developmental Medicine and Child Neurology* 34: 499–506.

Caplan, R.; Shields, W. D.; Mori, L.; and Yudovin, S. 1991. Middle childhood onset of interictal psychosis. *Journal of the American Academy of Child and Adolescent Psychiatry* 30: 893–96.

Cascino, G. D.; Luckstein, R. R.; Sharbrough, F. W.; and Jack, C. R. 1993. Facial asymmetry, hippocampal pathology, and remote symptomatic seizures: A temporal lobe epileptic syndrome. *Neurology* 43: 725–27.

Cendes, F.; Andermann, F.; Dubeau, F.; Gloor, P.; Evans, A.; Jones-Gotman, M.; Olivier, A.; Andermann E.; Robitaille, Y.; Lopes-Cendes, I.; Peters, T.; and Melanson, D. 1993. Early childhood prolonged febrile convulsions, atrophy and sclerosis of mesial structures, and temporal lobe epilepsy: An MRI volumetric study. *Neurology* 43: 1083–87.

Cendes, F.; Andermann, F.; Gloor, P.; Evans, A.; Jones-Gotman, M.; Watson, C.; Melanson, D.; Olivier, A.; Peters, T.; Lopes-Cendes, I.; and Leroux, G. 1993. MRI volumetric measurement of amygdala and hippocampus in temporal lobe epilepsy. *Neurology* 43: 719–25.

Cereghino, J. J. 1992. Clinical trial design for antiepileptic drugs. *Annals of Neurology* 32: 393–94.

Chee, M. W. L.; Kotagal, P.; Van Ness, P. C.; Gragg, L.; Murphy, D.; and Lüders,

H. O. 1993. Lateralizing signs in intractable partial epilepsy: Blinded multiple-observer analysis. *Neurology* 43: 2519–2525.

Chevrie, J. J., and Aicardi, J. 1972. Childhood epileptic encephalopathy with slow spike-wave: A statistical study of 80 cases. *Epilepsia* 13: 259–71.

Chugani, H. T.; Shewmon, D. A.; Sankar, R.; Chen, B. C.; and Phelps, M. E. 1992. Infantile spasms: II. Lenticular nuclei and brain stem activation on positron emission tomography. *Annals of Neurology* 31: 212–19.

Chugani, H. T.; Shields, W. D.; Shewmon, D. A.; Olson, D. M.; Phelps, M. E.; and Peacock, W. J. 1990. Infantile spasms: I. PET identifies focal cortical dysgenesis in cryptogenic cases for surgical treatment. *Annals of Neurology* 27: 406–13.

Cohen, M.; Prather, A.; Town, P.; and Hynd, G. 1990. Neurodevelopmental differences in emotional prosody in normal children and children with left and right temporal lobe epilepsy. *Brain and Language* 38: 122–35.

Commission on Classification and Terminology of the International League Against Epilepsy. 1989. Proposal for revised classification of epilepsies and epileptic syndromes. *Epilepsia* 30: 389–99.

Committee on Drugs. 1985. Behavioral and cognitive effects of anticonvulsant therapy. *Pediatrics* 76: 644–47.

Coulter, D. L. 1991. Carnitine, valproate, and toxicity. *Journal of Child Neurology* 6: 7–14.

Coulter, D. L., and Allen, R. J. 1981. Hyperammonemia with valproic acid therapy. *Journal of Pediatrics* 99: 317–19.

Cowan, L. D.; Bodensteiner, J. B.; Leviton, A.; and Doherty, L. 1989. Prevalence of the epilepsies in children and adolescents. *Epilepsia* 30: 94–106.

Dalla Bernardina, B.; Chiamenti, C.; Capovilla, G.; Treisan, E.; and Tassinari, C. A. 1985. Benign partial epilepsy with affective symptoms ("benign psychomotor epilepsy"). In J. Roger, C. Dravet, M. Bureau, F. E. Driefuss, and P. Wolf (eds.), *Epileptic Syndromes in Infancy, Childhood, and Adolescence* (London: John Libbey), pp. 171–75.

Dalla Bernardina, B.; Sgrò, V.; Fontana, E.; Colamaria, V.; La Selva, L. (1992) Idiopathic partial epilepsies in children. In J. Roger, M. Bureau, C. Dravet, F. E. Dreifuss, A. Perret, and P. Wolf (eds.), *Epileptic Syndromes in Infancy, Childhood, and Adolescence* (2nd ed.) (London: John Libbey), pp. 173–88.

Dam, M. 1972. The density and ultrastructure of the Purkinje cells following diphenylhydantoin treatment in animals and man. *Acta Neurologica Scandinavica* 48(suppl. 49): 1–65.

———. 1990. Children with epilepsy: The effect of seizures, syndromes, and etiological factors on cognitive function. *Epilepsia* 31(suppl. 4): S26–S29.

Delgado-Escueta, A. V.; Greenberg, D.; Weissbecker, K.; Liu, A.; Treiman, L.; Sparkes, R.; Park, M. S.; Barbetti, A.; and Terasaki, P. I. 1990. Gene mapping in the idiopathic generalized epilepsies: Juvenile myoclonic epilepsy, childhood absence epilepsy, epilepsy with grand mal seizures, and early childhood myoclonic epilepsy. *Epilepsia* 31(suppl. 3): S19–S29.

Delgado-Escueta, A. V.; Serratosa, J. M.; Liu, A.; Weissbecker, K.; Medina, M. T.; Gee, M.; Treiman, L. J.; and Sparkes, R. S. 1994. Progress in mapping human epilepsy genes. *Epilepsia* 35(suppl. 1): S29–S40.

DeMarco, P., and Ghersini, L. 1985. Videogames and epilepsy. *Developmental Medicine and Child Neurology* 27: 519–21.

De Negri, M. 1993. Landau-Kleffner syndrome: Some suggestions. *Archives of Neurology* 50: 896.

Deonna, T. W. 1991. Acquired epileptiform aphasia in children (Landau-Kleffner syndrome). *Journal of Clinical Neurophysiology* 8: 288–98.

Deonna, T.; Peter, C.; and Ziegler, A.-L. 1989. Adult follow-up of acquired aphasia-epilepsy syndrome in childhood: Report of 7 cases. *Neuropediatrics* 20. 132–38.

Deonna, T.; Ziegler, A.-L.; Moura-Serra, J.; and Innocenti, G. 1993. Autistic regression in relation to limbic pathology and epilepsy: Report of two cases. *Developmental Medicine and Child Neurology* 35: 166–76.

Deuel, R. K., and Lenn, N. J. 1977. Treatment of acquired epileptic aphasia. *Journal of Pediatrics* 90: 959–61.

Devinsky, O.; Hafler, D. A.; and Victor, J. 1982. Embarrassment as the aura of a complex partial seizure. *Neurology* 32: 1284–85.

Devinsky, O.; Kelley, K.; Yacubian, E. M. T.; Sato, S.; Kufta, C. V.; Theodore, W. H.; and Porter, R. J. 1994. Postictal behavior: A clinical and subdural electroencephalographic study. *Archives of Neurology* 51: 254–59.

Devinsky, O.; Vazquez, B.; Perrine, K.; and Luciano, D. J. 1993. Ictal and postictal apraxia. *Neuropsychiatry, Neuropsychology, and Behavioral Neurology* 6: 256–59.

Dodrill, C. B. 1986. Correlates of generalized tonic–clonic seizures with intellectual, neuropsychological, emotional and social function in patients with epilepsy. *Epilepsia* 27: 399–411.

———. 1992. Problems in the assessment of cognitive effects of antiepileptic drugs. *Epilepsia* 33(suppl. 6): S29–S32.

Dodrill, C. B., and Temkin, N. R. 1989. Motor speed is a contaminating factor in evaluating the "cognitive" effects of phenytoin. *Epilepsia* 30: 453–57.

Dodrill, C. B., and Troupin, A. 1977. Psychotropic effects of carbamazepine in epilepsy: A double-blind comparison with phenytoin. *Neurology* 27: 1023–28.

———. 1991. Psychotropic effects of carbamazepine in epilepsy: A reanalysis. *Neurology* 41: 141–43.

Dreifuss, F. E. 1987. Goals of surgery for epilepsy. In J. Engel, Jr. (ed.), *Surgical Treatment of the Epilepsies* (New York: Raven Press), pp. 31–49.

Dreifuss, F. E.; Langer, D. H.; Moline, K. A.; and Maxwell, J. E. (1989) Valproic acid hepatic fatalities: II. US experience since 1984. *Neurology* 39: 201–7.

Duchowny, M. 1987. Complex partial seizures of infancy. *Archives of Neurology* 44: 911–14.

Duchowny, M.; Jayakar, P.; Resnick, T.; Levin, B.; and Alvarez, L. 1994. Posterior temporal epilepsy: Electroclinical features. *Annals of Neurology* 35: 427–31.

Dugas, M.; Masson, M.; Le Heuzey, M. F.; and Regnier, N. 1982. Aphasie 'acquise' de l'enfant avec epilepsie (syndrome de Landau et Kleffner): Douze observations personnelles. *Revue Neurologique* 138: 755–80.

Duncan, J. S.; Shorvon, S. D.; and Trimble, M. R. 1990. Effects of removal of phenytoin, carbamazepine and valproate on cognitive function. *Epilepsia* 31: 584–91.

Earle, K. M.; Baldwin, M.; and Penfield, W. 1953. Incisural sclerosis and temporal lobe seizures produced by hippocampal herniation at birth. *Archives of Neurology and Psychiatry* 69: 27–42.

Echenne, B.; Cheminal, R.; Rivier, F.; Negre, C.; Touchon, J.; and Billiard, M. 1992. Epileptic electroencephalographic abnormalities and developmental dysphasias: A study of 32 patients. *Brain and Development* 14: 216–25.

Engel, J., Jr. 1988. Brain metabolism and pathophysiology of human epilepsy. In M. A. Dichter (ed.), *Mechanisms of Epileptogenesis: The Transition to Seizure* (New York: Plenum Press), pp. 1–16.

Engel, J., Jr.; Ludwig, B. I.; and Fetell, M. 1978. Prolonged partial complex status epilepticus: EEG and behavioral observations. *Neurology* 28: 863–69.

Farwell, J. R.; Dodrill, C. B.; and Batzel, L. W. 1985 Neuropsychological abilities of children with epilepsy. *Epilepsia* 26: 395–400.

Farwell, J. R.; Lee, J. L.; Hirtz, D. G.; Sulzbacher, S. I.; Ellenberg, J. H.; and Nelson, K. B. 1990. Phenobarbital for febrile seizures—Effects on intelligence and on seizure recurrence. *New England Journal of Medicine* 322: 364–69.

Feekery, C. J.; Parry-Fielder, B.; and Hopkins, I. J. 1993. Landau-Kleffner syndrome: Six patients including discordant monozygotic twins. *Pediatric Neurology* 9: 49–53.

Feindel, W., and Rasmussen, T. 1991. Temporal lobectomy with amygdalectomy and minimal hippocampal resection: Review of 100 cases. *Canadian Journal of Neurological Sciences* 18: 577–79.

Flor-Henry, P. 1969. Psychosis and temporal lobe epilepsy. *Epilepsia* 10: 363–95.

Fornazzari, L.; Farcnik, K.; Smith, I.; Heasman, G. A.; and Ichise, M. 1992. Violent visual hallucinations and aggression in frontal lobe dysfunction: Clinical manifestions of deep orbitiofrontal foci. *Journal of Neuropsychiatry and Clinical Neurosciences* 4: 42–44.

Forsythe, I.; Butler, R.; Berg, I.; and McGuire, R. 1991. Cognitive impairment in new cases of epilepsy randomly assigned to carbamazepine, phenytoin and sodium valproate. *Developmental Medicine and Child Neurology* 33: 524–34.

French, J. A.; Williamson, P. D.; Thadani, V. M.; Darcey, T. M.; Mattson, R. H.; Spencer, S. S.; and Spencer, D. D. 1993. Characteristics of medial temporal lobe epilepsy: I. Results of history and physical examination. *Annals of Neurology* 34: 774–80.

Gabr, M.; Lüders, H.; Dinner, D.; Morris, H.; and Wyllie, E. 1989. Speech manifestations in lateralization of temporal lobe seizures. *Annals of Neurology* 25: 82–87.

Gaillard, A. W. K. 1980. The use of task variables and brain potentials in the assessment of cognitive impairment. In B. M. Kulig, H. Meinardi, and G. Stores (eds.), *Epilepsy and Behaviour '79* (Lisse: Swets & Zeitlinger), pp. 104–10.

Gale, K. 1988. Progression and generalization of seizure discharge: Anatomical and neurochemical substrates. *Epilepsia* 29(suppl. 2): S15–S34.

Gastaut, H. 1982. A new type of epilepsy: benign partial epilepsy of children with occipital spike-waves. *Clinical Electroencephalography* 13: 13–22.

Genton, P. 1993. What differentiates Landau-Kleffner syndrome from the syndrome of continuous spikes and waves during slow sleep? *Archives of Neurology* 50: 1008.

Genton, P.; Maton, B.; Ogihara, M.; Samoggia, G.; Guerrini, R.; Medina, M. T.; Dravet, C.; and Roger, J. 1992. Continuous focal spikes during REM sleep in a case of acquired aphasia (Landau-Kleffner syndrome). *Sleep* 15: 454–60.

Gibbs, F. A., and Gibbs, E. L. 1952. *Atlas of Electroencephalography,* vol. 2, *Epilepsy* (Cambridge, Mass.: Addison-Wesley), pp. 56–57.

Gilman, J. T.; Alvarez, I. A.; and Duchowny, M. 1993. Carbamazepine toxicity resulting from generic substitution. *Neurology* 43: 2696–97.

Glaze, D. G.; Hrachovy, R. A.; Frost, J. D.; Kellaway, P.; and Zion, T. E. 1988. Prospective study of outcome of infants with infantile spasms treated during controlled studies of ACTH and prednisone. *Journal of Pediatrics* 112: 389–96.

Gloor, P.; Olivier, A.; Quesney, L. F.; Andermann, F.; and Horowitz, S. 1982. The role of the limbic system in experiential phenomenona of temporal lobe epilepsy. *Annals of Neurology* 12: 129–44.

Gloor, P.; Salanova, V.; Olivier, A.; and Quesney, L. F. 1993. The human dorsal hippocampal commissure: An anatomically identifiable and functional pathway. *Brain* 116: 1249–73.

Goddard, G.; McIntyre, D. C.; and Leech, C. K. 1969. A permanent change in brain function resulting from daily electrical stimulation. *Experimental Neurology* 25: 295–330.

Gomez, M. R.; and Klass, D. W. 1983. Epilepsies of infancy and childhood. *Annals of Neurology* 13: 113–24.

Goodridge, D. M. G., and Shorvon, S. D. 1983. Epileptic seizures in a population of 6000: I. Demography, diagnosis and classification, and role of the hospital services. *British Medical Journal* 287: 641–44.

Gordon, N. 1990. Acquired aphasia in childhood: The Landau-Kleffner syndrome. *Developmental Medicine and Child Neurology* 32: 270–74.

Grunewald, R. A.; Chroni, E.; and Panayiotopoulos, C. P. 1992. Delayed diagnosis of juvenile myoclonic epilepsy. *Journal of Neurology, Neurosurgery and Psychiatry* 55: 497–99.

Grunewald, R. A., and Panayiotopoulos, C. P. 1993. Juvenile myoclonic epilepsy: A review. *Archives of Neurology* 50: 594–98.

Guzzetta, F.; Crisafulli, A.; and Isaya Crinó, M. 1993. Cognitive assessment of infants with West syndrome: How useful is it for diagnosis and prognosis? *Developmental Medicine and Child Neurology* 35: 379–87.

Haas, K. Z.; Sperber, E. F.; and Moshé, S. L. 1990. Kindling in developing animals: Expression of severe seizures and enhanced development of bilateral foci. *Developmental Brain Research* 56: 275–80.

Haefely, W.; Pole, P.; Schaffner, R.; Keller, H.; Pieri, L.; and Möhler, H. 1979. Facilitation of GABA-ergic transmission by drugs. In P. Krogsgaard-Larsen, J. Scheel-Krüger, and H. Kofod (eds.), *GABA-Neurotransmitters* (New York: Academic Press), pp. 357–75.

Hanson, P. A., and Chodos, R. 1978. Hemiparetic seizures. *Neurology* 28: 920–23.

Hardiman, O.; Burke, T.; Phillips, J.; Murphy, S.; O'Moore, B.; Staunton, H.; and Farrell, M. A. 1988. Microdysgenesis in resected temporal neocortex: Incidence and clinical significance in focal epilepsy. *Neurology* 38: 1041–47.

Hasegawa, T.; Matsuoka, H.; Takahasi, T.; and Okuma, T. 1981. Myoclonic seizures induced by writing, calculation with fingers and constructive acts: With special reference to "neuropsychological EEG activation." *Psychiatrica et Neurologia Japonica (Seishin Shinkeigaku Zasshi)* 83: 199–210.

Heijbel, J.; Blom, S.; and Rasmuson, M. 1975. Benign epilepsy of childhood with centrotemporal EEG foci: A genetic study. *Epilepsia* 16: 285–93.

Heilman, K. H., and Gregory, J. H. 1980. Seizure-induced neglect. *Journal of Neurology, Neurosurgery, and Psychiatry* 43: 1035–40.

Henry, T. R.; Mazziotta, J. C.; and Engel, J. 1993. Interictal metabolic anatomy of mesial temporal lobe epilepsy. *Archives of Neurology* 50: 582–89.

Hermann, B. P. 1982. Neuropsychological functioning and psychopathology in children with epilepsy. *Epilepsia* 23: 545–54.

Hermann, B. P., and Seidenberg, M., eds. 1989. *Childhood Epilepsies: Neuropsychological, Psychosocial, and Intervention Aspects.* New York: Wiley.

Hirsch, E.; Marescaux, C.; Maquet, P.; Metz-Lutz, M. N.; Kiesmann, M.; Salmon, E.; Franck, G.; and Kurtz, D. 1990. Landau-Kleffner syndrome: A clinical and EEG study of five cases. *Epilepsia* 31: 756–67.

Holmes, G. L. 1993. Benign focal epilepsies of childhood. *Epilepsia* 34(suppl. 3): S49–S61.

Holmes, G. L.; McKeever, M.; and Saunders, Z. 1981. Epileptiform activity in aphasia of childhood: An epiphenomenon? *Epilepsia* 22: 631–39.

Holmes, G. L.; Thompson, J. L.; Marchi, T. A.; Gabriel, P. S.; Hogan, M. A.; Carl, F. G.; and Feldman, D. S. 1990. Effects of seizures on learning, memory, and behavior in the genetically epilepsy-prone rat. *Annals of Neurology* 27: 24–32.

Hrachovy, R. A.; Frost, J. D.; and Kellaway, P. 1981. Sleep characteristics in infantile spasms. *Neurology* 31: 688–93.

———. 1984. Hypsarrhythmia: Variations on the theme. *Epilepsia* 25: 317–25.

Hudson, L. P.; Munoz, D. G.; Miller, L.; McLachlan, R. S.; Girvin, J. P.; and Blume, W. T. 1993. Amygdaloid sclerosis in temporal lobe epilepsy. *Annals of Neurology* 33: 622–31.

Huttenlocher, P. R.; Taravath, S.; and Mojtahedi, S. 1994. Periventricular heterotopia and epilepsy. *Neurology* 44: 51–54.

Iadarola, M., and Gale, K. 1982. Substantia nigra: A site of anticonvulsant activity mediated by gamma-aminobutyric acid. *Science* 218: 1237–40.

Ichiba, N. 1990. West syndrome associated with hyperlexia. *Pediatric Neurology* 6: 344–48.

Jackson, G. D.; Kuzniecky, R. I.; and Cascino, G. D. 1994. Hippocampal sclerosis without detectable hippocampal atrophy. *Neurology* 44: 42–46.

Jackson, J. H. 1880–1881. On right- or left-sided spasm at the onset of epileptic paroxysms, and on crude sensation warnings and elaborate mental states. *Brain* 3: 192–306.

Janz, D. 1985. Epilepsy with impulsive petit mal (juvenile myoclonic epilepsy). *Acta Neurologica Scandinavica* 72: 449–59.

Jasper, H. 1958. Report of committee on methods of clinical exam in EEG. *Electroencephalography and Clinical Neurophysiology* 10: 370–75.

Jayakar, P.; Duchowny, M.; Resnick, T.; and Alvarez, L. 1992. Lateralizing significance of the pattern of head movement. *Neurology* 42: 1989–91.

Jayakar, P. B., and Seshia, S. S. 1991. Electrical status epilepticus during slow-wave sleep: A review. *Journal of Clinical Neurophysiology* 8: 299–311.

Jeavons, P. M.; Bishop, A.; and Harding, G. F. A. 1986. The prognosis of photosensitivity. *Epilepsia* 27: 569–75.

Jeavons, P. M.; Bower, B. D.; and Dimitrakoudi, M. 1973. Long-term prognosis of 150 cases of "West syndrome." *Epilepsia* 14: 153–64.

Jellinger, K. 1987. Neuropathological aspect of infantile spasms. *Brain Development* 9: 358–60.

Kasteleijn-Nolst Trenité, D. G.; Bakker, D. J.; Binnie, C. D.; and Buerman, A. 1988. Psychological effects of subclinical epileptiform EEG discharges: I. Scholastic skills. *Epilepsy Research* 2: 111–16.

Kasteleijn-Nolst Trenité, D. G.; Siebelink, B. M.; and Berends, S. G. 1990. Lateralized effects of subclinical epileptiform EEG discharges on scholastic performance in children. *Epilepsia* 31: 740–46.

Kasteleijn-Nolst Trenité, D. G.; Smit, A. M.; Velis, D. N.; Willemse, J.; and van Emde Boas, W. 1990. On-line detection of transient neuropsychological disturbances during EEG discharges in children with epilepsy. *Developmental Medicine and Child Neurology* 32: 46–50.

Ketter, T. A.; Malow, B. A.; Flamini, R.; White, S. R.; Post, R. M.; and Theodore, W. H. 1994. Anticonvulsant withdrawal-emergent psychopathology. *Neurology* 44: 55–61.

Koch, G., and Allen, J. P. 1987. Untoward effects of generic carbamazepine therapy. *Archives of Neurology* 44: 578–79.

Kulig, B., and Meinardi, H. 1977. Effects of antiepileptic drugs on motor activity and learned behavior in the rat. In H. Meinardi and A. J. Rowan (eds.), *Advances in Epileptology* (Amsterdam: Swets & Zeitlinger), pp. 98–104.

Kupke, T., and Lewis, R. 1985. WAIS and neuropsychological tests: Common and unique variance within an epileptic population. *Journal of Clinical and Experimental Neuropsychology* 7: 353–66.

Kurthen, M.; Helmstaedter, C.; Linke, D. B.; Solymosi, L.; Elger, C. E.; and Schramm, J. 1992. Interhemispheric dissociation of expressive and receptive language functions in patients with complex-partial seizures: An amobarbital study. *Brain and Language* 43: 694–712.

Kuzniecky, R.; de la Sayette, V.; Ethier, R.; Melanson, D.; Andermann, F.; Berkovic, S.; Robitaille, Y.; Olivier, A.; Peters, T.; and Feindel, W. 1987. Magnetic resonance imaging in temporal lobe epilepsy: Pathological correlations. Annals of Neurology 22: 341–47.

Lancman, M. E.; Asconapé, J. J.; Craven, W. J.; Howard, G.; and Penry, J. K. 1994. Predictive value of induction of psychogenic seizures by suggestion. *Annals of Neurology* 35: 359–61.

Landau, W. M., and Kleffner, F. R. 1957. Syndrome of acquired aphasia with convulsive disorder in children. *Neurology* 7: 523–30.

Landolt, H. 1953. Some clinical electroencephalographical correlations in epileptic psychoses (twilight states). *Electroencephalography and Clinical Neurophysiology* 5: 121.

Lee, S. I.; Sutherling, W. W.; Persing, J. A.; and Butler, A. B. 1980. Language induced seizures: A case of cortical origin. *Archives of Neurology* 37: 433–36.

Lencz, T.; McCarthy, G.; Bronen, R. A.; Scott, T. J.; Inserni, J. A.; Sass, K. J.; Novelly, R. A.; Kim, J. H.; and Spencer, D. D. 1992. Quantitative magnetic resonance imaging in temporal lobe epilepsy: Relationship to neuropathology and neuropsychological function. *Annals of Neurology* 31: 629–37.

Lenoir, P.; Ramet, J.; De Meirleir, L.; D'Allest, A.-M.; Desprechins, B.; and Loeb, H. 1989. Bathing-induced seizures. *Pediatric Neurology* 5: 124–25.

Leppik, I. E. 1988. Compliance during treatment of epilepsy. *Epilepsia* 29: (suppl. 2): S79–S84.

Lerman, P., and Kivity, S. 1991. The benign partial nonrolandic epilepsies. *Journal of Clinical Neurophysiology* 8: 275–87.

Lishman, W. A. 1987. *Organic Psychiatry*, 2d ed. London: Blackwell Scientific.

Loiseau, P., and Beaussart, M. 1973. The seizures of benign childhood epilepsy with rolandic paroxysmal discharges. *Epilepsia* 14: 381–89.

Loiseau, P.; Duche, B.; Cordora, S.; Dartigues, J. F.; and Cohadon, S. 1988. Prognosis of benign childhood epilepsy with centrotemporal spikes: A follow-up study of 168 patients. *Epilepsia* 29: 229–35.

Lüders, H.; Lesser, R. P.; Hahn, J.; Dinner, D. S.; Moris, H. H.; Wyllie, E.; and Godoy, J. 1991. Basal temporal language area. *Brain* 114: 743–54.

Maeda, Y.; Kurokawa, T.; Sakamoto, K.; Kitamoto, I.; Ueda, K.; and Tashima, S. 1990. Electroclinical study of video-game epilepsy. *Developmental Medicine and Child Neurology* 32: 493–500.

Marks, D. A.; Katz, A.; Hoffer, P.; and Spencer, S. S. 1992. Localization of extratemporal epileptic foci during ictal single photon emission computed tomography. *Annals of Neurology* 31: 250–55.

McDonald, J. W.; Garofalo, E. A.; Hood, T.; Sackellares, J. C.; Gilman, S.; McKeever, P. E.; Troncoso, J. C.; and Johnston, M. V. 1991. Altered excitatory and inhibitory amino acid receptor binding in hippocampus of patients with temporal lobe epilepsy. *Annals of Neurology* 29: 529–41.

McGuire, A. M.; Duncan, J. S.; and Trimble, M. R. 1992. Effects of vigabatrin on cognitive function and mood when used as add-on therapy in patients with intractable epilepsy. *Epilepsia* 33: 128–34.

McLachlan, R. S. 1987. The significance of head and eye turning in seizures. *Neurology* 37: 1617–19.

Meador, K. J.; Loring, D. W.; Huh, K.; Gallagher, B. B.; and King, D. W. 1990. Comparative cognitive effects of anticonvulsants. *Neurology* 40: 391–94.

Meinhard, E. A.; Oozeer, R.; and Cameron, D. 1988. Photosensitive epilepsy in children who set fires. *British Medical Journal* 296: 1773.

Merritt, H. H., and Putnam, T. J. 1938. Sodium diphenyl hydantoinate in treatment of convulsive disorders. *Journal of the American Medical Association* 111: 1068–73.

Metrakos, K., and Metrakos, J. D. 1961. Genetics of convulsive disorders: II. Genetic and electroencephalographic studies in centrencephalic epilepsy. *Neurology* 11: 474–83.

Milrod, L. M., and Urion, D. K. 1992. Juvenile fire setting and the photoparoxysmal response. *Annals of Neurology* 32: 222–23.

Morikawa, T.; Seino, M.; Watanabe, Y.; Watanabe, M.; and Yagi, K. 1989. Clinical relevance of continuous spike-waves during slow wave sleep. In J. Manelis, E. Bental, J. N. Loeber, and F. E. Dreifuss (eds.), *Advances in Epileptology: The XVII Epilepsy International Symposium*. vol. 17 (New York: Raven Press), pp. 359–63.

Murro, A. M.; Park, Y. D.; King, D. W.; Gallagher, B. B.; Smith, J. R.; Yaghmai, F.; Toro, V.; Figueroa, R. E.; Loring, D. W.; and Littleton, W. 1993. Seizure localization in temporal lobe epilepsy: A comparison of scalp-sphenoidal EEG and volumetric MRI. *Neurology* 43: 2531–33.

Nass, R., and Myerson, R. 1985. Bilateral language: Is the left hemisphere still dominant? *Brain and Language* 25: 342–56.

Nass, R., and Petrucha, D. 1990. Acquired aphasia with convulsive disorder: A pervasive developmental disorder variant. *Journal of Child Neurology* 5: 327–28.

Neumann, P. E., and Collins, R. L. 1991. Genetic dissection of susceptibility to audiogenic seizures in inbred mice. *Proceedings, National Academy of Science, USA* 88: 5408–12.

Niedermeyer, E.; Riggio, S.; and Santiago, M. 1988. Benign occipital lobe epilepsy. *Journal of Epilepsy* 1: 3–11.

Noriega-Sanchez, A., and Markand, O. N. 1976. Clinical and electroencephalographic correlation of independent multifocal spike discharges. *Neurology* 26: 667–72.

Ochs, R.; Gloor, P.; Quesney, F.; Ives, J.; and Olivier, A. 1984. Does head-turning during a seizure have lateralizing or localizing significance. *Neurology* 34: 884–90.

O'Dougherty, M.; Wright, F. S.; Cox, S.; and Walson, P. 1987. Carbamazepine plasma concentration: Relationship to cognitive impairment. *Archives of Neurology* 44: 863–67.

Ohtani, Y.; Endo, F.; and Matsuda, I. 1984. Carnitine deficiency and hyperammonia associated with valproate therapy. *Journal of Pediatrics* 101: 782–85.

Ojemann, G. A. 1983. Brain organisation for language from the perspective of electrical stimulation mapping. *Behavioral and Brain Sciences* 6: 189–230.

Ojemann, G. A., and Dodrill, C. B. 1985. Verbal memory deficits after left temporal lobectomy for epilepsy: Mechanisms and intraoperative prediction. *Journal of Neurosurgery* 62: 101–7.

Oles, K. S., and Gal, P. 1993. Bioequivalency revisited: Epitol versus tegretol. *Neurology* 43: 2435–36.

Pakalnis, A.; Drake, M. E.; John, K.; and Kellum, J. B. 1987. Forced normalization: Acute psychosis after seizure control in seven patients. *Archives of Neurology* 44: 289–92.

Palmini, A.; Andermann, F.; Olivier, A.; Tampieri, D.; Robitaille, Y.; Andermann, E.; and Wright, G. 1991*a*. Focal neuronal migration disorders and intractable partial epilepsy: A study of 30 patients. *Annals of Neurology* 30: 741–49.

Palmini, A.; Andermann, F.; Olivier, A.; Tampieri, D.; Robitaille, Y.; Melanson, D.; and Ethier, R. 1991*b*. Neuronal migration disorders: A contribution of modern neuroimaging to the etiologic diagnosis of epilepsy. *Canadian Journal of Neurological Sciences* 18: 580–87.

Palmini, A., and Gloor, P. 1992. The localizing value of auras in partial seizures: A prospective and retrospective study. *Neurology* 42: 801–8.

Palmini, A. L.; Gloor, P.; and Jones-Gotman, M. 1992. Pure amnestic seizures in temporal lobe epilepsy: Definition, clinical symptomatology and functional anatomical considerations. *Brain* 115: 749–69.

Panayiotopoulos, C. P. 1989. Benign childhood epilepsy with occipital paroxysms: A 15-year prospective study. *Annals of Neurology* 26: 51–56.

Panayiotopoulos, C. P.; Obeid, T.; and Tahan, A. 1994. Juvenile myoclonic epilepsy: A 5-year prospective study. *Epilepsia* 35: 285–96.

Paquier, P. F.; Van Dongen, H. R.; and Loonen, M. C. B. 1992. The Landau-Kleffner syndrome or "acquired aphasia with convulsive disorder": Long-term follow-up of six children and a review of the recent literature. *Archives of Neurology* 49: 354–59.

Patry, G.; Lyagoubi, S.; and Tassinari, C. A. 1971. Subclinical "electrical status epilepticus" induced by sleep in children. *Archives of Neurology* 24: 242–52.

Payton, J., and Minshew, N. 1987. Early appearance of partial complex seizures in children with infantile autism. *Annals of Neurology* 22: 408A–9A.

Penfield, W. 1975. *The Mystery of the Mind: A Critical Study of Consciousness and the Human Brain.* Princeton, N.J.: Princeton University Press.

Penfield, W.; von Santha, K.; and Cipriani, A. 1939. Cerebral blood flow during induced epileptiform seizures in animals and man. *Journal of Neurophysiology* 2: 257–67.

Penry, J. K.; Dean, J. C.; and Riela, A. R. 1989. Juvenile myoclonic epilepsy: Long-term response to therapy. *Epilepsia* 30(suppl. 4): S19–S23.

Perez, E. R.; Davidoff, V.; Despland, P-A.; and Deonna, T. 1993. Mental and behavioural deterioration of children with epilepsy and CSWS: Acquired epileptic frontal syndrome. *Developmental Medicine and Child Neurology* 35: 661–74.

Post, R. M. 1992. Transduction of psychosocial stress into the neurobiology of recurrent affective disorder. *American Journal of Psychiatry* 149: 999–1010.

Quesney, L. F.; Constain, M.; Fish, D. R.; and Rasmussen, T. 1990. The clinical differentiation of seizures arising in the parasagittal and anterolaterodorsal frontal convexities. *Archives of Neurology* 47: 677–79.

Rapin, I. 1991. Autistic children: Diagnosis and clinical features. *Pediatrics* 76: 751–60.

Rapin, I.; Mattis, S.; Rowan, A. J.; and Golden, G. G. 1977. Verbal auditory agnosia in children. *Developmental Medicine and Child Neurology* 19: 192–207.

Rausch, R.; Henry, T. R.; Ary, C. M.; Engel, J., Jr.; and Mazziotta, J. 1992. Hemispheric asymmetries of cerebral glucose metabolism related to cognitive performance in epileptic patients. *Journal of Clinical and Experimental Neuropsychology* 14: 99.

Regard, M.; Landis, T.; Wieser, H. G.; and Hailemariam, S. 1985. Functional inhibition and release: Unilateral tachistoscopic performance and stereoelectroencephalographic activity in a case with left limbic status epilepticus. *Neuropsychologia* 23: 575–81.

Ritaccio, A. L.; Hickling, E. J.; and Ramani, V. 1992. The role of dominant premotor cortex and grapheme to phoneme transformation in reading epilepsy: A neuroanatomic, neurophysiologic, and neuropsychological study. *Archives of Neurology* 49: 933–39.

Robertson, M. M. 1985. Depression in patients with epilepsy: An overview and clinical study. In M. R. Trimble (ed.), *The Psychopharmacology of Epilepsy* (New York: Wiley), pp. 65–82.

Rodin, E. A.; Schmaltz, S.; and Twitty, G. 1986. Intellectual functions of patients with childhood-onset epilepsy. *Developmental Medicine and Child Neurology* 28: 25–33.

Ronen, G. M.; Rosales, T. O.; Connolly, M.; Anderson, V. E.; and Leppert, M. 1993. Seizure characteristics in chromosome 20 benign familial neonatal convulsions. *Neurology* 43: 1355–60.

Roulet, E.; Deonna, T.; Gaillard, F.; Peter-Favre, C.; and Despland, P. A. 1991. Acquired aphasia, dementia, and behavior disorder with epilepsy and countinuous spike and waves during sleep in a child. *Epilepsia* 32: 495–503.

Rourke, B. P. 1985. *Neuropsychology of Learning Disabilities: Essentials of Subtype Analysis.* New York: Guilford Press.

Rutter, M.; Graham, P.; and Yule, W. 1970. *A Neuropsychiatric Study in Childhood.* (Clinics in developmental medicine Nos. 35–36). London: Heinemann Medical Books.

Sagar, H. J., and Oxbury, J. M. 1987. Hippocampal neuron loss in temporal lobe epilepsy: Correlation with early childhood convulsions. *Annals of Neurology* 22: 334–40.

Savard, G.; Andermann, F.; Olivier, A.; and Rémillard, G. M. 1991. Postictal psychosis after partial complex seizures: A multiple case study. *Epilepsia* 32: 225–31.

Scheibel, M.; Crandall, P.; and Scheibel, A. 1974. The hippocampal-dentate complex in temporal lobe epilepsy: A golgi study. *Epilepsia* 15: 55–80.

Schiffmann, R.; Mannheim, G. B.; Stafstrom, C. E.; Hamburger, S. D.; and Holmes, G. L. 1993. Posterior fossa abnormalities in children with infantile spasms. *Journal of Child Neurology* 8: 360–65.

Schubert, R., and Cracco, J. B. 1992. Familial rectal pain: A type of reflex epilepsy? *Annals of Neurology* 32: 824–26.

Segal, R. A.; Chapman, C.; and Barlow, J. 1991. Monozygotic twins with seizures: Shared characteristics. *Archives of Neurology* 48: 1041–45.

Shewmon, D. A., and Erwin, R. J. 1988. The effect of focal interictal spikes on perception and reaction time: II. Neuroanatomic specificity. *Electroencephalography and Clinical Neurophysiology* 69: 338–52.

Silfvenius, H.; Blom, S.; Nilsson, L. G.; and Christianson, S. A. 1984. Observations on verbal, pictorial and stereognostic memory in epileptic patients during intra-carotid Amytal testing. *Acta Neurologia Scandinavica* 99: 57–75.

Smith, D. B.; Mattson, R. H.; Cramer, J. A.; Collins, J. F.; Novelly, R. A.; Craft, B.; and Veterans Administration Epilepsy Cooperative Study Group. 1987. Results of a nationwide Veterans Administration cooperative study comparing the efficacy and toxicity of carbamazepine, phenobarbital, phenytoin and primidone. *Epilepsia* 28(suppl. 3): S50–S58.

Snead, O. C., III. 1990. Treatment of infantile spasms. *Pediatric Neurology* 6: 147–50.

Stores, G. 1978. School children with epilepsy at risk for learning and behaviour problems. *Developmental Medicine and Child Neurology* 20: 502–8.

Stores, G.; Williams, P. L.; Styles, E.; and Zaiwalla, Z. 1992. Psychological effects of sodium valproate and carbamazepine in epilepsy. *Archives of Disease in Childhood* 67: 1330–37.

Strauss, E.; Wada, J.; and Moll, A. 1992. Depression in male and female subjects with complex partial seizures. *Archives of Neurology* 49: 391–92.

Sutula, T.; Xiao-Xian, H.; Cavazos, J.; and Scott, G. 1988. Synaptic reorganization in the hippocampus induced by abnormal functional activity. *Science* 239: 1147–50.

Suzuki, I.; Shimizu, H.; Ishijima, B.; Tani, K.; Sugishita, M.; and Adachi, N. 1992. Aphasic seizure caused by focal epilepsy in the left fusiform gyrus. *Neurology* 42: 2207–10.

Theodore, W. H.; Sato, S.; Kufta, C.; Balish, M. B.; Bromfield, E. B.; and Leiderman, D. B. 1992. Temporal lobectomy for uncontrolled seizures: The role of positron emission tomography. *Annals of Neurology* 32: 789–94.

Thompson, P. J. 1987. Educational attainment in children and young people with epilepsy. In J. Oxley and G. Stores (eds.), *Epilepsy and Education, 1987* (London: Medical Tribune Group), pp. 15–24.

Todd, R. B. 1855. *Clinical Lectures on Paralysis, Disease of the Brain, and Other Affections of the Nervous System* (Philadelphia: Lindsay & Blakiston), pp. 196–210.

Trimble, M. R. 1990. Antiepileptic drugs, cognitive function and behavior in children: Evidence from recent studies. *Epilepsia* 31(suppl. 4): S30–S34.

van der Meij, W.; van Huffelen, A. C.; Willemse, J.; Schenk-Rootlieb, A. J. F.; and Meiners, L. C. 1992. Rolandic spikes in the inter-ictal EEG of children: Contribution to diagnosis, classification and prognosis of epilepsy. *Developmental Medicine and Child Neurology* 34: 893–903.

Velasco, M.; Velasco, F.; Velasco, A. L.; Juján, M.; and del Mercado, J. V. 1989. Epileptiform EEG activities of the centromedian thalamic nuclei in patients with intractible partial motor, complex partial, and generalized seizures. *Epilepsia* 30: 295–306.

Vining, E. P.; Mellits, E. D.; Dorsen M. M.; Cataldo, M. F.; Quaskey, S. A.; Spielberg, S. P.; and Freeman, J. M. 1987. Psychologic and behavioral effects of antiepileptic drugs in children: A double-blind comparison between phenobarbital and valproic acid. *Pediatrics* 80, 165–74.

Watanabe, K.; Yamamoto, N.; Negoro, T.; Takahashi, I.; Aso, K.; and Maehara, M. 1990. Benign infantile epilepsy with complex partial seizures. *Journal of Clinical Neurophysiology* 7: 409–16.

Waterman, K.; Purves, S. J.; Kosaka, B.; Strauss, E.; and Wada, J. A. 1987. An epileptic syndrome caused by mesial frontal lobe seizure foci. *Neurology* 37: 577–82.

West, W. J. 1841. On a peculiar form of infantile convulsions. *Lancet* 1: 724–25.

Wilkins, A. J.; Zifkin, B.; Andermann, F.; and McGovern, E. 1982. Seizures induced by thinking. *Annals of Neurology* 11: 608–12.

Williamson, P. D.; French, J. A.; Thadani, V. M.; Kim, J. H.; Novelly, R. A.; Spencer, S. S.; Spencer, D. D.; and Mattson, R. H. 1993. Characteristics of medial temporal lobe epilepsy: II. Interictal and ictal scalp electroencephalography, neuropsychological testing, neuroimaging, surgical results and pathology. *Annals of Neurology* 34: 781–87.

Williamson, P. D.; Spencer, D. D.; Spencer, S. S.; Novelly, R. A.; and Mattson, R. H. 1985. Complex partial seizures of frontal lobe origin. *Annals of Neurology* 18: 497–504.

Williamson, P. D.; Thadani, V. M.; Darcey, T. M.; Spencer, D. D.; Spencer, S. S.; and Mattson, R. H. 1992. Occipital lobe epilepsy: Clinical characteristics, seizure spread patterns, and results of surgery. *Annals of Neurology* 31: 3–13.

Willmore, L. J.; Triggs, W. J.; and Pellock, J. M. 1991. Valproate toxicity: Risk-screening strategies. *Journal of Child Neurology* 6: 3–6.

Wuarin, J. P.; Kim, Y. I.; Cepeda, C.; Tasker, J. G.; Walsh, J. P.; Peacock, W. J.; Buchwald, N. A.; and Dudek, F. E. 1990. Synaptic transmission in human neocortex removed for treatment of intractable epilepsy in children. *Annals of Neurology* 28: 503–11.

Wyllie, E.; Lüders, H.; Morris, H. H.; Lesser, R. P.; and Dinner, D. S. 1986. The lateralizing significance of versive head and eye movements during epileptic seizures. *Neurology* 36: 606–11.

Yamamoto, J.; Egawa, I.; Yamamoto, S.; and Shimizu, A. 1991. Reflex epilepsy induced by calculation using a "soroban," a Japanese traditional calculator. *Epilepsia* 32: 39–43.

Zung, A., and Margalith, D. 1993. Ictal cortical blindness: A case report and review of the literature. *Developmental Medicine and Child Neurology* 35: 921–26.

9

Head Trauma

Accidental head trauma is quite frequent in childhood and adolescence. While not all instances of head trauma lead to brain injury, many children experience behavioral changes following a head injury. These behavioral changes can affect various cognitive functions, achievement, psychological adjustment, and personal or social adaptive functioning (Fennell & Mickle 1992; Fletcher & Levin, 1988; Levin, Benton & Grossman 1982). In recent years, the number of studies of children who have suffered head trauma has increased. These investigations have permitted the clinician and family to better understand and cope with the problems a child may experience while recovering from a head injury. Most research has tended to focus on small groups of moderately to severely head-injured children. The type, extent, and duration of behavioral changes following minor and mild brain trauma remain less well described, despite the fact that most children who experience head trauma suffer these less severe injuries (Kraus, Rock & Hemyari 1990). Recent prospective studies of minor head injuries that included pediatric patients suggest that the vast majority of patients do not experience medical/neurologic symptoms sufficient to required neurosurgical intervention (Dacey & Dikmen 1987; Fletcher et al. 1990), and that most recover without specific medical intervention. Preliminary data from the UCLA studies of mild head injury suggest that premorbid risk factors may account for many of the purported deficits in the mildly injured group (Asarnow 1993; Satz 1993).

Sometimes the clinical neuropsychologist first encounters a more severely injured child when the child is transferred to a rehabilitation setting. More commonly, a child who has suffered a mild or moderate brain injury is seen in an outpatient setting before, or shortly after, the child's resumption of school activities. Rarely, a child may be referred to a neuropsychologist only after a lengthy history of school or adjustment problems, when the treating physician or family raises the possibility that these problems are due to the earlier head trauma. Finally, it is not uncommon for an evaluation of the child's functioning to occur in the context of a lawsuit involving claims of personal injury or suffering.

This chapter presents a brief review of the epidemiology of head injuries in children and discusses the pathophysiology of brain injuries. Characteristics of the hospital setting (inpatient and outpatient) and neurodiagnostic procedures that a child may undergo are briefly reviewed. Neurobehavioral changes observed in children who have experienced a head injury are described in connection with the severity of injury. Psychological and adaptive behavioral problems are also discussed. In the final section, rehabilitation strategies with children are reviewed.

EPIDEMIOLOGY OF PEDIATRIC HEAD INJURIES

Traumatic brain injuries are a leading cause of death and permanent disability in children and adolescents (Guyer & Ellers 1990). Estimates of the rate of such injuries among children vary from 193/100,000 to 367/100,000, with most researchers agreeing that the figure obtained depends on the type and severity of the injury reported. Among head-injured children, there are two peak incidences: in children of mid-to-late adolescence and in children younger than age 5 years (Kraus 1987; Kraus, Rock & Hemyari 1990). After children reach age 5, studies generally report a higher rate of head injuries among males than among females. For example, a study conducted in San Diego County, California, yielded a rate of 185/100,000 injuries in males age 15 years or younger, compared to 132/100,000 in same-age females (Kraus, 1987). Racial differences have also been reported. Blacks and other nonwhites suffer higher rates of head injuries than do whites; ethnic differences—specifically, Hispanic versus non-Hispanic—remain less clear (Rivara & Mueller 1986). Socioeconomic factors affect the rates of reported head injuries for all ages, including the pediatric age group. The highest rates of injuries are reported among the lowest socioeconomic classes (Kraus 1987).

Severity also varies among age groups. For example, Kraus, Rock, and Hemyari (1990) reported that, for pediatric cases (ages 0 to 15 years), only 5% of the injuries are fatal, 17% are severe or moderately severe, and 82% are mild. Estimates such as these are typically gathered from hospital emergency room or admission data, so they may not (and presumably do not) include children who are not taken to these facilities for treatment because of the mild or minor nature of the trauma sustained, or for other reasons (Casey, Ludwig & McCormick 1986).

CAUSES OF HEAD TRAUMA

Children sustain traumatic head injuries in various settings, with rates varying according to chronological age. Among infants, toddlers, and young children, the major causes of head trauma are falls (in the home or in a play area), pedestrian–motor vehicle accidents, bicycle–motor vehicle accidents, sports-related injuries, and child abuse. By late childhood and adolescence, the leading causes of head trauma include injuries suffered in accidents involving motor vehicles (such as cars or motorcycles) and injuries sustained in sports and recreational activities (Kraus 1987). Motor-vehicle-related injuries are often the most severe, and they account for a higher proportion of fatal injuries among pediatric cases. Among children younger than 4 years of age, 10.5% of all deaths were caused by injuries from motor vehicle accidents. Among children between the ages of 5 and 14 years, 8.9% of deaths were attributable to injuries suffered in motor vehicle accidents (Kraus 1987; Shapiro 1987). In recent years, the reported annual number of children who have suffered injuries, including fatal injuries, as a result of child abuse has risen dramatically (Christoffel 1990), as has the rate of assaults among inner-city youth gangs, giving rise to differences in incidence estimates according to reporting metropolitan areas (Cooper, Tabaddor & Hauser, 1983; Guyer & Ellers, 1990; Kraus, 1987). As a result of these statistics, a number of state and federal programs aimed at preventing child abuse, predicting the injury-prone child, increasing home safety, and reducing drunk driving have been initiated.

CLASSIFICATION OF HEAD INJURIES

Traumatic brain injuries can be grouped into two broad categories: penetrating head injuries, and nonpenetrating head injuries. In one type of penetrating injury, the head is forcefully hit by an object resulting in fracture of the skull and subsequent movement downward of the skull, tearing the dura and/or lacerating the brain underneath. In a second type, a missile (for instance, a BB pellet) passes through the skull and dura and lodges within a brain structure or passes through brain structures and exits the skull. Nonpenetrating head injuries, also termed *closed head injuries,* occur when the force of a blow to the head causes either a nondepressed or a linear skull fracture or when no fracture occurs but the force of the blow is transmitted to the brain contents within the cranial vault.

PATHOLOGY OF HEAD INJURIES

Both focal and diffuse effects of head trauma may be seen in either penetrating or closed head injuries (see Table 9–1). Focal effects of penetrating head injuries may include dural tears, injuries to blood vessels of the dura or meninges, focal injuries to brain structures underlying the depressed skull, or skull fragments penetrating underlying brain tissue. In missile injuries, additional damage due to pathway lesions from the missile trajectory through brain tissue or from penetration of the brain by bony skull fragments and contrecoup hemorrhagic lesions may also occur. In addition, more diffuse effects of trauma— including shearing and stretching of neurons, diffuse brain swelling, and cerebral edema—may be observed.

Brain injuries resulting from closed head trauma are attributable to the effects of the compression of the head against an object as well as to the shifting of brain structures within the cranial vault by the rapid acceleration/deceleration of the head as it encounters a moving or stationary object. At impact, the brain may shift forward, striking the undersurface of the skull *(coup),* then rebound

Table 9-1 Pathology of Brain Injury After Penetrating and
Nonpenetrating Head Trauma

Focal Effects (Primary Types of Damage)

Penetrating brain injury
    Tearing of dura
    Tearing of surface vasculature—epidural or subdural bleeds
    Focal compression/laceration of brain tissue
    Intracranial contusion (coup or contrecoup)
    Intracranial hemorrhage
    Focal fragmentary trajectory lesion to brain tissue

Nonpenetrating brain injury
    Intracranial contusion (coup or contrecoup)
    Tearing of surface vasculature
    Intracranial hemorrhage

Diffuse Effects of Brain Trauma of Either Type

Primary effects
    Axonal shearing/stretching
Secondary effects
    Cerebral edema
    Diffuse brain swelling
    Increased intracranial pressure
    Focal edema surrounding focal traumatic or hemorrhagic lesions
    Ischemic brain damage due to blood loss, cardiac disorders, or respiratory disorders
    Axonal degeneration following trauma to neurons
    Posttraumatic hydrocephalus

backward and injure a distant site in the brain *(contrecoup);* or injuries may result from side-to-side movement within the cranium. These movements can result in both focal and diffuse injuries to brain tissue. Focal effects of closed head injuries include intracranial hemorrhages (coup or contrecoup) and rupture of dural, meningeal, or cerebral vessels from the mechanical forces involved in the rapid acceleration or deceleration of the head. Similar diffuse effects are also reported in closed head injuries and include axonal shearing and tearing, diffuse brain swelling, and cerebral edema.

A number of secondary effects of head injury have also been described. These include increased intracranial pressure, focal edema (which may surround intracranial hemorrhages), and ischemic brain damage resulting from blood loss or decreased cardiac or respiratory function. Three later-appearing effects of head trauma of either type have also been reported in children: white matter degeneration; posttraumatic hydrocephalus; and posttraumatic epilepsy (Cooper 1991; Levin, Benton & Grossman 1982; Menkes & Batzdorf 1984). Children are more likely than adults to experience diffuse cerebral swelling following a head injury (Shapiro 1987), and they are also more prone to develop seizures in the early posttraumatic period. Unlike adult cases, these cases involving early seizures do not predict later-appearing epilepsy (Anneagars et al. 1980; Jennett 1975).

LEVELS OF CONSCIOUSNESS AFTER HEAD INJURY

Examiners encounter numerous difficulties in assessing level of consciousness in a head-injured child. While loss of consciousness has been used as an index of the severity of head injuries in adult patients (Lishman 1987), many children who sustain even a severe head injury may show only a transient loss of consciousness or none at all at the time of initial injury (Shapiro 1987). The most frequently used adult assessment tool, the Glasgow Coma Scale (Teasdale & Jennett 1974), presumes that the individual would, if uninjured or minimally injured, be able to communicate and comprehend questions posed by the examiner. However, many children are injured as infants or toddlers before they have developed complete language skills. Moreover, children's emotional response to trauma may include so much anxiety that they are unwilling or unable to respond to or cooperate with requests from a stranger. For this reason, recent efforts have been directed at developing an assessment tool for young children. Like the Glasgow Coma Scale, the Children's Coma Scale (CCS)(Hahn et al. 1988) assesses eye opening and best motor response, but the best verbal response has been modified to include behaviors (such as consolable crying) that do not depend on language. Table 9–2 presents a brief comparison of these two indices of levels of consciousness.

CONCUSSION

In its mildest form, a closed head injury may cause only a momentary change in neurologic functioning (Gennarelli 1987). There may be only a short period of confusion or disorientation. Concussion severity is commonly classified according to the length of time the patient experiences loss of consciousness, with classical concussion involving a period of up to six hours of continued nervous system disruption. During this period of disruption, other physical signs may be present, including changes in heart rate, blood pressure, muscle tone, and periphery responses. The patient may have no memory or faulty memory for this period of time (Gennarelli 1987). In a small number of pediatric patients, delayed onset of neurologic signs has been reported to occur minutes to hours after a head injury in which there was no clear loss of consciousness. This childhood concussion syndrome includes late onset of pallor, nausea, vomiting, and irritability from which the child fully recovers within 24 hours of onset (Shapiro 1987).

A number of behavioral changes have been reported by parents and teachers following uncomplicated concussions in children and adolescents. These include headaches, increased irritability, sleepiness, and lethargy, emotionality, disrupted sleep-walking cycles, memory problems, mild depressive symptoms, and academic difficulties (Casey, Ludwig & McCormick 1986; Lanser,

Table 9-2 Comparisons Between Glasgow Coma Scale (GCS) for Adolescents and Adults and Children's Coma Scale (CCS) for Young Children

Eye Openings (GCS, CCS)	*Best Motor Response (GCS, CCS)*
4. Spontaneous	6. Responds to verbal commands
3. Nonspecific reaction to speech	5. Localized movement to terminate painful stimulus
2. Response to painful stimulus	4. Withdrawal from painful stimulus
1. No response	3. Decorticate posture
	2. Decerebrate posture.
	1. No response
Best Verbal Response (GCS)	*Best Verbal Response (CCS)*
5. Oriented	5. Smiles, oriented to sound, interacts, follows objects
4. Confusion, disorientation	4. Consolable crying, but inappropriate interactions
3. No sustained or coherent conversation	3. Inconsistently consolable, moaning
2. No recognizable words	2. Inconsolable, restless and irritable
1. No response	1. No response

Modified and adapted from Teasdale & Jennett (1974), and, Hahn et al. (1988).

Jennekens-Schinkel & Peters 1988; Levin, Ewing-Cobbs & Fletcher 1989). Academic problems tend to involve difficulties with concentrating in the classroom, completing assignments within the required time, and (in some cases) maintaining prior test score levels. Unfortunately, the frequency, duration, and severity of these behavioral changes are not well-documented for pediatric patients, nor is the time course for resolution of these complaints well-described. In general, it would be very unusual for such complaints to persist beyond 6 months after concussion, in the absence of other neurologic complications (Levin, Eisenberg & Benton 1989).

THE HOSPITALIZED PATIENT

Most head injuries in children are minor or mild, with minimal or brief alteration of central nervous system function. In fact, recent epidemiological studies suggest that only about 50% of all patients who sustain head trauma of any severity are hospitalized, and that the average length of hospital stay is less than three days (Dacey & Dikmen 1987). The remainder of these patients go untreated, are seen in physicians' offices or are treated and released from hospital emergency rooms.

When a head-injured child is hospitalized, the length of stay and the degree of medical intervention beyond observation clearly depend on the severity of the child's injury. The intent of this chapter is not to discuss in detail the variety of treatments available, since a number of excellent texts do so. Rather, the discussion here will consist of a brief overview of the hospital setting and a description of relevant procedures pertaining to head-injured children.

The Intensive Care Unit (ICU)

The ICU is a specialized hospital unit designed to provide both comprehensive and intensive medical monitoring of the patient. Many hospitals do not have a separate pediatric ICU, or the ICU may include patients with various disorders, including head trauma. Typically, at least one nurse may be assigned to provide continuing intensive care to the patient for a shift period of up to 12 hours. Depending on the patient's status, this nurse will provide both routine physical care and specialized care to the patient. Commonly, ICU patients are hooked up to various telemetry devices that monitor the patient's vital signs (heart rate, respiratory rate, and blood pressure); these may include special devices for monitoring intracranial pressure (ICP), as discussed in the next section. Thus, the ICU setting is often replete with the sounds of these monitoring devices, and alarm signals may be heard intermittently. In monitoring head-injured patients, the nurse may check the level of consciousness as frequently as every 15 minutes, as well as overseeing fluid intake and output. Respiratory therapists may check on the functioning of devices designed to assist breathing or may check levels of blood gases to monitor respiratory functioning. Typically, parents and visitors have restricted access to the patient, although some facilities permit parents to remain near the stabilizing patient indefinitely. Length of stay in the ICU is usually dictated by the patient's medical or neurological status, but it is not always an index of the severity of the head injury itself. For example, pediatric patients are often moved from an ICU to a regular patient floor and then discharged within a day of this transfer to home care or to a rehabilitation facility. It is also common for children—even those with moderate head injuries—to be discharged to home care, rather than to be transferred to a rehabilitation facility. This is especially the case with younger children, who do not have requirements for specific medical treatments. Finally, many patients begin physical therapy while in the ICU, in order to maintain muscle tone and to begin training in needed skills.

The Pediatric Inpatient Setting

Once assessed as medically stable, the child may be transferred to a general-care pediatric inpatient floor. Depending on whether the hospital is a general community hospital, a specialized children's hospital, or a teaching hospital, different levels of medical and support services staffing may be available. The staffing of all medical facilities includes several levels of nursing personnel (nurse clinicians, registered nurses, licensed practical nurses, and nursing assistants) as well as specialty allied health services (respiratory care, physical and occupational therapy, and dietary services). Social workers are also commonly available. In specialty or teaching hospitals, physicians in training (students, interns, and residents) may be involved in patient care along with the primary attending physician. Specialties such as pediatric psychologists, neuropsychologists, and educators may also be available, but this is less commonly so. As a result, detailed neuropsychological evaluations of the pediatric patient may not occur until the patient is received by a rehabilitation facility or is seen in follow-up outpatient care. When there is a neuropsychologist on staff, this individual often serves to educate the patient's family about the specific behavioral problems of the patient, the general consequences of head injuries, and recovery from them. Social workers often assist the family in contacting local support groups for head-injured patients and their families, such as the National Head Injury Foundation. Social workers also often assist in the selection of and transfer of the patient to a rehabilitation facility. Where no transfer is anticipated, social workers may assist the family in obtaining needed outpatient services such as physical therapy or speech therapy. In many hospitals, professionals who work with head-injured patients are often organized into a team that works with both the patient and the family, from admission to the ICU or the patient floor through discharge and follow-up outpatient care.

NEURODIAGNOSTIC STUDIES

Following a physical examination of the head-injured patient, a number of routine neurodiagnostic studies may be ordered and consultation may be sought from specialized hospital diagnostic facilities. Commonly, radiologic examination of the skull (skull film) and other body structures (abdomen, chest, long bones) is ordered, to check for the presence of bone fractures or other soft-tissue trauma. Routine blood chemistries or assessments of blood arterial gases may be ordered, to assess the extent of hemorrhagic blood loss or compromised respiratory function. A lumbar puncture (LP) may reveal the presence of blood in the cerebrospinal fluid, indicating a brain bleed due to trauma; but this procedure is only selectively ordered, since it carries a risk of herniation. Often, an electroencephalogram (EEG) may be ordered, to check for the presence of generalized slowing or focal abnormalities, which can accompany cerebral trauma.

In addition, several neurodiagnostic imaging studies may be ordered. Computed tomography scans (CT scans) are routinely ordered to examine the head for the presence of epidural, subdural, intracranial, and intraventricular or parenchymal hemorrhagic lesions. These studies may include the use of a contrast dye to highlight suspected lesions and are often ordered within the first 8 to 24 hours of an injury. At many hospitals, magnetic resonance imaging (MRI) scans are also available. Recent studies comparing CT scans to MRI scans suggest that the MRI may better define the extent of intracranial hemorrhagic lesions, particularly those involving fronto-temporal structures (Levin et al. 1987; Wilberger, Deeb & Rothfus 1987). It takes longer to complete an MRI study, however, and the procedure often requires sedation of the pediatric patient. As a result, physicians who are caring for a head-injured child may be reluctant to submit the child to MRI study in the early phases of treatment. Recently, Levin et al. (1993) demonstrated that 40% of lesions demonstrated on MRIs conducted for a sample of mild and moderate-to-severe CHI pediatric patients were gray-matter lesions restricted to orbitofrontal and dorsolateral frontal regions. White-matter frontal lesions were the second most common finding. Analyses of extrafrontal and subcortical lesions were not conducted. At present, other neurodiagnostic procedures such as SPECT scanning, PET (positron emission tomography) scanning, and regional cerebral blood flow (rCBF) studies are not routinely used in assessing hospitalized adult or pediatric head-injured patients.

Intracranial Pressure (ICP) Monitoring

Normal intracranial pressure of circulating cerebrospinal fluid is below 15 mm Hg pressure. Sustained levels of ICP above 60 mm Hg are almost always fatal (Marmarou & Tabaddor 1987; Mickle 1990). One complication of head injury is a rise in ICP, which can interfere with cerebral blood flow and reduce oxygen and glucose needed to sustain neuronal functions. As a result, if the patient's ICP reaches levels above 15 to 20 mm Hg, neurosurgeons often initiate treatment to dissipate the increased pressure. These treatments may include drug therapy (with Mannitol, for instance) and ventriculostomy, in which an external drainage tube is inserted into the ventricular system to decrease ventricular fluid pressure. ICP can be monitored continuously by introducing a pressure gauge into the subdural subarachnoid, parenchymal, or ventricular space. Various types of monitoring devices have been developed, but they will not be discussed here. In head-injured patients, ICP changes have been found to occur prior to changes in the patient's clinical neurologic status (Wilkinson 1987).

Establishing a Baseline of Neuropsychological Functioning

In the immediate post-injury period, problems of fluctuating medical (nausea, neurologic problems, headaches, and attentional dysfunction) and behavioral (irritability) symptoms may interfere with the clinicians' ability to conduct an extensive neuropsychological assessment, particularly with regard to the moderately to severely injured child. Alternatively, early discharge of a child with minor or mild head injury may prevent the neuropsychologist from completing a comprehensive assessment. Thus, many neuropsychologists who see hospitalized pediatric head-injured patients utilize a briefer test battery, which they can give within a 1- to 2-hour window of time, to establish an index of baseline functioning for the child tested. The selection of tests employed must take into account the age of the child, the possibility of language or communication difficulties, and the potential confounding effects of fatigue on test results. In general, it is helpful to select a test battery that is easy to administer at bedside and that consists of several shorter subtests; this arrangement permits any needed rest periods to be interjected easily. The following six domains of functioning should be assessed: an index of general cognitive or intellectual functioning; memory and learning; attentional functions; motor functions; language; and constructional skills. These domains have been shown in studies of the pediatric age group to be the ones most likely to be affected by head injuries. (Specific findings relating to these areas of functioning are reviewed in later sections of this chapter.) Table 9–3 presents a representative brief assessment battery for baseline neuropsychological evaluations.

At the time of initial evaluation, the neuropsychologist should also obtain a detailed history of the child's developmental history before the injury. Academic functioning and any prior existing developmental disabilities—including language disabilities, attentional disorders, and learning disabilities—should also be ascertained. Prior head injuries, medical illnesses, and social or behav-

Table 9-3 Brief Assessment Battery for Baseline Neuropsychological Evaluation

Cognitive Functions
    Wechsler Intelligence Scale for Children-III[1] (selected subtests)
        Comprehension
        Similarities
        Vocabulary
        Picture Completion
Memory Functions[2]
    Verbal
        Digit Span (WISC-III)
        Verbal List Learning (e.g., CVLT-C[3])
        Story Recall (e.g., WRAML[4])
    Nonverbal
        Pointing Span[2]
        Visual Learning (e.g., WRAML)
Language[2]
    Visual Naming
    Verbal Fluency
Visuospatial Functions
    Object Assembly (WISC-III)
    Block Design (WISC-III)
    Beery Test of Visual Motor Integration[5]
Motor
    Finger Tapping[2]
Attention/Concentration
    Symbol Search (WISC-III)
    Trail Making Test[6]
    Go No-Go[7]

[1] Wechsler (1991).
[2] Spreen & Strauss (1991).
[3] Delis et al. (1989).
[4] Sheslow & Adams (1990).
[5] Beery (1989).
[6] Reitan & Davison (1974).
[7] Benton (1968).

ioral problems should be carefully documented and explored with the child's parent. Such preexisting disorders may interact with the effects of a mild to severe injury or may complicate the interpretation of symptoms and complaints that may arise in the post-injury recovery period. If the baseline evaluation is to occur in an outpatient setting, parents should be encouraged to bring *all* school and medical records to the evaluation, including any standardized achievement or behavioral assessments that may have antedated the injury. In the preschool age child, careful documentation of developmental milestones is helped if the parent can bring personal (that is, baby book) or physician records of growth and development. Finally, having the parent complete standardized developmental questionnaires (for example, the Child Developmental Inventory, or CDI), adaptive functioning interviews (such as the Vineland Adaptive Behavior Scale), and problem behavior checklists (such as the Child Behavior Checklist) often yields results that complement the findings from interview and testing data.

NEUROBEHAVIORAL EFFECTS OF HEAD INJURY

This section presents a brief review of the neurobehavioral effects of childhood head injuries. Areas to be reviewed include intellectual functioning, memory and learning, attention and concentration, language, motor skills, and achievement. Social and emotional behavior pathology that may follow head injury are also briefly reviewed.

The behavioral changes that can follow a head injury vary with the severity of the injury, as well as according to the time elapsed since the injury and the age at which the injury occurred. Most studies involving the pediatric age group have focused on the changes observed in children who have sustained a moderate or severe head injury with fewer studies investigating children with a minor or mild head injury. These studies often include children assessed within a relatively short time after their injury and involve cross-sectional data by ages. Other studies have followed children from 6 months through 2 or more years post-injury, assessing changes in dysfunction as the healing or recovery process proceeds. Finally, most studies have included children from a fairly wide age range (toddler through adolescence), with the majority focusing on school-age children. As a result, relatively few longitudinal studies span the course of development from preschool through high-school years.

Studies differ in whether they include control or contrast groups, in the measures they use to assess behavioral changes, and in the methods they use to classify the injury severity. Thus, the neuropsychologist who seeks to understand the clinical picture associated with head injuries in children is confronted with a wide variety of studies, many of which may yield disparate findings. In the following sections, a brief survey of the results of studies of the neurobehavioral effects observed in pediatric head injuries is presented. Within each section, studies (where available) are reported according to the general classification of mild, moderate, and severe head injuries. Table 9–4 presents a sum-

Table 9-4 Neuropsychological Changes
Following Closed Head Injuries

Intellectual and Cognitive Changes

Declines in full scale and performance IQ scores
Attention/concentration dysfunction
Memory disorder
Language dysfunction
Motor slowing
Achievement/academic declines

Emotional and Behavioral Changes

Development of new behavior problems
Exaggeration of preexisting behavior problems

---

mary overview of common neurobehavioral changes that have been reported to
follow closed head injury in children and adolescents.

Intellectual Functions

It is now generally accepted that some decline in scores on standardized intelligence tests may be observed following head injuries in children (Jaffe et al.
1992; Levin, Benton & Grossman 1982; Levin, Ewing-Cobbs & Fletcher
1989). Declines in performance IQ and full-scale IQ have been reported in
children with mild, moderate, and severe head injuries (Klonoff, Low & Clark
1977; Gulbrandsen 1984; Ewing-Cobbs et al. 1989). When compared to normal
controls or matched orthopedically injured control groups, the greatest declines
in performance IQ are observed among children with relatively severe injuries,
particularly in the early posttraumatic period (Chadwick et al. 1981; Winogron,
Knights & Bawden 1984). Some improvement in these measures has been observed over follow-up periods extending to 5 years, with the greatest improvement observed in the mildly head-injured groups (Bassett & Slater 1990; Bawden, Knights & Winogron 1985; Berger-Gross & Shakelford 1985). Declines
in verbal IQ are less commonly observed and when found, typically are found
only among the severely head-injured children (Brink et al. 1990; Filley et al.
1987). Long-term follow-up studies have suggested that persistent deficits in
verbal, performance, and full-scale IQ are most likely to occur among the severely injured (Klonoff, Low & Clark 1977; Mahoney et al. 1983).

However, some cautions must be raised in interpreting these data. For example, it is possible that differential attrition rates between children with good
recovery and children with poor recovery may have led to overrepresentation
of the severely impaired in longer-term studies. Large groups of mildly head-
injured children have rarely been studied for extended follow-up periods. Patients with minor head injuries are clearly not well-represented in the available

research. This second issue is particularly problematic, since the least amount of detailed information is available about the most common type of pediatric head injury (Cooper 1991). Finally, there have been few efforts to disentangle the possible confounding effects of socioeconomic factors or premorbid intellectual levels on the outcome of head trauma in children. Given these difficulties with group studies of intellectual changes following head injury in children, the clinician should be extremely cautious in using this research as a basis for predicting the effects in an individual case.

Memory Functions

Most studies of memory functioning following head injuries in children and adolescents have excluded the lower age ranges because of the difficulties in assessing memory in younger children (5 years or younger). In the ages examined, both verbal and nonverbal memory problems have been reported. In the following subsections, an overview of these findings is presented.

Verbal Memory Problems

The largest series of studies of verbal memory disorders resulting from mild, moderate, or severe head injuries in the pediatric patient have come from the collaborative work of Levin and colleagues in Galveston, Texas. In a series of studies published over the past 20 years, various verbal memory deficits have been observed in children. Utilizing a word list learning task, for example, the researchers found problems in the storage and retrieval of these words among mildly, moderately, and severely head-injured children at initial evaluation. By 6 months after the injury, improvements were noted in all groups, with greatest recovery noted for the mildly injured group (Levin & Eisenberg 1979a, 1979b). In contrast, Levin et al. (1988) reported that no memory deficits were observed in a group of mildly and moderately head-injured pediatric patients, either at initial resolution of posttraumatic amnesia or at 1-year follow-up. As in the earlier study, severely injured children had verbal memory deficits at both initial and follow-up evaluations. This same collaborative group has also observed problems in verbal recognition memory at initial assessment of mildly, moderately or severely injured children (Levin & Eisenberg 1979a, 1979b) which were resolved at six month follow-up and one year follow-up (Levin et al. 1988) for all but the severely injured group. Other investigators have reported problems in learning word pairs (Chadwick et al. 1981) and recall of storage passages in children who have sustained severe head injuries (Bassett & Slater 1990). More recently, Levin et al. (1993) and Jaffe et al. (1992) also demonstrated deficits in verbal learning on the children's version of the California Verbal Learning Test. In both studies, size and location of lesion (Levin et al.) or severity of injury (Jaffe et al.) was a predictor of worse performance.

Nonverbal Memory Problems

Compared to studies that have examined verbal memory performance following head trauma, much less information is available regarding nonverbal memory problems. Problems in remembering shapes in the Tactual Performance Test (TPT) of the Reitan battery for children (Reitan & Davison 1974) were reported by Klonoff, Low, and Clark (1977) in a study of a large group of children followed for up to 5 years after mild, moderate, or severe head injury. These problems were present for up to 3 years posttrauma in the younger children (<9 years) but for only 1 year posttrauma in the older children (>9 years). Problems in remembering locations on the TPT have also been observed in moderately and severely head-injured children, but not in mildly head-injured children (Gulbrandsen 1984; Winogron, Knights & Bawden 1984). Deficits in the ability to reproduce simple geometric figures from immediate memory and from delayed memory have also been reported, but only among severely head-injured pediatric patients tested for up to 1 year after injury (Bassett & Slater 1990; Berger-Gross & Shackelford 1985).

The preceding studies suggest that a child who sustains a severe head injury is at greatest risk to experience persistent problems in aspects of verbal and nonverbal memory functioning—at least for up to 1 year post-injury. Results of studies of mildly and moderately head-injured children are more controversial, with some studies reporting initial problems that resolve at follow-up examinations conducted at 6 months or 1 year posttrauma, while others report no differences or minimal differences initially between mildly injured children and control groups and none remaining at follow-up. These mixed findings may be due, at least in part, to the likelihood of co-existing problems in attention and concentration among head-injured children. In the next section, a brief review of the findings on head-injury-induced attentional difficulties is presented.

Attention and Concentration Functions

Early reports of problems in attention and concentration following severe pediatric head injuries were most commonly clinical descriptions provided by parents or contained in school reports (Black et al. 1969; Bruce et al. 1978). Later studies of groups of mildly, moderately, or severely head-injured children have employed various neuropsychological measures in attempting to describe, quantify, and observe recovery patterns among these patients. For example, Klonoff, Low, and Clark (1977), utilizing elements of the Reitan battery, observed that deficits in speed of responding could be observed at up to 5 years posttrauma for older (but not younger) children. Parental reports of problems in concentration and attention also persisted for up to 5 years of follow-up. More recent studies employing a continuous performance task (Chadwick et al. 1981), reaction-time paradigms (Gulbrandsen 1984), attentional span measures (Winogron, Knights & Bawden 1984; Bawden, Knights & Winogron 1985), and interpretation of problem behaviors on an adaptive functioning scale or in clinical interviews (Fletcher et al. 1990; Rutter, Chadwick & Shaffer 1983), as well as recent reviews of the risks of head injury in the pediatric age group (Ewing-Cobbs et al. 1989) offer a mixed picture. In general, the greatest risk for attention and concentration problems occurs in the initial posttraumatic period, for all degrees of severity; but then the risk shifts disproportionately toward the severely injured at short-term and long-term follow-up.

Language Functions

Aphasic disorders involve alteration or loss of function in the expression or comprehension of language, as well as related disorders with regard to reading or writing. Frank aphasia is not a common outcome of head injury in adults or in pediatric patients; subtle deficits in language may be observed, however, and these have been characterized as "aphasoid symptoms." In younger children, mutism followed by gradual recovery to normal speech has also been reported (Hecaen 1976; Levin, Benton & Grossman 1982; Ylvisaker 1986). Studies of children who have sustained a severe head injury suggest the presence of post-traumatic motor speech disturbances and acquired articulation problems (Brink et al. 1970) in these patients. Estimates of the incidence of these problems in the severely head-injured child range from 31% (Kaiser & Pfenninger 1984) to 63.1% (Gilchrist & Wilkinson 1979). In contrast, language problems reported among mildly or moderately head-injured children have tended to include problems in naming (Jordan, Ozanne & Murdock 1990), fluency (Slater & Bassett 1988), repetition (Levin & Eisenberg 1979a, 1979b), and written language (Ewing-Cobbs et al. 1989). These problems were present at the initial post-trauma evaluation and tended to show improvement at the follow-up examination 6 months to 1 year later.

Comparisons between younger and older head-injured children suggest that language deficits following head injury appear to have the greatest impact on language functions that are in development at the time of the injury (Ewing-Cobbs et al. 1989). Younger children seem more susceptible to problems on both expression and receptive language tasks, while older children are more selectively affected on tasks requiring comprehension or written expression of complex language. The persistence of these deficits and the recovery course of trauma-induced language dysfunction have not been widely studied in children, particularly among the mildly injured patients. Recently, reduced verbal fluency has also been reported (Levin, Culhane et al. 1993); it was found to be associated with left and right frontal MRI white- and gray-matter lesions, particularly those involving dorsolateral surfaces of the frontal lobes. The effect of coexisting intellectual problems or other cognitive deficits on severity of the language disorder is unclear, as is the potential impact of specific speech and language treatment techniques.

Motor Functions

Motor disabilities following a head injury in children are most commonly seen in the clinical neurological examination. Evidence of lateralized motor pathologies involving the limbs or facial muscles or of motor speech disorders is the most frequent finding in case studies of head-injured children (Shapiro 1987). Direct assessment of speed of finger tapping, of manual dexterity, and of performance on tasks involving visuomotor or tactuomotor skill and speed has also been included in some studies of mildly, moderately, and severely head-injured children and adolescents. Motor slowing is a common finding in the initial assessment of the head-injured child. But these deficits of motor speed are most likely to persist beyond 6 months only in severely injured children (Chadwick et al. 1981; Klonoff, Low & Clark 1977; Levin & Eisenberg 1979a, 1979b; Winogron, Knights & Bawden 1984). The prognosis for the mildly injured child is more positive, with resolution of these deficits possible within 6 months (Gulbrandsen 1984).

Deficits have also been reported among head-injured children on tasks that depend to some extent on the speed and accuracy of the motor expression of problem-solving skills (Levin, Benton & Grossman 1982; Levin, Eisenberg & Benton 1989). For example, lower scores on the performance IQ subtests have been interpreted in some studies to reflect, at least in part, visuomotor deficits (Chadwick, et al. 1981). Fine visuomotor copying deficits have also been observed among moderately and severely head-injured children (Bawden, Knights & Winogron 1985; Fletcher & Levin 1988; Levin & Eisenberg 1979b). However, the frequency, severity, and duration of these reported deficits are unclear from the research studies available. As in the areas reviewed earlier, it is quite difficult to use these studies as the basis for predicting the outcome in any individual case. Predictions regarding individual recovery would have to take into account an array of factors including premorbid abilities (often unavailable in these areas of neuropsychological functioning) and the impact of individual differences on the interpretation of test variations from the test normative data.

Achievement and Academic Performance

Almost as common as complaints of attentional problems or disruption of memory functions are reports of changes in academic performance following a head injury in childhood or adolescence (Fletcher & Levin 1988; Levin, Eisenberg & Benton 1989). Problems reported include reading, writing, and mathematics (Ewing-Cobbs et al. 1987; Fletcher et al. 1990). The literature in this area is somewhat sketchy, but it suggests that children or adolescents who sustain a severe head injury are at significant risk for academic performance problems, including school failure and the need for special educational interventions (Klonoff, Low & Clark 1977; Shaffer et al. 1980; Levin & Benton 1986; Ewing-Cobbs et al. 1987). The picture is clouded in the adolescent age group, where a substantial proportion of head-injured patients have a prior history of academic difficulties, including diagnosed learning disabilities (Prigatano et al. 1984). Similarly, assessing whether a learning disability in a younger child is a consequence of a specific head injury or reflects a familial tendency toward learning disabilities depends on a careful evaluation not just of the patient but also of the patient's family history. Finally, very scant research data are available that address the likelihood of significant and/or persistent academic achievement difficulties following a mild head injury, despite the fact that the vast majority of pediatric-age head injuries are minor and/or mild.

Psychological and Behavioral Problems

Parental reports of behavioral problems following mild head injury are not uncommon. As the severity of the injury increases, there is an increased likelihood that problematic behavioral changes will be observed by parents and teachers during both the initial and the later post-injury periods. Behavioral problems implicated include changes in temperament, increased irritability, temper outbursts, impulsivity, aggression, hyperactivity, and problems in inter-personal/social adaptation. In general, behavioral changes may occur even in cases of minor and mild head injury (Casey, Ludwig & McCormick 1986), but these tend to be transient and did not persist through extended follow-up periods (Gulbrandsen 1984; Levin, Eisenberg & Benton 1989). Severe head injuries are much more likely to lead to development of new problem behaviors, even among children who had a prior history of behavioral problems (Filley et al. 1987; Rutter, Chadwick & Shaffer 1983). In particular, long-term problems in social adjustment seem to be a considerable risk for the child or adolescent who sustains a severe head injury (Filley et al. 1987; Klonoff, Low & Clark 1977), as do problems in adaptive functioning and in participation in social or school activities (Fletcher et al. 1990). Among the severely head-injured, the constellation of problems in attention, impulsivity, and temperament may lead to a psychiatric diagnosis of attention deficit disorder (ADD) (Black et al. 1969; Klonoff, Low & Clark 1977).

It is important to recognize that parental response to any head injury, whether minor or severe, can influence the parent's perception of behavior disorder. This seems to be particularly important among the minor or mild head-injured groups, whose parents may unconsciously change their expectations of the child or become more permissive. The parents may then misattribute to brain damage changes in behavior more appropriately attributed to changes in parenting behaviors—particularly if these problems (for instance, the child forgets to do homework) persist beyond the first few months posttrauma in minor or mild head injuries. The clinician, therefore, needs to interview the parents of any head-injured child or adolescent carefully, in order to develop an accurate picture of the patient and of the responses of the patient's family to any perceived problems before and after a child's head injury.

Finally, the type of behavioral changes reported may differ according to the child's age at the time of the injury and the child's age at subsequent follow-up visits. Just as age-related factors influence the expression of cognitive pathology following head injuries in children and adolescents (Fletcher et al. 1987; Goldstein & Levin 1985), so too do they affect the expression of psychopathology or behavioral pathology (Chadwick et al. 1981; Rutter, Chadwick & Shaffer 1983; Fennell & Mickle 1992). For example, problems in sustaining effort at schoolwork might be attributed to dependency or immaturity in the younger-age child, but to poor motivation in the teenager. Each instance, however, could be the result of injury to frontal-executive function systems of the brain, which are frequently traumatized in closed head injuries (Ruff, Cullum and Luerssen, 1989). For this reason, it is essential that the clinician who evaluates head-injured children have a clear understanding of normal cognitive, behavioral, and emotional development. The relationship of brain development to behavioral development is critical to interpreting the pathologies that can arise following a traumatic injury.

REHABILITATION OF THE HEAD-INJURED CHILD

Since the early 1970s, publication of texts and journals focused on rehabilitation of the brain-injured patient has markedly increased. Most of these publications, however, continue to address the treatment of adult patients or contain only a chapter or an article or two about children's rehabilitation needs. Recent reviews of rehabilitation methods stress the importance of this developing field, particularly in the areas of cognitive and behavioral rehabilitation. The child or adolescent who suffers a closed head injury of sufficient magnitude to require outpatient or inpatient care may work with any or all of the following specialists: physical therapist, occupational therapist, speech therapist, recreational therapist, educator, cognitive rehabilitator, social worker, and behavioral counselor. Most commonly, however, the child or adolescent will be monitored by the physical, occupational, or speech therapist for a period of inpatient, transitional, or outpatient care. In many school districts, these specialty services are offered through exceptional student or special services housed in the school facility.

Children in homebound programs work with educators in their homes until they are able to return to a regular (or special) classroom setting. Each of these specialists can play a significant role in the recovery of physical, adaptive skills, language, and educational functioning of the brain-injured child. Typically, however, these types of services are indicated for the more severely injured patient. The child who sustains a minor or mild head injury often quickly returns to normal daily activities—including school—without the specific intervention of these specialists. Among adolescent patients, vocational counseling may be an important facet of the treatment process, although these services are not routinely offered. Instead, schools may be expected to provide the services of a vocational counselor through career or guidance counseling.

Therapies to intervene in the cognitive and behavioral pathologies that sometimes follow a closed head injury are frequently directed at both the patient and the patient's family. Two major models underlie most cognitive rehabilitation approaches: a *restorative model,* which directs efforts at the restoration of lost or impaired functions via relearning and practice; and a *substitution model,* which directs efforts at replacing or altering the means or pathways that underlie a given behavior in order to obtain a new approximation of that behavior. Examples of the former type are seen in many therapies designed to correct motor speech disorders. An example of the latter type involves training patients in the use of memory aides.

Approaches to correcting the behavioral pathologies that can follow a head injury often include several focuses: environmental adaptations; family interventions; and behavior therapies for specific problem behaviors. In the first instance, for example, the physical environment in a home may be modified to enhance mobility, or the routines of study efforts may be modified to address a shortened attention span. Family interventions may include counseling to cope with changes in role structure due to the physical needs of the patient, and developing changes in parental expectations or responses to problem behaviors such as temper outbursts. Behavior therapies may be employed to treat specific problem behaviors such as enuresis, nightmares, or poor study skills (Ylvisaker, Szekeres & Hartwick 1992).

Relatively few empirical studies have been conducted of rehabilitation efforts in large groups of pediatric head-injured patients (Jennett & Teasdale 1981), as opposed to such efforts in groups of adult patients (Benedict 1989; Levin, Grafman & Eisenberg 1987). Studies of acute trauma predominate (Jaffe & Hays 1986; McGuire & Sylvester 1987), and they tend to include mostly adolescent patients, as part of a larger group of adult patients. Few theoretical models are available to guide cognitive rehabilitation efforts in children, since most were developed from the perspective of the mature versus the developing brain (Fletcher et al. 1987; Finger et al. 1988). All too often, the rehabilitation approaches taken with regard to children are borrowed from adult models, and little attention is paid to age differences in brain development, memory, language, or problem-solving strategies of children (Kail 1985; Kolb & Whishaw 1990; Spreen et al. 1984).

The clinical neuropsychologist may play several different roles in working with the pediatric head-injured patient or the patient's family. As a diagnostician, the neuropsychologist may provide a careful and comprehensive assessment of the patient's strengths and deficits at the time of initial injury and during the course of recovery (Fennell & Bauer 1989). In this role, the neuropsychologist may recommend various types of rehabilitative approaches to the patient. As an educator, the neuropsychologist may provide information to the treating physician, to the patient's family, and to the school regarding specific problems or needs of the patient as assessed through examination. The neuropsychologist may work closely with rehabilitative therapists to provide information about intervention strategies or responses to treatment. When the child resumes schoolwork, the neuropsychologist may need to communicate with educators regarding specific residual disabilities of the child. As a clinician, the neuropsychologist may offer counseling services to the patient or the family, or may facilitate provision of these services through other providers such as psychiatry or social work services. The amount of time devoted to each of these activities will vary according to the setting in which the neuropsychologist practices. But regardless of the setting, the neuropsychologist may play a continuing or intermittent role in evaluating and treating pediatric patients who sustain a traumatic head injury.

CONCLUSION

In this chapter, different causes and types of head injuries and the pathophysiology of penetrating and closed head injuries were briefly presented. More detailed discussion of the neurobehavioral effects of closed head injuries followed. Review of the available research literature suggests that problems in intellectual, memory, visuomotor, language, and attentional functions may follow mild, moderate, or severe head injuries in children—particularly in the first six months following injury. However, persistent long-term deficits have been reported only among severely injured patients. Psychosocial, emotional, academic, and behavioral problems can follow head injuries in children, as well, although the type and duration of these difficulties may vary considerably according to the severity of the injury, the presence of preexisting problems, and the ability of the patient's family to adjust to the changes triggered by the injury. Finally, review of rehabilitation strategies among pediatric head-injury cases suggests that the majority of techniques are based on adult models of treatment, underscoring the tremendous need for empirical studies of the efficacy of different treatment interventions for head-injured children.

REFERENCES

Anneagars, J. F.; Grabow, J. D.; Groover, R. V.; Laws, E. R.; Elveback, L. R.; and Kurland, L. T. 1980. Seizure after head trauma: A population study. *Neurology* 30: 683–89.

Asarnow, R. 1993. Head injury in children and adolescents: Neurobehavioral outcome. Symposium at the 21st annual meeting of the International Neuropsychological Society, Galveston, Texas.

Bassett, S. S., and Slater, E. J. 1990. Neuropsychological function in adolescents sustaining mild closed head injury. *Journal of Pediatric Psychology* 15: 225–36.

Bawden, H. N.; Knights, R. M.; and Winogron, H. W. 1985. Speeded performance following head injury in children. *Journal of Clinical and Experimental Neuropsychology* 7: 39–54.

Beers, S. R. 1992. Cognitive effects of mild head injury in children and adolescents. *Neuropsychology Review* 3: 281–320.

Beery, K. 1989. *Manual for the Development Test of Visuo-Motor Integration,* 2d ed. Odessa, Fla.: Psychological Assessment Resources.

Benedict, R. N. 1989. The effectiveness of cognitive remediation strategies for victims of traumatic head injury: A review of the literature. *Clinical Psychology Review* 9: 39–54.

Benton, A. L. 1968. Differential behavioral effects of frontal lobe disease. *Neuropsychologia* 6: 53–60.

Berger-Gross, P., and Schackelford, M. 1985. Closed head injury in children: Neuropsychological and scholastic outcomes. *Perceptual and Motor Skills* 61: 254.

Black, P.; Jeffries, J. J.; Blumer, D.; Wellner, A.; and Walker, A. F. 1969. The posttraumatic syndrome in children. In A. M. Walker, W. F. Raveness, and M. Critchley (eds.), *Late Effects of Head Injury* (Springfield, Ill.: Charles C. Thomas), pp. 142–49.

Brink, J. D.; Garrett, A. L.; Hale, W. R.; Woo-Sam, J.; and Nickle, V. L. 1970. Recovery of motor and intellectual functions in children sustaining severe head injuries. *Developmental Medicine and Child Neurology* 12: 565–71.

Bruce, D. A.; Schut, L.; Bruno, L. A.; Wood, J. H.; and Sutton, L. N. 1978. Outcome following severe head injury in children. *Journal of Neurosurgery* 48: 679–88.

Casey, R.; Ludwig, S.; and McCormick, M. C. 1986. Morbidity following minor head trauma in children. *Pediatrics* 78: 497–502.

Chadwick, O.; Rutter, M.; Shaffer, D.; and Shrout, P. E. 1981. A prospective study of children with head injuries: IV. Specific cognitive deficits. *Journal of Clinical Neuropsychology* 3: 101–20.

Christoffel, K. K. 1990. Violent death and injury in U.S. children and adolescents. *American Journal of Diseases of Children* 144: 697–706.

Cooper, J. O.; Tabaddor, K.; and Hauser, W. A. 1983. The epidemiology of head injury in the Bronx. *Neuroepidemiology* 2: 70–88.

Cooper, P. R. 1991. *Head Injury.* 2d ed. Baltimore: Williams & Wilkins.

Dacey, R. G. 1989. Complications after apparently mild head injury and strategies of neurosurgical management. In H. S. Levin, H. M. Eisenberg, and A. L. Benton (eds.), *Mild Head Injury* (New York: Oxford University Press), pp. 83–101.

Dacey, R. G., and Dikmen, S. S. 1987. Mild head injury. In P. R. Cooper (eds.), *Head Injury* (Baltimore: Williams & Wilkins), pp. 125–42.

Delis, D. C.; Kramer, J. H.; Kaplan, E.; and Ober, B. A. 1989. *California Verbal Learning Test—Children's Version,* research ed. San Antonio: Psychological Corporation.

Ewing-Cobbs, L.; Miner, M.; Fletcher, J. M.; and Levin, H. S. 1989. Intellectual, motor and language sequelae following closed head injury in infants and preschoolers. *Journal of Pediatric Psychology* 14: 531–47.

Ewing-Cobbs, L. E.; Levin, H. S.; Eisenberg, H. M.; and Fletcher, J. M. 1987. Language functions following closed head injury in children and adolescents. *Journal of Clinical and Experimental Neuropsychology* 2: 575–92.

Fennell, E. B., and Bauer, R. M. 1989. Models of inference in evaluating brain–behavior relationships in children. In C. R. Reynolds and E. Fletcher-Janzen (eds.), *Handbook of Clinical Child Neuropsychology* (New York: Plenum Press), pp. 167–78.

Fennell, E. B., and Mickle, J. P. 1992. Behavioral effects of head trauma in children and adolescents. In M. B. Tramontana and S. R. Hooper (eds.), *Advances in Child Neuropsychology,* vol. 1 (New York: Springer-Verlag), pp. 24–49.

Filley, C. M.; Cranberg, L. D.; Alexander, M. P.; and Hart, E. J. 1987. Neurobehavioral outcome after closed head injury in childhood and adolescence. *Archives of Neurology* 44: 194–98.

Finger, S.; LeVere, T. E.; Almli, R.; and Stein, D. G. 1988. *Brain Injury and Recovery: Theoretical and Controversial Issues.* New York: Plenum Press.

Fletcher, J. M.; Ewing-Cobbs, L.; Miner, M. E.; Levin, H. S.; and Eisenberg, H. M. 1990. Behavioral changes after closed head injury in children. *Journal of Consulting and Clinical Psychology* 58: 93–98.

Fletcher, J. M., and Levin, H. S. 1988. Neurobehavioral effects of brain injury in children. In D. K. Routh (ed.), *Handbook of Pediatric Psychology* (New York: Guilford Press), pp. 258–95.

Fletcher, J. M.; Miner, M. E.; and Ewing-Cobbs, L. 1987. Age and recovery from head injury in children: Developmental issues. In H. S. Levin, J. Grafman, and H. M. Eisenberg (eds.) *Neurobehavioral Recovery from Head Injury* (New York: Oxford University Press), pp. 279–92.

Gennarelli, T. A. 1987. Cerebral concussion and diffuse brain injuries. In P. R. Cooper (ed.), *Head Injury* (Baltimore: Williams & Wilkins), pp. 108–24.

Gilchrist, E., and Wilkinson, M. 1979. Some factors determining prognosis in young people with severe head injuries. *Archives of Neurology* 36: 355–59.

Goldstein, F. C., and Levin, H. S. 1985. Intellectual and academic outcome following closed head injury in children and adolescents: Research strategies and empirical findings. *Developmental Neuropsychology* 1: 195–214.

Gulbrandsen, G. B. 1984. Neuropsychological sequelae of light head injuries in older children 6 months after trauma. *Journal of Clinical Neuropsychology* 6: 257–68.

Guyer, B., and Ellers, B. 1990. Childhood injuries in the United States. *American Journal of Diseases of Children* 144: 649–52.

Hahn, Y. S.; Chyung, C.; Barthel, M. J.; Bailes, J.; Flannery, A.; and McLone, D. G. 1988. Head injuries in children under 36 months of age. *Child's Nervous System* 4: 34–40.

Hecaen, H. 1976. Acquired aphasia in children and the ontogenesis of hemispheric functional specialization. *Brain and Language* 3: 114–34.

Jaffe, K. M.; Fay, G. C.; Polissar, N. L.; Martin, K. M.; Shurtleff, H.; Rivara, J. M.; and Winn, H. R. 1992. Severity of pediatric traumatic brain injury and early neurobehavioral outcome: A cohort study. *Archives of Physical Medicine and Rehabilitation* 73: 540–47.

Jaffe, K. M., and Hays, R. M. 1986. Pediatric head injury: Rehabilitative medical management. *Journal of Head Trauma Rehabilitation* 4: 30–40.

Jennett, B. 1975. *Epilepsy After Non-missile Head Injuries*. London: Heinemann.

Jennett, B., and Teasdale, G. 1981. *Management of Head Injuries*. Philadelphia: F. A. Davis.

Jordan, F. M.; Ozanne, A. E.; and Murdoch, B. E. 1990. Performance of closed head injured children on a naming task. *Brain Injury* 4: 27–32.

Kail, R. 1985. *The Development of Memory in Children,* 2d ed. San Francisco: W. H. Freeman.

Kaiser, G., and Pfenninger, J. 1984. Effect of neurointensive care upon outcome following severe head injuries in childhood: A preliminary report. *Neuropediatrics* 15: 68–75.

Klonoff, H.; Low, M. D.; and Clark, C. 1977. Head injuries in children: A prospective five year follow-up. *Journal of Neurology, Neurosurgery and Psychiatry* 40: 1211–19.

Kolb, B. 1989. Brain development, plasticity and behavior. *American Psychologist* 44: 1203–12.

Kolb, B., and Whishaw, I. Q. 1990. *Fundamentals of Human Neuropsychology* (2nd ed.). New York: Freeman.

Kraus, J. F. 1987. Epidemiology of head injury. In P. R. Cooper (ed.), *Head Injury* (Baltimore: Williams & Wilkins), pp. 1–19.

Kraus, J. F.; Rock, A.; and Hemyari, P. 1990. Brain injuries among infants, children, adolescents and young adults. *American Journal of Diseases of Children* 144: 684–91.

Lanser, J. B.; Jennekens-Schinkel, A.; and Peters, A. C. 1988. Headache after closed head injury in children. *Headache* 28: 176–79.

Levin, H. S.; Amparo, E.; Eisenberg, H. M.; Williams, D. H.; High, W. M.; McArdle, C. B.; and Weiner, R. L. 1987. Magnetic resonance imaging and computerized tomography in relation to the neurobehavioral sequelae of mild and moderate head injuries. *Journal of Neurosurgery* 66: 706–13.

Levin, H. S., and Benton, A. L. 1986. Developmental and acquired dyscalculia in children. In I. Flehmig and L. Stern (eds.), *Child Development and Learning Behavior* (Stuttgart: Gustav Fisher), pp. 317–22.

Levin, H. S.; Benton, A. L.; and Grossman, R. G. 1982. *Neurobehavioral Consequences of Closed Head Injury*. New York: Oxford University Press.

Levin, H. S.; Culhane, K. A.; Mendelsohn, D.; Lilly, M. A.; Bruce, D.; Fletcher, J. M.; Chapman, S. B.; Harward, H.; and Eisenberg, H. M. 1993. Cognition in relation to magnetic resonance imaging in head-injured children and adolescents. *Archives of Neurology* 50: 897–905.

Levin, H. S., and Eisenberg, H. M. 1979*a*. Neuropsychological impairment after closed head injury in children and adolescents. *Journal of Pediatric Psychology,* 4: 389–402.

———. 1979*b*. Neuropsychological outcome of closed head injury in children and adolescents. *Child's Brain* 5: 281–92.

Levin, H. S.; Eisenberg, H. M.; and Benton, A. L., eds. 1989. *Mild Head Injury.* New York: Oxford University Press.

Levin, H. S.; Eisenberg, H. M.; Wigg, N. R.; and Kobayashi, K. 1982. Memory and intellectual ability after head injury in children and adolescents. *Neurosurgery* 11: 668–73.

Levin, H. S.; Ewing-Cobbs, L.; and Fletcher, J. M. 1989. Neurobehavioral outcome of mild head injury in children. In H. S. Levin, H. M. Eisenberg, and A. L. Benton (eds.), *Mild Head Injury* (New York: Oxford University Press), pp. 189–213.

Levin, H. S.; Grafman, J.; and Eisenberg, H. M. 1987. *Neurobehavioral Recovery from Head Injury.* New York: Oxford University Press.

Levin, H. S.; Hugh. W. M.; Ewing-Cobbs, L.; Fletcher, J. M.; Eisenberg, H. M.; Miner, M.; and Goldstein, F. C. 1988. Memory functioning during the first year after closed head injury in children and adolescents. *Neurosurgery* 22: 1043–52.

Lishman, W. A. 1987. *Organic Psychiatry,* 2d ed. London: Blackwell Scientific Publications.

Mahoney, W. J.; D'Souza, B. J.; Haller, J. A.; Rogers, M. C.; Epstein, M. H.; and Freeman, J. M. 1983. Long-term outcome of children with severe head trauma and prolonged coma. *Pediatrics* 77: 756–62.

Marmarou, A., and Tabaddor, K. 1987. Intracranial pressure: Physiology and pathophysiology. In P. R. Cooper (ed.), *Head Injury* (Baltimore: Williams & Wilkins), pp. 159–76.

McGuire, T. L., and Sylvester, C. E. 1987. Neuropsychiatric evaluation and treatment of children with head injury. *Journal of Learning Disabilities* 20: 590–95.

Menkes, J. H., and Batzdorf, U. 1984. Postnatal trauma and injuries by physical agents. In J. H. Menkes (ed.), *Textbook of Child Neurology* (Philadelphia: Lea & Febinger), pp. 312–38.

Mickle, J. P. 1990. Acute head injuries in children. In *Conns Current Therapy* (Philadelphia: Saunders), pp. 841–44.

Prigatano, G. P.; Fordyce, D. J.; Zeiner, H. K.; Roueche, J. R.; Pepping, M.; and Wood, B. C. 1984. Neuropsychological rehabilitation after closed head injury in young adults. *Journal of Neurology, Neurosurgery and Psychiatry* 47: 505–13.

Reitan, R. M., and Davison, L. A., eds. 1974. *Clinical Neuropsychology: Current Status and Applications.* New York: Wiley.

Rivara, F. P., and Mueller, B. A. 1986. The epidemiology and prevention of pediatric brain injury. *Journal of Head Trauma Rehabilitation* 1: 7–15.

Ruff, R. M.; Cullum, C. M.; and Luerssen, T. G. 1989. Brain imaging and neuropsychological outcome in traumatic brain injury. In E. D. Bigler, R. A. Yeo, and E. Turkheimer (eds.), *Neuropsychological Function and Brain Imaging* (New York: Plenum Press), pp. 161–83.

Rutter, M.; Chadwick, O.; and Shaffer, D. 1983. Head injury. In M. Rutter (ed.), *Developmental Neuropsychiatry* (New York: Guilford Press), pp. 83–111.

Satz, P. 1993. Personal communication.

Shaffer, D.; Bijur, P.; Chadwick, O.; and Rutter, M. 1980. Head injury and later reading disability. *Journal of the American Academy of Child Psychiatry* 19: 592–610.

Shapiro, K. 1987. Special considerations for the pediatric age group. In P. R. Cooper (ed.), *Head Injury* (Baltimore: Williams & Wilkins), pp. 367–89.

Sheslow, D., and Adams, W. 1990. *Manual for the Wide Range Assessment of Memory and Language.* Wilmington, Del.: Jastak & Associates.

Slater, E. J., and Bassett, S. S. 1988. Adolescents with closed head injuries. *American Journal of Diseases of Children* 142: 1048–51.

Slater, E. J., and Kohr, M. A. 1989. Academic and intellectual functioning of adolescents with closed head injury. *Journal of Adolescent Research* 4: 371–84.

Spreen, O., and Strauss, E. 1991. *A Compendium of Neuropsychological Tests.* New York: Oxford University Press.

Spreen, O.; Tupper, D.; Risser, A.; Tuokko, H.; and Edgell, D. 1984. *Human Developmental Neuropsychology.* New York: Oxford University Press.

Stuss, D. T. 1987. Contribution of frontal lobe injury to cognitive impairment after closed head injury: Methods of assessment and recent findings. In H. S. Levin, J. Grafman, and H. M. Eisenberg (eds.), *Neurobehavioral Recovery from Head Injury* (New York: Oxford University Press), pp. 166–77.

Teasdale, G., and Jennett, B. 1974. Assessment of coma and impaired consciousness: A practical scale. *Lancet* 2: 81–84.

Wechsler, D. 1991. *Manual for the Wechsler Intelligence Scale for Children—III.* New York: Psychological Corporation.

Wilberger, J. F.; Deeb, Z.; and Rothfus, W. 1987. Magnetic resonance imaging in cases of severe head injury. *Neurosurgery* 20: 571–76.

Wilkinson, H. A. 1987. Intracranial pressure monitoring: Techniques and pitfalls. In P. R. Cooper (ed.), *Head Injury* (Baltimore: Williams & Wilkins), pp. 197–237.

Winogron, H. W.; Knights, R. M.; and Bawden, H. N. 1984. Neuropsychological deficits following head injury in children. *Journal of Clinical Neuropsychology* 6: 269–86.

Ylvisaker, M. 1986. Language and communication disorders following pediatric head injury. *Journal of Head Trauma Rehabilitation* 1: 48–56.

Ylvisaker, M.; Szekeres, S.; and Hartwick, P. 1992. Cognitive rehabilitation following traumatic brain injury in children. In M. Tramontana and S. E. Hooper (eds.), *Advances in Child Neuropsychology,* vol. 1 (New York: Plenum Press), pp. 168–218.

10

Cancer

This chapter deals with some important issues that confront a neuropsychologist who is seeing a pediatric hematology/oncology patient. Initial contact with a child on this service generally occurs soon after an acute, life-threatening disease has been diagnosed, at a time when many diagnostic procedures are being conducted to classify and differentiate the exact nature and severity of the illness in order to give the child appropriate treatment.

Until recently, most psychological care for children with cancer focused on acute effects, since survival rates were low. Psychosocial issues that were addressed included the emotional impact of having a fatal disease and supportive therapy and counseling for the dying child and surviving family members. Medical treatment aimed to increase longevity and to relieve symptoms. Long-term effects of disease and its treatment are a more recent focus.

Major advances in the treatment of most childhood cancers have been made in the last two decades. This is especially true with regard to acute lymphoblastic leukemia (ALL), the most common childhood cancer. With new treatments, a greater percentage of children with cancer survive longer or are considered cured. A shift toward quality-of-life issues has resulted. Researchers now attempt to determine which variables may identify patients who are at risk for adverse behavioral sequelae. Newer therapies attempt to harness the most effective combinations of treatments that will yield the least long-term sequelae. A brief discussion of pediatric cancer, diagnostic methods, and treatment choices will familiarize the psychologist with the pediatric oncology service.

CHILDHOOD CANCERS

The leukemias—specifically, ALL—are the most common childhood cancers, followed by brain tumors and other central nervous system (CNS) cancers (see Table 10-1). Other common childhood cancers include non-Hodgkins lymphoma, Hodgkins disease, Wilms tumor, rhabdomyosarcoma, osteogenic sarcoma, and Ewings sarcoma. Age at diagnosis is a distinguishing feature among these cancers. For example, the peak incidence of ALL occurs at be-

A major contributor to the reviews and ideas expressed in this chapter was co-author Pim Brouwers, Ph.D. of the National Cancer Institute, Bethesda, Maryland.

Table 10-1 Incidence of Cancer in Children Under 15 Years of Age

Site	Number of Cases	Percent of All Cases	Number of Deaths	Percent Surviving
Leukemias	2000	31	850	58
Brain and central nervous system	1230	19	550	55
Lymphomas	780	12	160	79
Sympathetic nervous system	525	8	250	52
Soft tissue	420	6	110	74
Kidney	410	6	75	82
Bone	320	5	85	73
Retinoblastoma	200	3	20	90
Other sites	665	10	75	89
All sites combined	6550	100	2175	67

Based on data in the United States, 1985; adapted from Young et al. 1986.

tween 1.5 and 5 years, that of retinoblastoma occurs at around 2 years, and that of lymphoma occurs at 10 to 14 years or older. Survival rates for these cancers vary considerably.

Staging (classification) of the disease is an important element of the initial diagnostic procedures. Staging determines whether the cancer places the child at low, medium, or high risk of dying. Staging also determines how aggressively the disease will be treated. Variables considered in staging include the child's age, tumor size, and number of neoplastic cells; the presence of metastasis; the cell types involved; and the tumor location(s). Staging variables are often called *prognostic factors* because they have been proved to be associated with disease outcome. Children are placed on different treatments according to these prognostic factors in clinical trials and in treatment protocols (Brouwers & Mohr 1991).

PROCEDURES

Besides common medical procedures—such as taking vital signs and blood for complete blood counts (CBC)—more complex and invasive procedures are used in cancer diagnosis and treatment. In hematologic cancers, such as the leukemias, a *bone marrow aspiration* is performed. In this procedure, a small amount of bone marrow is removed for laboratory examination by placing a needle into the marrow through the bone. The site of bone marrow aspiration is normally the hip or chest. Local anesthetics, as well as relaxation, self-hypnosis, and imagery techniques, have been developed to make this painful procedure more tolerable (Zeiltzer & LeBaron 1982).

A *spinal tap* or *lumbar puncture (LP)* involves placing a needle through the lower back and into the spinal canal within the spinal column. First, cerebrospinal fluid (CSF) pressure within the canal is examined. High pressure may indicate increased intracranial pressure (IICP), which may lead to cortical tissue damage. Second, the CSF is examined for evidence of neoplastic disease or other CNS abnormalities. A lumbar puncture can also be used to deliver chemotherapy, referred to as *intrathecal injection (IT)*. This administration route, directly into the CSF, has the significant advantage of bypassing the blood–brain barrier (BBB). This route is specifically needed for chemotherapeutic agents that cannot pass through the BBB or that may cross in too low a concentration to be effective. In a *biopsy,* a small amount of tissue is removed, by needle aspiration or through an incision, for further pathologic examination.

The location and extent of neoplastic disease may sometimes be determined without invasive procedures such as lumbar punctures or biopsies. Scanning with newer imaging instruments may be undertaken. There are a number of different scanning techniques: ultrasound, computerized axial tomography (CT or CAT), magnetic resonance imaging (MRI) scans, single-photon emission computed tomography (SPECT) scans, and other metabolic imaging procedures. Each of these techniques may provide information about the size, location, and structural effects of brain or body tumors and may help monitor the effects of cancer treatment. Because scanning techniques require the patient to lie unmoving for a period of time, many young children must be mildly sedated before the procedure. The type of cancer cells present, however, can only be determined by direct pathological examination of tissue samples from biopsy or aspiration.

TREATMENT

Three common treatments for pediatric cancer are surgery, radiotherapy, and chemotherapy. Although treatment is primarily directed specifically at the diseased tissue (site), preventive and adjuvant measures may also be used. Because cancers tend to spread and, on a microscopic level, may already have disseminated beyond the primary site, therapy has two goals: to eradicate the primary disease site, and to prevent metastasis to another body region.

Surgery is considered when a lesion or tumor can safely be reached and can be removed in near entirety, as is the case with solid tumors or bone tumors. However, a tumor's location may make surgery risky. Other treatments, such as radiotherapy or chemotherapy, may then be utilized. *Radiotherapy* (radiation therapy) may also be chosen if the cancer is widespread or if it has invaded other structures near the primary lesion site. Specific organs may also be irradiated if they are common sites for metastatic spread of the cancer. Prophylactic irradiation of the CNS in children with ALL is routine except for children below age 3 years.

Chemotherapy, as practiced currently, is almost exclusively a "combination" rather than a "single-agent" therapy. Chemotherapeutic agents are designed to attack reproducing cancer cells. Chemotherapeutic procedures now lead to significantly greater survival and disease-free survival rates for patients with many cancers. Table 10-2, based on Balis, Holcenberg & Poplack (1989), lists the

Table 10-2 Toxicities Associated with Commonly Used Chemotherapeutic Agents

Agent	Toxicities
Adriamycin (B)	N/V (F), HL (F), red/pink urine (F), cardiac (R)
Cytosine arabinoside (M)	N/V (F), drowsiness, lethargy, malaise, tremor, dizziness, paraplegia (R)
Cisplatin (A)	N/V (F), Ap (F), HL, hearing, taste, renal, neuropathy (R)
Cyclophosphamide (A)	N/V (F) HL (F), Ap (F), water retention, cardiac (R)
5-fluorouracil (M)	N/V, mild NL, cerebellar ataxia, slurred speech, nystagmus, dizziness, somnolence
L-Asparaginase (E)	N/V, Ap (F), lethargy (F), somnolence, confusion, behavior abnormalities, encephalopathy (R)
Methotrexate (M)	N/V (F), Ap, HL, motor dysfunction syndrome, encephalopathy (R), renal, jaundice (R)
6-Mercaptopurine (M)	N/V, Ap, jaundice
Prednisone (E)	mood alterations & behavioral abnormalities, psychosis (R), decreased growth
Vinblastine (PA)	HL, headache, mental depression, mild neurologic signs
Vincristine (PA)	peripheral motor and sensory neuropathy with muscular weakness, tremors, ataxia, hallucinations, mental depression

Abbreviations: A – alkylating agent; M – antimetabolite; B – antibiotic; PA – plant alkaloid; E – other agent; N/V – nausea & vomiting; HL – hair loss; Ap – appetite; F – frequent complication; R – rare complication.

most common chemotherapeutic agents and their potential side effects. These side effects are due, in part, to the action of these agents on rapidly reproducing noncancerous cells in the CNS or in other body sites (for instance, the gastrointestinal tract). While many side effects are acute, some agents, such as methotrexate (MTX), can produce long-term residual effects. Most agents are administered orally or intravenously (IV). For CNS therapy, however, some of these agents—specifically, MTX, cytosine arabinoside (ARA-C), and hydrocortisone—are administered intrathecally into the spinal canal.

Cancer treatment by chemotherapeutic agents is often divided into several stages. *Induction therapy,* the first phase in chemotherapy, is associated with the most aggressive treatment, which is administered to achieve remission of the cancer. Usually initiated in systemic cancers, this treatment may follow excision of a tumor or biopsy of a tumor, as well as when the type of tumor or the extent of the residual tumor requires additional treatment. *Consolidation therapy,* the second phase, is intended to ensure that the cancer is indeed in remission. *Maintenance therapy,* the third phase, is administered when the cancer is in remission, to prevent recurrence or relapse. A cancer is in remission when evidence indicates that the cancer is under control and when the cancer symptoms have partially or completely disappeared. A relapse occurs when evidence indicates renewed presence of cancer symptoms and/or neoplastic growth.

Tumors arising in the CNS may be treated in several ways. Physicians may surgically excise the tumor, or they may insert a ventriculoperitoneal shunt to relieve elevated intracranial pressure (ICP) in cases of partial excision, biopsy, or inoperable tumors. Surgery may be followed by irradiation of the tumor and surrounding tissue, by systemic chemotherapy or (occasionally) by intrathecal or intraventricular chemotherapy in very high-risk tumors. A new treatment involves bone marrow harvesting followed by high doses of chemotherapy for highly malignant inoperable tumors of the medulla or brainstem. Sometimes, if the tumor is nonmalignant, no further treatment is given after surgical excision; and the child may simply be followed with routine MRI or CT scanning.

PHYSIOLOGICAL EFFECTS OF CHEMOTHERAPY AND IRRADIATION TREATMENT

To understand the influences of childhood cancer and its treatment on neuro-psychological functioning, one must be familiar with the physiology of acute and late treatment effects of radiotherapy and chemotherapy.

Acute Effects

Acute effects are most frequent in the period from 5 to 8 weeks after completion of radiation therapy. They may last for 7 to 14 days and are characterized by nausea and vomiting, lethargy, weight loss, and increased irritability. Patients may also report tingling and electric-like discharges down their legs upon neck flexion (Jones 1964). These complaints are generally transient and are likely related to radiation damage sustained by myelin sheaths around nerve fibers or to disruption of myelin synthesis. Acute toxicities secondary to chemotherapeutic agents (see Table 10-2), transient EEG abnormalities (slowing), and the "somnolence syndrome" (Freeman, Johnston & Voke 1973) have been observed in 10% to 75% of patients, in association with their CNS treatment. In general, little relationship exists between acute effects and later appearing effects.

Late Effects

CNS therapy may lead to late-appearing brain abnormalities (Rottenberg 1991). Four types of delayed CNS abnormalities in ALL patients have been described (Crosley et al. 1978; Price & Birdwell 1978; Stehbens et al. 1991). Their incidence varies and more than one complication may be present in a given patient.

The first of these, *subacute leukoencephalopathy,* is a severe but uncommon form of neurotoxicity. Histopathologically, it is a white-matter disorder with necrosis of the myelin sheaths and neuronal processes and reactive astrocytosis. In later disease stages, focal areas become more confluent, and extensive white-matter degeneration and cavitation may be observed, particularly in the periventricular regions. Progressive dementia, seizures, decerebration, coma, and even death may follow. The second condition, *mineralizing microangiopathy* refers to a noninflammatory degenerative and mineralizing small-vessel disorder. It is accompanied by dystrophic calcifications of adjacent cortex, primarily in gray matter. In early stages, it frequently involves the vessels of the putamen. This abnormality appears later in the arterial border zone regions of the cortex and in subcortical regions such as the basal ganglia. The development of this pathology is associated with younger age, longer duration of survival following radiation therapy, relapse (particularly when the disease involves the CNS), and cumulative treatment administered. The third abnormality, *cortical atrophy,* is a gray-matter disorder characterized by irregular neuronal loss involving all six cortical layers. This is perhaps the most common histopathological change associated with CNS treatment leading to ventricular or subarachnoid space dilatation. The fourth pathology, *subacute necrotizing leukomyelopathy,* is a spinal cord involvement first identified by Price (1983). It is most likely related to cumulative administration of MTX and secondarily to prolonged folate deficiency. It is not associated with any clear neurologic signs. In the spinal cord, one sees myelin and axonal necrosis, macrophage infiltration, and gliosis in the most severe cases.

Most of these effects are related to cranial or cranio-spinal irradiation. Higher dosages (2400 rads [or cGy] and up) are associated with a higher incidence and greater severity of late effects. Some authors have also implicated intrathecal chemotherapy—particularly MTX—and cumulative systemic dosage MTX in the occurrence of these abnormalities. These pathologies are most frequent in patients who have suffered relapses, especially when these involved the CNS or were associated with additional CNS therapy. Similar changes have been reported in the brains of children undergoing irradiation for brain tumors, although major structural changes tend to be close to the tumor site rather than more widespread (Menkes 1990; Rottenberg 1991).

ASSESSMENT OF CHILDREN BEING TREATED FOR CANCER

As has been discussed elsewhere (Brouwers, Belman & Epstein 1991), three issues should be addressed in cross sectional and longitudinal evaluations of children treated for cancer:

1. What should be measured, and how should the measuring be done?
2. When and how frequently should testing be done?
3. How should unstandardized administration be handled?

These issues and how they pertain to the pediatric oncology/hematology setting will be reviewed in the following sections.

What to Measure and How to Measure It

The primary focus in assessing children should be on the psychological functions that one wants to assess; secondarily, one must decide which instruments to use to measure these functions. The tests most frequently used in studies of children with cancer are relatively standard and similar to those used with other chronically ill pediatric populations.

The stability of psychological functions over time has to be considered, since they may very well change with further development. For example, changes in memory with age may reflect not simply increased capacity but also the development of different strategies for remembering (Kail 1984).

In a neurobehavioral evaluation of therapy-related changes—particularly when associated with non-psychological interventions—it is important to recognize two types of evidence for the efficacy of the treatment: general markers and specific markers of change. To establish a general marker, the examiner must determine that criteria of interval change are clinically and/or ecologically significant. The general marker describes the child's current level of functioning and may not be intended to indicate the neuropsychological basis of this change (for instance, IQ levels). In assessing specific markers, one looks for the mechanisms underlying the observed change, at a more "microscopic" level. Neuropsychological evaluations of cancer treatments need to include both general and specific measures of the child's functioning.

For children, using an IQ from a standardized intelligence test as a general marker of cognitive functioning seems valid. Age-appropriate intelligence tests provide a measure that is reasonably stable over the time of follow-up, with acceptable predictive reliabilities over various time intervals and a fairly constant construct validity (Appelbaum & Tuma 1977). The Bayley Scales of Infant Development, the McCarthy Scales of Children's Abilities, the Wechsler Intelligence Scale for Children—III [WISC-III], and the Wechsler Adult Intelligence Scale—Revised [WAIS-R] are all examples of appropriate global-level measures.

Many of these composite measures also allow for some initial analysis at the specific level. Discrepancies in the profile of subtest scores or item content may provide an indication of the underlying mechanisms of impairment or change. Of particular interest for long-term survivors of childhood cancer are discrepancies in performance on the subtests that constitute the three components of the Wechsler IQ tests: the Verbal-Comprehension, which includes Information, Similarities, Vocabulary, and Comprehension; the Perceptual Organization factor, which includes Picture Completion, Picture Arrangement, Block Design, and Object Assembly; and the Freedom from Distractibility factor, which includes Arithmetic, Digit Span, and Coding (Kaufman 1979). Similarly, any observed difference in performance between timed and untimed subtests should be evaluated.

Specific neuropsychological tests should then be administered to develop a hypothesis-driven assessment of particular higher brain functions (Fennell & Bauer 1989). The comprehensive assessment (see Table 10-3) should include

Table 10-3 Comprehensive Test Battery for Oncology Patients

Function Measured	Test	Age Range
General Intelligence	Bayley Mental Scales (MDI)	{0–2½ y}
	McCarthy Scales	{2½–8 y}
	WPPSI-R	{4–7 y}
	WISC-III	{6–16 y}
	(Stanford-Binet IV)*	{2–23 y}
	(Merrill-Palmer)*	18–63 m}
Language	Peabody PVT-R	{2½–40 y}
	Gardner Naming	{2–16 y}
	Verbal Fluency	{>2½ y}
Visuospatial	Beery VMI	{4–18 y}
	Rey-Osterrieth	{>8 y}
Memory (Verbal)	Children's Auditory Verbal Learning Test	{5–12 y}
&	Rey Auditory Verbal	{>6 y}
	McCarthy Memory	{2½–8 y}
Learning (Nonverbal)	Rey-Osterrieth	{>8 y}
	(Wechsler Designs)*	
	(S-B IV Bead Memory)*	{2–23 y}
	Design Memory – WRAML*	
Attention	(Target Detection)*	
	(Trail Making Test)*	
	(Reaction Time)*	
Motor Function	Bayley Motor Scale (PDI)	{0–2½ y}
	Peabody Motor Scales	{½–6 y}
	Bruininks-Oseretsky Test	{>5½ y}
	Grip Strength	{>5 y}
	(Grooved Pegboard)*	{>5 y}
	(Finger Tapping)*	{>5 y}
Concept Formation	Ravens Matrices	{>5½ y}
Behavior/Personality	Vineland	{0–19 y}
	(Behavior Ratings)*	
	(Video Recordings)*	{2–3 y}
	(Achenbach)*	{4–16 y}

* = Optional or alternative tests
Age Range (y = years; m = months) refers to the range of ages for which the test is standardized.

measures of attention and executive functions, motor skills, language, visuo-constructional abilities, memory and learning, and affective symptoms (Fennell & Bauer 1989). This yields a more comprehensive picture of the patient, which may then be related to specific CT brain-scan abnormalities (Brouwers & Poplack 1990). Parent-reported measures of global social and psychological functioning and achievement testing may help define the impact that specific neurobehavioral deficits have on the child's general adaptive abilities.

When to Test and How Frequently

The reliability and validity of testing of medically ill patients is complicated by a number of potentially confounding factors. The timing of testing is critical if one wishes to obtain valid and reliable estimates of the child's optimal level of functioning. One must consider the child's concurrent medical status and/or the timing of the exam in relationship to other medical procedures that the child may be undergoing. Assessments should be scheduled either before a treatment cycle is initiated or between periods of different treatment regimens (for instance, postirradiation but prechemotherapy). The period when early development of late effects can be measured reliably and the period when enduring late sequelae may become apparent represent critical determinants of both testing frequency and the timing of scheduled testing. Interim monitoring with a subset of tests that are less sensitive to practice effects may also be utilized; this allows the neuropsychologist to monitor adverse treatment effects while minimizing the potential influence of repeated administrations of the same test.

Longitudinal follow-up of the child requires serial testing, often with the same test procedures. Unfortunately, few childhood psychological tests have multiple or alternate forms. Apparent improvements in test scores due to repeated administration of similar tests (practice effects) may overestimate the degree or pace of a child's recovery. The size of a practice effect is related to a number of factors including the test–retest interval, the health status of the child, the rate of development of the function being measured, the initial or baseline level of functioning, and the potential for latent learning. The neuropsychologist should be aware of test–retest changes that can occur in normal children. For example, studies of normal healthy children of average intelligence have demonstrated practice effects of 4.5 points on the McCarthy Scales (McCarthy 1972) and of 7 points on the WISC-III (Wechsler 1991) when these tests were readministered after one month. Practice effects are reduced when the test–retest interval is longer (from 6 to 12 months): approximately 5 points on the WISC-R (Tuma & Appelbaum 1980), 2 points on the McCarthy Scales (Bryant & Roffe 1978; Davis & Slettedahl 1976), and less than 1 point on the Bayley Scales (Horner 1980). Moreover, children with lower levels of general abilities have smaller practice effects on serial testing (Tuma & Appelbaum 1980), as do children with chronic medical conditions (Moss, Nannis & Poplack 1981; Farwell et al. 1990). Unfortunately, data on test–retest changes over a time period may not be available for specific neuropsychological measures that may be utilized (Fennell & Bauer 1989). For this reason, data derived from normal control children of comparable age may have to be developed by the examiner in order to permit interpretation of positive or negative changes on test scores over repeated testings. Recent revisions of many commonly used global cognitive measures, including the WPPSI-R (1989), the WISC-III (1991), the Stanford-Binet IV (1988), and the Bayley Mental Scales (1993), have yielded somewhat different estimates of functioning from those of earlier versions. The neuropsychologist may need to take these differences into account in long-term patient follow-up.

Obtaining a baseline measure before starting treatment is of great value in assessing both late and acute effects of CNS therapy. Appropriate testing at the start of most cancer therapy is often very difficult to accomplish. In many current treatment protocols for systemic cancers, a "baseline" measure is obtained at 6 months postdiagnosis. This has proved to be an appropriate starting point for clinical neuropsychological follow-up and care. Among pediatric brain-tumor patients, however, baseline assessment is usually obtained in the immediate postdiagnosis period, before initiation of therapy. If a child has undergone a biopsy as part of the diagnostic evaluation, it is best to wait until the acute effects of the surgery have resolved and the child is able to tolerate testing better. This may occur as early as 1 week post-operatively.

How to Handle Unstandardized Administration

Special problems are associated with assessing chronically ill, very young children. Because ill patients may be functioning below the level expected of them on the basis of their chronological age, "floor" effects are very common. It is not unusual to find that a reliable measure on a standardized test for a specific age cannot be obtained. Problems with floor effects frequently occur when the patient's chronological age coincides with the normal transition age from a test appropriate for a younger age group to one appropriate for an older age range. An alternative way to obtain an estimate of level of functioning is to employ a test normally administered to younger children. By estimating mental age or determining age equivalence on the basis of that specific test, one can obtain a ratio IQ (Ratio IQ = ({Mental age equivalent/Chronological age} × 100) rather than a deviation IQ (given in the manual). If no age equivalence values are given in the manual, these can be obtained by determining the age or age range for which the obtained raw score would constitute average performance (that is, the 50th percentile, a standard score of 100, or the like). That age— or the middle of that age range—then represents the age equivalent. Under such circumstances, follow-up testing should use the same test and ratio IQ for evaluation of interval change. Unfortunately, specific modifications in neuropsychological tests are less commonly available. As a strategy, the clinician may have greater success in following children by developing construct-driven rather than test-driven assessment batteries, as has been done in recent studies of pediatric HIV infection (Fennell 1993).

NEUROBEHAVIORAL STUDIES

Acute Effects

The acute effects of radiotherapy, chemotherapy, or surgery have been described in earlier sections. Psychological reactions to the diagnosis or to treatment are also important factors confronting the neuropsychologist (Stehbens

1988). The potential life-threatening situation associated with the diagnosis of most childhood cancers results in a set of highly charged emotional circumstances for pediatric patients and for their caregivers. The neuropsychologist must take these into consideration in timing and interpreting the assessments. Any life-threatening situation is emotionally charged because the parent or child may be very aware of the gravity of the situation. The magnitude of these emotions depends on the evaluation by the patient or the patient's family of the seriousness of the situation and how it may affect their life (Frijda 1986). Despite their illness, many pediatric oncology patients are enormously resilient. After a relatively short period of time, they begin coping with the disease and its implications—sometimes better than their parents and siblings do. Some of the stresses felt by patients during this period are associated with fears about acceptance by their peers. As treatment progresses, adaptation to changes resulting from the long-term sequelae of treatment may be necessary.

Late or Long-Term Effects

The number of long-term survivors of childhood cancer has dramatically increased in recent decades and will continue to rise (Poplack 1988). However, improvements in treatment have been associated with adverse, long-term sequelae, including brain-scan abnormalities, altered intellectual and psychological function, and neuroendocrine abnormalities for a small number of children (Dowell & Copeland 1987; Duffner & Cohen 1991; Poplack & Brouwers 1985).

Initial behavioral studies of childhood ALL survivors treated with CNS-preventive therapy that included cranial irradiation and intrathecal chemotherapy did not reveal any evidence of lasting behavioral or intellectual impairment (Holmes & Holmes 1975; Soni et al. 1975; Li & Stone 1976; Verzosa et al. 1976). Subsequently, more specialized studies reported significant functional deficits (Stehbens 1988). Younger patients have consistently shown more marked cognitive defects than older patients (Eiser & Lansdown 1977; Eiser 1978; Goff, Anderson & Cooper 1980; Meadows et al. 1981; Duffner & Cohen 1991). Moreover, even asymptomatic long-term ALL survivors in first continuous complete remission scored significantly lower than their healthy siblings on psychometric testing (Moss, Nannis & Poplack 1981). Some controversy remains, however, over whether intellectual declines actually occur in the majority of leukemia survivors who undergo cranial radiation therapy (Stehbens et al. 1991).

Studies of the cognitive effects of pediatric brain tumors rely on collections of cases that are followed in collaborative studies, as well as on reports of individual case studies. Most research on childhood brain tumors has focused on global assessments of intellectual functioning and academic achievement (Duffner & Cohen 1991; Ellenberg et al. 1987; Kun & Mulhern 1983; Mulhern & Kun 1985). These studies suggest that children with brain tumors may show significant deficits in full-scale IQ or in verbal or performance IQ. Often the long-term effects of surgery, irradiation, or chemotherapy is a reduction in IQ from baseline levels (Duffner, Cohen & Parker 1988). However, this effect varies according to the location of the tumor (cortical versus cerebellar versus posterior fossa), the presence or absence of hydrocephalus, and the age at treatment—all of which are often confounded with tumor type. For example, medulloblastomas commonly arise in younger patients, while cortical or cerebellar tumors may not become manifest until late childhood or early adolescence. Studies that have compared the effects of tumor location on intellectual functioning have generally found higher scores in children with cerebellar or cortical tumors (Bordeaux et al. 1988; Fennell et al. 1993; Dennis et al. 1992; Duffner, Cohen & Thomas 1983; Hirsch et al. 1979; Maria & D'Souza 1984).

So far, the late cognitive effects of age at treatment have not been studied systematically in large groups of children treated for brain tumors. Children with brain tumors at any age often undergo irradiation as a primary treatment when surgery is not possible. Advances in radiation oncology have led to the ability to treat more focused areas, the use of hyperfractionated irradiation treatments, and even the development of radiosurgical techniques, since young children's nervous systems are less tolerant of radiotherapy (Tomlinson et al. 1992). Cases involving patients undergoing these newer treatments are now being collected by the collaborative members of the Pediatric Oncology Group (POG) and the Children's Cancer Study Group (CCSG). Whether these treatments will reduce the extent or degree of cognitive decline following certain brain cancer treatments remains to be determined.

The following subsections review the various stages of neuropsychological functioning that seem to be affected in long-term survivors of childhood cancers. Where available, the relationship between neuropsychological deficits and brain-scan abnormalities and data on pediatric brain tumors is also presented.

Attention

The initial stage of cognitive processing requires attention to stimuli and is critical for further processing, since most psychological functions require focused and/or sustained attention. Studies examining simple reaction time (SRT) have indicated that leukemia patients with abnormal CT scans (cortical atrophy and calcifications) reacted significantly more slowly than did patients with normal head scans, and that their response latency was exaggerated by the increased length of the preparatory interval (Brouwers, Cox et al. 1984). These findings confirmed and extended other reports, based on psychometric testing (Goff et al. 1980; Last, van Veldhuizen & de Ridder-Sluiter 1982) or on observations in the school environment (Deasy-Spinetta, Spinetta & Oxman 1988), that suggested the presence of attentional deficits in long-term ALL survivors. In a recent review, Stehbens et al. (1991) found that 7 of 14 studies noted attentional problems in the leukemia patients compared to controls. Attentional problems have also been reported in studies of children treated for brain tumors (Duffner & Cohen 1991).

Attentional abnormalities may cause these children to perform tasks more slowly, to be more easily distracted, and to retain and incorporate information only when their attention is specifically directed. Performance may vary as attention varies, whether on specific tests or in different environments. When attentional processes are altered, interpretation of the nature and severity of other neuropsychological deficits may be confounded by the effects of the attentional disorder. Finally, a recent study of event-related potentials in long-term survivors of childhood cancer (Moore et al. 1992) may provide some insight into the neuropsysiological basis of the attentional problems noted in some children. These investigations revealed a prolonged latency in the P300 wave component and slower mean reaction times in children receiving IT chemotherapy compared to a group of children who did not receive IT therapy. Therefore, any complete neuropsychological evaluation of the pediatric cancer patient should include several measures of attentional abilities, including speed of processing, focused attention, and sustained attention. The model of attention recently proposed by Mirsky et al. (1991) identifies several such measures.

Memory

Initial studies noted that ALL patients did not benefit from previous test experiences, in contrast to normal controls (Soni et al. 1975). The suggestion that learning and memory processes might be affected by leukemia and its treatment has been confirmed in subsequent studies of leukemic patients (Eiser & Lansdown 1977; Goff et al. 1980; Eiser 1980; Walther, Gutjahr & Beron 1981; Mulhern et al. 1988). Stehbens et al. (1991) observed that about half of the studies that they reviewed found both verbal and nonverbal memory problems in long-term survivors of ALL. Brouwers et al. (1985) noted that long-term leukemia survivors with brain-scan abnormalities (calcifications and/or cortical atrophy) exhibited a global memory deficit. This deficit was larger for verbal than for nonverbal material, and long-term retention was affected more than was immediate recall. When verbal and nonverbal learning and memory were systematically studied in ALL patients (Brouwers & Poplack 1990), significant differences between CT-scan subgroups of ALL survivors were again noted on memory tasks employing verbal material, as compared to tests using nonverbal material. In addition, Brouwers and Poplack observed that the short-term memory and learning impairments of ALL patients were generally associated with problems in attentional functioning; that is, the differential memory impairments were significantly reduced or disappeared altogether when a correction for the attentional deficit of the patient was introduced. Attentional factors seemed to affect primarily the encoding stage of learning and memory, rather than the consolidation and retrieval stages. Part of the observed memory difficulties are an independent late effect. Finally, memory impairments have also been reported in the absence of IQ deficits in long-term survivors of childhood cancer (Mulhern et al. 1988; Tamaroff et al. 1984).

Only a few studies of pediatric brain tumors have assessed the specific effects of tumor location on memory functioning in affected children (Brookshire et al. 1990; Dennis, Spiegler, Hoffman et al. 1991; Dennis, Spiegler, Fitz et al. 1991; Dennis et al. 1992; Fennell et al. 1993). These studies all suggest that verbal memory functions may be adversely affected by tumors at various anatomical sites, from cortex to posterior fossa. Nonverbal memory has been specifically assessed less often, but presumably similar effects obtain. (Dennis, Spiegler, Hoffman et al. 1991; Fennell et al. 1993).

Language and Verbal Functions

A number of investigators have reported that younger long-term survivors of ALL tend to have more depressed verbal IQ (VIQ) compared to performance IQ (PIQ) (Moss et al. 1981; Stehbens et al. 1981), due in large part to low scores on the Vocabulary, Similarities, and Information subtests (Goff et al. 1980). Stehbens et al. (1991) reviewed the literature and found that receptive (rather than expressive) language deficits were more common in nine studies that examined language functioning in ALL survivors. Brouwers et al. (1987) compared patients with ALL who received high-dose intravenous methotrexate (HDMTX) to patients who received cranial irradiation (2400 cGy) and intrathecal MTX (CR+IT) as CNS preventive therapy. Serial measures of general intelligence indicated that CR+IT patients show a steady decrease in VIQ, while patients who received HDMTX showed a small increase (albeit insignificant) in VIQ. This difference between treatment groups progressively increased as a function of time. There were no significant differences in PIQ between the two treatment groups (Brouwers, Moss & Poplack 1992). These results confirmed the particular vulnerability of language-associated functions, as measured here by the verbal IQ, to the combination of cranial irradiation and intrathecal MTX. In addition to decrements in verbal IQ, a number of patients also demonstrated a specific language deficit (anomia). These patients had severe word-finding problems, shown on confrontation naming tests and underscored by impaired performance on a word fluency test.

Very limited data are available on the language performance of children with brain tumors. Reduced verbal fluency has been reported in children with cortical, diencephalic, brainstem, and cerebellar tumors (Bordeaux et al. 1988; Fennell et al. 1993). As noted earlier, lower verbal IQ scores have also been reported in brain tumor patients, reflecting similar effects on the Vocabulary, Similarities, and Comprehension subtests of the Wechsler Scales as has been reported for survivors of ALL (Duffner & Cohen 1991; Copeland 1992). To the extent that adverse language effects may be present in a child who has had a brain tumor, these subtle or overt language deficits may confound results on measures of verbal memory or may themselves be influenced by attentional difficulties (described earlier).

Executive Functions

Most intracerebral calcifications that occur after CNS therapy are located in the basal ganglia—a set of subcortical nuclei, including the caudate nucleus, that have extensive connections to the frontal lobes. Damage to this region may produce neuropsychological profiles similar to those seen in patients with frontal lobe abnormalities. Indeed, large discrepancies on tests that are sensitive to frontal lobe dysfunctioning—such as word fluency and the Wisconsin card sorting task—were found among ALL patients with calcifications (Brouwers, Riccardi et al. 1984).

Frontal lobe lesions in adults have often been associated with changes in behavior such as lack of initiative, loss of motivation, increased distractibility, flat affect, and irritability (Stuss & Benson 1984). These traits have also been described among the personality changes observed in some long-term childhood leukemia survivors (Einsiedel, Weigl & Gutjahr 1979; Ross 1982; Stehbens et al. 1991). The observed social and personality changes in long-term survivors of childhood cancer may therefore be related to patterns of cerebral dysfunctioning (Poplack & Brouwers 1985). Unfortunately, little to no data are available regarding the pediatric brain tumor patient, although recent studies suggest that behavioral complaints may be similar in some focal tumors (Maria et al. 1993).

Academic Achievement

Academic problems are common in school-age children who survive ALL or other childhood cancers, including brain tumors (Copeland 1992; Stehbens 1988). For example, in a recent study, academic achievement was analyzed in ALL patients who received CR+IT and in those who received HDMTX (Brouwers et al. 1988). Preliminary findings indicated significant underachievement (p<.01) on reading, spelling, and arithmetic for the CR+IT group, whereas the HDMTX group showed a modest underachievement on only one subtest: the arithmetic subtest. This suggests that, in addition to experiencing a progressive decrement in IQ, ALL patients treated with CR+IT manifested significant impairments in academic achievement.

The data on achievement among children who survive brain tumors are still unclear. In part, this is due to the failure to control for the effects of IQ deficits on school functioning, as well as the failure to analyze groups of children according to the site of the lesion and according to tumor type. Children who survive brain tumors are frequently described as suffering from various learning disabilities (Ellenberg et al. 1987; Kun & Mulhern 1983; Kun, Mulhern & Crisco 1983). In addition to finding language-related problems in reading and spelling, one recent study found specific deficits in arithmetic abilities in children with posterior fossa as compared to children with cortical tumors (Fennell et al. 1993). Therefore, the pediatric neuropsychologist should include a comprehensive assessment of academic functioning in any evaluation of the pediatric brain-tumor patient. Any premorbid history of academic problems in the school-age child and a family history of learning disabilities are important in order to understand more completely the current effects of the brain tumor or its treatment on academic functioning.

Summary

The results of both retrospective and prospective longitudinal studies have demonstrated the adverse effects of cranial irradiation and intrathecal chemotherapy on intellectual and neuropsychological function in childhood cancers. Attention difficulties play an important role in the pattern of cognitive deficits seen in ALL and pediatric brain-tumor patients. The particular vulnerability of language-associated functions and attentional processes to CNS therapy has also been identified. Other long-term sequelae include some problems in speed of responding, in memory and learning, in motor skills, and in academic achievement.

These studies have also provided evidence of a clear relationship between CT brain-scan abnormalities and neuropsychological deficits in long-term survivors of childhood cancer. The major CT brain-scan abnormalities—intracerebral calcifications—tended to be located bilaterally in the basal ganglia, an area of the brain that has been associated with attentional functioning (Howes & Boller 1975) and with language functions, particularly expressive language (Wallesch et al. 1983; Metter et al. 1988). Verbal memory and learning impairments, as well as deficits in attentional processing, are therefore consistent with the anatomical location of observed CT brain-scan abnormalities. Moreover, the progressive decline in IQ, as time from initiation of CNS treatment with CR+IT increases (Jannoun 1983; Brouwers, Moss & Poplack 1992), seems associated with previously reported findings of a similar delayed effect in the development of CT brain-scan abnormalities (Riccardi et al. 1985). Notwithstanding the variability in types of cancers, in locations, and in modes of treatment, the major point is that, when certain CT brain-scan abnormalities are present in long-term survivors, they may signify substantial underlying impairment in neuropsychological functioning. These findings support the notion that adverse late sequelae—whether in personality functioning or in neuropsychological and cognitive/intellectual changes—are largely associated with CNS disease and/or therapy (Brouwers 1987; Dowell & Copeland 1987). Although the influence of psychosocial factors on neuropsychological functioning should not be neglected, physical factors have more impact and exert their greater effects in the acute stages of the disease.

TEAM APPROACH

This section focuses on the individual patient who may not be participating in a research protocol; it discusses the assessment, consulting, and liaison issues that are involved in treating such a child. Children who experience late adverse sequelae of childhood cancer and who are seen in the outpatient clinic for long-term follow-up may present in a number of ways. On routine medical follow-up examination, a large number of such children fall within normal limits, but some may have started to show decreased school performance. The inconsistencies in school performance—particularly with respect to mathematics—may concern some children enough to prompt them to express apprehensions about this problem. Other patients or their caregivers, however, may see these changes as possible precursors to relapse and consequently may be reluctant to admit to—or may even deny—such problems. Thus, a thorough interview is required.

Many centers that specialize in treating childhood cancers have a multidisciplinary "late-effects team" to evaluate late sequelae comprehensively and to provide guidance and counseling for patients and their parents. This team may include a radiation oncologist, a neurosurgeon, and a neuroradiologist, among others (see Table 10-4). The aims of the team are to assess the patient's problems comprehensively, to suggest appropriate remedial courses of action, and to communicate the findings to the patient and/or to responsible persons in their environment.

Typically, the child is seen by every team member individually. Significant others (parents, caregivers, teachers) are seen by selected members of the team. Afterward, in a team meeting, members summarize their assessments individually. A holistic approach is taken, with emphasis on the child's current and previous medical and psychological status, indicators of improvement or deterioration, the child's living environment, the social/family situation, and the child's current educational or vocational circumstances.

PATTERNS OF NEUROPSYCHOLOGICAL FUNCTIONING

Childhood cancer may take any of a great variety of forms, each of which has different characteristics with regard to median age at diagnosis, type of treatment and length of treatment. This obviously supports numerous types of late adverse sequelae and differing frequencies of occurrence (Copeland 1992). At the most basic level of distinction, however, two general patterns of neuropsychological functioning have been seen in long-term survivors of childhood leukemias (Brouwers 1987). Patients with the first type of profile are impaired compared to their healthy siblings, but in general they score within normal limits on standard psychological tests. Patients with the second type of profile are more severely impaired, may show deterioration over baseline levels, and perform in the below-normal range.

Type 1

With respect to the natural history of their disease, children with the first type of profile normally have an uneventful course, achieve complete remission, and remain in continuous remission. No evidence of spread of the disease to the CNS is documented. In the clinic, these children are often considered medical success stories. In the outpatient clinical environment, they seem very much at home and have good interpersonal contact with other patients. Their familiarity with medical procedures gives them a limited form of authority or expertise in relation to the other patients. They tend to have no problem coming back to the clinic, which is a familiar place and can even become a "second home." Parents may complain about the child's level of school achievement, and the child may indicate that hard work is not resulting in good grades. Further, the child may express concern about failing to meet the parents' expectations. These complaints and concerns should be taken by professionals as a sign that the child may be experiencing late effects of their treatment. These children are typically very likable and socially appropriate: they voice their concerns and

Table 10-4 Late-effects Team in Pediatric Hematology/Oncology

Professional	Team Function
Pediatric oncologist and Nurse practitioner	Primary providers of medical care, serving as the stable contact in the clinic for the patient and forming the liaison with the late-effects team.
Neurologist	Neurological exam, interpretation of special procedures (e.g., CT brain scans, EEG), and medication advice.
Psychiatrist	Psychiatric evaluation of patient and family (e.g., depression, independence).
Endocrinologist	Assessment of neuroendocrine function, evaluation of growth and fertility, integrity of hypothalamic–pituitary function.
Clinical psychologist	General assessment of intelligence, personality, and social behavior.
Neuropsychologist	Evaluation of brain–behavior relationships.
Social worker	Family situation assessment, identification of resources in the home community.
Occupational therapist	Vocational assessment and consultation.
Educator	Assessment of school performance, type of school attended, and possibilities for help within that school system.

aspirations when prompted; and they often display a desire for autonomy, wanting to be treated as an adult and to be as independent from their parents as possible.

Psychometrically, children in this group have suffered some cognitive loss but seem less affected neuropsychologically as a result of their disease and its treatment. The reliable discrepancy between the child's IQ and the IQs of siblings offers evidence of their loss in intellectual potential. Nevertheless, their IQs remain at least within the normal range—that is, above 90. The overall profile of IQ subtests, although showing a somewhat larger degree of scatter than usual, does not reveal individual subtest scores that are significantly above or below their average. On the factorial components of the IQ test, there may be comparatively lower scores on the Freedom from Distractibility and Perceptual Organization factors and higher scores on the Verbal Comprehension factor. With longitudinal psychometric testing, appropriate intellectual development without deterioration is typically observed. On the other hand, academic achievement testing, when assessed formally with, for example, the Wide Range Achievement Test—3 (WRAT-3) (Jastak & Wilkinson 1993), may reveal discrepancy between the scores on the Reading, Spelling, and (particularly) Arithmetic subtests and the obtained full-scale IQ. This may indicate a certain degree of underachievement that is not due to absenteeism or lack of effort.

The neurological examination, including EEG and CSF measures, is unremarkable in most cases. On brain scans, no clear signs of gross brain abnormalities are noted. The majority of these children have normal scans, although some may show evidence of minimal cortical atrophy. In general, these children do not present with short stature or have problems with infertility or failure to develop secondary sex characteristics—problems that have been associated with neuroendocrinological abnormalities.

On neuropsychological testing, these children tend to perform in the low normal rather than in the normal range on tests of attention and memory and when using nonverbal, visuospatial material. No evidence, however, can be found to relate these patterns of functioning to specific (focal) cerebral structural abnormalities.

Psychiatric status is also considered. The psychiatrist and social worker on the late-effects team are often instrumental in establishing close communication among team members, the patient, and the parents. Evaluations by these team members often reveal that the children have problems in social interactions with peers. In part this may be due to their poorer school performance, which sets them apart from their peers and leads to adjustment problems and social isolation. In addition, these children may have difficulty regaining autonomy after having depended on physicians, nurses, and parents for a long time during their illness. Parents may become overprotective, based on their perception of the child as being extremely vulnerable to many environmental influences. The family must learn to accept that, although the child has suffered from a disease and its treatment, the child may be fully functional psychologically. Another problem is that the child may develop a fear of failure in the school system that generalizes to other social situations, leading to passivity and lack of initiative. Furthermore, a negative self-image may develop. To alleviate this and the anxiety associated with academic performance, psychotherapy in combination with relaxation techniques may be appropriate for some of these long-term survivors. Some parents, confronted by the intellectual and emotional limitations of the long-term survivor, may need professional help in adjusting their hopes for and expectations about their child's future.

The discrepancy in school performance between the child, healthy siblings, and neighborhood friends may result in adjustment problems. Some children may have been placed in an academic environment that is too competitive or in a school that lacks the appropriate resources to cope with the minimal learning difficulties that some long-term cancer survivors may experience. Sometimes it is better to place the child in a different school from the one that a sibling attends, to avoid comparisons. This also gives the child a better chance to develop a separate identity. Long-term survivors are perfectly capable of finding a satisfying vocation and of leading an independent life, even though they may not reach the same academic goals as their siblings. Expecting excellence in academics may not be realistic. When indicated, teachers and the school principal may also be included in the team meetings to delineate further the child's areas of strength, to exchange information, and to promote future rehabilitative efforts. Again, relaxation techniques may prove helpful if the child becomes anxious about tests. The psychologist, together with the oncologist or psychiatrist, may request that the child be given untimed examinations or that an extended time period be allowed. As reviewed earlier, medical and psychological evidence suggests that these children may have attentional difficulties secondary to their disease or its treatment. Attentional problems may place an unfair burden on a child faced with taking a timed standardized examination, such as the Scholastic Aptitude Test. An explanatory letter to the examination center often permits a variation in the standard testing condition.

The late-effects team's occupational therapist or vocational specialist may provide additional input about the child's current status, or guidance about appropriate vocational goals and training possibilities. In general, however, Type 1 patients do not require adjunctive occupational therapy when they have been in a stable remission. Still, vocational assessment and planning as the adolescent patient enters high school can be helpful in realistically assessing post-secondary-school educational and occupational training opportunities.

Type 2

With respect to the natural history of their disease, children with the second type of profile frequently have a more eventful course, including one or more relapses. They often receive more aggressive therapy and may experience significant acute and long-term side effects of their treatments. In this group, one often finds children in whom the brain was a primary site of neoplastic disease or of metastasis. These children often need especially careful monitoring of adverse effects, and they may require the integrated intervention of several different medical disciplines, such as neurology, neurosurgery, and psychiatry. Persistent neurological sequelae such as weakness or aphasia may necessitate occupational therapy, physical therapy, and speech therapy to help the child adapt to functional losses. In more severe cases, adaptive devices may be needed for ambulation, feeding, communication, or other aspects of daily living skills.

Psychometrically, children in this group are not only impaired relative to their healthy siblings; they are often below the normal range. Since they tend to fall behind their normally developing peers, and since their development is slowed, they typically demonstrate an IQ decline over time. Subtest scatter on IQ tests is more pronounced than that seen in test results for type 1 patients. On the factorial components of the IQ test, they tend to show lowered scores on the Freedom from Distraction factor—most frequently on the Arithmetic, Coding, and Digit Span (Backward) subtests. They also have lower scores on the Information subtest. In contrast to the scores of children in the type 1 group, their scores on the Verbal Comprehension factor tend to be lower than their scores on the Perceptual Organization factor.

On formal academic achievement evaluation, these children tend to perform below grade-level expectations on arithmetic, spelling, and reading. These academic deficits are evident beyond their already lowered scores on intelligence tests. The discrepancies between academic achievement and full-scale IQ might result in a classification of Learning Disabled, particularly for arithmetic.

Neurological examination may reveal "soft" or localizing focal neurological signs (see Chapter 4). A number of children may require treatment for more serious neurologic disorders, such as epilepsy. In addition, the electroencephalographic study may show mild irregularities or frank abnormality. Most of these children have evidence of brain lesions on CT scan, such as intracerebral calcifications, multiple areas of decreased attenuation coefficient, or more severe cortical atrophy. For children with primary CNS involvement, the scans may show evidence of residual brain tumor, surgical intervention, and other treatments.

These children frequently present with short stature that is associated with abnormalities in their "pulsatile" growth-hormone levels (Duffner & Cohen 1991). Development of secondary sex characteristics (facial and pubic hair, breasts) may also be affected. If so, the child should undergo thorough evaluation by an endocrinologist, who may suggest hormonal treatment. These effects may lead to a distorted body self-image. A special case involves boys and young men with metastatic or primary disease of the testes. Treatment-related infertility is likely under these circumstances. The possibility of freezing semen obtained before initiation of therapy for later use must be addressed, but it is associated with a host of ethical, moral, and psychiatric issues (van Asperen 1992).

On neuropsychological evaluation, type 2 children often demonstrate attentional deficits—particularly in their ability to sustain focused attention, but also in their ability to divide attention. These patients also present with global learning and memory impairments. These learning, memory, and attentional impairments are distinct deficits, noted in addition to an IQ deficit, and are likely to be associated with specific CT brain-scan abnormalities. In contrast to results for the type 1 group, the learning and memory impairments of type 2 children are often more pronounced for verbal–linguistic than for nonverbal, visuospatial material. Careful clinical testing may demonstrate the presence of a word-finding deficit (anomia). Residual CNS abnormalities may help account for the social and personality changes that are observed in these children.

On the other hand, these children often appear to be functioning at a much higher level than formal test results would seem to predict. This also has to be taken into consideration when discussing placement. A child with acquired neuropsychological and intellectual deficits may be very different from a child who has always functioned at a below-normal level.

Examination of the child's psychiatric status may reveal significant adjustment and personality problems, although they may appear less obvious to the casual observer. Frequently, these children are quiet, do not exhibit any overt behavioral problems, and are polite and obedient. They may seem minimally affected by either positive or negative events in their life and may show flattened affect. Not uncommonly, parents complain that the child sits in front of a TV for long periods of time, or that the child does not seem able to initiate recreational play activities, complete homework, or perform household chores. In addition, these children may demonstrate obsessive–compulsive characteristics. They often want to do things in the same organized way in which they responded before, and they may become upset by any changes in their schedule or routine. This is probably related to inflexibility, difficulty shifting mental set, and increased perseveration due to frontal lobe deficiencies.

Because of their learning, memory, and attentional deficits, as well as their personality changes, type 2 patients are often unable to maintain acceptable school performance in a regular classroom or work environment. Their need for special resources may exceed what is offered in the average school. For example, they may need an environment providing continuous supervision and a low teacher-to-student ratio. Instruction may have to be given in simple language, and repetition may be especially helpful. Being susceptible to distraction, the child must be shielded from outside stimulation as much as possible, and multiple rest breaks and short instruction periods are recommended. In addition, teachers need to be aware of the difficulty these children have in shifting from one idea to another, so they can allow for appropriate transitions between subjects. It is also likely that the ability of these children to learn new information or skills is limited. Generalization to other situations cannot be expected, and they may need external help to make correct associations.

It is important that the education of these children emphasize their strengths and that a positive self-image be maintained. Since the children's deficits are often associated with structural brain changes, it is unlikely that the underlying reason for their cognitive weakness can be improved, although the practical applications can be altered favorably. Mathematics, for example, is an area of relative weakness: even with great effort, only minimal improvements can generally be achieved. But practical arithmetic skills can be improved so that the child is able to function adaptively (for instance, making change or balancing a checkbook). External supports, such as a calculator, can be employed. The advice of a vocational specialist during the secondary-school years is often helpful in further delineating career opportunities.

CONCLUSION

Establishing a team approach for the pediatric cancer patient provides a comprehensive way to care for the long-term survivor of childhood cancer. Interactions between team members and children (and their parents or caregivers) support optimum decision making about interventions, often producing excellent compliance and a more successful outcome. The multidisciplinary approach also creates a clinical research setting in which team members learn a great deal from each other about the sequelae of childhood cancer and its treatment, the interrelationships between behavioral changes and brain pathology, and the opportunities available for improving a child's outcome at many different levels.

REFERENCES

Appelbaum, A. S., and Tuma, J. M. 1977. Social class and test performance: Comparative validity of the Peabody with the WISC and WISC-R for two socioeconomic groups. *Psychology Reports* 40: 139–45.

Balis, F. M.; Holcenberg, J. S.; and Poplack, D. G. 1989. General principles of chemotherapy. In P. A. Pizzo & D. G. Poplack (eds.), *Principles and Practice of Pediatric Oncology* (Philadelphia: Lippincott), pp. 165–205.

Bordeaux, J. D.; Dowell, R. E.; Copeland, D. R.; Fletcher, J. M.; Francis, D. J.; and Van Eys, J. 1988. A prospective study of neuropsychological sequelae in children with brain tumors. *Journal of Child Neurology* 3: 63–68.

Brookshire, B.; Copeland, D. R.; Moore, B. D.; and Ater, J. 1990. Pretreatment neuropsychological status and associated factors in children with primary brain tumors. *Neurosurgery* 27: 887–91.

Brouwers, P. 1987. Neuropsychological abilities of long-term survivors of childhood leukemia. In M. K. Aaronson and J. Bechman (eds.), *The Quality of Life of Cancer Patients* (New York: Raven Press), pp. 153–66.

Brouwers, P.; Belman, A.; and Epstein, L. 1991. Organ specific complications: Central nervous system involvement: Manifestations and evaluation. In P. A. Pizzo and C. M. Wilfert (eds.), *Pediatric AIDS: The Challenge of HIV Infection in Infants, Children and Adolescents* (Baltimore: Williams & Wilkins), pp. 318–35.

Brouwers, P.; Cox, C.; Martin, A.; Chase, T.; & Fedio, P. 1984. Differential perceptual-spatial impairment in Huntington's and Alzheimer's dementias. *Archives of Neurology* 41: 1073–76.

Brouwers, P., and Mohr, E. 1991. Design and clinical trials. In E. Mohr and P. Brouwers (eds.), *Handbook of Clinical Trials: The Neurobehavioral Approach* (Amsterdam: Swets & Zeitlinger), pp. 45–66.

Brouwers, P.; Moss, H.; and Poplack, D. 1992. Retrospective and prospective studies of the effect of preventive central nervous system therapy on neuropsychological functioning in long-term survivors of childhood cancer. In B. F. Last and A. M. van Veldhulzen (eds.), *Developments in Pediatric Psychosocial Oncology* (Lisse: Swets & Zeitlinger), pp. 79–89.

Brouwers, P.; Moss, H.; Reaman, G.; McGuire, T.; Trupin, E.; Libow, J.; Tarnowski, K.; Bleyer, W.; Feusner, J.; Ruymann, F.; Miser, J.; Hammond, D.; and Poplack, D. 1987. Central nervous system preventive therapy with systemic high-dose methotrexate versus cranial radiation and intrathecal methotrexate: Longitudinal comparison of effects of treatment on intellectual function of children with acute lymphoblastic leukemia. (Abstract #622.) *Proceedings: Twenty-third Annual Meeting, American Society of Clinical Oncology Abstracts* 6: 158.

————. 1988. Central nervous system preventive therapy with systemic high-dose methotrexate versus cranial radiation and intrathecal methotrexate: Comparison of effects of treatment on academic achievement in children with acute lymphoblastic leukemia. (Abstract #678.) *Proceedings: Twenty-fourth Annual Meeting, American Society of Clinical Oncology* 7: 176.

Brouwers, P., and Poplack, D. 1990. Memory and learning sequelae in long-term survivors of acute lymphoblastic leukemia: Association with attention deficits. *American Journal of Pediatric Hematology/Oncology* 12(2): 174–81.

Brouwers, P.; Riccardi, R.; Fedio, P.; and Poplack, D. 1985. Long-term neuropsychological sequelae of childhood leukemia: Correlation with CT brain scan abnormalities. *Journal of Pediatrics* 106: 723–738.

Brouwers, P.; Riccardi, R.; Poplack, D.; and Fedio, P. 1984. Attentional deficits in long-term survivors of childhood acute lymphoblastic leukemia (ALL). *Journal of Clinical Neuropsychology* 6: 325–36.

Bryant, C. K., and Roffe, M. W. (1978). A reliability study of the McCarthy Scales of Children's Abilities. *Journal of Clinical Psychology* 34: 401–6.

Copeland, D. R. (1992). Neuropsychological and psychosocial effects of childhood leukemia and its treatment. *Cancer Journal for Clinicians* 42(5): 283–95.

Crosley, C. J.; Ronke, L. B.; Evans, A.; and Nigro, M. 1978. Central nervous system lesions in childhood leukemia. *Neurology* 28: 678–85.

Davis, E. E., and Slettedahl, R. W. 1976. Stability of the McCarthy Scales over a 1-year period. *Journal of Clinical Psychology* 32: 798–800.

Deasy-Spinetta, P.; Spinetta, J. J.; and Oxman, J. B. 1988. The relationship between learning deficits and social adaptation in children with leukemia. *Journal of Psychosocial Oncology* 6: 109–21.

Dennis, M.; Spiegler, B. J.; Fitz, C. R.; Hoffman, H. J.; Hendrick, E. B.; Humphreys, R. P.; and Chuang, S. 1991. Brain tumors in children and adolescents: II. The neuroanatomy of deficits in working, associative and serial-order memory. *Neuropsychologia* 29: 829–47.

Dennis, M.; Spiegler, B. J.; Hoffman, H. J.; Hendrick, E. B.; Humphreys, R. P.; and Becker, L. E. 1991. Brain tumors in children and adolescents: I. Effects on working, associative and serial-order memory of IQ, age at tumor onset and age of tumor. *Neuropsychologia* 29: 813–27.

Dennis, M.; Spiegler, B. J.; Obonsawin, M. C.; Maria, B. L.; Colwell, C.; Hoffman, H. J.; Hendrick, E. B.; Humphreys, R. P.; Bailey, J. D.; and Ehrlich, R. M. 1992. Brain tumors in children and adolescents: III. Effects of radiation and hormone status on intelligence and on working, associative and serial-order memory. *Neuropsychologia* 30: 257–75.

Dowell, R. E., and Copeland, D. R. 1987. Cerebral pathology and neuropsychological effects: Differential effects of cranial radiation as a function of age. *American Journal of Pediatric Hematology/Oncology* 9: 68–72.

Duffner, P. K., and Cohen, M. E. 1991. The long-term effects of central nervous system therapy on children with brain tumors. In D. A. Rottenberg (ed.), *Neurological Complications of Cancer Treatment* (Boston: Butterworth-Heinemann), pp. 479–495.

Duffner, P. K.; Cohen, M. E.; and Parker, M. S. 1988. Prospective intellectual testing in children with brain tumors. *Annals of Neurology* 23: 575–79.

Duffner, P. K.; Cohen, M. E.; and Thomas, P. L. 1983. Late effects of treatment on the intelligence of children with posterior fossa tumors. *Cancer* 51: 233–37.

Einseidel, E.; Weigl, I.; and Gutjahr, P. 1979. The psycho-social status of children surviving a long time with acute lymphoblastic leukemia. *Therapiewoche* 29: 8669–73.

Eiser, C. 1978. Intellectual abilities among survivors of childhood leukemia as a function of CNS irradiation. *Archives of Disease in Childhood* 53: 391–95.

———. 1980. Effects of chronic illness on intellectual development. *Archives of Disease in Childhood* 55: 766–70.

Eiser, C., and Lansdown, R. 1977. A retrospective study of intellectual development in children treated for acute lymphoblastic leukemia. *Archives of Disease in Childhood* 52: 525–29.

Ellenberg, L.; McComb, J. G.; Siegel, S. E.; and Stowe, S. 1987. Factors affecting intellectual outcome in pediatric brain tumor patients. *Neurosurgery* 21: 638–44.

Farwell, J. R.; Lee, Y. J.; Hirtz, D. G.; Sulzbacher, S. I.; Ellenberg, J. H.; and Nelson, K. 1990. Phenobarbital for febrile seizures—Effects on intelligence and on seizure recurrence. *New England Journal of Medicine* 322: 364–69.

Fennell, E. B. 1993. Assessing neurobehavioral changes in HIV+ infants and children: A methodological approach. *Annals of the New York Academy of Science* 693: 141–50.

Fennell, E. B., and Bauer, R. M. 1989. Models of inference in evaluating brain–behavior relationships in children. In C. R. Reynolds and E. Fletcher-Janzen (eds.), *Handbook of Clinical Child Neuropsychology* (New York: Plenum Press), pp. 167–78.

Fennell, E. B.; Mann, L.; Maria, B.; Fiano, K.; Booth, M.; Mickle, J. P.; and Quisling, R. 1993. Neuropsychology of posterior fossa versus other focal brain tumors in children. *Journal of Clinical and Experimental Neuropsychology* 15: 58 [abstract].

Freeman, J. E.; Johnston, P. G.; and Voke, J. M. 1973. Somnolence after prophylactic cranial radiation in children with acute lymphoblastic leukemia. *British Medical Journal* 4: 523–25.

Frijda, N. H. 1986. *The Emotions*. London/Paris: Bambridge University Press/Editions de la Maison des Sciences de l'Homme.

Goff, J. R.; Anderson, H. R.; and Cooper, P. F. 1980. Distractibility and memory deficits in long-term survivors of acute lymphoblastic leukemia. *Developmental and Behavioral Pediatrics* 1: 158–63.

Hirsch, J. F.; Renier, D.; Czernichow, P.; Benveniste, L.; and Pierre-Kahn, A. 1979. Medulloblastoma in childhood: Survival and functional results. *Acta Neurochirwigy* 48: 1–15.

Holmes, H. A., and Holmes, F. F. 1975. After ten years, what are the handicaps and lifestyles of children treated for cancer? *Clinical Pediatrics* 14: 819–23.

Horner, T. M. 1980. Test–retest and home–clinic characteristics of the Bayley Scales of Infant Development on nine- and fifteen-month-old infants. *Child Development* 51: 751–58.

Howes, D., and Boller, F. 1975. Simple reaction time: Evidence for focal impairment from lesions of the right hemisphere. *Brain* 8: 317–32.

Jannoun, L. 1983. Are cognitive and educational development affected by age at which prophylactic therapy is given in acute lymphoblastic leukemia? *Archives of Disease in Childhood* 58, 953–58.

Jastak, S., and Wilkinson, G. 1993. *Wide Range Achievement Test—3*. Wilmington, Del.: Jastak Associates.

Jones, A. 1964. Transient radiation myelopathy (with reference to Lhermitte's sign of electrical paresthesia). *British Journal of Radiology* 37: 727–44.

Kail, R. 1984. *The Development of Memory in Children*. San Francisco: W. H. Freeman.

Kaufman, A. S. 1979. *Intelligent Testing with the WISC-R*. New York: Wiley.

Kun, L. E., and Mulhern, R. K. 1983. Neuropsychological function in children with brain tumors. *American Journal of Clinical Oncology* 6: 651–56.

Kun, L. E.; Mulhern, R. K.; and Crisco, J. J. 1983. Quality of life in children treated for brain tumors. *Journal of Neurosurgery* 58: 1–6.

Last, B. F.; van Veldhuizen, A. M.; and de Ridder-Sluiter, J. G. 1982. Intelligentie en concentratievermogen van kinderen met leukemie en hun aanpassing op school. *Tydschrift voor Kindergeneeskunde* 50: 76–82.

Li, F. P.; and Stone, R. 1976. Survivors of cancer in childhood. *Annals of Internal Medicine* 84: 551–53.

Maria, B. L., and D'Souza, B. J. 1984. Brain stem glioma. *Contemporary Neurosurgery* 6(18): 1–6.

Maria, B. L.; Rehder, K.; Eskin, T. A.; Harred, L. M.; Fennell, E. B.; Quisling, R.; Mickle, J. P.; Marcus, R. B.; Drane, W. E.; Mendenhall, N. P.; McCollough, W. M.; and Kedar, A. 1993. Brainstem glioma: I. Pathology, clinical features and therapy. *Journal of Child Neurology* 8: 112–28.

McCarthy, D. 1972. *Scales of Children's Abilities.* New York: Psychological Corporation.

Meadows, A.; Massari, D.; Fergusson, J.; Gordon, J.; Littman, P.; and Moss, K. 1981. Declines in IQ scores and cognitive dysfunctions in children with acute lymphocytic leukemia treated with cranial irradiation. *Lancet* 1: 1015–18.

Menkes, J. H. 1990. *Textbook of Child Neurology,* 4th ed. Philadelphia: Lea & Febinger.

Metter, E. J.; Riege, W. H.; Hanson, W. R.; Jackson, C. A.; Kempler, D.; and van Lancker, D. 1988. Subcortical structures in aphasia: An analysis based on (F-18)-fluorodeoxyglucose, positron emission tomography, and computed tomography. *Archives of Neurology* 45: 1229–34.

Mirsky, A. F.; Anthony, B. J.; Duncan, C. C.; Ahearn, M. B.; and Kellam, S. G. 1991. Analysis of the elements of attention: A neuropsychological approach. *Neuropsychology Review* 2: 109–46.

Moore, B. D.; Copeland, D. R.; Ried, H.; and Levy, B. 1992. Neurophysiological basis of cognitive deficits in long-term survivors of childhood cancer. *Archives of Neurology* 49: 809–17.

Moss, H. A.; Nannis, E. D.; and Poplack, D. G. 1981. The effects of prophylactic treatment of the central nervous system on the intellectual functioning of children with acute lymphocytic leukemia. *American Journal of Medicine* 71: 47–52.

Mulhern, R. K., and Kun, L. E. 1985. Neuropsychologic function in children with brain tumors: III. Interval changes in the six months following treatment. *Medicine in Pediatric Oncology* 13: 318–24.

Mulhern, R. K.; Wasserman, A. L.; Fairclough, D.; and Ochs, J. 1988. Memory function in disease free survivors of childhood acute lymphocytic leukemia given CNS prophylaxis with or without 1800 cGy cranial irradiation. *Journal of Clinical Oncology* 6: 315–20.

Poplack, D. G. 1988. Acute lymphoblastic leukemia. In P. A. Pizzo and D. G. Poplack (eds.), *Principles and Practice of Pediatric Oncology* (Philadelphia: Lippincott), pp. 323–66.

Poplack, D. G., and Brouwers, P. 1985. Adverse sequelae of central nervous system therapy. *Clinics in Oncology* 4: 263–85.

Price, R. A. 1983. Therapy related central nervous system diseases in children with acute lymphocytic leukemia. In R. Mastrangelo, D. G. Poplack, and R. Riccardi (eds.), *Central Nervous System Leukemia: Prevention and Treatment* (Boston, Martinus Nyhoff), pp. 71–81.

Price, R. A., and Birdwell, D. A. 1978. The central nervous system in leukemia: III. Mineralizing microangiopathy and dystrophic calcification. *Cancer* 42: 717–28.

Riccardi, R.; Brouwers, P.; Di Chiro, G.; and Poplack, D. 1985. Abnormal computed tomography brain scans in children with acute lymphoblastic leukemia: Serial long-term follow-up. *Journal of Clinical Oncology* 3: 12–18.

Ross, J. W. 1982. The role of the social worker with long-term survivors of childhood cancer and their families. *Social Work Health Care* 7: 1–13.

Rottenberg, D. A. 1991. *Neurological Complication of Cancer Treatment.* Boston: Butterworth-Heinemann.

Soni, S.; Marten, G.; Pitner, S.; Duenas, L. D. A.; and Powazek, M. 1975. Effects of central nervous system irradiation on neuropsychological functioning of children with acute lymphocytic leukemia. *New England Journal of Medicine* 293: 113–18.

Stehbens, J. A. 1988. Childhood cancers. In D. K. Routh (ed.), *Handbook of Pediatric Psychology* (New York: Guilford Press), pp. 135–61.

Stehbens, J. A.; Ford, M.; Kisker, C.; Clarke, W. R.; and Strayer, F. 1981. WISC-R Verbal/Performance discrepancies in pediatric cancer patients. *Journal of Pediatric Psychology* 6: 61–68.

Stehbens, J. A.; Kaleita, T. A.; Noll, R. B.; MacLean, W. E.; O'Brien, R. T.; Waskerwitz, M. J.; and Hammond, G. D. 1991. CNS prophylaxis of childhood leukemia: What are the long-term neurological, neuropsychological and behavioral effects? *Neuropsychology Review* 2: 147–78.

Stuss, D. T., and Benson, D. F. 1984. Neuropsychological studies of the frontal lobes. *Psychology Bulletin* 95: 3–28.

Tamaroff, M.; Salwen, R.; Miller, D. R.; Murphy, M. L.; and Nir, Y. 1984. Comparison of neuropsychologic performance in children treated for acute lymphoblastic leukemia (ALL) with 1800 rads cranial radiation plus intrathecal methotrexate or intrathecal methotrexate alone. *Proceedings of the American Society of Clinical Oncology* 3: 198.

Tomlinson, F. H.; Scheithauer, B. W.; Meyer, F. B.; Smithson, W. A.; Shaw, E. G.; Miller, G. M.; and Groover, R. V. 1992. Medulloblastoma: I. Clinical, diagnostic and therapeutic overview. *Journal of Child Neurology* 7: 142–55.

Tuma, J. M., and Appelbaum, A. S. 1980. Reliability and practice effects of WISC-R IQ estimates in a normal population. *Education and Psychological Measurement* 40: 671–678.

van Asperen, T. 1992. Treatment-related infertility and its alternatives: A moral dilemma. In B. F. Last and A. M. van Veldhulzen (eds.), *Developments in Pediatric Psychosocial Oncology* (Lisse: Swets & Zeitlinger), pp. 79–89.

Verzosa, M.; Aur, R.; Simone, J.; Hustu, H. D.; and Pinkel, D. P. 1976. Five years after central nervous system irradiation of children wit leukemia. *International Journal of Radiation Oncology and Biological Physics* 1: 209–15.

Wallesch, C.; Kornhuber, H.; Brunner, R.; Kunz, T.; Hollerback, B.; and Suger, G. 1983. Lesions of the basal ganglia, thalamus, and deep white matter: Differential effects on language functions. *Brain and Language* 20: 286–304.

Walther, B.; Gutjahr, P.; and Beron, G. 1981. Therapiebeglettende und uberdauernde neurologische und neuropsychologische diagnostik bei akuter lymphoblastischer leukamie im kindesalter. *Klinische Padiatrie* 193: 177–83.

Wechsler, D. 1991. *Manual for the Wechsler Intelligence Scale for Children—III.* New York: Psychological Corporation.

Young, J. L., Jr.; Ries, L. G.; Silverberg, E. et al. 1986. Cancer incidence, survival and mortality in children younger than 15 years. *Cancer* 58: 598–602.

Zeitzer, L., and LeBaron, S. 1982. Hypnosis and nonhypnotic techniques for reduction of pain and anxiety during procedures in children and adolescents with cancer. *Journal of Pediatrics* 101: 1032–35.

11

Cardiovascular Disease

This chapter deals with the pediatric cardiac disorders most commonly seen by neuropsychologists in medical settings. The fundamentals of cardiac anatomy and circulation, diagnosis, treatment, and outcome described here in relation to congenital heart defects can be applied to a considerably broader range of cardiac conditions.

PRESENTATION OF CONGENITAL CARDIAC DEFECTS

Congenital heart defects (CHDs) occur in 6 to 8 per 1000 liveborn children (Behrman & Vaughan 1992; Clark 1992; Perry et al. 1993) and another small percentage develop acquired heart disease in childhood. Congenital heart defects are largely unexplained structural *in-utero* aberrations. Between 5% and 12% of CHDs are believed to result from gross chromosomal abnormalities (Behrman & Vaughan 1992; Clark 1992), and 3% from classically inherited Mendelian gene effects (Hoffman 1990). Environmental risk factors include maternal illness (for example, rubella), maternal age, and noxious influences such as anoxia or vitamin deficiency (Nadas & Fyler 1972) and cardiac teratogens (such as alcohol, anticonvulsants, organic solvents, pesticides, and retinoic acid (Behrman & Vaughan 1992; Clark 1992; Perry et al. 1993). Among children with CHDs, 28% have associated noncardiac abnormalities (Perry et al. 1993).

Cardiac palliative measures and medical and surgical refinements enable many children with CHD to survive longer, with a markedly improved quality of life. Various interim surgical and pharmacological interventions allow delay of repair until the child's body can better tolerate more invasive procedures. In some cases, the cardiac defect resolves spontaneously or becomes hemodynamically insignificant, and surgery is avoided. However, more than one-third of all infants born with cardiac defects require surgical correction during their first year of life (Ferry 1987; Perry et al. 1993). The prevalence of critical CHD requiring repair in infancy is 3.5 per 1000 live births (Ferry 1990). Lifelong medical follow-up is often required, and secondary heart problems such as en-

The technical, editorial, and scholarly advice of Lowell W. Perry, M.D., of the Department of Pediatrics of Georgetown University School of Medicine in the preparation of this chapter is greatly appreciated.

343

docarditis (an infection of the heart lining) must be anticipated and prevented.

To shed some light on the population of children diagnosed as having CHD, the following sections present a review of heart function, diagnostic procedures, the range of common anatomic anomalies, and various treatment options.

HEART ANATOMY AND CIRCULATION

The heart is a four-chambered pumping organ (see Figure 11-1). The two upper chambers are the left atrium and the right atrium, and the two lower chambers are the left and right ventricles. A system of one-way valves permits blood to flow from one chamber to the next in a specific series of steps. Deoxygenated (venous) blood returns from the body through the inferior and superior vena cavae, enters the right atrium and flows to the right ventricle through the tricuspid valve. The right ventricle pumps the blood, via the pulmonary artery, into the lungs, where it is oxygenated. The pulmonary valve is situated between the right ventricle and the pulmonary artery. Oxygenated (arterial) blood returns via the pulmonary veins into the left atrium. From there it flows through the mitral valve into the left ventricle, which pumps it through the aortic valve and to the aorta—the main artery carrying blood to the body. The four cardiac valves are all one-way valves that allow antegrade flow but prevent retrograde flow.

The fetal circulatory pattern differs from the circulatory pattern of the newborn. *In utero,* fetal blood is oxygenated in the placenta, since the lungs are not functional until birth. Blood bypasses the lungs by flowing through the *foramen ovale* (the opening between the two atria) and the *ductus arteriosus* (a vessel between the pulmonary artery and the aorta). Normally, the ductus arteriosus closes hours after a term birth, or within the first weeks or months in a low-birthweight infant (Behrman & Vaughan 1992).

The right side of the heart pumps blood to the lungs, and the left side of the heart pumps blood to the body. The right ventricle pumps under lower pressure than does the left ventricle, because less force is required to pump to the lungs than to the body. Pressure is the product of flow and resistance ($P = F \times R$). Increased pressure may be due to increased flow, to increased resistance or to increases in both flow and resistance. Over the first few weeks of life, pulmonary vascular resistance (resistance to blood flow within the small blood vessels of the lungs) falls, and a congenital heart defect may become clinically apparent.

EVALUATION AND TREATMENT OF CARDIAC DEFECT AND DISEASE

A heart murmur detected on routine neonatal or pediatric evaluation may be the first indication of a cardiac defect. Some murmurs are innocent (benign)

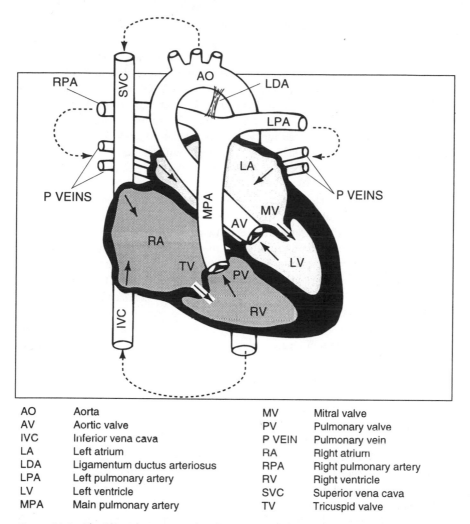

AO	Aorta	MV	Mitral valve
AV	Aortic valve	PV	Pulmonary valve
IVC	Inferior vena cava	P VEIN	Pulmonary vein
LA	Left atrium	RA	Right atrium
LDA	Ligamentum ductus arteriosus	RPA	Right pulmonary artery
LPA	Left pulmonary artery	RV	Right ventricle
LV	Left ventricle	SVC	Superior vena cava
MPA	Main pulmonary artery	TV	Tricuspid valve

Figure 11-1   The Normal Heart (Used with permission of Ross Products Division, Abbott Laboratories, Columbus, OH 43216. From Clinical Education Aid, © 1987 Ross Products Division, Abbott Laboratories.)

and of no clinical concern. A functional murmur is not associated with anatomic defect, but it may have physiological significance; for instance, it may be associated with anemia or fever. In such a case, treatment of the underlying condition eliminates the functional murmur. A pathological murmur indicates underlying structural abnormality and is often the first evidence of CHD (in 50% to 75% of cases involving infants and children) (Perry 1969).

More obvious signs and symptoms may also alert the physician to the presence of a cardiac defect. For example, poor feeding, excessive irritability, tachycardia (fast heart rate), tachypnea (respiration rate greater than 60/minute while sleeping), central cyanosis, and sweating may signal cardiac distress.

Other signs include slow growth or failure-to-thrive. In many cases, however, a child is asymptomatic.

A number of diagnostic techniques are available when cardiac defect is suspected. Noninvasive techniques, associated with few complications, assist in defining CHD. An *electrocardiogram* (EKG or ECG) provides information about electrical conduction within the heart. A *Holter monitor* is worn for continuous electrocardiogram monitoring, to detect intermittent rate or rhythm abnormalities. A *chest roentgenogram* (X-ray) provides gross estimates of the heart's size and its relationship to the lungs, information about pulmonary blood flow, and data that help to distinguish between pulmonary and cardiac disease.

The echocardiogram is among the most important noninvasive tools. High-frequency (2- to 5-million-Hz) sound beams reflect from the heart whenever a change in acoustical impedance occurs. The sound signals are reconstructed by a computer to give an accurate picture of the anatomy of the heart. Three types of echocardiograms are currently used: M-mode (to measure cardiac dimensions), two-dimensional (to demonstrate heart anatomy), and Doppler (to detect shunts and obstructed or leaky valves). Transthoracic echocardiograms are obtained from the chest wall. Transesophageal echocardiograms are obtained by passing a small transducer down the esophagus. The information provided by noninvasive techniques often renders more invasive cardiac procedures unnecessary.

Sometimes invasive procedures are required for precise diagnosis. Cardiac catheterization provides information about type and severity of a cardiac defect, including size, hemodynamics (pressure, flow, and resistance), and anatomy. This technique involves inserting a thin tube into a vein or artery and, in association with compatible X-ray techniques, moving the catheter through the heart while blood samples and blood pressures are taken. Diagnostic catheterization carries risks of neurological and cardiac complications that are greater in the newborn period than for the older child (Lock 1987). Catheterization is undertaken only if noninvasive procedures cannot provide an exact diagnosis or if additional diagnostic details are required. The overall risk of complications is less than 1% at all ages. These risks range from minimal (low-grade fever, hematoma at the catheterization site, transient occlusion of the catheterized vessel, transient arrhythmias) to more serious problems (cardiac perforation, seizures, infarction, and allergic reaction) and even to death. Prevention of cerebrovascular complication is often accomplished by means of systemic anticoagulation and a refined catheter placement technique (Grossman 1986). The cardiologist must take care not to inject air into the blood system during the procedure.

Percutaneous balloon valvuloplasty (Dotter & Judkins 1964) can avert or delay the need for surgery in certain cases. This procedure involves passing a catheter (under fluoroscopic guidance) to an area of obstruction and inflating a balloon there to stretch the constricted area. Balloon valvotomy has been successfully performed in children (Keane & Lock 1987) with aortic, mitral, and pulmonary valve stenosis (Rupprath & Neuhaus 1986) and in recurrent coarctation of the aorta. Balloon septostomy uses a similar procedure to enlarge an atrial septal defect in children who have transposition of the great arteries. Transcatheter closure of atrial and ventricular septal defects is under development. Stainless steel stents can be placed inside certain obstructed vessels to permit permanent dilatation. Conversely, certain hemangiomas can be closed with catheter embolization techniques.

Reparative Surgery

Congenital heart defects can be corrected with "closed-heart" or "open-heart" techniques. The procedure selected depends on the underlying problem. Introduction of the cardiopulmonary bypass (CPB) procedure in 1953 allowed physicians to support the circulation and to open the heart to correct major malformations by operations that previously led to death or serious morbidity. An external machine artificially maintains heart and lung function, so that well-oxygenated arterial blood circulates to all organ systems while the heart is stopped. The optimal procedure avoids ischemic damage, maintains cerebral blood flow and cerebral metabolic rate, and thus preserves brain function. Relaxing the heart for delicate surgery reduces the time required for surgery and permits efficient exploration of the surgical field during repair (Haka-Ikse, Blackwood & Steward 1978).

The CPB apparatus, or heart–lung machine, consists of a machine to pump blood, an oxygenator to supply needed gases and remove dispelled gases, and a heat exchanger to regulate temperature. Arterial filters remove particles released by the machine components that might result in emboli. Some centers favor membrane oxygenators to avoid risk of damage to blood components associated with bubble oxygenators (Ferry 1990; Gilman 1990). Corrective heart surgery can now be performed on infants who weigh as little as 2.0 kilograms.

With profound hypothermia—a procedure used frequently in surgeries for small infants—the body temperature is reduced to 17 to 18°C, to protect central nervous system function. All blood is drained from the body, and the heart is stopped. The surgeon then has a bloodless field and a quiet heart to work on, but must complete the repair within 60 minutes; otherwise, severe CNS damage may occur. At the end of the operation, the blood is returned to the infant's body, the heart–lung machine is restarted, and the body temperature is raised back to normal. Even in cases where profound hypothermia lasts less than 1 hour, significant neurological impairment can occur.

Rates of mortality and morbidity due to severe neonatal cardiorespiratory complications have fallen dramatically since the introduction of extracorporeal membrane oxygenation (ECMO) in the 1970s. The procedure involves irreversible ligation of the right common carotid artery and the right internal jugular vein. External control of heart and lung function is maintained without opening the infant's chest. Infants with meconium aspiration, diaphragmatic hernia, or pneumonia, for example, may benefit from ECMO. The procedure is usually not performed on premature infants, however, because of the increased risk of intraventricular hemorrhage.

TYPES OF CARDIAC ABNORMALITIES

Heart disease may be congenital (present at birth) or acquired (occurring sometime after birth). Congenital heart defects may involve valve function, chamber separation, or vessel anomaly. Often, the natural system for separating oxygenated and deoxygenated blood is not maintained. CHDs are commonly classified by the presence or absence of cyanosis.

Cyanosis is a physical sign referring to a slate blue color of the mucous membranes, lips, nail beds, and skin (Driscoll 1990). Cyanosis is present whenever the proportion of reduced (nonoxygenated) hemoglobin is more than approximately 5 g/100 cc and the level of oxygen saturation is less than 85%. Normal oxygen saturation is 95% to 100%. The amount of oxygen delivered to body tissues may be normal if the amount of hemoglobin in the blood is high. If the amount of hemoglobin is not elevated, the diminished blood oxygen saturation may lead to diminished perfusion of oxygen in body tissues. Functional status depends on the degree of desaturation. For example, at 85% saturation, a person's ability to exercise is somewhat decreased. At 60% saturation, the individual may be severely compromised. Cyanosis is usually produced by a mixing of unoxygenated systemic venous blood with fully oxygenated pulmonary venous blood—that is, *right-to-left shunt*. This can occur at any level—atrial, ventricular, or great vessel—within the heart.

A *left-to-right shunt* occurs when oxygenated blood from the left side of the heart is pumped to the right side, instead of through the aorta and to the body. This increases pulmonary blood flow and (consequently) the heart's workload. Depending on the size of the shunt, the heart may enlarge (cardiomegaly), and pulmonary blood vessels may be subjected to much higher pressures than normal (pulmonary hypertension). The more common defects associated with this type of circulation abnormality are described in the section that follows. Most of these defects are not associated with cyanosis.

CONGENITAL ACYANOTIC DEFECTS

In the following subsections, the most common cyanotic and acyanotic defects are discussed. Table 11-1 presents prevalence rates for both cyanotic and acyanotic CHDs.

Ventricular Septal Defect

Ventricular septal defect (VSD) is the most common form of congenital heart defect. A hole in the septum (wall) separating the ventricles allows some oxy-

Table 11-1 Prevalence of Selected Congenital
Cardiac Defects*

Cardiac Defect	Percentage†
Ventricular septal defect	32.1%
Pulmonary stenosis	9.0%
Atrial septal defect	7.7%
Atrioventricular canal defect	7.4%
Tetralogy of fallot	6.8%
Transposition of the great arteries	4.7%
Coarctation of the aorta	4.6%
Hypoplastic left heart syndrome	3.7%
Aortic stenosis	2.9%
Patent ductus arteriosus	2.4%
Total anomalous pulmonary venous return	1.4%
Pulmonary atresia (intact septum)	1.7%
Truncus arteriosus	1.2%
Ebstein's malformation of the tricuspid valve	1.0%
Tricuspid atresia	0.7%

*Data obtained from the *Baltimore–Washington Infant Study, 1981–1989* (N = 4390) (Perry et al. 1993).

†Percentage represents the percentage of all CHDs that consist of the named cardiac defect.

genated blood, which is under high pressure in the left ventricle, to be forced across the defect to the right side (left-to-right shunt), where pressure is lower, with each pumping action rather than being pumped out to the body through the aorta. Normally, sufficient oxygenated blood exits the aorta to preserve bodily functions. In the presence of a VSD, some oxygenated blood, mixed with venous blood, is sent back to the lungs and then to the left side of the heart again. As a result, the right ventricle may carry a much heavier load of blood than usual, if the defect is large.

Ventricular septal defects vary by size and location in the septal wall. The smaller the VSD, the fewer the problems. A VSD may not be detected until several weeks after birth, when pulmonary vascular resistance and right ventricular pressure decrease. Since most patients with VSD have no symptoms, VSDs are frequently discovered at a well-baby checkup by the presence of a heart murmur. Surgery is required in less than 10% of cases; 50% to 80% of VSDs close spontaneously, and the rest are so small that they are of no hemodynamic significance.

Atrial Septal Defect

Atrial septal defect (ASD) is a hole in the wall between the atria. Like a VSD, an ASD causes left-to-right shunting, congestion of the pulmonary circuit and an increased heart workload, but generally it produces fewer symptoms than does a VSD. Some oxygenated blood from the lungs that enters the left atrium is shunted to the right atrium, instead of being directed through the aorta and to the body. An ASD closes spontaneously in 20% to 40% of cases. Open-heart surgery is often required.

Patent Ductus Arteriosus

A patent ductus arteriosus (PDA) results from persistence of the ductus arteriosus—a communication between the aorta and the pulmonary artery that is normally patent (open) in the fetus but that closes shortly after birth. In the fetus, the ductus arteriosus allows a *right-to-left shunt* of blood to bypass the lungs (which are not used until birth). When the ductus does not close after birth, some oxygenated blood pumped out of the left ventricle (and normally destined for the body) flows back into the lungs through the ductus, a left-to-right shunt. Premature infants are at risk for PDA. The greater the degree of prematurity, the more likely PDA becomes. Clinically significant PDA is found in over 80% of infants who weigh less than 1000 grams and in 10% to 15% of infants who weigh 1500 to 2000 grams (Sikes 1986). Term infants may not show signs of PDA until 2 to 3 weeks of age, and older children may be asymptomatic (Clark 1992). Most patients with PDA have no symptoms, and the lesion is detected by the presence of the typical murmur.

Pharmacologic treatment with indomethacin, an inhibitor of prostaglandin synthesis, often obviates the need for surgery, if given to the premature infant during the first 10 to 12 days of life. Surgical ligation of the PDA is performed when medical treatment is unsuccessful. Patent ductus arteriosus, which does not require open-heart techniques, may be ligated in a premature infant as small as 400 to 500 grams. Transcatheter occlusion of PDA can be performed in selected older children.

Pulmonary Stenosis

Pulmonary stenosis, a narrowing of the pulmonary valve, results in mild to severe obstruction of the flow of blood from the right ventricle into the pulmonary circuit. The right ventricle must then pump harder. Surgical treatment may be necessary when the obstruction is severe. This may be accomplished with balloon valvuloplasty at catheterization or with surgery. The child may be cyanotic when stenosis is severe enough to produce elevated right-atrial pressures and right-to-left shunt *via* a valve-incompetent patent foramen ovale. Pulmonary stenosis also may be supravalvar or subvalvar.

Aortic Stenosis

Aortic stenosis may occur at the valvar, supravalvar, or subvalvar level. Valvar aortic stenosis consists of obstruction of the aortic valve. This obstruction may be due to a dysplastic valve, to fusion of the commissures, to an inadequate number of commissures (unicuspid or bicuspid valves), or to valve degeneration (calcification). The degree of stenosis may vary from minimal to severe.

Correction is performed only in cases of moderate or severe obstruction. Balloon valvuloplasty generally improves valve function, as long as the valve is not dysplastic. Surgical valvotomy or valve replacement may be required if severe restriction is involved, if a subaortic membrane is present, or if the coronary blood vessels just above the valve are compromised.

Coarctation of the Aorta

Coarctation of the aorta is a localized constriction of the aorta. Since blood vessels that supply different body regions arise along the aortic arch, blood supply to body parts is differentially affected by coarctation site. Blood pressure is elevated in blood vessels that arise proximal to the constriction, and it is lowered below the constriction. Coarctation often occurs at the level of the ligamentum arteriosum—the remnant of the closed ductus arteriosus. Rarely, infants may present dramatically at 10 to 14 days of age with sudden onset of severe congestive heart failure. In milder forms, however, symptoms may be absent and the condition may not be detected until older childhood or adolescence—for instance, as a result of leg pain or weakness after exercise. Disparities in pulsations and limb blood pressures or a murmur may be the only clinical manifestation. Techniques of surgical correction may include resection–reanastomosis, patch aortoplasty, or subclavian flap arterioplasty. Balloon angioplasty generally is used only for recoarctation, because of the risk of intimal (innerlining) tears. Limitations on physical activity depend on the severity of the obstruction prior to or following a corrective procedure. Patients with severe coarctation may suffer upper extremity or central nervous system hypertension. A berry aneurysm, with or without central nervous system bleeding, is occasionally encountered.

Atrioventricular Canal Defect

Atrioventricular (AV) canal defect is also known as *endocardial cushion defect* and *atrioventricular septal defect*. In the complete atrioventricular canal defect, a large hole exists at the center of the heart, where all four chambers meet, and the lower portion of the atrial septum and the upper posterior part of the ventricular septum are involved. This defect involves the chambers and the tricuspid and mitral valves. A single large valve crosses the defect and allows oxygen-rich blood from the left side of the heart to pass into the right side where it is returned to the lungs commingled with oxygen-poor blood. The resulting excessive workload and increased blood flow to the lungs leads to heart enlargement and pulmonary hypertension. One early treatment involved using a pulmonary artery banding procedure to constrict the pulmonary artery, thereby reducing pulmonary blood flow and protecting the lungs so that definitive repair could occur when the child was better able to tolerate surgery. Currently, surgical correction requires two steps that are performed during a single operation. First, the defect is patched. Second, two valves are created from the single valve. This defect is often associated with Down syndrome.

Since infants with complete AV canal defects are at risk for developing pulmonary vascular obstructive disease, corrective surgery is performed at between 6 and 12 months of age, to minimize that complication. Incomplete or partial AV canal defects include low-lying ASDs and high posterior VSDs.

CONGENITAL CYANOTIC DEFECTS

Tetralogy of Fallot

Tetralogy of Fallot has four components: a VSD that allows venous blood to pass from the right ventricle to the left ventricle and out the aorta to the body without passing through the lungs, associated with cyanosis; pulmonary stenosis at or just beneath the pulmonary valve that blocks the flow of venous blood into the lungs; an overriding aorta, lying directly over the VSD; and right ventricular hypertrophy that is secondary to the pulmonary stenosis. Full repair of this condition is usually possible when the patient is between 1 and 2 years of age, and often it is performed before the patient is 1 year of age. A palliative shunt—the Blalock-Taussig procedure—can be used to connect the subclavian artery to the pulmonary artery, to improve blood flow to the lungs temporarily; this measure may be necessary if the condition is not amenable to early correction.

Transposition of the Great Arteries

Complete transposition of the great arteries (TGA) means that the great vessels arise from the wrong ventricle; that is, they are transposed. The aorta, instead of arising from the anatomic left ventricle, arises from the anatomic right ventricle. The pulmonary artery, instead of arising from the anatomic right ventricle, arises from the anatomic left ventricle.

In TGA, systemic venous blood enters the aorta via the right atrium and ventricle, and pulmonary venous blood recirculates to the pulmonary artery via the left atrium and ventricle. Thus, deoxygenated blood is directed to the aorta and oxygenated blood is directed to the pulmonary artery. Profound cyanosis generally occurs soon after birth. Since survival depends on having oxygenated blood reach the body, prostaglandin is used initially to maintain ductal patency. Balloon atrial septostomy during heart catheterization enlarges the opening or defect between the atria, increasing the mixing of the two circulations and reducing cyanosis. Surgery follows within days.

Two surgical procedures are considered. In the older procedure, a tunnel is created inside the atria to redirect oxygenated blood to the right ventricle and aorta and venous blood to the left ventricle and pulmonary artery via an intraatrial baffle. This repair, known as a *venous switch,* is performed by using one of two techniques: the Senning procedure or the Mustard procedure. Venous switch operations dramatically improve the early prognosis of babies born with

TGA, but long-term prognosis is complicated by life-threatening arrhythmias, baffle obstruction, and right ventricle failure. Currently, most centers use the arterial switch procedure, in which the major arteries and coronary arteries are severed and then reconnected, resulting in connection of the aorta to the left ventricle and connection of the pulmonary artery to the right ventricle.

Pulmonary Atresia

Pulmonary atresia refers to an aplasia or complete obstruction of the pulmonary valve. This absent pulmonary valve syndrome produces problems because of pulmonary insufficiency. The right ventricle usually is poorly developed and small. Often the tricuspid valve is also small. An ASD allows venous blood to exit the right atrium and mix with oxygenated blood in the left atrium. This poorly oxygenated mixture is then pumped by the left ventricle into the aorta and to the body. The only source of blood flow to the lungs is through the PDA, which allows blood from the aorta to pass into the pulmonary artery and thence into the lungs. Drugs (for example, prostaglandin) are prescribed to maintain ductal patency. Surgical creation of a shunt (the Blalock-Taussig procedure) between the aorta and the pulmonary artery increases blood flow to the lungs. Complete repair depends on the size of the pulmonary artery and of the right ventricle. If the latter is too small, the right atrium must be surgically connected directly to the pulmonary artery, and the atrial defect must be closed; that is the Fontan procedure. There are several modifications of the Fontan procedure, but all are associated with late development of life-threatening arrhythmias.

Tricuspid Atresia

Tricuspid atresia results from absence of a functional tricuspid valve. As a result of this defect, no direct communication between the right atrium and the right ventricle exists, and the latter may be small and undeveloped; this condition is termed a *hypoplastic right ventricle*. Tricuspid atresia may be associated with normally related or transposed great vessels, and may arise with or without a VSD. Normally related great vessels exist in about two-thirds of all instances, while transposition of the great vessels is found in the remaining one-third of cases. In infancy, pulmonary blood flow is inadequate to maintain satisfactory systemic arterial saturation. A shunt is therefore required, to increase pulmonary blood flow. If pulmonary blood flow is excessive, a pulmonary artery band may be required, to limit pulmonary blood flow. Implanting a bidirectional Glenn shunt is often the first step. A bidirectional Glenn shunt, connecting the superior vena cava to the side of the right pulmonary artery, removes venous return from the superior vena cava and thus decreases the left ventricle's workload and improves its functional life. Subsequently (usually at 3 to 5 years of age), a fenestrated Fontan is performed: a connection is created between the right atrium and pulmonary artery and the atrial defect closed, the "corrective" procedure.

Total Anomalous Pulmonary Venous Return

Total anomalous pulmonary venous return (TAPVR) consists of inappropriate pulmonary venous drainage to the systemic venous system, rather than to the left atrium. Thus, both systemic and pulmonary venous drainages connect with the pulmonary artery via the right atrium and ventricle. Oxygenated blood from the lungs mixes with venous blood returning from the body. Blood reaches the body by passing through an ASD or patent foramen ovale into the left atrium and then via the left ventricle to the aorta. The greater the pulmonary flow, the higher the systemic saturation. The remainder of the blood is directed through the right ventricle, to the pulmonary artery, and thence to the lungs. TAPVR may occur at the cardiac, supracardiac, or infracardiac level. Infracardiac TAPVR often is obstructed and requires emergency surgery. Surgical repair involves reconnecting the pulmonary veins to the left atrium and closing the ASD.

Truncus Arteriosus

Truncus arteriosus is a defect in which one great artery arises from the heart. There is a large VSD. Blood enters the lungs via one or more vessels arising from the abnormal arterial trunk. Surgery involves closing the VSD, detaching the pulmonary arteries from the large common artery and connecting the pulmonary arteries to the right ventricle with a graft.

Ebstein's Malformation of the Tricuspid Valve

Ebstein's malformation of the tricuspid valve involves displacement of the origin of the anterior leaflet of the tricuspid valve from the atrioventricular junction into the cavity of the right ventricle, abnormal distal attachment of the valve leaflets, and valve dysplasia. Early detection is common because of the systolic murmur of tricuspid regurgitation and the presence of cyanosis due to arterial right-to-left shunt. There may also be right ventricular outflow-tract obstruction by the displaced redundant tricuspid valve. If the malformation is mild, hemodynamics are unaltered. Severe malformation results in functional impairment of the right side of the heart. Electrocardiographic changes of the Wolff-Parkinson-White syndrome occur in about one-third of cases.

Hypoplastic Left Heart Syndrome

Hypoplastic left heart syndrome (HLHS) refers to a spectrum of congenital anomalies, including underdeveloped left ventricle, aorta, aortic arch, and mitral valve. Incidence is 3.7% of all CHDs, with more males than females affected (Perry et al. 1993). Genetic and chromosomal anomalies are associated with HLHS, so affected infants often have other organ anomalies. Brain anomalies, such as agenesis of the corpus callosum, holoprosencephaly, and other migrational anomalies often coexist. A rare form of autosomal recessive inheritance may exist, in addition to the more common multifactorial inheritance. The 15% prevalence of occurrence of congenital heart defect in siblings of children with hypoplastic left heart suggests an autosomal recessive trait (Perry et al. 1993). HLHS accounts for about 15% of all neonatal CHD deaths in the first month of life. Presentation is often marked by abrupt onset of congestive heart failure, after the PDA closes. Surgical treatment is only modestly success-ful and often is only palliative. Heart transplantation may be an option.

LATE-ONSET OR ACQUIRED CARDIAC DISEASE

Cardiac defects may exist without overt symptomatology. The myocardium may be progressively injured by increased volume or pressure associated with an undetected CHD. Structural abnormalities are eventually detected when symptoms appear. For example, coronary artery anomalies may cause anginal chest pain after exercise, due to poor coronary artery blood flow that creates an imbalance between myocardial oxygen supply and demand. Other anomalies may remain undetected for years or may develop after birth—for instance e.g., left ventricular outflow tract obstructive lesions (coarctation of the aorta, aortic stenosis) and lesions producing ischemic myocardial dysfunction (valve or sub-valve stenosis, hypertrophic obstructive cardiomyopathy).

Acquired myopericardial disease may be caused by various viral, bacterial, autoimmune, and rickettsial diseases; arteritis associated with other systemic disease; parasitic and fungal infections; tumor metastasis; or pulmonary embo-lus. Although rare now, rheumatic fever was a common form of acquired bac-terial heart disease until the mid-1970s. Carditis, one manifestation of this multisystem disease, results from the body's delayed response to systemic in-fection by certain strains of Group A beta hemolytic streptococcus organisms, which crossreact immunologically with the heart. Each part of the heart—the endocardium (inner lining), myocardium (heart muscle), and pericardium (outer heart lining)—may be involved, in that order.

Cardiovascular involvement is the most common and most severe (poten-tially fatal) complication of mucocutaneous lymph node syndrome, Kawasaki syndrome, which occurs in about 20% of untreated cases. Suspected causes of this childhood inflammatory illness of unknown origin include viral infection and chemical exposure (Daniels & Specker 1991). Clinical presentation in-cludes persistent fever, a truncally distributed polymorphous rash, distal limb swelling, eye irritation and redness (bilateral bulbar conjunctivitis), cervical lymphadenopathy, and irritation and inflammation of the mouth, lips, and throat. Therapy includes administering hyperimmune gammaglobulin (Stiehm 1991) and salicylates during acute stages (Neches 1988). The second to fourth week of illness is the most likely time for serious complication, due to necrotiz-ing coronary arteritis, aneurysm formation, and thrombosis of the aneurysm with subsequent myocardial infarction or rupture. Hyperimmunogammaglo-bulin reduces the risk of cardiac involvement to 3% to 6% of treated cases.

About 30% of cases involving systemic lupus erythematosus present with pericarditis, endocarditis, myocarditis, or coronary arteritis. Infants born to mothers who have systemic lupus erythematosus may have complete heart block.

NEUROLOGICAL TREATMENT SEQUELAE

Neurological sequelae of surgical treatment for CHD may limit the positive prognosis following cardiac repair. Prevalence of neurological sequelae as high as 9% has been reported for adults; the rate for children is unknown (McConnell et al. 1990). Neurological changes reported in the operative or perioperative period include: nystagmus, diplopia, paresis, hemiplegia secondary to cerebrovascular accident, dyskinetic movement disorder secondary to anesthetic hypothermia and cardiac arrest (Hesz & Clark 1988), extensor–plantar response, and seizures (Gilman 1965; Tufo, Ostfeld & Shekelle 1970; Sotaniemi 1980). Prevalence of neurologic and neuropsychologic disturbances in the early postoperative period has not declined with procedural and management improvements (Townes et al. 1989). Since many CHDs are accompanied by associated CNS abnormalities, one should not assume that all neurological sequelae are related to treatment (Aram, Ekelman, Ben-Shachar & Levinsohn 1985; Medlock et al. 1993).

Neurological and neuropsychological damage after open-heart surgery (OHS) may result from a number of pathogenetic factors. Neuronal injury can occur due to microembolization, air embolism, hypoxia, hypoperfusion, inadequate cerebral perfusion, or biochemical and metabolic disturbances. Air embolism is a significant risk despite technical advances; and the risk is particularly great when air collected in the heart during reparative surgery is replaced with blood to allow resumption of spontaneous function. Embolism and severely reduced cerebral blood flow, due to hypotension or prolonged time on CPB intraoperatively, are etiological factors that were recognized early in adult pathological studies (Gilman 1965) and were considered primary causes of postoperative neurological and neuropsychological sequelae (Grote et al. 1992). Microembolization of tiny air bubbles, fibrin, tissue elements, or platelet thrombi is associated with prolonged CPB (Moody 1990); and neurologic sequelae of OHS have a high association with ischemic events secondary to microemboli (Gilman 1990). Procedural intraoperative factors that affect outcome include cooling (prolonged hypothermia, which reduces oxygen consumption and results in cardiorespiratory slowing), extracorporeal circulation (perfusion time), anticoagulation, and anesthesia. Associated noncardiac abnormalities or other congenital problems may contribute.

While many children do well, and their brain structure is presumed to remain intact, a number of adult brains have gone to autopsy with interesting results. Neuropathological studies confirm the presence of widely distributed brain lesions following OHS. Bilateral cortical necrosis may be prominent in the arterial boundary zones (Gilman 1965). This results in a characteristic pattern of cortical injury on the lateral side of the hemisphere, between the areas supplied by the anterior, middle, and posterior cerebral arteries. Microscopic white- and gray-matter abnormalities, anoxic damage in the hippocampal formation (Tufo, Ostfeld & Shekelle 1970), and intracranial hemorrhage and hematoma are common (Hungxi et al. 1982). Serum and cerebrospinal fluid adenylate kinase levels—markers of ischemic brain injury—increased in 59% of adults undergoing OHS (Aberg et al. 1984). In addition to brain effect, spinal cord infarction (Puntis & Green 1985) and peripheral nervous system lesions have been reported among children (Ferry 1987).

Assumptions about central nervous system anomalies associated with CHD had to await postmortem examination in early investigations. For example, Veith & Ziegler (1965) found very high rates of developmental brain anomalies in CHD patients. Currently, sophisticated neurodiagnostic and imaging techniques allow for investigation of morphologic characteristics of brain pre-, peri-, and post-operatively. These techniques have confirmed unsuspected sequelae of OHS in childhood, including infarction, diffuse ischemia, atrophy, edema, gliosis, subacute hemorrhages, and loss of differentiation between gray and white matter. Despite normal preoperative electroencephalographic (EEG) assessments, frequent postoperative cerebral abnormalities were detected in a group of children who had hypothermic open-heart surgery for VSD (Shida et al. 1981). EEG abnormalities were distinguished from changes specifically associated with hypothermia and CPB, and immediate treatment was provided (Hicks & Poole 1981). Results of a prospective brain-imaging study of 12 acyanotic and 6 cyanotic children with CHD, who were undergoing moderate hypothermic CPB with a nonpulsatile membrane oxygenator, revealed that one-third had ventriculomegaly and dilatation of the subarachnoid spaces on pre-operative magnetic resonance images. Post-operatively, bicaudate and third ventricular diameters increased. Four patients developed small subdural hematomas, without mass effect. One patient developed cerebral infarction (McConnell et al. 1990). Given the wide range of possible pathogenetic factors, sensitive neuropsychological testing may be expected to result in discovery of a varied range of deficits subsequent to OHS.

COGNITIVE/NEUROPSYCHOLOGICAL TREATMENT SEQUELAE

Many early pediatric outcome studies of OHS were hampered by design and methodological weaknesses. Early studies were often retrospective; instrumentation was limited, or behavioral description sufficed (Settergren et al. 1982; Wright et al. 1979); results were not correlated with type of cardiac defect; cyanotic and acyanotic groups were combined (Fyler, Silbert & Rothman 1976); neurological and genetic evaluations were not routine; and age at testing varied, and socioeconomic factors were not considered. Most researchers excluded children with congenital abnormalities associated with mental retardation (Linde, Rasof & Dunn 1967), but not all did so (Fyler, Silbert & Rothman 1976). IQ tests were often the only measure used, and sometimes different IQ measures were compared within a single study—although later investigation supported this procedure (Aram, Ekelman, Ben-Shachar & Levinsohn 1985).

Descriptive analysis sometimes supplanted statistical analysis (Fyler, Silbert & Rothman 1976).

Perhaps because of the complexity of caring for a seriously ill child, neurodevelopmental abnormalities associated with cardiac defect were only slowly recognized. Recently, cognitive and neuropsychological profiles and course in the pediatric cardiac population have received increased attention, although the literature remains quite limited in scope. Diagnostic and treatment interactions and their impact on developmental cerebral functioning continue to be largely unknown. Still, it is becoming clearer that some early assumptions about cognitive integrity must be dismissed. Delayed physical growth (Rosenthal & Castaneda 1975) and delayed cognitive development characterize the cardiac population (Aisenberg et al. 1982; Brunberg, Reilly & Doty 1974). This population is small for gestational age at birth, due in part to restricted cardiac reserve and chronic hypothermia. It has been proposed that protective parental restriction on activity (Hesz & Clark 1988) may be a factor; but in the absence of confirmatory data, such a conclusion remains debatable.

EFFECTS OF CYANOSIS

Generally, children with cyanotic CHD have fared more poorly than those with acyanotic CHD (Feldt et al. 1969; Fyler, Silbert & Rothman 1976; Linde, Rasof & Dunn 1967; O'Dougherty et al., 1983; Silbert et al., 1969). The majority of early studies examined children with acyanotic defects and found IQ scores falling within average limits (Dickinson & Sambrooks 1979; Fyler, Silbert & Rothman 1976, Whitman 1973).

Fyler, Silbert & Rothman (1976) reported on 126 children who had OHS for mixed diagnoses as infants, 118 of whom had later taken the Wechsler Preschool and Primary Scale of Intelligence Test and 8 of whom had later taken the Leiter International Scale of Intelligence, a nonverbal measure. A distribution similar to that of the normal population was reported, with a median IQ of 98. Children with congenital central nervous system abnormalities (N = 14) had a mean IQ of 85. A slightly higher average IQ was reported for boys than for girls. Comparison between cyanotic (26%) and acyanotic (74%) groups found median IQs of 93 and 98, respectively.

Silbert et al. (1969) found that cyanotic children differed in intelligence level from acyanotic children, independent of activity level. Feldt et al. (1969) found more frequent cognitive difficulties and motor developmental delays among cyanotic than among acyanotic children. Severity of cyanosis, size of shunt, presence of pulmonary vascular disease, previous palliative surgery, and history of cardiac failure were not correlated with negative effects on mental development of a full group of 411 children. Small head circumference was identified as one factor highly correlated with lowered intelligence when associated with congenital cardiac disease. The authors proposed that the association of small head size, growth failure, and CHD could be a result of simultaneous teratogenic effects on the fetus's developing organ systems, and that infant malnutrition associated with cardiac abnormality might be the etiological factors responsible for abnormal brain development. Of interest, given the consistency with which these studies found IQ scores within average limits, are clinical indications that these scores may be misleading. For example, scores were more widely dispersed about the mean in the sample than would be expected for the normal population, and a significant proportion of survivors were retarded (Dickinson & Sambrooks 1979).

Whether certain types of cyanotic heart disease entail poorer cognitive outcome as a result of structural defect or degree of cyanosis was addressed by Haka-Ikse, Blackwood & Steward (1978). Drawing conclusions from a small number of patients examined retrospectively—17 subjects and 7 sibling controls—they suggested that the type of structural defect may have more influence on outcome than the degree of cyanosis. Children with VSD had the highest developmental quotient scores, TAPV drainage patients had the midrange scores, and children with TGA had the lowest scores.

Newburger et al. (1984) investigated duration of cyanosis and hypoxemia. The authors reviewed data on children who had had corrective surgery for TGA. They evaluated the cognitive outcome of surgical correction instituted at progressively earlier ages. The 5-year span of retrospective analysis resulted in data from 38 children who survived to 5.5 years of age. The WPPSI mean IQ was consistent with the population mean. The researchers found a significant inverse relationship between age at correction and cognitive function. All patients had had repeat cardiac catheterization before their corrective Mustard procedure. Systemic arterial oxygen saturation and performance of atrial septectomy did not confound the relationship between cognitive function and age at repair. The cumulative effects of hypoxemia were interpreted as being responsible for the cyanotic group's lower cognitive function compared to an acyanotic group, who had had palliative surgery for correction of VSD. Children with TGA and VSD both had significantly lower mean scores on the Wechsler Preschool and Primary Scales of Intelligence geometric design subtest than the expected population mean; their means on this subtest were also lower than their mean on the other six subtest scores.

Aram, Ekelman, Ben-Shachar, and Levinsohn (1985) evaluated 82 neurologically normal children who had no history of prior cardiac surgery, to correct for subject selection weaknesses of previous studies. Two classification groups were based on clinical and cardiac catheterization data indicating whether their cardiac illness would—or would not—be expected to interfere with test performance. Cyanotic and acyanotic children were included in both groups. Intelligence testing preceded catheterization and other laboratory measures. Sex, race, and socioeconomic status did not differ between the cyanotic and acyanotic groups. Significantly more cyanotic children were classified as sick, and these children were younger than the acyanotic group, although no significant differences were found in comparisons of these variables within cyanotic and acyanotic groups. While both groups had mean IQs within normal limits, the acyanotic group's IQ was significantly higher. No significant differences were found among scores on the four different IQ tests administered to assess intelligence across the wide age-span represented by the full group. Younger and older cyanotic groups performed equally, suggesting no influence of a longer period of hypoxemia. Sickness level was not found to be factor of greater significance than cyanosis. Degree of cyanosis was identified as the critical factor related to intelligence score.

REPARATIVE SURGERY AND COGNITIVE/ NEUROPSYCHOLOGICAL OUTCOME

The presence of patent ductus arteriosus and the need for pharmacologic treatment or surgical correction appear to be unassociated with long-term adverse cognitive effects (Merritt et al. 1982). The authors studied preschoolers who had been treated as neonates with either therapy. While psychomotor performance was significantly lower among surgically treated children for the first 18 months of life, later analyses (up to 30 months) found these children's psychomotor (Bayley Scale) and receptive language (Peabody Picture Vocabulary Test) performances within normal ranges.

Presence or absence of cyanosis is an important variable. The significance of this discrimination may be changing, however, now that earlier reparative surgery is possible. Early surgical correction means that a child must endure hypoxia, congestive heart failure, and pulmonary hypertension for a shorter time. In addition, the effect of surgical and anesthetic technique on a child's developmental course is difficult to measure, because of the multiple risk factors inherent in a pediatric cardiac group. Chronic hypoxemia or congestive heart failure, poor nutrition, polycythemia, right-to-left shunting with risk of embolic events or brain abscess, arrhythmia episodes, cardiac arrest, and other organ anomalies complicate interpretation (Bellinger et al. 1991). In an early study, Haka-Ikse, Blackwood & Steward (1978) reported developmental quotients that were significantly lower for a CPB group than for a small sibling control group, but they obtained scores within the average range for 16 of 17 patients who responded to a written request for follow-up evaluation. The researchers' failure to include sensitive measures of neuropsychological status, however, undermines their conclusions that using CPB and profound hypothermia during the correction of cardiac defects in infants can be done safely and without adversely affecting neurological or psychomotor functioning.

Circulatory arrest time and correlation with intellectual test performance has been of interest to a number of investigators. The relationship between length of deep hypothermic arrest and mental and motor integrity was considered preliminarily by Wright, Hicks & Newman (1979). Closure of VSD in infancy under conditions of continuous perfusion or deep hypothermic arrest was followed by motor and intellectual compromise—principally with the latter procedure. However, clinical observations (primarily parental report) were the only reported post-operative behavioral data. Intra-operative electroencephalographic recordings provided information indicating the current status of perfusion parameters, but these did not correlate with later developmental abnormality. Clarkson et al. (1980) could not demonstrate post-operative IQ score correlation with any operative technique. IQ was the only behavioral measure employed, and this is likely the reason that subtle deficit or change could not be measured. Others have found no serious psychomotor disturbance but have acknowledged subtle deficit (for example, motor deficit) (Settergren et al. 1982).

Duration of time on pump may be an excellent predictor of post-operative cerebral dysfunction in adult and pediatric cardiac patients. Early data suggested that a longer time on CPB was associated with smaller subsequent intellectual gains (Frank et al. 1972) and a greater incidence of neurological damage (Branthwaite 1972). Duration of perfusion was the most significant operative variable reported for adult patients. Less than 2 hours perfusion time correlated with only 19.6% cerebral disorder, in contrast to 51.9% after longer bypass duration (Sotaniemi 1980). Advances in pump technology may improve overall cognitive outcome. In one study, the use of a pulsatile pump was noted to be the likely significant factor for lack of correlation between post-operative deficit in adults and duration of CPB (Hammeke & Hastings 1988). More recently, other perfusion variables have taken precedence over pulsatile blood flow as influences on cardiovascular hemodynamics (Louagie et al. 1992). Careful attention to these variables may decrease the prevalence of post-operative neuropsychological deficit (Grote et al. 1992).

In another study, intelligence test scores of children who had CPB with profound hypothermia in infancy were associated with normal IQ scores and effective brain protection when periods of arrest did not exceed 60 minutes (Dickinson & Sambrooks 1979). Caution about exceeding 60 minutes was also expressed by Settergren et al. (1982), who found a negative correlation between duration of circulatory arrest and cerebral blood flow measured directly after surgery. Seizures were more likely to occur when the CPB procedure lasted more than 60 minutes (Ferry 1987). Intellectual test performance declined for each minute of increased circulatory arrest time in a group of children who underwent profound hypothermia and total circulatory arrest, compared to a sibling control group, on tests conducted five years post-operatively (Wells et al. 1983). These researchers suggested that the young human brain is able to conceal early changes with an arrest time of less than 45 minutes. Despite complications and concerns about long-term neurological sequelae and quality of life, survival rates associated with OHS have increased dramatically with the introduction of the CPB procedure.

Concern exists about a critical period for duration of profound hypothermia for CPB. A range of purportedly "safe" times are recommended, although cerebral tissue vulnerability cannot easily be detected with currently available techniques. Stevenson et al. (1974) assessed development for 32 children who underwent surgery with surface-induced hypothermia and circulatory arrest. They found no significant correlation between late mean IQ and minimum temperature or duration of circulatory arrest, but they noted more frequent post-operative problems with arrest times of longer than 50 minutes. They concluded that the hypothermic technique did not cause neurologic or intellectual impairments.

The relationships of deep hypothermia and core cooling before circulatory arrest were explored by Bellinger et al. (1991). They found that 10 children who had TGA repair in infancy with deep hypothermia and cardiac arrest had more impaired performance IQ than 7 children with ventricular septal defects (acyanotic heart disease). The TGA children also had an increase in somatic complaints and aggressive behavior (Hesz & Clark 1988). There was a trend toward lowered achievement, compared to sibling control groups, for both cardiac groups. Duration of deep hypothermic circulatory arrest (DHCA) was not associated with cognitive performance in a TGA group, but lower scores were associated with shorter core cooling periods before the DHCA. These data suggested that core cooling time needs to be sufficient to ensure that brain metabolism has slowed in all—not just in some—brain areas.

Studies of adult patients undergoing OHS have revealed neuropsychological deficits involving sensation, language, motor function, memory, and mental status in general after surgery (Lee et al. 1971; Sotaniemi 1980). Few pediatric neuropsychological studies have used pre-operative baseline assessments. However, Dabek (1983) examined the pre-operative intellectual and neuropsychological status of 18 children, between 5 and 14 years of age, who were to undergo OHS to repair a CHD. She found that, while pre-operative IQ scores did not differ significantly from either a normal orthopedic surgery population (O) or a neurologically impaired (ventriculomegaly) (V) control group, the cardiac defect group (CD) did differ significantly on several neuropsychological measures. Specifically, CD was significantly worse on tests of grip strength, tapping speed, and sensory integration for tactile stimuli than O, but significantly better than V on tests of sensory-perceptual integration, tactile form discrimination, kinesthesis, coordination of movement of upper extremities, and manual dexterity. CD did not differ significantly from V on strength and speed. These findings were interpreted as demonstrating the presence of subtle preexisting neuropsychological deficits, none of which had been noticed previously by researchers who chose more global measures of integrity to evaluate the cardiac population or who assumed presurgical integrity of cerebral functions. The mean length of time on pump for CD was 53.3 minutes. No significant alteration in intellectual or neuropsychological functioning was observed 6 weeks postsurgery. Transient cognitive decline, as commonly observed in adult studies, was not found. These data suggested that children are less vulnerable to, or better protected from, the deleterious effects of OHS.

CONCLUSIONS AND FUTURE DIRECTIONS

The effects of cardiac disease and treatment on developmental course constitute an important area for neuropsychological investigation in children; they have only been addressed minimally to date. Prospective, well-controlled, longitudinal studies investigating the correlation between cardiac variables and cognitive development are needed.

Comparability of existing studies has been complicated by experimental design limitations—for instance, whether baseline evaluation was conducted, whether investigators selected homogeneous diagnostic groups, the choice of test instrumentation, whether appropriate statistical methodology was utilized, whether appropriate control groups were included, and the timing of post-operative assessments (particularly important for a population that may have transient abnormalities that dissipate over time following treatment).

Interpretation of results has also been confounded by diverse operative variables that may strongly influence outcome, such as anesthesia, frequency of catheterization, type of surgical procedure(s), and whether there is prolonged hypothermia or total circulatory arrest with or without profound hypothermia. Duration of cyanosis, relationship of cognitive function to the presence, duration, and degree of hypoxemia, and complications of hypoxemia in diverse forms of cardiac disease are further complicating variables. The increased use of cerebral protection agents, improved equipment modifications, and improved monitoring of intra-operative cerebral functioning (Ferry 1990) hold promise for future understanding of the variables affecting neuropsychological outcome of cardiac disease and treatment.

The test instrumentation most appropriate for this population has yet to be determined. General intelligence measures alone do not detect subtle difficulties and do not measure responses to condition and treatment with sufficient precision (Aram, Ekelman, Rose & Whitaker 1985). Therefore, a broad range of assessment instruments may be most useful for detecting subtle deficits in neuropsychological functioning. Clinical reports suggest that motor and psychomotor development, attention/concentration, memory, new learning, and executive functioning may be especially compromised in this population.

Importantly, cognitive deficiencies may antedate treatment, possibly as a consequence of physiological factors related to the underlying pathology. Improved diagnostic techniques, less invasive pre-operative treatments, earlier correction, improved intra-operative myocardial protection, and better post-operative care (Bircks 1991) enhance the likelihood that a child will now survive with more intact cerebral functioning than was likely before these medical advances. Investigations of adult patients have not yet identified the variables that permit discrimination between adversely affected adult patients and those who recover rapidly (O'Brien et al. 1992), nor have these variables been well addressed in pediatric studies.

Studies of adult patients suggest a tendency toward a sparing of left-hemisphere functions and a susceptibility of right-hemisphere functions (Sota-niemi 1980). Such a dissociation has been recognized with diverse pediatric populations, particularly among children with chronic medical conditions (Baron & Goldberger 1993), and including pediatric cardiac disease (Newburger et al. 1984). Further, the particular vulnerability of hippocampal damage, as documented in adult animal and adult human studies, raises questions about the pre-operative and post-operative integrity of these regions in children. While there are no conclusive answers, memory retention tests may be especially sensitive measures of this capacity (Bethune 1980). Yet different memory tests distinguish subtle outcome variably (O'Brien et al. 1992), limiting the conclusions one may draw from single measures or from limited behavioral sampling.

The importance of emotional factors in considerations of neuropsychological outcome and the influence of age at time of treatment on personality development have only partly been investigated. Modifications of peri-operative care have been instituted to lessen the anxiety and disorientation associated with the surgical experience—for instance, through preoperative behavioral sensitization techniques (Jay 1988; Peterson & Mori 1988). Personality characteristics have received some attention. Baer, Freedman & Garson (1984) studied young adults who underwent corrective surgery in childhood for complete repair of tetralogy of Fallot. Two groups differed on age at surgery. Significantly different personality traits and relationships with parents were found between children having late surgery (preadolescent) and those having early surgery (6 years or younger). The authors suggested that invalidism imposed between the ages of 6 and 12 years had long-term consequences on personality trait development. Extended invalidism in childhood resulted in an invalid role in adulthood.

Future research directions are expected to include prospective studies of the effects of heart transplantation for severe cardiac defect (Backer et al. 1991), and the sequelae of intrauterine CPB (Fenton, Heineman & Hanley 1993) and of extracorporeal membrane oxygenation (ECMO) (Hofkosh et al. 1991).

The issue of neuronal migration is especially important when one considers any pediatric cardiac diagnosis. What is the status of the brain? If it is not normal, why not? Is there a differential migrational deficit related to type of lesion? What are the influences of acquired insults, such as cyanosis and other neuropathogenetic factors? What are the influences of catheterization and other invasive procedures used for palliation, and of surgical technique and corrective procedures? Answers to these questions may be central to understanding the effects of pediatric cardiac defects specifically and of chronic childhood disease in general.

REFERENCES

Aberg, T.; Ronquist, G.; Tyden, H.; Brunnkvist, S.; Hultman, J.; Bergstrom, K.; and Lilja, A. 1984. Adverse effects on the brain in cardiac operations as assessed by biochemical, psychometric, and radiologic methods. *Journal of Thoracic and Cardiovascular Surgery* 87: 99–105.

Aisenberg, R. B.; Rosenthal, A.; Nadas, A. S.; and Wolff, P. H. 1982. Developmental delay in infants with congenital heart disease. *Pediatric Cardiology* 3: 133–37.

Aram, D. M.; Ekelman, B. L.; Ben-Shachar, G.; and Levinsohn, M. W. 1985. Intelligence and hypoxemia in children with congenital heart disease: Fact or artifact? *Journal of the American College of Cardiology* 6: 889–93.

Aram, D. M.; Ekelman, B. L.; Rose, D. F.; and Whitaker, H. A. 1985. Verbal and cognitive sequelae following unilateral lesions acquired in early childhood. *Journal of Clinical and Experimental Neuropsychology* 7: 55–78.

Backer, C. L.; Zales, V. R.; Harrison, H. L.; Idriss, F. S.; Benson, D. W.; and Mavroudis, C. 1991. Intermediate term results of infant orthotopic cardiac transplantation from two centers. *Journal of Thoracic and Cardiovascular Surgery* 101: 826–32.

Baer, P. E.; Freedman, D. A.; and Garson, A. 1984. Long-term psychological follow-up of patients after corrective surgery for tetralogy of Fallot. *Journal of the American Academy of Child Psychiatry* 23: 622–25.

Baron, I. S., and Goldberger, E. 1993. Neuropsychological disturbances of hydrocephalic children with implications for special education and rehabilitation. *Neuropsychological Rehabilitation* 3: 389–410.

Behrman, R. E., and Vaughan, V. C. 1992. The cardiovascular system. In R. E. Behrman and V. C. Vaughan (eds.), *Nelson Textbook of Pediatrics,* 13th ed. (Philadelphia: W. B. Saunders), pp. 943–1032.

Bellinger, D. C.; Wernovsky, G.; Rappaport, L. A.; Mayer, J. A.; Castaneda, A. R.; Farrell, D. M.; Wessel, D. L.; Lang, P.; Hickey, P. R.; Jonas, R. A.; and Newburger, J. W. 1991. Cognitive development of children following early repair of transposition of the great arteries using deep hypothermic circulatory arrest. *Pediatrics* 87: 701–7.

Bethune, D. W. 1980. The assessment of organic brain damage following open-heart surgery. In H. Speidel and G. Rodewald (eds.), *Proceedings of an International Symposium: Psychic and Neurological Dysfunctions after Open-heart Surgery* (Stuttgart: Georg Thieme Verlag), pp. 100–106.

Bircks, W. 1991. Cardiac surgery: Past, present and future. *Journal of Cardiovascular Surgery* 32: 217–24.

Branthwaite, M. A. 1972. Neurological damage related to open heart surgery. *Thorax* 27: 748–53.

Brunberg, J. A.; Reilly, E. L.; and Doty, D. B. 1974. Central nervous system consequences in infants of cardiac surgery using deep hypothermia and circulatory arrest. *Circulation* 50(suppl. 2): 60.

Clark, E. B. 1992. Congenital heart disease. In R. A. Hoekelman (ed.), *Primary Pediatric Care,* 2d ed. (St. Louis, Mo.: Mosby Year Book), pp. 1195–1200.

Clarkson, P. M.; MacArther, B. A.; Barratt-Boyes, B. G.; Whitlock, R. M.; and Neutze, J. M. 1980. Developmental progress after cardiac surgery in infancy using hypothermia and circulatory arrest. *Circulation* 62: 855–61.

Dabek, R. F. 1983. Neuropsychological consequences of open heart surgery with cardiopulmonary bypass in children. Unpublished dissertation. *Dissertation Abstracts International* 44(4-B): 1233.

Daniels, S. R., and Specker, B. 1991. Association of rug shampooing and Kawasaki disease. *Journal of Pediatrics* 118(3): 485–88.

Dickinson, D. F., and Sambrooks, J. E. 1979. Intellectual performance in children after circulatory arrest with profound hypothermia in infancy. *Archives of Diseases of Children* 54: 1–6.

Dotter, C. T., and Judkins, M. P. 1964. Transluminal treatment of arteriosclerotic obstruction. *Circulation* 30: 654–79.

Driscoll, D. J. 1990. Evaluation of the cyanotic newborn. In P. C. Gillette (ed.), *The Pediatric Clinics of North America: Congenital Heart Disease* (Philadelphia: W. B. Saunders), pp. 1–23.

Feldt, R. H.; Ewert, J. C.; Stickler, G. B.; and Weidman, W. H. 1969. Children with congenital heart disease. *American Journal of Diseases of Children* 117: 281–87.

Fenton, K. N.; Heineman, M. K.; and Hanley, F. L. 1993. Exclusion of the placenta during fetal cardiac bypass augments systemic flow and provides important information about the mechanism of placental injury. *Journal of Thoracic and Cardiovascular Surgery* 105: 502–12.

Ferry, P. C. 1987. Neurologic sequelae of cardiac surgery in children. *American Journal of Diseases of Children* 141: 309–12.

———. 1990. Neurologic sequelae of open-heart surgery in children *American Journal of Diseases of Children* 144: 369–73.

Frank, K. A.; Heller, S. S.; Kornfeld, D. S.; and Malm, J. R. 1972. Long-term effects of open-heart surgery on intellectual functioning. *Journal of Thoracic and Cardiovascular Surgery* 64: 811–15.

Fyler, D. C.; Silbert, A.; and Rothman, K. 1976. Five year follow-up of infant cardiacs: Intelligence quotient. In B. S. L. Kidd and R. D. Rowe (eds.), *The Child with Congenital Heart Disease after Surgery* (New York: Futura), pp. 409–19.

Gilman, S. 1965. Cerebral disorders after open-heart operations. *New England Journal of Medicine* 272(10): 489–98.

———. 1990. Neurological complications of open heart surgery. *Annals of Neurology* 28: 475–76.

Grossman, W. 1986. Complications of cardiac catheterization: Incidence, causes and prevention. In W. Grossman (ed.), *Cardiac Catheterization and Angiography*, 3d ed. (Philadelphia: Lea & Febiger), pp. 30–42.

Grote, C. L.; Shanahan, P. T.; Salmon, P.; Meyer, R. G.; Barrett, C.; and Lansing, A. 1992. Cognitive outcome after cardiac operations: Relationship to intraoperative computerized electroencephalographic data. *Journal of Thoracic and Cardiovascular Surgery* 104: 1405–9.

Haka-Ikse, K.; Blackwood, M. J. A.; and Steward, D. J. 1978. Psychomotor development of infants and children after profound hypothermia during surgery for congenital heart disease. *Developmental Medicine and Child Neurology* 20: 62–70.

Hammeke, T. A., and Hastings, J. E. 1988. Neuropsychological alterations after cardiac surgery. *Journal of Thoracic and Cardiovascular Surgery* 96: 326–31.

Hesz, N., and Clark, E. B. 1988. Cognitive development in transposition of the great vessels. *Archives of Diseases of Children* 63: 198–200.

Hicks, R. G., and Poole, J. L. 1981. Electroencephalographic changes with hypothermia and cardiopulmonary bypass in children. *Journal of Thoracic and Cardiovascular Surgery* 81: 781–86.

Hoffman, J. I. E. 1990. Congenital heart disease: Incidence and inheritance. In P. C. Gillette (ed.), *The Pediatric Clinics of North America: Congenital Heart Disease* (Philadelphia: W. B. Saunders), pp. 25–43.

Hofkosh, D.; Thompson, A. E.; Nozza, R. J.; Kemp, S. S.; Bowen, A.; and Feldman, H. M. 1991. Ten years of extracorporeal membrane oxygenation: Neurodevelopmental outcome. *Pediatrics* 87: 549–55.

Hungxi, S.; Xiaoqin, H.; Kongsoon, L.; Jiaquiang, G.; and Letien, X. 1982. Intracranial hemorrhage and hematoma following open-heart surgery. In R. Becker, J. Katz, M.-J. Polonius, and H. Speidel (eds.), *Psychopathological and Neurological Dysfunctions Following Open Heart Surgery* (New York, Springer-Verlag), pp. 293–99.

Jay, S. M. 1988. Invasive medical procedures: Psychological intervention and assessment. In D. K. Routh (ed.), *Handbook of Pediatric Psychology* (New York: Guilford Press), pp. 401–25.

Keane, J. F., and Lock, J. E. 1987. Catheter intervention: Balloon valvotomy. In J. E. Lock, J. F. Keane, and K. E. Fellows (eds.), *Diagnostic and Interventional*

Catheterization in Congenital Heart Disease (Boston: Martinus Nijhoff), pp. 111–22.

Lee, W. H.; Brady, M. P.; Rowe, J. M.; and Miller, W. C. 1971. Effects of extracorporeal circulation upon behavior, personality and brain function: II. Hemodynamic, metabolic, and psychometric correlations. *Annals of Surgery* 173: 1013–23.

Linde, L. M.; Rasof, B.; and Dunn, O. J. 1967. Mental development in congenital heart disease. *Journal of Pediatrics* 71: 198–203.

Lock, J. E. 1987. Evaluation and management prior to catheterization. In J. E. Lock, J. F. Keane, and K. E. Fellows (eds.), *Diagnostic and Interventional Catheterization in Congenital Heart Disease* (Boston: Martinus Nijhoff), pp. 1–9.

Louagie, Y. A.; Gonzalez, M.; Collard, E.; Mayne, A.; Gruslin, A.; Jamart, J.; Buche, M.; and Schoevaerdts, J.-C. 1992. Does flow character of cardiopulmonary bypass make a difference? *Journal of Thoracic and Cardiovascular Surgery* 104: 1628–38.

McConnell, J. R.; Fleming, W. H.; Chu, W.; Hahn, F. J.; Sarafian, L. B.; Hofschire, P. J.; and Kugler, J. D. 1990. Magnetic resonance imaging of the brain in infants and children before and after cardiac surgery. *American Journal of Diseases of Children* 144: 374–78.

Medlock, M. D.; Cruse, R. S.; Winek, S. J.; Geiss, D. M.; Horndasch, R. L.; Schultz, D. L.; and Aldag, J. C. 1993. A 10-year experience with postpump chorea. *Annals of Neurology* 34: 820–26.

Merritt, T. A.; White, C. L.; Coen, R. W.; Friedman, W. F.; Gluck, L.; and Rosenberg, M. 1982. Preschool assessment of infants with a patent ductus arteriosus: Comparison of ligation and indomethacin therapy. *American Journal of Diseases of Children* 136: 507–12.

Moody, D. M.; Bell, M. A.; Challa, V. R.; Johnston, W. E.; and Prough, D. S. 1990. Brain microemboli during cardiac surgery or aortography. *Annals of Neurology* 28: 477–86.

Nadas, A. S., and Fyler, D. C. 1972. *Pediatric Cardiology,* 3d ed. Philadelphia: W. B. Saunders.

Neches, W. H. 1988 Kawasaki Syndrome. In R. H. Anderson, W. H. Neches, S. C. Park, and J. R. Zuberbuhler (eds.), *Perspectives in Pediatric Cardiology,* vol 1. (New York: Futura), pp. 411–24.

Newburger, J. W.; Silbert, A. R.; Buckley, L. P.; and Fyler, D. C. 1984. Cognitive function and age at repair of transposition of the great arteries in children. *New England Journal of Medicine* 310(23): 1495–99.

O'Brien, D. G.; Bauer, R. M.; Yarandi, H.; Knauf, D. G.; Bramblett, P.; and Alexander, J. A. 1992. Patient memory before and after cardiac operations. *Journal of Thoracic and Cardiovascular Surgery* 104: 1116–24.

O'Dougherty, M.; Wright, F. S.; Garmezy, N.; Loewenson, R. B.; and Torres, F. 1983. Later competence and adaptation in infants who survive severe heart defects. *Child Development* 54: 1129–42.

Perry, L. W. 1969. The innocent murmurs in children. *Medicine Today* 3: 1–9.

Perry, L. W.; Neill, C. A.; Ferencz, C.; Rubin, J. D.; and Loffredo, C. A. 1993. Infants with congenital heart disease: The cases. In C. Ferencz, J. D. Rubin, C. A. Lofredo, and C. A. Magee (eds.), *Epidemiology of Congenital Heart Disease: The Baltimore–Washington infant study, 1981–1989* (New York: Futura), pp. 33–62.

Peterson, L. J. and Mori, L. 1988. Preparation for hospitalization. In D. K. Routh (ed.), *Handbook of Pediatric Psychology* (New York: Guilford Press), pp. 460–91.

Puntis, J. W., and Green, S. H. 1985. Ischaemic spinal cord injury after cardiac surgery. *Archives of Diseases of Children* 60: 517–20.

Rosenthal, A., and Castaneda, A. R. 1975. Growth and development after cardiovascular surgery in infants and children. *Progress in Cardiovascular Disease* 18: 27–37.

Rupprath, G., and Neuhaus, K. L. 1986. Percutaneous balloon aortic valvuloplasty in infancy and childhood. In E. F. Doyle, M. A. Engle, W. M. Gersony, W. J. Rashkind, and N. S. Talner (eds.), *Pediatric Cardiology: Proceedings of the Second World Congress* (New York: Springer-Verlag), pp. 331–33.

Settergren, G.; Ohqvist, G.; Lundberg, S.; Henze, A.; Bjork, V. O.; and Persson, B. 1982. Cerebral blood flow and cerebral metabolism in children following cardiac surgery with deep hypothermia and circulatory arrest: Clinical course and follow-up of psychomotor development. *Scandinavian Journal of Thoracic and Cardiovascular Surgery* 16: 209–15.

Shida, H.; Morimoto, M.; Inokawa, K.; Ikeda, Y.; Tsugane, J.; and Yuzuriha, H. 1981. Somatic and psychomotor development of children after hypothermic open-heart surgery. *Japanese Journal of Surgery* 11: 154–61.

Sikes, C. L. 1986. Care of the child in the neonatal intensive care unit: Role of PDA in the very low birth weight infant. In E. F. Doyle, M. A. Engle, W. M. Gersony, W. J. Rashkind, and N. S. Talner (eds.), *Pediatric Cardiology: Proceedings of the Second World Congress* (New York: Springer-Verlag), pp. 783–86.

Silbert, A.; Wolff, P. H.; Mayer, B.; Rosenthal, A.; and Nadas, A. 1969. Cyanotic heart disease and psychological development. *Pediatrics* 43: 192–200.

Sotaniemi, K. A. 1980. Brain damage and neurological outcome after open heart surgery. *Journal of Neurology, Neurosurgery and Psychiatry* 43: 127–35.

Stevenson, J. G.; Stone, E. F.; Dillard, D. H.; and Morgan, B. C. 1974. Intellectual development in children subjected to prolonged circulatory arrest during hypothermic open heart surgery in infancy. *Circulation* 49: 54–59.

Stiehm, E. R. 1991. New pediatric indications for IVIG. *Contemporary Pediatrics* 8: 29–52.

Townes, B.; Bashein, G.; Hornbein, T. F.; Coppel, D. B.; Goldstein, D. E.; Davis, K. B.; Nessly, M. L.; Bledsoe, S. W.; Veith, R. C.; Ivey, T. D.; and Cohen, M. A. 1989. Neurobehavioral outcomes in cardiac operations. *Journal of Thoracic and Cardiovascular Surgery* 98: 774–82.

Tufo, H. M.; Ostfeld, A. M.; and Shekelle, R. 1970. Central nervous system dysfunction following open-heart surgery. *Journal of the American Medical Association* 212(8): 1333–40.

Veith, G., and Ziegler, H. K. 1965. Fehlbildungen des gehirnes bei endokardfibroelastose. *Beitraege Zur Pathologischen Anatomie und Zur Allgemeinen Pathologie* 132: 160–87.

Wells, F. C.; Coghill, S.; Caplan, H. L.; and Lincoln, C. 1983. Duration of circulatory arrest does influence the psychological development of children after cardiac operations in early life. *Journal of Thoracic and Cardiovascular Surgery* 86: 823–31.

Whitman, V.; Drotar, D.; Lambert, S.; VanHeeckeren, D. W.; Borkat, G.; Ankeney, J.; and Liebman, J. 1973. Effects of cardiac surgery with extracorporeal circulation on intellectual function in children. *Circulation* 48: 160–63.

Wright, J. S.; Hicks, R. G.; and Newman, D. C. 1979. Deep hypothermic arrest: Observations on later development in children. *Journal of Thoracic and Cardiovascular Surgery* 77(3): 466–68.

Zuberbuhler, J. R., and Anderson, R. H. 1988. Ebstein's malformation of the tricuspid valve: Morphology and natural history. In R. H. Anderson, W. H. Neches, S. C. Park, and J. R. Zuberbuhler (eds.), *Perspectives in Pediatric Cardiology,* vol. 1 (New York: Futura), pp. 99–112.

12

Renal Disease

Approximately 3 children per 1 million in the general population develop end-stage renal disease (ESRD) each year. Most of these children receive services to ameliorate the side effects of renal insufficiency, to preserve life through dialysis, and to restore function through kidney transplantation. Programs for managing children and adolescents with chronic renal failure (CRF) have a major impact both financially and logistically on healthcare delivery systems. Diagnosis, medical management, and treatment of children with CRF involves a number of healthcare professionals, including neuropsychologists and neurologists. This chapter reviews the physiology of the kidneys, describes common causes of chronic renal disease and failure, outlines treatment procedures, and discusses neuropsychological effects of chronic renal disease and its treatment.

PHYSIOLOGY OF THE KIDNEYS

The kidney is a paired organ located in the retroperitoneal space. At the most general level, the kidney consists of an outer cortex and an inner medulla. The ureters propel urine produced in the kidney to the bladder. The kidneys' major function is to filter the waste products of protein metabolism out of the blood. During this process, electrolytes are reclaimed, water is conserved or excreted, acid (hydrogen ions) is secreted, and sodium bicarbonate is regenerated, providing the body with its major buffering system.

The structure responsible for filtration, reclamation, secretion, conservation, and regeneration is the *nephron,* of which there are more than 1 million per kidney. Structurally, the nephron consists of the glomerulus, the proximal tubule, the loop of Henle, the distal tubule and collecting ducts. The glomerulus and some portions of the tubules are located in the kidney complex; the loops of Henle, the tubules, and the collecting ducts are located in the medulla. Initial filtration occurs in the glomeruli. The rate of filtration is called the *glomerular filtration rate (GFR)* and is usually measured in terms of *creatinine clearance*—the amount of plasma cleared of creatinine, in milliliters per minute, corrected to the surface area of an adult (1.73 m^2). Normal creatinine clearance

Significant portions of this chapter reflect the scholarly thinking and writing of its co-author, Robert S. Fennell, III, M.D. of the Department of Pediatrics, University of Florida, Gainesville, Florida.

is 100 to 120 ml/min/1.73 m^2. Infants do not develop adult levels of clearance until 18 to 24 months of age. The energy for glomerular filtration is provided by the heart. Thus, creatinine clearance is related to cardiac output and, by extension, to mean arterial blood pressure.

The glomeruli are really a system of specially adapted capillaries. The kidney regulates glomerular filtration through a wide range of blood pressures through a process of autoregulation. Only at very low mean arterial pressures does glomerular filtration cease. An afferent arteriole leads to the glomerulus, and an efferent arteriole emerges from the glomerulus. The tone in each of these arterioles allows for autoregulation and maintains a uniform pressure gradient between the glomerular capillary space and the urinary space. The basement membrane system separates the blood side from the urinary space. Waste products, water, and electrolytes must pass across this barrier, which serves as an ultrafilter. Proteins, such as immunoglobulins and albumin, are retained on the blood side because of their size and their electrical charge.

The proximal tubule is responsible for reabsorbing most of the ultrafiltrate. Energy is expended locally to generate concentration and electrical gradients that allow sodium bicarbonate, water, potassium, phosphorus, amino acids, glucose, calcium, and magnesium to be reabsorbed. Approximately 66% to 75% of the filtered load is reabsorbed in the proximal tubule. The loop of Henle, as it dips into the renal medulla in a hairpin fashion, provides a countercurrent multiplier system for electrolytes and osmolality (solute concentration). Depending on its location in the kidney cortex, a nephron may have a long loop of Henle that extends into the center of the medulla or a short loop with a very short medullary loop. This loop preferentially reabsorbs sodium and chloride, making the ultrafiltrate very dilute and making the medulla of the kidney very hyperosmolar. Hence, the concentration of salts in the medulla of the kidney progressively increases as the ultrafiltrate progresses deeper into the medulla. A special configuration of arterioles and venules called the *vasa recta* prevents the rapid washout of the hyperosmolor medulla. The ultrafiltrate progresses through the loop of Henle into the distal convoluted tubule and collection duct, where acid (hydrogen ion) and potassium are secreted and sodium is reabsorbed.

For every molecule of hydrogen ion secreted, one molecule of bicarbonate is produced, thus replenishing the body's buffer stores. Water is reabsorbed in the collecting duct, depending on the amount of vasopressin (antidiuretic hormone) secreted by the posterior pituitary gland. The posterior pituitary secretes vasopressin in response to the osmolality of the blood. When water is in excess, vasopressin is not produced and the collecting duct does not reabsorb water. When the individual is water-deprived, vasopressin is produced, and water is reabsorbed because of the hyperosmolality of the renal medulla.

Endocrine Function of the Kidney

The kidney has an endocrine function in addition to a secretory function. The kidney produces a hormone called *erythropoietin* that stimulates the production of red cells by the bone marrow. Without this hormone, the patient develops a severe anemia. Vitamin D_3, another hormone produced by the kidney, increases calcium, magnesium, and phosphorous absorption from the intestines. Patients with renal failure who produce insufficient amounts of this hormone may exhibit *renal osteodystrophy* (failure to produce normal bone and loss of existing bone due to reabsorption). This is especially true when they develop secondary hyperparathyroidism in response to low serum calcium and high serum phosphorus levels. The parathyroids are four small glands in the neck behind the thyroid gland. They become active in response to low levels of serum calcium and high levels of serum phosphorus. Vitamin D_3 increases calcium absorption from bone and decreases phosphorus absorption by the kidneys, thereby tending to maintain serum calcium and phosphorus levels within a certain range.

ETIOLOGY OF CHRONIC RENAL FAILURE IN CHILDREN

Tubular Interstitial Disease

Children may develop renal failure for a number of different reasons. Renal failure occurring in early infancy usually involves tubular interstitial disease, which results from a mechanical obstruction of urine flow or from a failure of the kidneys to develop properly *(renal dysplasia)*. Since the process primarily involves the interstitium (structure surrounding the nephrons) and the portion of the nephron that reabsorbs the filtered load, children with this group of diseases present with an inability to concentrate their urine, polyuria (large urine volume), and the loss of electrolytes such as sodium, calcium, potassium, and bicarbonate. Polyuria is exhibited by frequent voiding and incontinence. Obstruction of urine flow leads to urinary stasis (urine pooling in the bladder or ureters) and urinary tract infections. Signs of a poor urine stream (such as dribbling), abnormal voiding patterns, or abdominal masses (due to a distended bladder or kidney pelvis) may be evident. The body may be depleted of electrolytes, leading to deficiencies in sodium, potassium, or bicarbonate. The kidney may not be able to secrete hydrogen ions and to regenerate bicarbonate, leading to acidosis. The bones act as a buffer for the acidosis and thus, in conjunction with the electrolyte loss, become demineralized. Renal rickets (osteodystrophy) can result, leading to deformities and pathologic features (fractures of bone already weakened by disease when subjected to minimal trauma). The child also may exhibit growth failure, resulting in poor weight gain and (eventually) short stature.

Glomerulonephritis

Glomerulonephritis is the major cause of renal failure in older children and adolescents. The term *glomerulonephritis* refers to inflammation of the glomeruli of the kidney, which results in damage to the basement membrane. This damage may be manifested by proteinuria (protein in the urine), hematuria (blood in the urine), and the retention of salt and water. Hypertension may result, and renal failure may rapidly develop. Fortunately, many forms of glomerulonephritis are reversible, and the kidney is able to repair itself completely. However, some forms persist and result in permanent kidney damage.

Children may present to physicians with headaches and (in some cases) seizures, as the result of hypertension. The children and their families may have noted the blood in the urine—either bright red or "cola colored." The child may appear puffy, especially around the eyes. The abdomen may be protuberant; the legs and ankles may be swollen. This edema may be from salt and water retention, as well as from low serum proteins (due to protein loss in the urine). When the edema is massive because of low serum proteins and high loss of urinary proteins (approximately 3 grams per day or more), the child is said to have *nephrotic syndrome*. Nephrotic syndrome, when combined with hematuria, hypertension, and renal failure, is an especially bad sign and usually results in permanent loss of renal function. Sometimes, glomerulonephritis can present with a minimum of symptoms. As a result, patients may approach end-stage renal disease before the disease is detected.

Hereditary Kidney Disease

One group of diseases is not associated with urinary obstruction, renal dysplasia, or glomerluonephritis. Diseases of this group are best described as hereditary. Polycystic kidneys, cystinosis, congenital nephrotic syndrome, and Alport's syndrome are examples. The presentation of these diseases depends on what portion of the kidney is initially affected. In Alport's syndrome, where the glomerular basement membrane is abnormal, proteinuria and hematuria are the usual manifestations of the disease. In cystinosis, the proximal tubular epithelium is initially affected. Patients suffering from cystinosis present with acidosis, electrolyte losses, and polyuria. These disease are inherited and have characteristic modes of transmission.

Adult-onset polycystic disease is autosomal dominant. Therefore, one parent and approximately half the offspring can be expected to have the disease. Cystinosis is autosomal recessive. Consequently, 25% of the children of two adults who are unaffected carriers can be expected to have the disease.

Progression of Renal Failure

As renal function deteriorates, all patients, regardless of cause, begin to exhibit similar symptomatology. When patients develop moderate renal failure (creatinine clearances of less than 35% of normal), they begin to show signs of hyperparathyroidism and renal osteodystrophy. Anemia, due to decreased erythropoietin production, may become a problem. Acidosis may occur. Hypertension, which can occur at any time, is more likely to become a problem. As renal failure progresses, the child stops growing. Acidosis, hyperparathyroidism and decreased caloric intake all tend to exaggerate growth failure. With careful management, many children can continue to grow until their renal function falls below 10% of normal. At this point, the child's ability to excrete a sodium load and to maintain a normal calcium-phosphorus balance becomes increasingly more difficult. The child's nutritional state becomes progressively more tenuous, and he or she loses fat and muscle stores more rapidly. Growth all but ceases.

By the time renal function has dropped to 5% of normal, most children have been placed on dialysis or have received a kidney transplant. Both dialysis and transplantation are widely accepted therapies for infants and children with end-stage renal disease. Newborn and premature infants can be placed on chronic peritoneal dialysis. Infants weighing more than 7 to 10 kilograms may receive kidney transplants. There is no evidence that infants and children are any less appropriate candidates for end-stage therapy (dialysis or transplantation) than adults. The type of dialysis chosen depends on the age of the child, the disease duration (acute or chronic), the ability of the child's family to comply with different dialysis procedures, and the availability of a suitable kidney donor.

END-STAGE THERAPY

Chronic Dialysis

There are two types of chronic dialysis: hemodialysis and peritoneal dialysis. Hemodialysis is performed by cycling the patient's blood through an external filtering device, called an *artificial kidney*. Excess water and waste products are removed from the blood by the process of ultrafiltration and diffusion across a biologically inert semipermeable membrane into a dialysate. The *dialysate* is a fluid designed to match proportionately the electrolyte content of the patient's blood. Heparinizing the blood to prevent coagulation is usually necessary. Access to the circulatory system (vascular access) is always necessary and can be accomplished by creating a fistula (connection) between an artery and vein or by placing a semipermanent catheter in a large vein (usually subclavian). In the former, cannulation of the fistula is necessary to initiate dialysis, using large-bore dialysis needles. Children often find this disconcerting because of the pain and their fear of needles. Dialysis sessions usually last 3 to 4 hours and are necessary three times per week. Most children require artificial kidneys and blood lines that hold much smaller volumes of blood. Since higher nurse-to-patient ratios are necessary, most children are dialyzed in specialized pediatric dialysis units.

Infection and clotting of the fistula are all too frequent complications in children undergoing hemodialysis. In addition, hemostasis after needle removal may be a problem. Infection is yet another frequent complication of the semipermanent catheters. Clotting may be avoided by irrigating the line with heparin. Rarely, the catheter may erode through the venous wall, and uncontrollable bleeding may result.

Peritoneal dialysis is performed through a catheter surgically inserted through the wall of the abdominal cavity and into the peritoneum. Dialysate fluid is infused into the cavity. Waste products and water diffuse across the peritoneal membrane and are removed when the dialysate is drained. At least four exchanges of dialysate are made each day. If a machine is used to deliver the dialysate, as many as 20 exchanges may be performed. The manual method of making exchanges is called *continuous ambulatory peritoneal dialysis (CAPD),* and dialysis by the cycling device is called *continuous cycling peritoneal dialysis (CCPD).*

Both methods are done daily, but CCPD is usually done while the patient (normally) sleeps. CAPD and CCPD are done at home and are especially adaptable to infants and children. With CAPD and CCPD, smaller volumes are necessary, and they are more easily managed than hemodialysis with its attendant specialized equipment. The children do not have to be heparinized with CAPD and CCPD, and vascular access is not necessary. Dialysis occurs daily rather than episodically (as in hemodialysis) and therefore comes closer to replicating the normal physiology of the kidneys. Peritonitis, due to bacterial or fungal contamination, remains the major complication of peritoneal dialysis.

Children receiving either type of dialysis therapy must face the same complications of renal failure, including acidosis, hyperparathyroidism, anemia, poor appetite, poor nutrition, hypertension, and growth failure. It is usually necessary to use calcium carbonate as a phosphorus binder; and dietary supplementation is frequently required. Sometimes, nasogastric tube feedings become necessary if food intake is poor. Erythropoietin and vitamin D_3 therapy can be used to ameliorate the anemia and bone disease of renal failure. Not infrequently, antihypertensive medication is necessary; but often, simple fluid removal (ultrafiltration) adequately controls blood pressure. Growth hormone has been administered (with some positive results) to children with advanced renal failure, once nutrition, acidosis, and hyperparathyroidism have been adequately controlled.

Renal Transplantation

Renal transplantation is considered the preferred mode of therapy for end-stage renal disease in children. Kidneys may be obtained from two sources: a family member, or a cadaver donor. Kidneys donated by a family member have the advantage of being immunologically more compatible with the patient than kidneys from a cadaver. The more immunologically compatible the donated kidney is, the less likelihood there is of rejection. Kidney transplantation involves major surgery, typically in two stages. Initial surgery removes the malfunctioning kidneys and makes the patient fully dependent on dialysis. The patient then either is placed on a waiting list to receive a donated organ or undergoes a second surgical procedure, in which the donor kidney is placed in the abdominal cavity for easy access should rejection occur. Following transplantation, the child is followed closely for signs of rejection and undergoes systemic immunosuppression therapy to prevent rejection of the new organ.

Kidney Rejection and Immunosuppressant Treatment

Rejection is the body's process of destroying foreign tissue. A heart, liver, or kidney transplanted to replace a diseased organ is subject to this process. The primary cell involved in rejection is the T-lymphocyte. Immunosuppressive agents are given to the organ recipient to control rejection. The agents in widest use are prednisone, azathioprine, and cyclosporine. Antibodies to lymphocytes, either polyclonal or monoclonal, may be given at the time of transplantation to prevent rejection from occurring or to reverse an ongoing rejection episode. Steroids, given orally or intravenously, may also be used to reverse a rejection episode. Rejection may be either acute or chronic. Acute rejections usually occur in the first six months after a transplant. The symptoms are a rapid decrease in renal function, decreased urine output, hypertension, salt retention, and sometimes fever and graft tenderness; but these are potentially reversible. Chronic rejection is more insidious. It is associated with the gradual loss of renal function, hypertension and proteinuria. Chronic rejection is much more difficult to treat and often results in allograft loss. If the blood vessels are primarily involved in the rejection, it is called *vascular rejection*. This type of rejection, whether acute or chronic, is usually more difficult to treat and may cause more rapid loss of the grafted kidney.

Immunosuppression therapy may have significant side effects. Steroids cause cataracts, hirsutism, truncal obesity, osteopenia, osteonecrosis, glucose intolerance, hypertension, and growth failure. Azathioprine may cause low white blood cell counts, anemia, alopecia, and liver dysfunction. Cyclosporine may cause hirsutism, hypertension, renal dysfunction, gastroenteritis, headaches, tremors, and (occasionally) seizures. All three agents make patients more prone to infections and increase the risk of certain cancers.

Noncompliance with Medical Management of Chronic Renal Failure and Transplantation

Many patients who have received kidney transplants become noncompliant with their medications. Various social and psychological factors are associated with noncompliance. Some factors involve the adverse side effects of the medications, but many other factors involve family organization, social support, and stability. Noncompliance with immunosuppressive therapy is a major factor in loss of a transplanted kidney. Often, the noncompliant patient develops progressive rejection, reduction in allograft function, and the necessity to return to dialysis. Retransplantation may be attempted, but about half of all such noncompliant patients repeat the same behavior, resulting in irreversible allograft rejection and loss. Unfortunately, patient education alone is not effective in preventing this behavior, and no approach has been proved to prevent noncompliant behavior.

Children who receive renal transplants usually have the best chance for rehabilitation. They have the opportunity to return to school and are freed from the problems of dialysis. Linear growth and even accelerated growth may be achieved if good allograft function is preserved. Steroid dosage must be low to achieve growth; but with the addition of the newer immunosuppressive drugs such as cyclosporine, steroid dosage may be reduced to lower levels relatively rapidly without increasing the danger of rejection. Therefore, children are more likely to exhibit accelerated or normal growth and are less likely to be dwarfed by chronic renal failure. As immunosuppressive regimens improve, allograft functioning is likely to be extended for longer periods of time. At present, adverse side effects of these medications continue to be problematic.

NEUROPSYCHOLOGICAL STUDIES OF PEDIATRIC CHRONIC RENAL FAILURE AND TRANSPLANTATION

A chronic medical illness such as renal disease can cause brain and neuropsychological dysfunction in several ways. (Tarter, Van Thiel & Edwards 1988). Unlike disorders that arise directly from the CNS, chronic organ system failure can have several indirect but still potent effects on the functional integrity of the brain (Tarter, Edwards & Van Thiel, 1988). For example, the diseased organ may function suboptimally, depriving the brain of sufficient quantities of one or more substances necessary for normal functioning. Increased levels of blood plasma urea secondary to end-stage renal disease have been invoked to explain the increased predominance of EEG slow waves and delayed evoked potential responses in some patients (Ginn et al. 1975). Another possible disruption of higher brain functioning is through disequilibrium of target organ activity, leading to pathological overactivity or underactivity of that organ, which in turn affects brain functioning. Polyurea associated with glomerulonephritis may lead to metabolite and plasma parathyroid hormone imbalance and to subsequent alteration of brain neuronal firing (Arieff 1981). Finally, the diseased organ system may be unable to perform all of its metabolic or physiological functions, resulting in secondary CNS pathology. Chronic renal failure can lead to various neurological complications (Uysal et al. 1990). Untreated end-stage renal disease has been shown to produce a severe encephalopathic state, called *uremic encephalopathy*, that results in structural brain lesions, behavioral deterioration, and ultimately death if left untreated (Arieff 1981; Ginn 1975).

In the following sections, studies of the neuropsychological effects of chronic renal failure, end-stage renal disease, dialysis, and kidney transplantation in children are briefly reviewed. Many of the studies reviewed contain a number of methodological problems. These problems, which are also present in studies of adult renal patients (Hart & Kreutzer 1988; Stewart et al. 1993), include absence of appropriate normal or medical control groups; failure to exclude children with confounding medical or developmental problems; and absence of long-term follow-up studies. Despite these weaknesses, some general conclusions can be discerned, and these are discussed in the following subsections. The final subsection addresses psychosocial functioning and behavioral problems in children with chronic renal disease.

Studies of the Cognitive Effects of Chronic Renal Failure in Children

Hemodialysis was first made available to children in the 1960s, followed shortly thereafter by kidney transplantation. Although both diagnosis and treatment have improved since then, renal failure has been shown to damage the developing nervous system, resulting in various cognitive and motor impairments (Baluarte et al. 1977; McGraw & Haka-Ikse 1985; Geary & Haka-Ikse 1989; Bock et al. 1989). Infants and young children with chronic renal failure have been described as manifesting both normal growth and a range of developmental delays in mental and motor skills. As they age, they obtain lower performance IQ scores on the Wechsler intelligence tests and lower overall intelligence scores, even on tests that emphasize verbal abilities over timed motor tasks, such as the Stanford-Binet scales (Crittenden et al. 1980; Fennell et al. 1984; Rasbury, Fennell & Morris 1983). Age-related deficits in visuomotor copying skills, in visuospatial constructional skills, and in verbal learning and memory have also been described in children with chronic renal failure. Problems in visual and auditory vigilance—including slowed reaction times, inattention, and impulsivity—have also been described (Fennell et al. 1990a, 1990b; Fennell et al. 1986).

These deficits have been reported when children with chronic renal failure were compared to age-matched normal controls (Fennell et al. 1990a, 1990b) and in identical twins discordant for renal disease (Fennell & Rasbury 1980; Morris et al. 1985). These neurocognitive deficits have been attributed to electrophysiological (Lewis et al. 1980; Teschan 1975), structural (Geary et al. 1980; Steinberg et al. 1985), and toxic (Rotundo et al. 1982) changes in the brains of children with chronic renal failure.

Studies of Neuropsychological Effects of Dialysis Treatment

A number of studies have compared the cognitive performance of pediatric patients before and after hemodialysis. These studies suggest that dialysis can improve performance on tests of attention, of immediate short-term memory, and of long-term retrieval in children undergoing hemodialysis (Rasbury et al. 1986). These effects may last for up to 24 hours after dialysis, but they may not be observed in all children who undergo dialysis (Davidovicz, Iacoriello & McVicar 1981). Several studies have suggested that higher levels of performance can be obtained when children undergo CAPD as compared to intermittent hemodialysis (Baum et al. 1982; Fennell et al. 1986). In these studies, no children were included who had suffered any complications during the dialysis treatment (such as dialysis disequilibrium or aluminum toxicity). In addition, children who had suffered neurological complications of their renal disease (for example, stroke) or who were too mentally impaired to cooperate in the testing procedures were excluded. Longitudinal studies of children on CAPD compared to children on intermittent hemodialysis suggest that children on CAPD generally do better on tests of attention and memory than do children on hemodialysis, while few differences exist between these treatment groups on measures of general verbal abilities and visuospatial constructional tasks (Fennell et al. 1990a, 1990b). Finally, children who undergo CAPD appear to show better rates of physical growth and development than do children on hemodialysis (Warady et al. 1988), although they often remain behind normal growth trajectories.

Studies of Renal Transplantation in Children and Adolescents

Renal transplantation is among the most common kinds of organ transplantations in children, and it has been routinely available since the late 1960s. Despite this, relatively few large-scale studies have investigated the effects of renal transplantation in children's neuropsychological functioning. Some studies have simply described short-term before-and-after transplantation scores among clinical cases (Najarian et al. 1990), while others have attempted to compare children with kidney transplants both to normal controls and to children whose renal failure was medically managed or treated with dialysis procedures (Fennell et al. 1986; Fennell et al. 1984). In general, transplantation appears to improve performance on tests of attention, visual vigilance, simple and choice reaction time, short-term memory, and verbal learning (Fennell et al. 1986; Fennell et al. 1990a). In some instances, the scores of children with renal transplants did not differ from those obtained by age- and sex-matched normal controls. Some problems in visuomotor skills, however, do not appear to respond to renal transplantation (Fennell et al. 1990a). The observed impairments in neuropsychological functioning are correlated with each other, suggesting some general neurocognitive change factor (Fennell et al. 1990c), as well as being linked to general improvements in physical growth and maturation (Davis, Chang & Nevins 1990).

Fennell et al. (1990a) have suggested that renal disease can have two types of effects on the developing brain. The first, a traitlike effect, interferes with and may even prevent the acquisition of new skills as the disease progresses. As a result, the child is unable to acquire newly emerging skills adequately, and neuropsychological testing of the child yields age-related deficits. The second effect is state-dependent; that is, it is linked to the level of physiological activity of the CNS, it may be metabolically dependent, and it can be altered by restoration of normal or near-normal renal function. Consequently, results of tests (such as memory and reaction-time tasks) that depend on attention, processing speed, and response speed—although initially impaired—improve with dialysis and transplantation. This model of the effects of renal disease and of its treatment on neurocognitive performance in children and adolescents has been developed only for renal diseases that are congenital or that have been acquired in infancy or early childhood. To date, no model has been described that explains the observed dissociation in neuropsychological studies of chronic renal diseases acquired in later childhood or adolescence.

Psychological Factors in Chronic Renal Failure and Transplantation

Chronic medical illness in children can have effects on the psychological adjustment of the ill child, on that child's sibling, and on the family as a whole (Frank et al. 1991; Siegel & Hudson 1992). Effects on the family of a chronic childhood medical illness such as chronic renal failure include economic stresses associated with the costs of treatment; role changes for parents and siblings; disruption of family routines due to frequent doctor or hospital visits; emotional reactions to the child's illness, such as developing depression or anxiety in response to initial diagnoses and treatment; and problems in adapting to or coping with changes in family functioning because of the child's illness (Johnson 1991; Korsch, Fine & Francis-Negrete 1978; Shulman 1983). A number of studies have also focused on problems that the affected child experiences, including coping with changes in body appearance in response to various medical treatments; noncompliance with medical treatments; adjustment reaction with behavior and mood disorders; school problems; and vocational limitations due to physical limitations or neuropsychological problems, such as learning disabilities or memory disorder (Beck et al. 1980; Foulkes et al. 1993, LaGreca 1988; Varni & Babani 1986). Different types of problems may be experienced by the child or the family, depending on the child's age, the frequency of hospitalizations and treatments, and the child's and family's conceptualization of the illness (Kaplan-DeNour 1979; Siegel & Hudson 1992).

Given the likelihood that the child with chronic renal disease and the child's family may experience a number of different types of psychological, psychosocial, and behavioral difficulties along the course of the illness from diagnosis through treatment, the neuropsychologist who works with such children should be prepared to amplify the neuropsychological examination to include measures of psychological adjustment, emotional symptoms, and problem behaviors. A number of well-standardized tests assess emotional complaints, behavior complaints, family coping, self-esteem, and response to illness for children from early childhood through adolescence (Goldman, Stein & Guerry 1984; Johnson & Goldman 1990). In addition, several recent texts provide fairly comprehensive reviews of diagnosis and intervention in children's chronic illnesses (Krasnegor, Arasteh & Cataldo 1986; Routh 1988; Walker & Roberts 1992).

Despite the number of studies that have reported emotional or neuropsychological problems among children who are treated for chronic renal failure or who undergo transplantation, no current studies appear to have attempted to examine closely the interactions between these factors. In the future, investigators may wish to examine the relationship between degree of neuropsychological impairment and stresses or emotional symptoms in the affected child and family.

CONCLUSION

Chronic renal failure has both direct and indirect effects on the development and function of the child's brain. Problems that have been reported in children with chronic renal failure and end-stage renal disease include developmental delay, intellectual impairment, and delayed physical growth. Specific neuropsychological impairments that have been reported include immediate short-term memory problems, problems in verbal learning and long-term recall of newly learned verbal material, attentional disorder, slowed cognitive processing speed, slowed reaction time, and difficulties in visuospatial constructional tasks and problem solving. Language abilities appear to be relatively spared. Treatment of renal failure by hemodialysis, CAPD, and kidney transplantation improves many of these neuropsychological impairments, with successful transplantation providing the greatest improvements. The chronicity of renal failure, the intensity of medical management, and the stresses of kidney transplantation can lead to psychological problems for the affected child and family. The neuropsychologist who undertakes a consultative role with a pediatric renal service or pediatric dialysis unit should be familiar with the emotional and behavioral factors that can complicate the management and care of the child who has chronic renal failure or end-stage renal disease.

REFERENCES

Arieff, A. I. 1981. Neurological complications of uremia. In B. Brennan and F. Rector (eds.), *The Kidney* (Philadelphia: W. B. Saunders), pp. 2307–43.

Baluarte, H. J.; Gruskin, A. B.; Hiner, L. B.; Foley, C. M.; and Grevor, W. D. 1977. Encephalopathy in children with chronic renal failure. *Proceedings of Clinical Dialysis and Transplantation Forum* 7: 95 [abstract].

Baum, M.; Powell, D.; Calvin, S.; McDaid, T.; McHenry, K.; Mar, H.; and Potter, D. 1982. Continuous ambulatory peritoneal dialysis in children: Comparisons with hemodialysis. *New England Journal of Medicine* 307: 1537–42.

Beck, D. D.; Fennell, R. S.; Yost, R. L.; Robinson, J. D.; Geary, M. B.; and Richard, G. A. 1980. Evaluation of an educational program on compliance with medication regimens in pediatric patients with renal transplants. *Journal of Pediatrics* 96: 1094–97.

Bock, G. H.; Conners, K.; Ruley, J.; Samango-Sprouse, C. A.; Conry, J. A.; Weiss, I.; Eng. G.; Johnson, E. L.; and David, C. T. 1989. Disturbances of brain maturation and neurodevelopment during chronic renal failure in infancy. *Journal of Pediatrics* 114: 231–38.

Crittenden, M.; Holliday, M.; Potter, D.; Piel, C.; and Salvatierra, O. 1980. IQ in children with renal failure. *Pediatric Research* 14: 617 [abstract].

Davidovicz, H.; Iacoviello, J.; and McVicar, M. 1981. Cognitive functions (CF) in children on chronic intermittent hemodialysis (CH). *Pediatric Research* 15: 692 [abstract].

Davis, I. D.; Chang, P. N.; and Nevins, T. E. 1990. Successful renal transplantation accelerates development in young uremic children. *Pediatrics* 86: 594–600.

Fennell, E. B.; Fennell, R. S.; Mings, E.; and Morris, M. K. 1986. The effect of various modes of therapy on cognitive performance in a pediatric population: Preliminary data. *International Journal of Pediatric Nephrology* 7: 107–12.

Fennell, R. S.; Fennell, E. B.; Carter, R. L.; Mings, E.; Klausner, A. B.; and Hurst, J. R. 1990a. A longitudinal study of the cognitive function of children with renal failure. *Pediatric Nephrology* 4: 11–15.

———. 1990b. Association between renal function and cognition in childhood chronic renal failure. *Pediatric Nephrology* 4: 16–20.

———. 1990c. Correlations between performance on neuropsychological tests in children with chronic renal failure. *Child Nephrology and Urology* 10: 199–204.

Fennell, R. S., III, and Rasbury, W. C. 1980. Cognitive functioning of identical twins discordant for Prune Belly syndrome and end stage renal failure. *Journal of Pediatrics* 90: 41–44.

Fennell, R. S., III; Rasbury, W. C.; Fennell, E. B.; and Morris, M. K. 1984. The effects of kidney transplantation on cognitive performance in a pediatric population. *Pediatrics* 74: 273–78.

Foulkes, L. M.; Boggs, S. R.; Fennell, R. S.; and Skibinski, R. 1993. Social support, family variables, and compliance in renal transplant children. *Pediatric Nephrology* 7: 185–88.

Frank, S. J.; Olmsted, C. L.; Wagner, A. E.; Lamb, C. C.; Freeark, K.; Breitzer, G. M.; and Peters, J. M. 1991. Child illness, the parenting alliance and parenting stress. *Journal of Pediatric Psychology* 16: 361–72.

Geary, D. F.; Fennell, R. S., III; Andriola, M.; Gudat, J.; Rodgers, B. M.; and Richard, G. A. 1980. Encephalopathy in children with chronic renal failure. *Journal of Pediatrics* 90: 41–44.

Geary, D. F., and Haka-Ikse, K. 1989. Neurodevelopmental progress of young children with chronic renal disease. *Pediatrics* 84: 68–72.

Ginn, H. E. 1975. Neurobehavioral dysfunction in uremia. *Kidney International* 7: 217–21.

Ginn, H. E.; Teschan, P. E.; Walker, P. J.; Bourne, J. R.; Fristoe, M.; Ward, J. W.; McLain, L. W.; Johnston, H. B., Jr.; and Hamel, B. 1975. Neurotoxicity in uremia. *Kidney International* 7: 357–60.

Goldman, J. R.; Stein, C. L'E.; and Guerry, S. 1984. *Psychological Methods of Child Assessment.* New York: Bruner/Mazel.

Hart, R. P., and Kreutzer, J. S. 1988. Renal system. In R. E. Tarter, D. H. Van Thiel, and K. L. Edwards (eds.), *Medical Neuropsychology* (New York: Plenum Press), pp. 99–120.

Johnson, J. H., and Goldman, J. R. 1990. *Developmental Assessment in Clinical Child Psychology.* New York: Pergamon.

Johnson, S. B. 1991. Compliance in pediatric psychology. In J. H. Johnson and S. B. Johnson (eds.), *Advances in Child Health Psychology* (Gainesville, Fla.: University of Florida Press), pp. 249–64.

Kaplan De-Nour, A. 1979. Adolescents' adjustments to chronic hemodialysis. *American Journal of Psychiatry* 136: 430–33.

Korsch, B. M.; Fine, R. N.; and Francis-Negrete, V. 1978. Noncompliance in children with renal transplants. *Pediatrics* 61: 872–76.

Krasnegor, N. A.; Arasteh, J. D.; and Cataldo, M. F. 1986. *Child Health Behavior: Behavioral Pediatrics Perspective.* New York: Wiley.

LaGreca, A. M. 1988. Adherence to prescribed medical regimens. In D. K. Routh (ed.), *Handbook of Pediatric Psychology* (New York: Guilford Press), pp. 299–320.

Lewis, E. G.; O'Neill, W. M.; Dustman, R. E.; and Beck, E. G. 1980. Temporal effects of hemodialysis on measures of neural efficiency. *Kidney International* 17: 357–63.

McGraw, M. S., and Haka-Ikse, K. 1985. Neurologic-developmental sequelae of chronic renal failure in infancy. *Journal of Pediatrics* 106: 579–83.

Morris, M. K.; Fennell, E. B.; Fennell, R. S., III; and Rasbury, W. C. 1985. A case study of identical twins discordant for renal failure: Longterm neuropsychological deficits. *Developmental Neuropsychology* 1: 81–92.

Najarian, J. S.; Frey, D. J.; Matas, A. J.; Gillingham, K. J.; So, S. S. K.; Cook, M.; Chavers, B.; Mauer, S. M.; and Nevins, T. E. 1990. Renal transplantation in infants. *Annals of Surgery* 212: 353–65.

Rasbury, W. C.; Fennell, R. S., III; Fennell, E. B.; and Morris, M. K. 1986. Cognitive functioning in children with end stage renal disease, pre- and post-dialysis sessions. *International Journal of Pediatric Nephrology* 7: 45–50.

Rasbury, W. C.; Fennell, R. S., III; and Morris, M. K. 1983. Cognitive functioning of children with end stage renal disease before and after successful transplant. *Journal of Pediatrics* 102: 589–92.

Rotundo, A.; Nevins, T. E.; Lipton, M.; Lockman, L. A.; Mauer, S M.; and Michael, A. F. 1982. Progressive encephalopathy in children with chronic renal insufficiency in infancy. *Kidney International* 21: 486–91.

Routh, D. K., ed. 1988. *Handbook of Pediatric Psychology*. New York: Guilford Press.

Shulman, J. L. 1983. Coping with major disease—Child, family and pediatrician. *Pediatrics* 102: 988–91.

Siegel, L. J., and Hudson, B. O. 1992. Hospitalization and medical care of children. In C. E. Walker and M. C. Roberts (eds.), *Handbook of Clinical Child Psychology*, 2d ed. (New York: Wiley), pp. 845–58.

Steinberg, A.; Efrat, R.; Pomeranz, A.; and Drukker, A. 1985. Computerized tomography of the brain in children with chronic renal failure. *International Journal of Pediatric Nephrology* 6: 121–26.

Stewart, S. M.; Kennard, B. D.; Waller, D. A.; and Fixler, D. 1993. Cognitive function in children who receive organ transplantation. *Health Psychology*, (In press).

Tarter, R. E.; K. L.; and Van Thiel, D. H. 1988. Perspective and rationale for neuropsychological assessment of medical disease. In R. E. Tarter, D. H. Van Thiel, and K. L. Edwards (eds.), *Medical Neuropsychology* (New York: Plenum Press), pp. 1–10.

Tarter, R. E.; Van Thiel, D. H.; and Edwards, K. L., eds. 1988. *Medical Neuropsychology*. New York: Plenum Press.

Teschan, P. E. 1975. Electroencephalographic and other neurophysiological abnormalities in uremia. *Kidney International* 7: 210–16.

Uysal, S.; Renda, Y.; Saatci, U.; and Yaiaz, K. 1990. Neurological complications in chronic renal failure: A retrospective study. *Clinical Pediatrics* 29: 510–14.

Varni, J. W., and Babani, L. 1986. Long-term adherence to health care regimens in pediatric chronic disorders. In N. A. Krashegor, J. D. Arasteh, and M. F. Cataldo (eds.), *Child Health Behavior: A Behavioral Pediatrics Perspective* (New York: Wiley), pp. 502–20.

Walker, C. E., and Roberts, M. C., eds. 1992. *Handbook of Clinical Child Psychology*, 2d ed. New York: Wiley.

Warady, B. A.; Kriley, M.; Lovell, H.; Farrell, S. E.; and Hellerstein, S. 1988. Growth and development of infants with end-stage renal disease receiving long-term peritoneal dialysis. *Journal of Pediatrics* 112: 714–19.

13

Neuropsychiatric Disorders

Genetic, neurodevelopmental, and environmental factors may contribute to the development of symptoms of psychiatric disorder in children and adolescents. The term *neuropsychiatry* refers to psychiatric evaluation and treatment approaches that focus on medical (including genetic and neurological) factors that may lead to disorders of mental development, to mood disorders, and to other forms of psychopathology. Although the specific patterns of brain dysfunction underlying many psychiatric disorders are still being researched, increasing evidence links some psychiatric disorders with specific neuropathology among adult patients (Yudofsky & Hale 1992). Although relatively few neurobehavioral studies of neuropsychiatric syndromes in children and adolescents have been conducted, several disorders discussed in this chapter are likely to be encountered by a pediatric neuropsychologist in a medical setting. These include mood disorder, Tourette's syndrome, obsessive compulsive disorder, schizophrenia, and autism. The reader is referred to the *Diagnostic and Statistical Manual of Mental Disorders,* fourth edition (DSM-IV) (American Psychiatric Association 1994) for the detailed diagnostic criteria of each disorder. This chapter reviews what is known about the neuroanatomy of these disorders (see Table 13-1), as elaborated in relevant neurobehavioral studies. Where appropriate, co-morbid conditions are also discussed.

MOOD DISORDER

The DSM-IV (American Psychiatric Association 1994) nosology identifies two major types of mood disorder: depressive disorder and bipolar disorder. Depressive disorder is itself subdivided into major depression, dysthymia (a history of predominantly depressed mood during the last two years), and major depressive disorder not otherwise specified. Bipolar disorder involves manic or hypomanic episodes. *Cyclothymic disorder* refers to a 1-year history of hypomanic symptoms and numerous episodes of depressed mood or loss of interest or pleasure that nonetheless do not qualify as major depressive episodes under established criteria.

Table 13-1 Brain Regions and Neurotransmitters Implicated in Common
Neuropsychiatric Disorders of Childhood

Disorder	Anatomic Region	Neurotransmitter
Depression	*Cortical:* right hemisphere (?) *Subcortical:* basal ganglia; hypothalamus–pituitary–adrenal axis	Serotonin, Norepinepherine
Bipolar disorder	*Cortical:* left-hemisphere temporal basal poles (?) *Subcortical:* limbic system; thalamus	Norepinepherine
Tourette syndrome	*Cortical:* frontotemporal regions *Subcortical:* basal ganglia; CSNTC loops–putamen, caudate nuclei; limbic system; striatum	Dopamine
Obsessive compulsive disorder	*Cortical:* orbitofrontal *Subcortical:* globus pallidus; basal ganglia; caudate; nucleus accumbens, ventral pallidum; dorsal medial nucleus of thalamus	Serotonin
Schizophrenia	*Cortical:* dorsolateral frontal lobes; prefrontal, hippocampus, entorhinal cortex *Subcortical:* anterior cingulate; parahippocampal gyrus; basal ganglia; ventricular enlargement	Dopamine, Glutamate, Serotonin
Autism	*Cortical:* frontal *Subcortical:* cerebellum; limbic system	Dopamine

Depressive Disorder

Several studies of children diagnosed with depressive disorders suggest that the mean length of a first episode of depression is 8 to 9 months, and that the mean duration of subsequent episodes is 32 weeks (Kovacs et al. 1984a, 1984b) or 35 weeks (McCauley et al. 1993). While duration of depression did not differ between males and females, episodes of depression may be longer in adolescent girls than in same-age boys (Kovacs et al. 1984a, 1984b). Kovacs et al. also noted that younger children had longer initial episodes, but this was not reported by McCauley et al. (1993).

Previously, the proposition that children and adolescents could suffer from depression was questioned on the ground that a child's "immature" cognitive system might not be able to support true depressive disorder. According to the alternative theory, dysphoric experiences and mood alterations were due to transitory developmental stressors. However, clinical studies have provided strong support for the existence of childhood depression (Rutter 1987), even in preschoolers (Kashani & Carlson 1985). By adolescence, depression may become especially serious—in some cases even leading to suicide (Rao et al. 1993; Kovacs Goldston & Gatsonis 1993).

Although major depressive disorder (MDD) does occur in childhood, it is uncommon and hard to diagnose. Prevalence was estimated at 1.8% for major depression and 2.5% for minor depression in a population of 9-year-olds (Kashani et al. 1983). Diagnostic criteria are similar for children and for adults, requiring the presence of at least five of the following symptoms for a minimum of two consecutive weeks: depressed mood, anhedonia, weight loss or weight gain, alteration in sleep pattern (insomnia or hypersomnia), psychomotor agitation or retardation, fatigue or energy loss, feelings of worthlessness or guilt, decreased concentration, and/or suicidal ideation. In addition, the mood disturbance cannot be due to a known organic disorder, to the effects of a substance or of a general medical condition, or to an uncomplicated grief reaction; and it cannot be superimposed on schizophrenia or another psychotic disorder. Age-specific associated features may include somatic complaints, separation anxiety, phobias, and hallucinations. Compared to younger children, adolescents are more likely to exhibit conduct disturbance, anhedonia, weight changes, and substance abuse (Ryan et al. 1987). Irritable mood may substitute for depressed mood, and failure to make expected weight gains may substitute for decreased appetite. Dysthymia in children is defined as a mood disturbance present for at least 1 year (2 years in adults) that is not sufficiently severe to meet the criteria for major depression.

Diagnosis depends on the histories obtained from the child and from the parent. Children are capable of providing valid self-reports about mood in an interview or play setting and by questionnaire. Useful measures include the Child Depression Inventory (CDI) (Kovacs 1985; Smucker et al. 1986) and the Schedule for Affective Disorders and Schizophrenia for School Age Children (K-SADS-P) (Puig-Antich & Chambers 1986). Systematic interviews that apply adult research criteria may identify depressed children more successfully than traditional interview techniques. Some authorities contend that diligent interviews "unmask" behavior disorders that initially bring the child to the attention of mental health professionals, and that these disorders may overshadow existing depression. Exclusive reliance on parent report may be inadequate, since parents often have difficulty assessing their child's internal emotional state accurately, and they may focus on externalizing conditions such as hyperactivity or defiant, aggressive behavior.

Studies of the prevalence of depression within families have demonstrated that there is a strong genetic component and probably several genetic subtypes. The presence of depressive disorder (unipolar or bipolar) in a parent substantially increases a child's risk of experiencing a depressive episode by adolescence (Hammen et al. 1990). Although negative environmental factors increase the incidence of depressive events in children, the emergence of symptoms may also be under genetic control and may be related to maturation and/or hormonal events around puberty. Children with depressive disorders may also be at increased risk for co-morbid conditions such as attention deficit hyperactivity disorder (ADHD) and generalized anxiety (Biederman et al. 1991; Biederman et al. 1992).

Studies of depressed adults suggest that depression can cause profound changes in a number of biological markers related to the activity of the hypothalamic–pituitary–adrenal axis (Rubinow et al. 1984; Siever & Davis 1985). Among the reported changes are increased cortisol excretion; early escape from dexamathasone suppression of corticotropin, beta-endorphin, and cortisol; hypersecretion of corticotropin-releasing factor; and increased sensitivity of corticotropin receptors (Nemeroff et al. 1992). Depressed patients may have blunted growth hormone response and reduced rapid-eye-movement (REM) sleep as a manifestation of noradrenergic dysregulation (Schittecatte et al. 1992). Sleep cycle alterations observed in depressed patients include early onset of the first REM sleep period (Taub 1984). Impaired immune function during depressive episodes may occur (particularly in severely depressed older subjects) as a result of alteration in corticotropin or beta endorphin levels.

Some biological markers of the hypothalamic–pituitary–adrenal axis noted in depressed adults have been found in depressed children. Weller and Weller (1988) summarized findings of dexamethasone suppression test studies in children and adolescents with major depression. As in depressed adults, increased baseline cortisol secretion and nonsuppression of cortisol after dexamethasone administration were found. REM sleep abnormalities have not been reported in depressed children and adolescents (Puig-Antich et al. 1982). Studies of growth hormone secretion have yielded mixed results, with both hypo- and hypersecretion of growth hormone reported in depressed children. An important question is whether these markers are present before adolescence or are related to neural development and/or hormonal events at puberty. In a recent study of prepubertal children with MDD and their controls, depressed children secreted less cortisol and depressed girls secreted more prolactin when their serotonergic systems were stimulated (Ryan et al. 1992). Depressed children have also shown alterations in circadian activity rhythm, similar to those seen in depressed adults (Teicher et al. 1993).

Neuroanatomy of Depression

Few systematic studies have examined the neuroanatomy of depression and mania in children and adolescents. Inferences about the anatomic basis of these disorders are based on adult studies and implicate cortical and subcortical structures. Basal ganglia involvement was suggested when smaller caudate volumes were found in depressed adults (Krishnan et al. 1992). An association between left cerebral hemisphere damage—particularly the left frontal region—and depression has been reported (Robinson et al. 1984; Starkstein & Robinson 1989). Patients with left basal ganglia or left frontal cortex lesions had more frequent episodes of major depression than did patients with left posterior cortical or subcortical lesions (Starkstein, Robinson & Price 1987). These studies may have significance for understanding the effects of lateralized lesions in depressed children. In contrast to adult studies, however, studies investigating the neuroanatomical basis of depression in children have suggested that, in children, major depression may represent a reversible physiological disturbance of right brain function. This right brain disorder may also lead to attentional deficits and learning disorder symptoms (Staton, Wilson & Brumback 1981; Weinberg & Emslie 1988).

Lesion-induced depressive episodes have been reported as being indistinguishable from endogenous depression, and both groups of patients responded well to antidepressant medication (Lipsey et al. 1984). Drug treatment studies have also provided some evidence of the role of norepinephrine and serotonin in depression. Drugs that increase biogenic amines have antidepressant effects. Drugs that reduce biogenic amines and serotonin encourage depression. Whether decreased levels of metabolites of serotonin (5-HIAA) and norepinephrine (MHPG) in the cerebrospinal fluid (CSF) of depressed subjects reflects decreased production or decreased uptake of these neurotransmitters is still controversial.

Bipolar Disorder and Mania

Mania—including hypomanic and cyclothymic episodes—is relatively uncommon in childhood, but it does occur. Individuals affected typically have high rates of familial affective disorder. Bipolar disorder typically emerges in late childhood and adolescence in susceptible individuals. Mania may present as irritability, extreme emotional lability, hyperactivity, inattention, impulsivity, or extreme excitability, in association with aggressive, antisocial behavior and verbal abuse (Nieman and Delong 1987). Psychosis may be present during severe attacks (Ballenger, Reus & Post 1982). Hyperactivity may be episodic rather than continuous, mimicking ADHD (Weinberg & Brumback 1976).

Mania may also occur following psychostimulant treatment. The use of antidepressants may result in *switching*—the development of mania during treatment for a depressive episode. A high prevalence of bipolar disorder was observed in relatives of children treated with tricyclic antidepressants. Children treated with tricyclic antidepressants also developed mania (rather than hypomania) at a higher rate than did those who went untreated (Geller, Fox & Fletcher 1993).

Neuroanatomy of Mania

Right cerebral hemisphere injuries—particularly those involving anterior temporal regions—have been linked to manic symptoms in adults, although mania may not evolve until several years after a lesion is sustained (Shukla et al. 1987). Presenting symptoms included irritability, sleeplessness, grandiosity, and assaultiveness. Manic episodes were reported following cortical (Bakchine et al. 1989), limbic (Starkstein et al. 1987), and other subcortical lesions, such as thalamic lesions (Cummings & Mendez 1984; Kulsievsky, Berthier & Pujol 1993; Migliorelli et al. 1993). Temporal basal polar lesions were reported to produce secondary mania (Jorge et al. 1993). Contrary to reports in the adult literature of mania following right hemisphere damage, childhood mania may involve left-hemisphere limbic system dysfunction. For example, abnormal right-limb motor signs have been reported in children during the manic state that disappeared with recovery (Weinberg & Brumback 1976; Weinberg & Emslie 1988).

Conditions Co-Morbid with Mood Disorder

Co-morbid psychiatric disorder is present in many children diagnosed with mood disorders. For example, additional psychiatric diagnoses are present in 80% of depressed children and in more than 90% of those with dysthymia (Biederman et al. 1991; Biederman et al. 1992; Kovacs et al. 1984*a,* 1984*b*). Another common combination is *double depression*—a major depressive episode superimposed on chronic dysthymia.

Depressed children often present with symptoms that are features of other childhood psychiatric conditions, for example, acting-out, negativism, social discomfort, withdrawal, attentional variability. These symptoms may not be sufficient to warrant a second (co-morbid) diagnosis. There are two childhood conditions that are frequently co-morbid with depression, ADHD and conduct disorder (CD).

Attention Deficit Hyperactivity Disorder

Attention deficit hyperactivity disorder is a heterogeneous disorder characterized by inattention, impulsivity, and hyperactivity occurring to a greater degree than would be expected for a child of that age (American Psychiatric Association 1987). ADHD is frequently co-morbid with mood disorder (Brumback 1988). Nearly 60% of depressed children show attentional deficits (Staton, Wilson & Brumback 1981). Relatives of children with ADHD and ADHD plus mood disorder are at higher risk for affective disorder (Biederman et al. 1991). Bipolar disorder may be manifested in childhood as hyperactivity and disruptive behavior disorder, mimicking ADHD (Bowring & Kovacs 1992; Nieman & Delong 1987). Children with ADHD may evolve into depressed adolescents.

Conduct Disorder

Conduct disorder (CD) is characterized by "a persistent pattern of conduct in which the basic rights of others and major age-appropriate societal norms or rules are violated" (American Psychiatric Association, 1987, p. 53). Depression occurs in conduct-disordered adolescents at a rate higher than that expected for the general population. Reportedly, 23% of 13- to 15-year-olds in a correctional facility met research criteria for major depression (Chiles, Miller & Cox 1980). High rates of CD also occur in adolescents with major depression. In a group of depressed prepubertal males, 37% also met full criteria for CD (Puig-Antich et al. 1982).

A careful history can help determine whether the conduct disorder or the mood disturbance occurred first. In primary CD, antisocial acts are the initial event and are usually more chronic and severe. In primary mood disorder, CD usually begins after the onset of affective symptoms, and there is a better prognosis than with primary CD. Adolescents with CD may be at higher risk for suicidal behavior, because of increased impulsivity and aggressivity, even though they do not appear to be as depressed as do purely affectively ill children.

Neuropsychological Studies of Mood Disorder

Early studies of the neuropsychology of childhood mood disorders suggested that symptoms in children differed from those seen in adults. More recent conceptualizations suggest that similar processes are involved in children and adults, although specific aspects pertinent to the developing child are still being delineated.

The general intellectual ability of depressed children does not differ from that of normal children (Kashani et al. 1983; Weinberg et al. 1973; Weiner & Pfeffer 1986), but weak negative correlations between severity of depression and intelligence have been found in epidemiological studies (Lefkowitz & Tesiny 1985; Tesiny, Lefkowitz & Gordon 1980). Longitudinal studies of childhood-onset depression found evidence of persistent cognitive and social problems into adulthood (Kovacs & Goldston 1991).

Depression may selectively affect certain neuropsychological functions (for instance, attention, psychomotor speed, and coordination) while leaving other functions (such as verbal skills) relatively intact (Kaslow et al. 1983). Lowered performance (visuomotor/visuospatial) subtest scores on the Wechsler Intelligence Scale for Children during depressive episodes have been reported (Kovacs & Goldston 1991). Depressed children were especially impaired on block design and anagram tasks (Kaslow et al. 1983; Mullins, Siegel & Hodges 1985). A higher error rate on the Matching Familiar Figures Test has also been found (Schwartz et al. 1982). Depressed children often exhibit impaired academic performance, proportionate to the severity of their depression (Brumback 1988; Lefkowitz & Tesiny 1985). While depressed adolescents may appear to process social cues and solve social problems competently, they may be hampered by a negative self-evaluation (Marton et al. 1993).

Childhood depression has been reported in children with a left hemisyndrome—that is, left-sided neurological signs, clumsiness, visuospatial skill deficit, and impaired processing of nonverbal social signals (Brumback 1988; Brumback, Jackoway & Weinberg 1980). Interestingly, specific cognitive deficits noted during depressive episodes may resolve following treatment or predict a good response to treatment. In particular, the relationship of verbal IQ to performance IQ has been shown to predict treatment response to electroconvulsive therapy (Warneke 1975), as well as response to pharmacologic treatment (Ossofsky 1974; Wilson & Staton 1984).

TOURETTE'S SYNDROME

Tourette's syndrome (TS), first described in 1885 by Georges Gilles de la Tourette, was initially considered to be a rare condition. Prevalence rates of 1 per 1000 for boys and 1 per 10,000 for girls (Apter et al. 1993; Comings, Himes & Comings 1990; Shapiro et al. 1988) may be underestimates, however, since some individuals have subtle signs or may be unaware of the significance of their symptoms. For example, in a kindred of 159 members, Kurlan et al. (1987) identified 54 who had either vocal or motor tics. Of those affected, 30% were unaware of their tics, and only 18.5% sought medical attention.

The genetic pattern of TS is consistent with autosomal dominant inheritance, with incomplete, sex-specific penetrance and variable expression (Pauls & Leckman 1986; van de Wetering & Heutink 1993; see also Chapter 3). The male-to-female ratio of incidence is approximately 3:1. Penetrance is nearly complete for males, considering only tics. Tics occur in about 50% of females. If symptoms of obsessive compulsive disorder (OCD) are included, penetrance estimates increase to 70%. Over 50% of the human genome has been searched for the TS gene (Pakstis et al. 1991). Epigenetic prenatal factors also appear correlated with tic severity (Leckman et al. 1990).

The disorder first appears in childhood, at around the age of 7 years. Head and facial muscles are affected in a waxing and waning fashion, followed by the emergence of vocal tics months or years later. Vocal tics may be simple phenomena (for instance, sniffing, hissing, humming, or coughing) or they may take more complex forms involving repetition of sounds, words, and phrases. Coprolalia (obscenity utterance), once considered a hallmark of the disorder, is present in only about 30% of diagnosed cases. Various instruments with good interrater reliability and concurrent validity have been developed for measuring tic severity (Walkup et al. 1992). A tic disorder classification has recently been published (Tourette Syndrome Classification Study Group 1993). Tourette syndrome is not purely a motor phenomenon. Some 75% to 90% of TS patients report premonitory sensations ("sensory tics") that are temporarily relieved by performing the tic.

Spontaneous exacerbations and remissions characterize TS. Symptoms typically increase during periods of increased stress and anxiety. Tics can be suppressed voluntarily for short periods of time. These periods may be associated with a distinct internal experience of mounting inner tension, with short-lived feelings of relief occurring after ticing (Kurlan, Lichter & Hewitt, 1989). TS symptoms are generally most severe during adolescence and decrease in severity by early adulthood. Goetz et al. (1992) reported that, although tics persisted in 58 adults studied, they were rated moderate/severe in only 24% as opposed to 60% at time of worst function (adolescence for most subjects). The rate of coprolalia declined from 22% in adolescence to 4% among adults. Even severe tics during childhood did not predict adult tic severity. However, severe tics in late adolescence were associated with severe adult tics.

Conditions Co-Morbid With Tourette's Syndrome

Attention deficit hyperactivity disorder occurs in about half of TS patients—more commonly in males than in females. ADHD symptomatology appears earlier than TS and may be more impairing. Comings and Comings (1984) proposed that TS and ADHD might be varying expressions of the same genetic condition, but it is currently thought that ADHD is genetically distinct from TS (Pauls et al. 1986).

Although TS and OCD have different clinical symptomatologies, they may be closely linked genetically and/or be different manifestations of the same neural dysfunction; for instance, they co-occur in families and are frequently co-morbid in the same individual. Significantly more first-degree relatives of TS patients had OCD than were found in the general population or in a control sample of adoptive relatives (Pauls, Towbin & Leckman 1986). Leonard et al. (1992) followed 54 children initially diagnosed as having OCD (excluding those with diagnosed TS) for 2 to 7 years. Six of these children later developed TS. The group with OCD and TS differed in three ways from those with OCD alone: more symptoms of anxiety; a greater baseline ratio of CSF 5-hydroxyindoleacetic acid to homovanillic acid (suggesting a disturbance in the serotonin/dopamine ratio); and a younger age of onset of OCD.

Neuroanatomy of Tourette's Syndrome

Basal ganglia dysfunction or the cortical–striatal–nigral–thalamocortical (CSNTC) loops may underly TS (Alexander, DeLong & Strick, 1988). These multiple, precisely somatotopically mapped circuits give rise to a "vast range of behavior, thoughts and feelings that are somewhat fragmentary in character when considered in isolation" (Leckman et al. 1991, p. 94). Stereotypies resembling TS tics have been produced in animals by electrical stimulation of the putamen, and by application of amphetamine to this region (Kelley, Lang & Gauthier 1988). Neurosurgical lesions that interfere with CSNTC circuits have been used to control tics (de Divitiis, D'Errico & Cerillo 1977), but risks are associated with this treatment method (Leckman et al. 1993). Tics can be effectively controlled with neuroleptics (such as haloperidol) that selectively block dopamine-2 (D_2) receptors (Seignot 1961).

TS movements involve complex motor programs that may be subserved by subcortical areas, without cortical representation of the movement sequences. For example, a young woman who had TS/OCD exhibited markedly suppressed tics while she was learning sign language. As she became proficient, however, sign language gestures began to be incorporated into her tic repertoire. Initially, the sign-tics were related to her thinking at the moment, but later they became unrelated. Thus, the motor programs generating signs might be voluntary (used with communicative intent) or involuntary (occurring without intention) (Lang, Consky & Sandor 1993). Longstanding, simple tics do not have the premovement cortical readiness electrophysiological potential that is noted in voluntary movements (Obcso, Rothwell & Marsden 1981).

Support for the notion that basal ganglia pathology is involved in TS comes from both postmortem and neuroradiological studies. Hypoplasia of the putamen and caudate nuclei and increased numbers of neuronal cell bodies in the basal ganglia, with small nuclei that resemble those found in young infants, have been found in autopsied TS patients (Haber et al. 1986; Richardson 1982). A significant increase in the number of striatal presynaptic dopamine carrier sites, attributed to an excessive number of dopamine afferent terminals in the striatum, has also been reported in postmortem studies (Singer, Hahn & Moran 1991).

Hypofunction of the basal ganglia and the frontal and temporal regions in TS was demonstrated by single-photon emission computed tomography (SPECT) techniques (Hall et al. 1990) and by positron emission tomography (PET) techniques (Stoetter et al. 1992). In a SPECT study of 9 TS subjects, researchers found a reduction in ,CBF in the left lenticular nucleus and in the right frontal cortex (Riddle et al. 1992). Normal controls had a left-greater-than-right basal ganglia asymmetry that was not present in TS patients (Peterson et al. 1993; Singer et al. 1993).

Kurlan (1992) proposed a neuropathological model for TS. He noted that the brain regions affected in TS (striatum and limbic structures) are involved in reproductive behaviors. These brain areas are highly influenced by sex hormones. This may explain licking, sucking, smelling, and pelvic thrusting tics, obscene gestures, and obscene language. Kurlan suggested that sex hormones enhance neuronal damage caused by excitotoxic amino acids, resulting in neuronal damage and decreased neuronal numbers. Autopsy studies (described earlier) that found numerous small neurons resembling those seen early in development and evidence of excessive dopamine innervation within the striatum support this theory.

OBSESSIVE COMPULSIVE DISORDER

A century ago, Tuke (1894) recognized that obsessive compulsive disorder lies at the borderland of psychiatry and neurology, and that it involves a neural mechanism. Understanding the pathophysiology of OCD may provide important insight into the neurobiology of cognition.

The two core diagnostic features of OCD are *obsessions* (ideas, thoughts, or impulses experienced as intrusive and ego-dystonic, which the affected person often tries to ignore, suppress, or resist) and *compulsions* (repetitive, intentional behaviors, performed in stereotypical fashion, often in response to obsessive thoughts or to ward off dreaded events). Three common obsessions in children are worries over body secretions, dirt, germs, or environmental toxins, with contamination themes predominating; fears that something terrible might happen to self or to loved ones; and preoccupation with symmetry, exactness, or order. Less common symptoms include preoccupation with special numbers; sexual and aggressive thoughts or impulses; and intrusive music or words. Common compulsions include excessive washing or grooming (often in response to obsessions about contamination); checking behaviors; ritualized touching, ordering, and rearranging (often in response to obsessions about orderliness); and various measures to prevent harm to self or to loved ones. The washing and grooming behaviors can be viewed as phylogenetically old (Swedo 1989). When symptoms in an individual were observed longitudinally, the specific symptom *content* was found to be quite variable (Rettew et al. 1992).

Symptoms may become severe enough to lead to functional impairment in family relationships, in schoolwork, or in social relationships with peers. Rituals may consume several hours every day. Concern about contamination may lead to an agoraphobic, housebound state. Since it may be difficult to obtain a full history and description of symptoms from a child in such cases, parent interview is essential in the beginning stages of an OCD evaluation. Several structured questionnaires for the diagnosis of OCD are available. These include the Leyton Obsessional Inventory, Child Version (LOI-CV) (Cooper 1970); a 44-item structured diagnostic interview with a 20-item survey form (Berg, Rapoport & Flament 1985); and the Yale-Brown Obsessive Compulsive Scale Symptom Checklist (Y-BOCS) (Goodman, Price, Rasmusson, Mazure, Delgado et al. 1989; Goodman, Price, Rasmusson, Mazure, Fleischman et al. 1989).

Prevalence of OCD in children and adolescents has been estimated to fall in the range of 0.2% to 1.9% (Flament et al. 1988). The frequency of this disorder may be underestimated, however, since adolescents may hide their symptoms. An estimate more likely to be accurate is in the 1.9% to 3.3% range (Karno et al. 1988). Rates of OCD are higher than normal in first-degree relatives of patients with OCD (Swedo, Rapoport et al. 1989) and among monozygotic twins (81%) versus dizygotic twins (47%) (Carey & Gottesman 1981). Subclinical symptoms (but not OCD proper) are increased in first-degree relatives (Hoover & Insel 1984). Co-morbid psychiatric conditions in OCD include depression, secondary depression in response to distress generated by OCD, anxiety disorder, and ADHD.

Several different treatment approaches are used for OCD: behavioral, pharmacological, and surgical. Behavioral therapies that employ principles of exposure and response prevention are of value in some cases. Psychopharmacological treatment involves using drugs that affect the neurotransmitter serotonin. Inhibitors of serotonin reuptake, such as clomipramine and fluoxetine (DeVeaugh-Geiss 1991), act to prevent the reuptake of serotonin at the postsynaptic junction (Rapoport 1991). However, OCD remains a chronic disorder despite the availability of these treatments. Surgical procedures such as cingulotomy may be of benefit in intractable cases (Kanner et al. 1993).

Neuroanatomy of Obsessive Compulsive Disorder

What brain structures are implicated in OCD behaviors? OCD-like behaviors occur in other neurological disorders, such as postencephalitic parkinsonism (Schilder 1938), Sydenham's chorea (Swedo, Rapoport et al. 1989), Huntington's chorea (Cummings & Cunningham 1992), bilateral globus pallidus necrosis (Laplane et al. 1984), orbital-frontal cortical damage (Eslinger & Damasio 1985), and frontal and basal ganglia lesions (Insel 1992). Electrophysiological, neuroimaging, and clinical observations suggest that OCD involves dysfunction in the neural circuit involving the orbital-frontal lobe, the head of the caudate, the nucleus accumbens, the ventral pallidum, and the dorsal medial nucleus of the thalamus (which projects to orbital frontal cortex) (Modell et al. 1989).

Although not all computerized tomographic (CT) and magnetic resonance imaging (MRI) studies have revealed structural pathology in OCD, one CT scan study found decreased caudate volume (Luxenberg et al. 1988). An MRI study suggested frontal cortical abnormalities, particularly right frontal (Garber, Ananth et al. 1989).

A number of PET scan studies in untreated OCD patients found increases in orbital frontal activity (left and/or right) (Baxter et al. 1988; Nordahl et al. 1989; Swedo, Schapiro et al. 1989; Sawle et al. 1991). Changes in SPECT and PET in response to both pharmacologic *and* behavioral treatment of OCD (Baxter et al. 1992), while interesting, do not completely agree with PET studies of untreated patients. With treatment, activity in various frontal lobe areas and in the basal ganglia decreased. At $2\frac{1}{2}$ to 4 months into therapy, changes in the caudate were observed (Baxter et al. 1992); changes occurred in the frontal regions after 12 months of treatment (Swedo et al. 1992). OCD subjects, compared to controls, had increased uptake in orbital-frontal cortex, in mesial aspects of the frontal lobes, in left posterofrontal cortex, in the dorsal parietal region, and in cingulate cortex (Machlin et al. 1991; Rubin et al. 1992). Caudate and orbital changes were found after 16 weeks of treatment (Benkelfat et al. 1990). After 20 months of treatment, orbital-frontal cortex changes were found (Swedo, Schapiro et al. 1989).

Neuropsychological Studies of TS and OCD

Neuropsychological studies of patients with TS or OCD found cognitive set shifting and visual-spatial deficits, consistent with right frontal dysfunction. Deficits in visuospatial function and praxis have been reported in TS patients (Bornstein, Carroll & King 1986; Bornstein, King & Carroll 1983; Incagnoli & Kane 1981; Sutherland et al. 1982) and in OCD patients (Hollander ct al. 1991; Boone et al. 1991; Christensen et al. 1992). In a study of 10 nonmedicated TS children, 5 had significant performance IQ > verbal IQ differences and decreased written and verbal arithmetic scores (Ferrari, Matthews & Barabas 1984). Performances on the Bender-Gestalt and Draw-a-Person tests were also impaired. Scores were significantly impaired on the Peabody Picture Vocabulary Test—Revised, a receptive language test. Head, Bolton & Hymas (1989) reported that OCD subjects, who had significantly higher ventricular–brain ratios than normal, also had deficits on the Rey-Osterrieth Complex Figure, stylus maze learning, and Money Road Map tests. "Soft" signs implicating greater right hemisphere than left hemisphere involvement have also been reported (Behar et al. 1984; Hollander et al. 1990; Hollander et al. 1991). Hollander et al. (1991) found a correlation between the severity of the soft signs and the severity of obsessions.

Children with TS who were of normal intelligence, but on neuroleptics or clonidine for TS, were divided into high-severity and low-severity OCD groups. Although both groups' Halstead-Reitan battery performance was within normal limits, the high OCD group had significantly lower Categories Achieved and significantly higher Perseverative Error scores on the Wisconsin

Card Sorting Test than the low OCD group. These differences were unaccounted for by demographic measures, concurrent medication, or full-scale IQ (Bornstein 1991). Devinsky et al. (1993) studied a small sample of patients with severe TS and found that these patients showed better than average skills for processing social signals.

SCHIZOPHRENIA

The diagnosis of schizophrenia is based on several characteristic psychotic symptoms: bizarre delusions, hallucinations, incoherence or marked loosening of associations, catatonia, and flat or inappropriate affect (American Psychiatric Association, 1994). These must represent a decline from a previous level of functioning, must be present continuously for at least 6 months, and cannot be attributable to schizoaffective disorder, mood disorder with psychotic features, or specific organic causes.

Schizophrenic symptomatology may be divided into positive symptoms (florid psychotic hallucinations and delusions) and negative symptoms (flat affect, social withdrawal, lack of initiative and motivation, poor insight, and poor judgment). Heterogeneity of clinical presentation is emphasized by those who consider it a syndrome rather than a disease (Carpenter et al. 1993). Heterogeneity is relevant to the neuropsychologist because it holds out the possibility that researchers may eventually be able to define clinical subtypes that have different neuropsychological test profiles reflecting different patterns of brain dysfunction. Several different subtypes have been proposed, including schizophrenics with primary versus transient negative symptoms (Carpenter et al. 1991; Carpenter, Heinrichs & Wagman 1988) and deficit versus nondeficit (Buchanan et al. 1990); and subtypes based on test evidence of psychomotor poverty versus disorganization versus reality distortion (Liddle 1987; Liddle & Morris 1991).

The prevalence of schizophrenia in the general population is about 1%. This rises to 12% among children who have one schizophrenic parent, to 40% among children who have two affected parents, and to 47% among monozygotic twins of schizophrenic subjects. Twins reared by adoptive parents develop schizophrenia at the same rate as siblings raised by biological parents. Genetic predisposition is apparent in patients with full-blown psychotic disorder and in a spectrum of schizotypal personality disorders (social isolation, oddness, aloofness, and cold demeanor) in relatives (Kendler 1988; Parnas et al. 1993). Pre-, peri-, and postnatal encephalopathic factors may increase the risk of disorder in genetically susceptible individuals (Andreasen et al. 1986; Cannon, Mednick & Parnas 1989).

Peak age of onset of schizophrenia occurs at about age 26 years for men and age 30 years for women (Lewine 1988). Prodromal symptoms include social isolation, impaired social functioning, peculiar behavior, poor personal hygiene, blunted affect, communication disturbance, odd beliefs, unusual perceptual experiences, and/or marked lack of initiative (American Psychiatric Association 1994).

Neuroanatomy of Schizophrenia

Considerable evidence indicates that the underlying neuropathology of schizophrenia is related to neural networks involving the dorsolateral prefrontal region, anterior cingulate, parietal association areas, the temporal lobe, and the caudate and ventral striatum. These regions are widely distributed and extensively interconnected. The neuropathological changes observed are consistent with a perturbation of normal brain development in the fetus. A detailed review of this area is beyond the scope of this chapter, but the following brief review of selected neurobiological and neuropsychological issues in adults is relevant to a discussion of childhood schizophrenia.

Neuropathological Findings in Adult Schizophrenics

Neuropathological studies have demonstrated a number of changes in the brain of schizophrenics: decreased cell density in the anterior cingulate and prefrontal cortices (Benes, Davidson & Bird 1986; Benes & Bird 1987); increased numbers of long, vertical, association axons in the anterior cingulate cortex (Benes et al. 1987); enlargement of the temporal horns (Brown et al. 1986); decreased volume of the hippocampus and disorientation of hippocampal pyramidal cells (Falkai & Bogerts 1986; Kovelman & Scheibel 1984); decreased thickness of the parahippocampal gyrus (Brown et al. 1986); and decreased neuronal cell count and cytoarchitectural changes in the entorhinal cortex (Jakob & Beckmann 1986; Falkai, Bogerts & Rozumak 1988). In addition to limbic system changes, basal ganglia regions that are interconnected with the limbic cortex show evidence of anomalous development (Bogerts, Meertz & Schonfeldt-Bausch 1985). Only the rostral and intermediate portions of the entorhinal cortex showed anomalous development. These areas receive input from higher-order sensory association areas and prefrontal areas, and project to the hippocampus and to an array of subcortical structures, as well as to orbital-frontal cortex. Since the entorhinal cortex is one of the earliest to develop, investigators have postulated that disruption of entorhinal cortical neurons results in a rerouting of incoming fibers from association areas (see Chapter 2), with resulting anomalous prefrontal system development. This leads to disrupted reality testing and impaired neuropsychological function. Feinberg (1987) proposed that the onset of psychotic symptoms during adolescence is related to the age-related decline in synaptic proliferation that occurs in frontal cortex.

CT studies in adults have found consistent differences between the brains of schizophrenics and the brains of controls. Schizophrenics—even first-episode, drug-naive patients—had enlarged third and lateral ventricles and increased sulcal size, suggesting decreased brain mass (Nyback, Berggren & Hindmarsh 1982; Schulz et al. 1983), particularly in the prefrontal region (Shelton &

Weinberger 1986). Enlarged ventricle-to-brain ratios in the frontal region were correlated with deficits in intelligence, conceptual thinking, immediate verbal memory, and psychomotor speed (Keilp et al. 1988). In contrast, the ventricle-to-brain ratio posteriorly was associated only with deficits in verbal memory and motor speed. Correlations between ventricular enlargement and perinatal encephalopathic insult (Williams et al. 1985) and poor premorbid social adjustment (Weinberger et al. 1980) have been reported. These changes were not secondary to institutionalization or neuroleptic medication (Illowsky et al. 1988), suggesting chronicity antedating the initial clinical episode, and unrelated to the disease process and treatment.

Magnetic resonance imaging and CT scan studies have been positively correlated (Kelsoe et al. 1988). Temporal lobe gray-matter volume in schizophrenics was 20% less than in controls; no differences were found in prefrontal areas (Suddath et al. 1989). Subtle abnormalities were detected in a study of monozygotic twins discordant for schizophrenia. Smaller anterior hippocampi and enlarged lateral and third ventricles in the schizophrenics suggested that extragenetic factors were involved (Suddath et al. 1990).

Franzen and Ingvar (1975) found that cerebral blood flow ($_r$CBF) was decreased in schizophrenics in the resting state compared to cerebral blood flow in controls. They found a more profound decrease for the more withdrawn and impaired patient. Subsequent $_r$CBF and PET scan studies have produced inconsistent results. Methodological differences between studies may have contributed to this failure to replicate findings. For example, using the Wisconsin Card Sorting Test (WCST)—a task associated with dorsolateral, prefrontal cortex function—Weinberger, Berman, and Zec (1986) found substantial cerebral metabolic activity differences between schizophrenics and controls. An inverse correlation existed between ventricular size and rCBF during WCST administration that was not seen during control cognitive tasks. Schizophrenics with enlarged ventricles also had diffusely lower cortical gray-matter blood flow (Berman et al. 1987). Another PET study found that actively psychotic schizophrenics had lower regional cerebral metabolic rates of glucose utilization in the hippocampus and anterior cingulate, but not in neocortical areas or extrapyramidal regions (Tamminga et al. 1992). A subgroup of deficit syndrome patients manifested thalamic, frontal, and parietal hypometabolism, whereas the nondeficit patients had normal metabolic patterns.

Neurotransmitter Studies in Adult Schizophrenics

The "dopamine hypothesis" of schizophrenia (Meltzer & Stahl 1976; see review by Davis et al. 1991) postulated that the dopaminergic system was dysregulated in the direction of *hyper*dopaminergia. The initial formulation was based on the clinical observation that neuroleptics that block the dopamine receptor constitute one of the most effective classes of drugs for controlling schizophrenic symptoms. Their clinical potency is directly proportional to striatal dopamine receptor binding in vitro (Creese, Burt & Snyder 1976). Not all schizophrenics, however, respond to neuroleptics; and some schizophrenic symptoms, such as deficit symptoms, do not improve with neuroleptic treatment. New drugs such as clozapine have a weak affinity for D_2 receptors but are highly effective in schizophrenia treatment. Furthermore, the metabolite of dopamine, homovanillic acid (HVA) is either normal or low in schizophrenics. The density of dopamine D_2 receptors was shown to be consistently elevated in postmortem specimens of schizophrenic brains (Seeman et al. 1987)—even in schizophrenics who were never exposed to neuroleptics (Joyce et al. 1988). Finally, since the initial dopamine hypothesis was formulated, it has become apparent that not one but several "dopamine systems" exist (including nigrostriatal, mesolimbic, and mesocortical), each with different cell bodies and a different anatomical distribution. Moreover, an array of dopamine receptors (D_3, D_4, and D_5) have now been cloned, each with different patterns of distribution and drug affinities. For example, clozapine targets the D_4 receptor. Seeman et al. (1993) demonstrated that the level of D_4 receptor was six times higher in the schizophrenic brain than in controls.

The most significant factor weighing against simple hyperdopaminergia is the finding of *hypo*dopaminergia in the prefrontal cortex (mesocortical dopaminergic system) of schizophrenics (Weinberger 1987). Thus, a new formulation of the dopamine hypothesis in schizophrenia asserts that there is relative hyperdominergia subcortically and hypodominergia at the cortical level. This apparent paradox can be resolved by recent clinical observations and experimental studies that suggested that lesioning or otherwise decreasing cortical dopamine results in increased subcortical dopamine (Pycock, Kerwin & Carter 1980; Haroutunian, Knott & Davis 1988). Weinberger (1987) postulated that the dorsolateral prefrontal cortical hypofunction (which causes negative or deficit symptoms) results in disinhibition of mesolimbic dopaminergic neurons. This triggers an increase in subcortical dopamine, leading to psychotic symptoms attributable to hyperdopaminergia. Davis et al. (1991) also emphasized that the heterogeneity of schizophrenic symptoms, coupled with patient age, might result in differences in dopaminergic activity. Thus, there may be differences between young schizophrenics with prominent positive symptoms and old schizophrenics with predominantly negative/deficit symptoms.

Other neurotransmitters have also been implicated in schizophrenia. For example, glutamate plays an important role in learning and memory (Collingridge 1987) and is markedly lower in prefrontal cortex in untreated schizophrenics compared to controls (Deutsch et al. 1989) Laruelle et al. (1993) reported that serotonin$_2$ receptors and uptake sites were decreased in prefrontal cortex of chronic schizophrenics, compared to their presence in occipital cortex in the same subjects and in both prefrontal and occipital cortices in controls. Norepinephrine activity was shown to be increased in a subgroup of schizophrenics (van Kammen and Gelernter 1987), and GABA was reported to be decreased.

While deficit symptoms are linked to hypofunction of prefrontal cortex, hallucinations (a positive symptom) may involve diminished activity in cortical language areas and increased activity in striatal regions. Cleghorn et al. (1992) studied schizophrenics who did and did not experience auditory hallucinations. All were unmedicated at initial study, and a subgroup on medication was reexamined one year later. Patients who experienced hallucinations had lower meta-bolic rates in the posterior superior temporal regions of both cerebral hemi-spheres, and higher left striatal metabolic rates than did nonhallucinators. This pattern differed from that seen during processing of incoming external lan-guage, with activation of left perisylvian cortex (Mazziotta, Phelps & Carson 1982). Neuroleptic treatment resulted in increased cortical metabolic rates and decreased striatal metabolic rates.

Smooth-pursuit eye tracking (see Chapter 4) is often impaired in schizo-phrenics (Abel et al. 1991) and was considered sufficiently specific to represent a biological marker. Children of schizophrenics have shown impairment (Holz-man et al. 1988), although it was not possible to separate the effects of age-related task difficulty from incipient pathology (Ross, Radant & Hommer 1993). It may be that intrusive saccades—possibly a manifestation of prefrontal cortex dysfunction (Paus et al. 1991)—rather than impaired smooth pursuit, were responsible for these findings (Radant & Hommer, 1992). Another mani-festation of prefrontal dysfunction was the difficulty schizophrenics had in in-hibiting response to a stimulus (Freedman et al. 1983).

Neuropsychological Studies of Schizophrenia

Most schizophrenics are intellectually impaired (Goldberg & Weinberger 1986) and thus experience difficulty on many different tasks. A large body of litera-ture suggests that prefrontal and limbic deficits are prominent (Gray et al. 1991). Schizophrenics had difficulty performing on attribute- and rule-learning paradigms (Bourne et al. 1977). Fey (1951) first noted that young schizophren-ics achieved fewer categories and made more perseverative errors than controls on the WCST. Since then, the impaired WCST performance of schizophrenics has been well studied and replicated (Kolb & Whishaw 1983; Stuss et al. 1983). Goldberg et al. (1987) found that, despite attempts to teach the WCST to attentive schizophrenic patients who could repeat instructions, the schizo-phrenics were unable to master the task. They had no difficulty learning a selective reminding test, suggesting that their WCST failure was not the result of a more general learning or memory deficit. Schizophrenics also had diffi-culty suppressing interference and inappropriate mental activity on the Stroop Interference Task (Stroop 1935; Golden 1978). Liddle (1987) reported that schizophrenics failed to maintain attention and to operate at an abstract level. Language and some memory functions were another area of deficit (Levin, Yurgelun-Todd & Craft, 1989). Verbal memory deficits include impaired ver-bal recall (Koh 1978), accelerated forgetting (Calev, Venables & Monk 1983), and impaired new learning (Calev, Berlin & Lerer 1987). The clinical blunting and dysregulation of emotional displays in schizophrenics is mirrored in im-paired performance on neuropsychological tests that assess facial affect recog-nition (Kline, Smith & Ellis 1992) and facial affective displays (Pitman et al. 1987).

One problem that confronts the neuropsychologist in any attempt to evaluate cognitive performance in schizophrenia is the difficulty of disentangling specific deficit from more general cognitive deficit. It is also necessary to equate different cognitive tasks in terms of psychometric properties. This can be done with standardized residual scores or by manipulating test conditions. Neuropsychological studies that employ such techniques have found selective differences in semantic memory, visual memory, and verbal learning in schizophrenic patients compared to matched normal controls (Saykin et al. 1991). Whether such methods overcome baseline differences between schizophrenics and controls remains controversial (Blanchard & Neale 1994).

Schizophrenia in Childhood

Early-onset ("prepubertal") schizophrenia is rare. From 1960 to 1980, the term *schizophrenia* was used for other severe childhood psychoses. The DSM-IV diagnosis of schizophrenia in children is based on the same criteria as are used for adults, except that among children the expected level of social development is not achieved (American Psychiatric Association 1994). The early-onset type differs from the later-appearing form in several ways: the persons affected are predominantly boys; onset is somewhat more insidious; a tighter association exists with more neurodevelopmental abnormalities; more strikingly "odd" premorbid personalities tend to emerge; delusions are less well-formed; resistance to antipsychotic drug treatment is greater; outcome is usually poorer; and a more obvious family history of schizophrenia is present (Beitchman 1985). Careful follow-up to validate diagnosis is necessary, since childhood schizophrenia can easily be confounded with other forms of psychosis.

Eggers (1978) reported on retrospective and follow-up data (for a median length of 15 years) on 57 schizophrenic children. About half (46.5%) had unremarkable early development, while 54.4% experienced difficulties with adaptive behavior, self-assertiveness, and relatedness. Premorbid personality development was related to outcome. In this study, 20% of patients recovered completely, 30% reached good social adjustment, and 50% continued to have problems.

Precursors of Schizophrenia in Childhood:
Identification of the Child at Risk

If schizophrenia is the result of a genetically programmed disturbance in neurogenesis and typically does not become clinically apparent until adolescence or early adulthood, certain markers might be present before the appearance of the full-blown syndrome. The term *pandysmaturation (PDM)* has been used to describe these precursors. It has been postulated that individuals at risk for schizophrenia—the offspring of schizophrenics who inherit the gene—also inherit a neurointegrative defect that is apparent early in infancy (Fish et al., 1992). This postulated neurointegrative defect does not predict the evolution of full-blown psychosis, but rather supports a spectrum of behaviors related to schizotypal personality disorder. Bender and Freedman (1952) identified three criteria that define PDM and occur within the first 2 years of life (usually appearing by 9 months): transient retardation of gross motor and/or visuomotor development, followed by an accelerated developmental rate back into the normal growth curve; an abnormal profile of function on a single developmental examination and, therefore, a spotty pattern of successes and failures (characteristically, the child fails simple items and succeeds on more complicated ones); and an accompanying retardation of skeletal growth. This combination of varied cognitive profile and fluctuating developmental quotient, coupled with skeletal growth lag, is characteristic of PDM.

Children at risk of developing schizophrenia have a higher incidence of deficits on tasks requiring manual dexterity and fine-motor coordination (Walker & Emory 1983). Evidence indicates that affective disturbances may be present within the first 6 months of life. For example, home movies of the infancy of 32 schizophrenic patients and of 31 healthy siblings were scored objectively. The preschizophrenic group had fewer facial expressions of happiness than controls (Walker et al. 1993). Using ratings of social competence, affective flattening, poverty of speech, and formal thought disorder, Dworkin et al. (1991) noted that children at risk for schizophrenia had more evidence of impaired social competence than did controls by early adolescence. Fish (1986) suggested that schizotypal symptoms may identify some preschizophrenics in early adolescence and pointed out the significance of regressions in academic and cognitive functions, including drops in IQ scores, as indicators of increasing psychopathology.

Longitudinal studies of infants at risk suggested that early signs of developmental disorder are present in some infants. For example, a long-term prospective study evaluated the early appearance of neurointegrative disorder in infants of schizophrenic parents (Fish 1984, 1986). These children (12 at risk and 12 controls) were followed for over 30 years; 7 at-risk infants and 1 control had PDM. The groups did not differ in their proportion of infants with low normal birthweights, but infants with PDM had smaller head circumferences. When seen between ages 27 and 34 years, 6 of the at-risk group had had severe social-affective symptoms since age 3 to 6 years, requiring prolonged treatment.

Neuropsychologists are in a unique position to contribute to the identification of children at risk for schizophrenia. One would expect these children to have impaired attentional capacity (Neuchterlein & Dawson 1984; Rutschmann, Cornblatt & Erlenmeyer-Kimling 1986) and a disturbance in smooth-pursuit eye movements (Holzman et al. 1988). Additional prefrontal, language, and memory deficits and impairment on tests of social competence might be seen. Caplan and colleagues (1989, 1990) reported on a formal thought disorder scale for children that involves systematic analysis of verbal output; this scale may contribute to language impairment analyses in these children. Incipient impaired social competence can also be identified by appropriate tests.

AUTISM

Autism is a life-long developmental impairment resulting in language and non-verbal social communication deficits and a restricted repertoire of activities. Described by Kanner in 1943, when psychodynamic etiologies ("refrigerator parents") were prominent, autism is now considered a result of brain dysfunction although the responsible neural systems involved have yet to be definitively identified. In DSM-IV (American Psychiatric Association 1994), autism is included under the heading Pervasive Developmental Disorder. To be diagnosed as autistic, an individual must meet criteria involving impairment in reciprocal social interaction; impairment in communication; restricted, repetitive, and stereotypic behavior patterns, interests, and activities; and delays or abnormal functioning in at least one of three areas (social interaction, language as social communication, and symbolic or imaginative play), with onset prior to age 3 years. Very few autistic children develop symptoms resembling schizophrenia. This depends, in part, on definitional criteria and the examiner's willingness to accept caretaker interpretations of behaviors (Howells & Guirguis 1984).

Asperger (1944) described a group of patients with "autistic psychopathy" who had seriously impaired interpersonal relationships; idiosyncratic, concrete, perseverative responding; deficient processing of nonverbal, visuospatial stimuli; pedantic, monotonic, and/or exaggerated speech patterns; and motor dysfunction. Arithmetic skill deficits, lack of humor, and gestural comprehension deficits were common (Wing 1981). Asperger's syndrome is recognized in DSM-IV, with estimates ranging from .6 per 10,000 among retarded children to 10–26 per 10,000 among children with normal intelligence.

Prevalence of autism is estimated at 4 to 5 per 10,000 children, and it is 4 or 5 times more common in males than in females. Autism has a genetic basis: siblings of autistic children have an incidence of autism of 2%—a prevalence 50 times greater than that in the general population (Rutter & Schopler 1987). Twin concordance rates strongly suggest a genetic etiology (Steffenberg et al. 1989). Parents of autistics have a greater lifetime prevalence rate of anxiety disorder than do controls, have impaired ability to process social cues (Piven et al. 1991), and have deficits in pragmatic aspects of language (Landa et al. 1992).

Autistic behavior also occurs as a secondary symptom following various encephalopathic insults (Ritvo et al. 1990). The incidence of autism associated with early encephalopathic (hypoxic–ischemic) damage is 7%. Autism was reported to be associated with neurometabolic disorders (such as phenylketonuria) and some acquired brain lesions (such as viral encephalopathy and tuberous sclerosis). Epilepsy occurs in 10% to 30% of autistic children (Deykin & MacMahon 1979; Olsson, Steffenburg & Gillberg 1988; Volkmar & Nelson 1990). Using strict definitional criteria and a limited, 4-year follow-up period, Wong (1993) reported that epilepsy occurred in 6.5% of autistic children. Autistic regression can occur in normally developing children, timed with the onset of seizures. Deonna et al. (1993) described two boys with tuberous sclerosis and seizures involving the limbic system whose autistic behaviors emerged with the seizures and decreased when the seizures were controlled. Chromosomal anomalies are also implicated. Autistic behaviors were described in some fragile-X males (Brown et al. 1982) but not in the majority (Bregman, Leckman & Ort 1988; Reiss & Freund 1990). Gillberg et al. (1991) reported partial trisomy of chromosome 15 in association with autistic behavior.

From a neurobehavioral standpoint, the major deficits in autism may involve several different domains. These children are unable to form reciprocal social relationships, to use language effectively for communication, to engage in symbolic play, and to represent the emotional states of others. They also have motor system disturbances, reflected by the difficulty they experience in programming motor acts and their tendency to engage in motor stereotypies. They have difficulty in adapting to environmental change. Dysfunction of the attentional systems is also likely. Various sites of possible neurological dysfunction have been proposed to explain this constellation of behaviors, ranging from the neocortex (Hauser, DeLong & Rosman 1975; Piven et al. 1990) to the limbic system (Damasio & Maurer 1978) to subcortical structures (diencephalon–brainstem and cerebellum) (Courchesne et al. 1988; Gaffney et al. 1987, Ritvo et al. 1986).

Neuroanatomy of Autism

Neuropathological studies of autistic individuals have revealed abnormalities in limbic structures and in the cerebellum. Microscopic abnormalities, consisting of reduced neuronal size and increased cell density (features of brain immaturity) in limbic structures, together with decreased Purkinje cell counts in the cerebellum, were reported with coexisting mental retardation and epilepsy (Bauman & Kemper 1985). Similar alterations in Purkinje cells were reported in nonepileptic autistics (Ritvo et al. 1986).

Although neuropathological studies found replicable cerebellar abnormalities at a microscopic level, MRI studies demonstrating structural abnormalities of posterior fossa structures were inconsistent until recently. Courchesne and colleagues (Courchesne et al. 1987; Courchesne et al. 1988; Murakami et al. 1989) described hypoplasia of cerebellar vermal lobules VI and VII and of the cerebellar hemispheres in autistic children. Gaffney et al. reported fourth ventricle enlargement (1987) and hypoplasia of the brainstem, particularly in the region of the pons (1988). However, not all investigators were able to replicate these findings (Ritvo & Garber 1988; Garber et al. 1989; Rumsey et al. 1988; Kleiman, Neff & Rosman 1992). To resolve conflicting results regarding cerebellar size in autism, Courchesne, Townsend, and Saitoh (1994) reanalyzed MRI data on 78 autistic patients and 91 controls from six different laboratories and found two types of cerebellar abnormalities: those with *hypo*plasia of posterior vermal lobules VI and VII; and those with *hyper*plasia of the same lobules. Thus, with small samples, some authors may report one abnormality while others may report another. Neocortical abnormalities are also reported in MRI studies. For example, Piven et al (1990) found a much larger proportion

(53.8%) of neuromigrational anomalies involving the cortex (polymicrogyria, schizencephaly, and macrogyria) in a group of high-functioning male autistic subjects (n = 13) than in an equal number of controls matched for age and nonverbal IQ.

PET scan studies of autistic patients have yielded variable findings, due to rapid evolution of technology, to subject selection issues, and to the methodological issue of whether studies were conducted under resting conditions or with activation procedures. Rumsey et al. (1985) reported an overall *increase* in glucose utilization in autistic subjects compared to controls, in the resting condition. Other studies have found otherwise (De Volder et al. 1987; Horwitz et al. 1988). For example, DeVolder et al. (1987) did not note any group differences between autistic subjects and controls, although they noted different patterns of correlations between various brain regions in these subjects. Six autistic children showed increased metabolism in the frontal area, while two did not. In a resting metabolism study, Horwitz et al. (1988) noted fewer large positive correlations between frontal and parietal regions, and negative correlations between various subcortical structures and the interconnected cortical regions (these were typically positive in controls). This study suggested that normal patterns of cortical-subcortical integration were absent. Activation studies have also suggested that differences existed between autistic subjects and normal controls. In a study of high-functioning adults with a history of childhood autism, asymmetries were noted on a visual vigilance continuous-performance task: autistic patients had a left-greater-than-right gyrus rectus asymmetry, in contrast to the right-greater-than-left asymmetry seen in controls. In some brain regions, metabolic rates were more than three standard deviations above the mean of normals (Siegel et al. 1992).

Neurophysiological studies, such as brainstem auditory evoked responses (BAER), have also contributed to the understanding of brain function in autistic individuals. For example, prolonged interpeak latencies have been found in autistic patients (Rumsey et al. 1984), suggesting that neurological deficits in auditory processing were involved. Thivierge et al. (1990) noted similar deficits and suggested that, although BAER were by no means pathognomonic of autism, their use—particularly with masking procedures—might help identify dysfunctional maturational processes in the higher brainstem of 50% of autistic subjects.

Thus, although several different central nervous system regions have been considered as sites of the pathology of autism, it remains difficult to integrate these into a single model. Recently, the cerebellum has been shown to play a role in cognitive as well as motor functions (Leiner, Leiner & Dow 1986; Bracke-Tolkmitt et al. 1989). In a review article, Schmahmann (1991) noted that, although the pathways that reciprocally link cortical regions to the cerebellum (the cortico–ponto–cerebellar and cerebellar–dentate–thalamic projections) are incompletely understood, the cerebellum may correlate motor acts with mood states and unconscious motivation and thus may play a role in nonverbal communication. He suggested that a "dysmetria of thought" may result in a mismatch between reality and its perception—an erratic pattern of over-

and undercorrection of thought and behavior. A relationship between the time course of development of the cerebellum and the neurodevelopmental disturbance in autism may exist (Courchesne et al. 1988). Whatever is disrupting Purkinje cell migration to the posterior vermis may also affect limbic system areas (such as the amygdala, portions of the hippocampal formation, and septum) that are undergoing important developmental processes at the same time.

Damasio and Maurer (1978) noted that the behavioral, motoric, sensory, and communication abnormalities of autistic persons resemble the abnormalities that follow frontal-subcortical and limbic system damage. For example, communication disturbance resembles that seen in cases involving mesial frontal lesions. Limbic system disturbance might underlie social impairments. Studies in primates suggest that limbic system damage in early infancy results in behavioral abnormalities reminiscent of autism (Bachevalier 1991; Merjanian et al. 1986; Merjanian, Pettigrew & Mishkin 1988). Kinesiologic analysis of gaits in autistic children compared to gaits in controls found reduced stride lengths, increased stance times, increased hip flexion at "toe-off," and decreased knee extension and ankle dorsiflexion at ground contact (Vilensky, Damasio & Maurer 1981). The involuntary movements, postural disturbances, and gait disturbances were like those noted in basal ganglia dysfunction (for instance, Parkinson's disease). However, these findings were disputed in a recent study. Gait was analyzed in a highly quantified manner; and gait velocity, step length, vertical forces, and stance time were found to be normal, supporting arguments against basal ganglia dysfunction (Hallett et al. 1993).

The anatomical areas implicated in autism form the "mesolimbic cortex," which possesses distinct characteristics of cell structure and vascular supply and is primarily dopaminergic. Thus, a disturbance in dopamine metabolism in mesolimbic cortex may be involved in the pathogenesis of autism. Serum levels of the enzyme dopamine beta hydroxylase (which converts dopamine to norepinephrine) is decreased in autistic children and their relatives (Lake, Ziegler & Murphy, 1977). Higher cerebrospinal fluid levels of homovanillic acid were found in autistic children who responded to psychostimulant treatment with increased activity and stereotypes. Autistic children had *elevated* blink rates (a measure of central dopaminergic activity), suggesting hyperactivity of the dopaminergic system (Goldberg et al. 1987).

Neuropsychological Studies of Autism

The spectrum of cognitive abilities in autism ranges from retardation to superior intellectual functions. Since most autistic individuals (about 70%) are mentally retarded (American Psychiatric Association 1980), however, it is often difficult to discriminate between specific cognitive deficits due to autism and those secondary to mental retardation. For this reason, most neuropsychological studies have focused on high-functioning autistics. Some general cognitive patterns have been observed in these studies. Autistic individuals perform better on visuoperceptual–motor tasks than they do on verbal abstraction tasks (Bartak, Rutter & Cox 1975). Lord and O'Neil (1983) found autistic individuals impaired in verbal and nonverbal reasoning, concept formation, and comprehension. Indeed, autistics had a remarkable stability of this pattern across a wide age span. Lincoln et al. (1988) studied 33 autistic subjects ranging in age from 8 to 29 years. They also evaluated 47 other children aged 8 to 12 years (autistic children and children with receptive developmental problems, oppositional disorder, and dysthymic disorder). There were highly significant differences between the autistic children and all others. Using Wechsler IQ tests, the researchers found a highly significant verbal < performance difference, with particularly poor scores on Comprehension and Vocabulary and near normal scores on Block Design and Object Assembly. Autistic children were most efficient at processing information that was nonverbal, unrelated to social behaviors, and noncontextual. Tasks such as Object Assembly and Block Design do not appear to require integration of previously learned information, but instead depend on immediate feedback and have modest reliance on visual short- and long-term memory. In contrast, subtests such as Picture Arrangement and Picture Completion require the integration of nonverbal, social, and context-relevant information.

Autistic children who speak may have relatively fluent output, with preservation of articulation and syntax. Nevertheless, the pragmatics of their language are quite deviant, reflecting a more general disturbance of social communication characterized by poverty of spontaneous speech; idiosyncratic word use; stereotypies; echolalia; abnormal intonation, speed, and rhythm; and disturbance in the social use of language. Whether these language deficits differ from those in children with specific language impairment (SLI) has been addressed. Bartack, Rutter, and Cox (1975) addressed this issue in a study of autistic and SLI boys who had nonverbal IQs of at least 70. Discriminate function analysis was conducted on a large number of language, behavioral, and cognitive variables. Although some specific items were found to be in common, the groups were discrete and non-overlapping when the total pattern of characteristics was analyzed. Pragmatics of language were much more disordered in the autistic group. Other atypical language behaviors, such as echolalia, appeared to be related to language impairment—particularly in comprehension—rather than being specific to autism.

Some children with autistic features demonstrate hyperlexia—the ability to read aloud utilizing both phonologic and lexical routes (Aram, Rose & Horowitz 1984; Welsh, Pennington & Rogers 1987; Healy et al. 1982). This unusual skill is often manifested at an early age and may occur in a child whose language is otherwise quite undeveloped and echolalic. The presence of hyperlexia often carries with it a much better long-range prognosis for function, compared to that among nonhyperplexic autistic children (Burd et al. 1987).

Analysis of social-emotional information is particularly difficult for autistic persons. This is evident in tasks that specifically assess affect processing (Hobson 1986) and in more complex social behaviors such as gaze (Dawson et al. 1990). High-functioning autistic adults had affective flattening (and did not differ in this regard from schizophrenic controls), poverty of speech and content of speech, and perseveration. They had less evidence of "positive thought disorder" than either schizophrenics or manics (Rumsey, Andreasen & Rapoport 1986). Vineland Social Quotients are often low, particularly relative to IQs (Rumsey, Rapoport & Sceery 1985). Particular difficulty with higher-level items, including initiative, self-direction, socialization, and relative independence, are reported.

Results of neuropsychological testing of high-functioning men with infantile autism suggested that the pragmatics of language are impaired (Rumsey & Hamburger 1988). These researchers also reported evidence of prefrontal dysfunction, based on the WCST. Memory was intact, except for aspects related to frontal dysfunction. More recently, Rumsey and Hamburger (1990) compared high-functioning autistic adults with severe dyslexics and normal controls. The autistic subjects performed better only on forward digit span. They had difficulty on the WCST and on the Binet verbal and picture absurdities and problem situations. The latter test correctly classified 80% of the autistic subjects and all of the controls (dyslexics did not differ from controls). Three variables discriminated the groups: digits forward, Binet verbal absurdities, and Binet problem situations.

Studies of learning have revealed that autistic patients experience specific difficulties. For example, Frith (1970) compared young autistic children to normals and mentally retarded children on a task that involved learning to organize colored counters into a specific pattern with explicit examiner feedback. Once a pattern was completed, it was hidden from sight, thus requiring reliance on internal working memory and understanding of the organizing principle. Normal and autistic children did not differ in the total number of correct choices they made, but there was a significant learning effect and an interaction of group by pattern effect. Error analysis indicated that the errors of normal children were consistent with the dominant rule of the given pattern. In contrast, autistic children had difficulty with feature extraction, or dominant rule learning. Similarly, Minshew and Goldstein (1993) administered neuropsychological tests to non-mentally retarded autistics and matched controls. Differences were noted on measures of complex learning and memory, conceptual flexibility, abstraction, verbal and social problem solving, reading comprehension, and semantic–pragmatic language comprehension. They suggested that the deficits involved a distributed network of structures that subserved function of complex information analysis, rather than involving specific cognitive functions.

Although Kanner originally identified the characteristic impairment in affective contact of autistic children, this deficit was considered secondary to a more general cognitive disorder. However, Fein et al. (1986) suggested that the impaired ability to develop social relationships was a primary dysfunction. In addition to having difficulty expressing emotion, autistic children have impaired ability to discriminate emotional signals and to represent the intentional states of others. These impairments in eye contact and emotional expression are seen early in infancy (Adrien et al. 1991). Baron-Cohen, Leslie & Frith (1986) compared high-ability autistics, low-ability Down syndrome children, and normal preschoolers on picture-sequencing tasks with mechanical (person–object), behavioral (person–person), and interpersonal intentional contents. Autistic children had equal or superior ability on the first two tasks but performed worse on the interpersonal intentional task. They rarely used language expressing any understanding of mental or emotional states in their story telling. The authors suggested that autistics have a specific deficit in the establishment of a "theory of mind," with disturbance of meta-representations (which normally develops around the end of the second year of life) as manifested by the child's inability to pretend play or share pretence with others (Frith, Morton & Leslie 1991).

SUMMARY

In this chapter, the neurobiological, genetic, and neuropsychological aspects of common psychiatric syndromes in children were reviewed. There is an emerging understanding of the psychiatric, neurological, and neuropsychological aspects of these disorders, although it remains unclear how underlying genetic mechanisms translate into neurocognitive and psychiatric disorders. Researchers now appear to be on the threshold of learning how genetic mechanisms are translated into normal and anomalous brain development. Basic neuroscience research, together with relevant clinical studies, will lead to increased understanding about human psychopathology.

REFERENCES

Abel, L.; Friedman, L.; Jesberger, J.; Malki, A.; and Meltzer, H. Y. 1991. Quantitative assessment of smooth pursuit gain and catch-up saccades in schizophrenia and affective disorders. *Biological Psychiatry* 29: 1063–72.

Adrien, J. L.; Faure, M.; Perrot, A.; Hameury, L.; Garreau, B.; Barthelemy, C.; and Sauvage, D. 1991. Autism and family home movies: Preliminary findings. *Journal of Autism and Developmental Disorders* 21: 43–49.

Alexander, G. E.; DeLong, M. R.; and Strick, P. L. 1988. Parallel organization of functionally segregated circuits linking basal ganglia and cortex. *Annual Review of Neuroscience* 9: 357–81.

American Psychiatric Association 1980. *Diagnostic and Statistical Manual of Mental Disorders,* 3rd ed. Washington, D.C.: American Psychiatric Association.

American Psychiatric Association 1987. *Diagnostic and Statistical Manual of Mental Disorders-III-R,* 3rd ed. Washington, D.C.: American Psychiatric Association.

American Psychiatric Association, Committee on Nomenclature and Statistics. 1994. *Diagnostic and Statistical Manual of Mental Disorders:* DSM-IV, 4th ed. Washington, D.C.: American Psychiatric Association.

Andreasen, N.; Nasrallah, H. A.; Dunn, V.; Olson, S. C.; Grove W. M.; Ehrhardt, J. C.; Coffman, J. A.; and Crossett, J. H. W. 1986. Structural abnormalities in the frontal system in schizophrenia: A magnetic resonance imaging study. *Archives of General Psychiatry* 43: 136–44.

Apter, A.; Pauls, D. L.; Bleich, A.; Zohar, A. H.; Kron, S.; Ratzoni, G.; Dycian, A.; Kotler, M.; Weizman, A.; Gadot, N.; and Cohen, D. J. 1993. An epidemiologic study of Gilles de la Tourette's syndrome in Israel. *Archives of General Psychiatry* 50: 734–38.

Aram, D. M.; Rose, D. F.; and Horowitz, S. J. 1984. Hyperlexia: Developmental reading without meaning. In R. H. Malatesha and H. A. Whitaker (eds.), *Dyslexia: A global issue*. NATO ASI Series (The Hague: Martinus Nijhoff), pp. 517–31.

Asperger, H. 1944. Die 'autistischen psychopathen' im kindesalter. *Archiv für Psychiatrie und Nervenkrankheiten* 117: 76–136.

Bachevalier, J. 1991. An animal model for childhood autism: Memory loss and socioemotional disturbances following neonatal damage to the limbic system in monkeys. In C. A. Tamminga and S. C. Schulz (eds.), *Advances in Neuropsychiatry and Psychopharmacology,* vol. 1, *Schizophrenia Research* (New York: Raven Press), pp. 129–40.

Bakchine, S.; Lacomblez, L.; Benoit, N.; Parisot, D.; Chain, F.; and Lhermitte, F. 1989. Manic-like state after bilateral orbitofrontal and right temporoparietal injury: Efficacy of clonidine. *Neurology* 39: 777–81.

Ballenger, J. C.; Reus, V. I.; and Post, R. M. 1982. The "atypical" clinical picture of adolescent mania. *American Journal of Psychiatry* 139: 602–6.

Balthasar, K. 1956. Uber das anatomische Substrat der generalisierten Tic-krankheit (maladie des tics, Gilles de la Tourette): Entwicklungshemmung des corpus striatum. *Archiv fur Psychiatrie und Zeitschrift fur des gesamte Neurologie* 195: 531–49.

Baron-Cohen, S.; Leslie, A. M.; and Frith, U. 1986. Mechanical, behavioural and intentional understanding of picture stories in autistic children. *British Journal of Developmental Psychology* 4: 113–25.

Bartak, L.; Rutter, M.; and Cox, A. 1975. A comparative study of infantile autism and specific developmental receptive language disorder: I. The children. *British Journal of Psychiatry* 126: 127–45.

Bauman, M. and Kemper, T. L. 1985. Histoanatomic observations of the brain in early infantile autism. *Neurology* 35: 866–74.

Baxter, L. R.; Schwartz, J. M.; Bergman, K. S.; Szuba, M. P.; Guze, B. H.; Mazziotta, J. C.; Alazraki, A.; Selin, C. E.; Ferng, H.-K.; Munford, P.; and Phelps, M. E. 1992. Caudate glucose metabolic rate changes with both drug and behavior therapy for obsessive-compulsive disorder. *Archives of General Psychiatry* 49: 681–89.

Baxter, L. R.; Schwartz, J. M.; Mazziotta, J. C.; Phelps, M. E.; Pahl, J. J.; Guze, B. H.; and Fairbanks, L. 1988. Cerebral glucose metabolic rates in nondepressed patients with obsessive-compulsive disorder. *American Journal of Psychiatry* 145: 1560–63.

Behar, D.; Rapoport, J. L.; Berg, C. J.; Denckla, M. B.; Mann, L.; Cox, C.; Fedio, P.; Zahn, T.; and Wolfman, M. G. 1984. Computerized tomography and neuropsychological test measures in adolescents with obsessive-compulsive disorder. *American Journal of Psychiatry* 141: 363–69.

Beitchman, J. H. 1985. Child schizophrenia: A review and a comparison with adult-onset cases. *Psychiatric Clinics* 8: 793–814.

Bender, L., and Freedman, A. M. 1952. A study of the first three years in the maturation of schizophrenic children. *Quarterly Journal of Child Behavior* 1: 245–72.

Benes, F. M., and Bird, E. D. 1987. An analysis of the arrangement of neurons in the cingulate cortex of schizophrenic patients. *Archives of General Psychiatry* 44: 608–16.

Benes, F. M.; Davidson, J.; and Bird, E. D. 1986. Quantitative cytoarchitectural studies of the cerebral cortex of schizophrenics. *Archives of General Psychiatry* 43: 31–35.

Benes, F. M.; Majocha, R.; Bird, E. D.; and Marotta, C. A. 1987. Increased vertical axon numbers in cingulate cortex of schizophrenics. *Archives of General Psychiatry* 44: 1017–21.

Benkelfat, C.; Nordahl, T. E.; Semple, W. E.; King, A. C.; Murphy, D. L.; and Cohen, R. M. 1990. Local cerebral glucose metabolic rates in obsessive-compulsive disorder: Patients treated with clomipramine. *Archives of General Psychiatry* 47: 840–48.

Berg, C.; Rapoport, J.; and Flament, M. 1986. The Leyton Obsessional Inventory, Child Version. *Journal of the American Academy of Child Psychiatry* 25: 84–91.

Berman, K. F.; Weinberger, D. R.; Shelton, R. C.; and Zec, R. F. 1987. A relationship between anatomical and physiological brain pathology in schizophrenia: Lateral cerebral ventricular size predicts cortical blood flow. *American Journal of Psychiatry* 144: 1277–82.

Biederman, J.; Faraone, S. V.; Keenan, K.; Benjamin, J.; Krifcher, B.; Moore, C.; Sprich-Buckminster, S.; Ugaglia, K.; Jellinek, M. S.; Steingard, R.; Spencer, T.; Norman, D.; Kolodny, R.; Kraus, I.; Perrin, J.; Keller, M. B.; and Tsuang, M. T. 1992. Further evidence for family-genetic risk factors in attention deficit hyperactivity disorder: Patterns of comorbidity in probands and relatives in psychiatrically and pediatrically referred samples. *Archives of General Psychiatry* 49: 728–38.

Biederman, J.; Faraone, S. V.; Keenan, K.; and Tsuang, M. T. 1991. Evidence of familial association between attention deficit disorder and major affective disorders. *Archives of General Psychiatry* 48: 633–42.

Blanchard, J. J., and Neale, J. M. 1994. The neuropsychological signature of schizophrenia: Generalized or differential deficit. *American Journal of Psychiatry* 151: 40–48.

Bogerts, B.; Meertz, E.; and Schönfeldt-Bausch, R. 1985. Basal ganglia and limbic system pathology in schizophrenia: A morphometric study of brain volume and shrinkage. *Archives of General Psychiatry* 42: 784–91.

Boone, K. B.; Ananth, J.; Philpott, L.; Kaur, A.; and Djenederedjian, A. 1991. Neuropsychological characteristics of nondepressed adults with obsessive-compulsive disorder. *Neuropsychiatry, Neuropsychology, and Behavioral Neurology* 4: 96–109.

Bornstein, R. A. 1991. Neuropsychological correlates of obsessive characteristics in Tourette's syndrome. *Journal of Neuropsychiatry and Clinical Neurosciences* 3: 157–62.

Bornstein, R. A.; Carroll, A.; and King, G. 1986. Relationship of age to neuropsychological deficits in Tourette's syndrome. *Journal of Developmental and Behavioral Pediatrics* 6: 284–86.

Bornstein, R. A.; King, G.; and Carroll, A. 1983. Neuropsychological abnormalities in Gilles de la Tourette's syndrome. *Journal of Nervous and Mental Disease* 171: 497–502.

Bourne, L. E., Jr.; Justesen, D. R.; Abraham, T.; Beeker, C.; Brauchi, J. T.; Whitaker, L. C.; and Yaroush, R. A. 1977. Limits to conceptual rule-learning by schizophrenic patients. *Journal of Clinical Psychology* 33: 324–34.

Bowring, M. A., and Kovacs, M. 1992. Difficulties in diagnosing manic disorders among children and adolescents. *Journal of the American Academy of Child and Adolescent Psychiatry* 31: 611–14.

Bracke-Tolkmitt, R.; Linden, A.; Canavan, A. G. M.; Rockstroh, B.; Scholz, E.; Wessel, K.; and H.-C. Diener 1989. The cerebellum contributes to mental skills. *Behavioral Neuroscience* 103: 442–46.

Bregman, J. D.; Leckman, J. F.; and Ort, S. I. 1988. Fragile X syndrome: Genetic predisposition to psychopathology. *Journal of Autism and Developmental Disorders* 18: 343–54.

Brown, R.; Colter, N.; Corsellis, J. A.; Crow, T. J.; Frith, C. D.; Jagoe, R.; Johnstone, E. C.; and Marsh, L. 1986. Postmortem evidence of structural brain changes in schizophrenia: Differences in brain weight, temporal horn area, and parahippocampal gyrus compared with affective disorder. *Archives of General Psychiatry* 43: 36–42.

Brown, W. T.; Jenkins, E. C.; Friedman, E.; Brooks, J.; Wisniewski, K.; Raguthu, S.; and French, J. 1982. Autism is associated with the fragile-X syndrome. *Journal of Autism and Developmental Disorders* 12: 303–8.

Brumback, R. A. 1988. Childhood depression and medically treatable learning disability. In D. L. Molfese and S. J. Segalowitz (eds.), *Brain Lateralization in Children: Developmental Implications* (New York: Guilford Press), pp. 463–505.

Brumback, R. A.; Jackoway, M. K.; and Weinberg, W. A. 1980. Relation of intelligence to childhood depression in children referred to an educational diagnostic center. *Perceptual Motor Skills* 50: 11–17.

Buchanan, R. W.; Kirkpatrick, B.; Heinrichs, D. W.; and Carpenter, W. T., Jr. 1990. Clinical correlates of the deficit syndrome of schizophrenia. *American Journal of Psychiatry* 147: 290–94.

Burd, L.; Fisher, W.; Knowlton, D.; and Kerbeshian, J. 1987. Hyperlexia: A marker for improvement in children with pervasive developmental disorder? *Journal of the American Academy of Child Psychiatry* 26: 407–12.

Calev, A.; Berlin, H.; and Lerer, B. 1987. Remote and recent memory in long-hospitalized chronic schizophrenics. *Biological Psychiatry* 22: 79–85.

Calev, A.; Venables, P. H.; and Monk, A. F. 1983. Evidence for distinct verbal memory pathologies in severely and mildly disturbed schizophrenics. *Schizophrenia Bulletin* 9: 247.

Cannon, T. D.; Mednick, S. A.; and Parnas, J. 1989. Genetic and perinatal determinants of structural brain deficits in schizophrenia. *Archives of General Psychiatry* 46: 883–89.

Caplan, R.; Guthrie, D.; Fish, B.; Tanguay, P.; and David-Lando, G. 1989. The kiddie formal thought disorder rating scale (K-FTDS): Clinical assessment, reliability, and validity. *Journal of the American Academy of Child and Adolescent Psychiatry* 28: 408–16.

Caplan, R.; Perdue, S.; Tanguay, P.; and Fish, B. 1990. Formal thought disorder in childhood onset schizophrenia and schizotypal personality disorder. *Journal of Child Psychology and Psychiatry* 28: 208–16.

Carey, G., and Gottesman, I. I. 1981. Twin and family studies of anxiety, phobic, and obsessive disorders. In D. F. Klein and J. Rabkin (eds.), *Anxiety: New Research and Changing Concepts* (New York: Raven Press), pp. 117–36.

Carpenter, W. T.; Buchanan, R. W.; Kirkpatrick, B.; Tamminga, C.; and Wood, F. 1993. Strong inference, theory testing, and the neuroanatomy of schizophrenia. *Archives of General Psychiatry* 50: 825–31.

Carpenter, W. T.; Heinrichs, D. W.; Buchanan, R. W.; Hanlon, T. E.; Kirkpatrick,

B.; and Summerfelt, A. 1991. Dr. Carpenter and associates reply. *American Journal of Psychiatry* 148: 1612–13.

Carpenter, W. T.; Heinrichs, D. W.; and Wagman, A. M. I. 1988. Deficit and non-deficit forms of schizophrenia: The concept. *American Journal of Psychiatry* 145: 578–83.

Chiles, J. A.; Miller, M. L.; and Cox, G. B. 1980. Depression in an adolescent delinquent population. *Archives of General Psychiatry* 37: 1179–84.

Christensen, K. J.; Kim, S. W.; Dysken, M. W.; and Hoover, K. M. 1992. Neuropsychological performance in obsessive-compulsive disorder. *Biological Psychiatry* 31: 4–18.

Cleghorn, J. M.; Franco, S.; Szechtman, B.; Kaplan, R. D.; Szechtman, H.; Brown, G. M.; Nahmias, C.; and Garnett, E. S. 1992. Toward a brain map of auditory hallucinations. *American Journal of Psychiatry* 149: 1062–69.

Collingridge, G. 1987. The role of NMDA receptors in learning and memory. *Nature* 330: 604–5.

Comings, D. E., and Comings, B. G. 1984. Tourette's syndrome and attention deficit disorder with hyperactivity: Are they genetically related? *Journal of the American Academy of Child Psychiatry* 23: 138–46.

Comings, D. E.; Himes, J. A.; and Comings, B. G. 1990. An epidemiological study of Tourette's syndrome in a single school district. *Journal of Clinical Psychiatry* 51: 463–69.

Cooper, J. 1970. The Leyton Obsessional Inventory. *Psychological Medicine* 1: 48–64.

Courchesne, E.; Hesselink, J. R.; Jernigan, T. L.; and Yeung-Courchesne, R. 1987. Abnormal neuroanatomy in a nonretarded person with autism: Unusual findings with magnetic resonance imaging. *Archives of Neurology* 44: 335–41.

Courchesne, E.; Townsend, J.; and Saitoh, O. 1994. The brain in infantile autism: Posterior fossa structures are abnormal. *Neurology* 44: 214–22.

Courchesne, E.; Yeung-Courchesne, R.; Press, G.; Hesselink, J. R.; and Jernigan, T. L. 1988. Hypoplasia of cerebellar vermal lobules VI and VII in autism. *New England Journal of Medicine* 318: 1349–54.

Creese, I.; Burt, D. R.; and Snyder, S. H. 1976. Dopamine receptor binding predicts clinical and pharmacological potencies of antischizophrenic drugs. *Science* 192: 481–83.

Cummings, J. L., and Cunningham, K. 1992. Obsessive-compulsive disorder in Huntington's disease. *Biological Psychiatry* 31: 263–70.

Cummings, J. L., and Mendez, M. F. 1984. Secondary mania with focal cerebrovascular lesions. *American Journal of Psychiatry* 141: 1084–87.

Damasio, A. R., and Maurer, R. G. 1978. A neurological model for childhood autism. *Archives of Neurology* 35: 777–86.

Davis, K. L.; Kahn, R. S.; Ko, G.; and Davidson, M. 1991. Dopamine in schizophrenia: A review and reconceptualization. *American Journal of Psychiatry* 148: 1474–86.

Dawson, G.; Hill, D.; Spencer, A.; Galpert, L.; and Watson, L. 1990. Affective exchanges between young autistic children and their mothers. *Journal of Abnormal Child Psychology* 18: 335–45.

de Divitiis, E.; D'Errico, A.; and Cerillo, A. 1977. Stereotactic surgery in Gilles de la Tourette syndrome. *Acta Neurochirugia* (1977, Suppl. 24): 73.

Deonna, T.; Ziegler, A.-L.; Moura-Serra, J.; and Innocenti, G. 1993. Autistic regression in relation to limbic pathology and epilepsy: Report of two cases. *Developmental Medicine and Child Neurology* 35: 166–76.

Deutsch, S. I.; Mastropaolo, J.; Schwartz, B. L.; Rosse, R. B.; and Morihisa, J. A. 1989. A "glutamatergic hypothesis" of schizophrenia: Rationale for pharmacotherapy with glycine. *Clinical Neuropharmacology* 12: 1–13.

DeVeaugh-Geiss, J. 1991. Pharmacologic treatment of obsessive-compulsive disorder. In J. Zohar, T. Insel, and S. Rasmussen (eds.), *The Psychobiology of Obsessive-Compulsive Disorder* (New York: Springer-Verlag), pp. 187–207.

De Volder, A.; Bol, A.; Michel, C.; Congneau, M.; and Goffinet, A. M. 1987. Brain glucose metabolism in children with autistic syndrome: Positron tomography analysis. *Brain and Development* 9: 581–87.

Devinsky, O.; Bear, D.; Moya, K.; and Benowitz, L. 1993. Perception of emotion in patients with Tourette's syndrome. *Neuropsychiatry, Neuropsychology, and Behavioral Neurology* 6: 166–69.

Deykin, E. Y., and MacMahon, B. 1979. The incidence of seizures among children with autistic symptoms. *American Journal of Psychiatry* 136: 1310–12.

Dworkin, R. H.; Bernstein, G.; Kaplansky, L. M.; Lipsitz, J. D.; Rinaldi, A.; Slater, S. L.; Cornblatt, B. A.; and Erlenmeyer-Kimling, L. 1991. Social competence and positive and negative symptoms: A longitudinal study of children and adolescents at risk for schizophrenia and affective disorder. *American Journal of Psychiatry* 148: 1182–88.

Eggers, C. 1978. Course and prognosis of childhood schizophrenia. *Journal of Autism and Childhood Schizophrenia* 8: 21–36.

Eslinger, P. J., and Damasio, A. R. 1985. Severe disturbance of higher cognition after bilateral frontal lobe ablation: Patient EVR. *Neurology* 35: 1731–41.

Falkai, P., and Bogerts, B. 1986. Cell loss in the hippocampus of schizophrenics. *European Archives of Psychiatry and Neurological Sciences* 236: 154–61.

Falkai, P.; Bogerts, B.; and Rozumek, M. 1988. Limbic pathology in schizophrenia: The entorhinal region: A morphometric study. *Biological Psychiatry* 24: 515–21.

Fein, D.; Pennington, B.; Markowitz, P.; Braverman, M.; and Waterhouse, L. 1986. Toward a neuropsychological model of infantile autism: Are the social deficits primary? *Journal of the American Academy of Child Psychiatry* 25: 198–212.

Feinberg, I. 1987. Adolescence and mental illness. *Science* 236: 507–8.

Ferrari, M.; Matthews, W. S.; and Barabas, G. 1984. Children with Tourette syndrome: Results of psychological tests given prior to drug treatment. *Journal of Developmental and Behavioral Pediatrics* 5: 116–19.

Fey, E. T. 1951. The performance of young schizophrenics and young normals on the Wisconsin Card Sorting Test. *Journal of Consulting Psychology* 15: 311–19.

Fish, B. 1984. Characteristics and sequelae of the neurointegrative disorder in infants at risk for schizophrenia (1952–1982). In N. F. Watt, E. J. Anthony, L. C. Wynne, and J. E. Rolf (eds.), *Children at Risk for Schizophrenia* (New York: Cambridge University Press), pp. 423–39.

————. 1986. Antecedents of an acute schizophrenic break. *Journal of the American Academy of Child Psychiatry* 25: 595–600.

Fish, B.; Marcus, J.; Hans, S. L.; Auerbach, J. G.; and Perdue, S. 1992. Infants at risk for schizophrenia: Sequelae of a genetic neurointegrative defect. *Archives of General Psychiatry* 49: 221–35.

Flament, M. F.; Whitaker, A.; Rapoport, J. L.; Davies, M.; Berg, C. Z.; Kalikow, K.; Sceery, W.; and Shaffer, D. 1988. Obsessive compulsive disorder in adolescence: An epidemiological study. *Journal of the American Academy of Child Psychiatry* 27: 764–71.

Franzén, G., and Ingvar, D. H. 1975. Absence of activation in frontal structures during psychological testing of chronic schizophrenics. *Journal of Neurology, Neurosurgery and Psychiatry* 38: 1027–32.

Freedman, R.; Adler, L. E.; Waldo, M. C.; Pachtman, E.; and Franks, R. D. 1983. Neurophysiological evidence for a defect in inhibitory pathways in schizophrenia: Comparison of medicated and drug-free patients. *Biological Psychiatry* 18: 537–52.

Frith, U. 1970. Studies in pattern detection in normal and autistic children: II. Reproduction and production of color sequences. *Journal of Experimental Child Psychology* 10: 120–35.

Frith, U.; Morton, J.; and Leslie, A. M. 1991. The cognitive basis of a biological disorder: Autism. *Trends in Neuroscience* 14: 433–38.

Gaffney, G.; Kuperman, S.; Tsai, L.; and Minchin, S. 1988. Morphological evidence for brainstem involvement in infantile autism. *Biological Psychiatry* 24: 578–86.

Gaffney, G.; Kuperman, S.; Tsai, L.; Minchin, S.; and Hassanein, K. 1987. Midsagittal magnetic resonance imaging of autism. *British Journal of Psychiatry* 151: 831–33.

Garber, H. J.; Ananth, J. V.; Chiu, L. C.; Griswold, V. J.; and Oldendorf, W. H. 1989. Nuclear magnetic resonance study of obsessive-compulsive disorder. *American Journal of Psychiatry* 146: 1001–5.

Garber, H. J.; Ritvo, E.; Chiu, L.; Griswold, V. J.; Kashanian, A.; Freeman, B. J.; and Oldendorf, W. H. 1989. A magnetic resonance imaging study of autism: Normal fourth ventricle size and absence of pathology. *American Journal of Psychiatry* 146: 532–34.

Geller, B.; Fox, L. W.; and Fletcher, M. 1993. Effect of tricyclic antidepressants on switching to mania and on the onset of bipolarity in depressed 6- to 12-year-olds. *Journal of the American Academy of Child and Adolescent Psychiatry* 32: 43–50.

Gillberg, C.; Steffenburg, S.; Wahlström, J.; Gillberg, I. C.; Sjöstedt, A.; Martinsson, T.; Liedgren, S.; and Eeg-Olofsson, O. 1991. Case study: Autism associated with marker chromosome. *Journal of the American Academy of Child and Adolescent Psychiatry* 30: 489–94.

Goetz, C. G.; Tanner, C. M.; Stebbins, G. T.; Leipzig, G.; and Carr, W. C. 1992. Adult tics in Gilles de la Tourette's syndrome: Description and risk factors. *Neurology* 42: 784–88.

Goldberg, T. E., and Weinberger, D. R. 1986. Methodological issues in the neuropsychological approach to schizophrenia. In H. A. Nasrallah and D. R. Weinberger (eds.), *The Neurology of Schizophrenia* (Amsterdam: Elsevier Science Publishers), pp. 141–56.

Goldberg, T. E.; Weinberger, D. R.; Berman, K. F.; Pliskin, N. H.; and Podd, M. H. 1987. Further evidence for dementia of the prefrontal type in schizophrenia? *Archives of General Psychiatry* 44: 1008–14.

Golden, J. C. 1978. *Stroop Color and Word Test*. Chicago. Stoelting.

Goodman, W. K.; Price, L. H.; Rasmussen, S. A.; Mazure, C.; Delgado, P.; Heninger, G. R.; and Charney, D. S. 1989. The Yale-Brown Obsessive Compulsive Scale: II. Validity. *Archives of General Psychiatry* 46: 1012–16.

Goodman, W. K.; Price, L. H.; Rasmussen, S. A.; Mazure, C.; Fleischmann, R. L.; Hill, C. L.; Heninger, G. R.; and Charney, D. S. 1989. The Yale-Brown Obsessive Compulsive Scale: I. Development, use, and reliability. *Archives of General Psychiatry* 46: 1006–11.

Gray, J. A.; Feldon, J.; Rawlins, J. N. P.; Hemsley, D. R.; and Smith, A. D. 1991. The neuropsychology of schizophrenia. *Behavioral and Brain Sciences* 14: 1–84.

Haber, S. N.; Kowall, N. W.; Vonsattel, J. P.; Bird, E. D.; and Richardson, E. P. 1986. Gilles de la Tourette's syndrome: A postmortem neuropathological and immunohistochemical study. *Journal of Neurological Science* 75: 225–41.

Hall, M.; Costa, D. C.; Shields, J.; Heavens, J.; Robertson, M.; and Ell, P. J. 1990. Brain perfusion patterns with Tc-99mHMPAO/SPECT in patients with Gilles de la Tourette syndrome. *European Journal of Nuclear Medicine* 16: 56 [abstract].

Hallett, M.; Lebiedowska, M. K.; Thomas, S. L.; Stanhope, S. J.; Denckla, M. B.; and Rumsey, J. 1993. Locomotion of autistic adults. *Archives of Neurology* 50: 1304–8.

Hammen, C.; Burge, D.; Burney, E.; and Adrian, C. 1990. Longitudinal study of diagnoses in children of women with unipolar and bipolar affective disorder. *Archives of General Psychiatry* 47: 1112–17.

Haroutunian, V.; Knott, P.; and Davis, K. L. 1988. Effects of mesocortical dopaminergic lesions upon subcortical dopaminergic function. *Pharmacological Bulletin* 24: 341–44.

Hauser, S.; DeLong, G.; and Rosman, N. 1975. Pneumographic findings in the infantile autism syndrome: A correlation with temporal lobe disease. *Brain* 98: 667–88.

Head, D.; Bolton, D.; and Hymas, N. 1989. Deficit in cognitive shifting ability in patients with obsessive-compulsive disorder. *Biological Psychiatry* 25: 929–37.

Healy, J. M.; Aram, D. M.; Horwitz, S. J.; and Kessler, J. W. 1982. A study of hyperlexia. *Brain and Language* 17: 1–23.

Hobson, R. P. 1986. The autistic child's appraisal of expressions of emotion: A further study. *Journal of Child Psychology and Psychiatry* 27: 671–80.

Hollander, E.; DeCaria, C. M.; Aronowitz, B.; Klein, D. F.; Liebowitz, M. R.; and Shaffer, D. 1991. A pilot follow-up study of childhood soft signs and the development of adult psychopathology. *Journal of Neuropsychiatry and Clinical Neurosciences* 3: 186–89.

Hollander, E.; Schiffman, E.; Cohen, B.; Rivera-Stein, M. A.; Rosen, W.; Gorman, J. M.; Fyer, A. J.; Papp, L.; and Liebowitz, M. R. 1990. Signs of central nervous system dysfunction in obsessive-compulsive disorder. *Archives of General Psychiatry* 47: 27–32.

Holzman, P. S.; Kringlen, E.; Matthysse, S.; Flanagan S. D.; Lipton, R. B.; Cramer, G.; Levin, S.; Lange, K.; and Levy, D. L. 1988. A single dominant gene can account for eye tracking dysfunctions and schizophrenia in offspring of discordant twins. *Archives of General Psychiatry* 45: 641–47.

Hoover, C. F., and Insel, T. R. 1984. Families of origin in obsessive-compulsive disorder. *Journal of Nervous and Mental Disease* 172: 207–15.

Horwitz, B.; Rumsey, J. M.; Grady, C. L.; and Rapoport, S. I. 1988. The cerebral metabolic landscape in autism: Intercorrelations of regional glucose utilization. *Archives of Neurology* 45: 749–55.

Howells, J. G., and Guirguis, W. R. 1984. Childhood schizophrenia 20 years later. *Archives of General Psychiatry* 41: 123–28.

Illowsky, B. P.; Juliano, D. M.; Bigelow, L. B.; and Weinberger, D. R. 1988. Stability of CT scan findings in schizophrenia: Results of an 8-year follow-up study. *Journal of Neurology, Neurosurgery and Psychiatry* 51: 209–13.

Incagnoli, T., and Kane, R. 1981. Neuropsychological functioning in Gilles de la

Tourette's syndrome. *Journal of Clinical and Experimental Neuropsychology* 3: 165–69.

Insel, T. R. 1992. Toward a neuroanatomy of obsessive-compulsive disorder. *Archives of General Psychiatry* 49: 739–44.

Jakob, H., and Beckmann, H. 1986. Prenatal developmental disturbances in the limbic allocortex in schizophrenics. *Journal of Neural Transmission* 65: 303–26.

Jorge, R. E.; Robinson, R. G.; Starkstein, S. E.; Arndt, S. V.; Forrester, A. W.; and Geisler, F. H. 1993. Secondary mania following traumatic brain injury. *American Journal of Psychiatry* 150: 916–21.

Joyce, J. N.; Lexow, N.; Bird, E.; and Winokur, A. 1988. Organization of dopamine D_1 and D_2 receptors in human striatum: Receptor autoradiographic studies in Huntington's disease and schizophrenia. *Synapse* 2: 546–57.

Kanner, A. M.; Morris, H. H.; Stagno, S.; Chelune, G.; and Luders, H. 1993. Remission of an obsessive-compulsive disorder following a right temporal lobectomy. *Neuropsychiatry, Neuropsychology, and Behavioral Neurology* 6: 126–29.

Kanner, L. 1943. Autistic disturbances of affective contact. *Nervous Child* 2: 217–50.

Karno, M.; Golding, J. M.; Sorenson, S. B.; and Burnam, M. A. 1988. The epidemiology of obsessive-compulsive disorder in five US communities. *Archives of General Psychiatry* 45: 1094–99.

Kashani, J. H., and Carlson, G. A. 1985. Major depressive disorder in a preschooler. *Journal of the American Academy of Child Psychiatry* 24: 490–94.

Kashani, J. H.; McGee, R. O.; Clarkson, S. E.; Anderson, J. C.; Walton, L. A.; Williams, S.; Silva, P. A.; Robins, A. J.; Cytryn, L.; and McKnew, D. H. 1983. Depression in a sample of 9-year-old children: Prevalence and associated characteristics. *Archives of General Psychiatry* 40: 1217–23.

Kaslow, N. J.; Tanenbaum, R. L.; Abramson, L. Y.; Peterson, C.; and Seligman, M. E. P. 1983. Problem-solving deficits and depressive symptoms among children. *Journal of Abnormal Child Psychology* 11: 497–502.

Keilp, J. G.; Sweeney, J. A.; Jacobsen, P.; Solomon, C.; St. Louis, L.; Deck, M.; Frances, A.; and Mann, J. J. 1988. Cognitive impairment in schizophrenia: Specific relations to ventricular size and negative symptomatology. *Biological Psychiatry* 24: 47–55.

Kelley, A. E.; Lang, C. G.; and Gauthier, A. M. 1988. Induction of oral stereotypy following amphetamine microinjection into a discrete subregion of the striatum. *Psychopharmacology* 95: 556–59.

Kelsoe, J. R.; Cadet, J. L.; Pickar, D.; and Weinberger, D. R. 1988. Quantitative neuroanatomy in schizophrenia: A controlled magnetic resonance imaging study. *Archives of General Psychiatry* 45: 533–41.

Kendler, S. K. 1988. The genetics of schizophrenia: An overview. In M. T. Tsuang and J. C. Simpson (eds.), *Handbook of Schizophrenia*, vol. 3, *Nosology, Epidemiology and Genetics* (New York: Elsevier Science Publishers), pp. 437–62.

Kleiman, M. D.; Neff, S.; and Rosman, N. P. 1992. The brain in infantile autism: Are posterior fossa structures abnormal? *Neurology* 42: 753–60.

Kline, J. S.; Smith, J. E.; and Ellis, H. C. 1992. Paranoid and nonparanoid schizophrenic processing of facially displayed affect. *Journal of Psychiatric Research* 26: 169–82.

Koh, S. D. 1978. Remembering of verbal materials by schizophrenic young adults. In S. Schwartz, (ed.), *Language and Cognition in Schizophrenia* (Hillsdale, N.J.: Lawrence Erlbaum), pp. 55–99.

Kolb, B., and Whishaw, I. Q. 1983. Performance of schizophrenic patients on tests sensitive to left or right frontal, temporal, or parietal function in neurological patients. *Journal of Nervous and Mental Disease* 171: 435–43.

Kovacs, M. 1985. The Children's Depression Inventory (CDI). *Psychopharmacological Bulletin* 21: 995–1000.

Kovacs, M.; Feinberg, T. L.; Crouse-Novak, M. A.; Paulauskas S. L.; and Finkelstein, R. 1984*a*. Depressive disorders in childhood: I. A longitudinal prospective study of characteristics and recovery. *Archives of General Psychiatry* 41: 229–37.

Kovacs, M.; Feinberg, T. L.; Crouse-Novak, M. A.; Paulauskas S. L.; Pollock, M.; and Finkelstein, R. 1984*b*. Depressive disorders in childhood: II. A longitudinal study of the risk for a subsequent major depression. *Archives of General Psychiatry* 41: 643–49.

Kovacs, M., and Goldston, D. 1991. Cognitive and social cognitive development of depressed children and adolescents. *Journal of the American Academy of Child and Adolescent Psychiatry* 30: 388–92.

Kovacs, M.; Goldston, D.; and Gatsonis, C. 1993. Suicidal behaviors and childhood-onset depressive disorders: A longitudinal investigation. *Journal of the American Academy of Child and Adolescent Psychiatry* 32: 8–20.

Kovelman, J. A., and Scheibel, A. B. 1984. A neurohistological correlate of schizophrenia. *Biological Psychiatry* 19: 1601–21.

Krishnan, K. R. R.; McDonald, W. M.; Escalona, P. R.; Doraiswamy, P. M.; Na, C.; Husain, M. M.; Figiel, G. S.; Boyko, O. B.; Ellinwood, E. H.; and Nemeroff, C. B. 1992. Magnetic resonance imaging of the caudate nuclei in depression: Preliminary observations. *Archives of General Psychiatry* 49: 553–57.

Kulisevsky, J.; Berthier, M. L.; and Pujol, J. 1993. Hemiballismus and secondary mania following a right thalamic infarction. *Neurology* 43: 1422–24.

Kurlan, R. 1992. The pathogenesis of Tourette's syndrome: A possible role for hormonal and excitatory neurotransmitter influences in brain development. *Archives of Neurology* 49: 874–76.

Kurlan, R.; Behr, J.; Medved, L.; Shoulson, I.; Pauls, D.; and Kidd, K. K. 1987. Severity of Tourette's syndrome in one large kindred: Implication for determination of disease prevalence rate. *Archives of Neurology* 44: 268–69.

Kurlan, R.; Lichter, D.; and Hewitt, D. 1989. Sensory tics in Tourette's syndrome. *Neurology* 39: 731–34.

Lake, C. R.; Ziegler, M. G.; and Murphy, D. L. 1977. Increased norepinephrine levels and decreased dopamine-beta-hydroxylase activity in primary autism. *Archives of General Psychiatry* 34: 553–56.

Landa, R.; Piven, J.; Wzorek, M. M.; Gayle, J. O.; Chase, G. A.; and Folstein, S. E. 1992. Social language use in parents of autistic individuals. *Psychological Medicine* 22: 245–54.

Lang, A. E.; Consky, E.; and Sandor, P. 1993. "Signing tics"—Insights into the pathophysiology of symptoms in Tourette's syndrome. *Annals of Neurology* 33: 212–15.

Laplane, D.; Baulac, M.; Widlöcher, D.; and Dubois, B. 1984. Pure psychic akinesia with bilateral lesions of basal ganglia. *Journal of Neurology, Neurosurgery and Psychiatry* 47: 377–85.

Laruelle, M.; Abi-Dargham, A.; Casanova, M. F.; Toti, R.; Weinberger, D. R.; and Kleinman, J. E. 1993. Selective abnormalities of prefrontal serotonergic receptors in schizophrenia: A postmortem study. *Archives of General Psychiatry* 50: 810–18.

Leckman, J. F.; de Lotbinieère, A. J.; Marek, K.; Gracco, C.; Scahill, L.; and Cohen, D. J. 1993. Severe disturbances in speech, swallowing, and gait following stereotactic infrathalamic lesions in Gilles de la Tourette's syndrome. *Neurology* 43: 890–94.

Leckman, J. F.; Dolnansky, E. S.; Hardin, M. T.; Clubb, M.; Walkup, J. T.; Stevenson, J.; and Pauls, D. L. 1990. Perinatal factors in the expression of Tourette's syndrome: An exploratory study. *Journal of the American Academy of Child and Adolescent Psychiatry* 29: 220–26.

Leckman, J. F.; Knorr, A. M.; Rasmusson, A. M.; and Cohen, D. J. 1991. Basal ganglia research and Tourette's syndrome. *Trends in Neuroscience* 14: 94.

Lefkowitz, M. M., and Tesiny, E. P. 1985. Depression in children: Prevalence and correlates. *Journal of Consulting and Clinical Psychology* 53: 647–56.

Leiner, H. C.; Leiner, A. L.; and Dow, R. S. 1986. Does the cerebellum contribute to mental skills? *Behavioral Neuroscience* 100: 443–54.

Leonard, H.; Lenane, M.; Swedo, S.; Rettew, D.; Gershon, E.; and Rapoport, J. L. 1992. Tics and Tourette's disorder: A 2- to 7-year follow-up of 54 obessive-compulsive children. *American Journal of Psychiatry* 149: 1244–51.

Levin, S.; Yurgelun-Todd, D.; and Craft, S. 1989. Contributions of clinical neuropsychology to the study of schizophrenia. *Journal of Abnormal Psychology* 98: 341–56.

Lewine, R. R. J. 1988. Gender and schizophrenia. In M. T. Tsuang and J. C. Simpson (eds.), *Handbook of Schizophrenia*, vol. 3, *Nosology, Epidemiology and Genetics* (New York: Elsevier Science Publishers), pp. 379–97.

Liddle, P. F. 1987. Schizophrenic syndromes, cognitive performance and neurological dysfunction. *Psychological Medicine* 17: 49–57.

Liddle, P. F., and Morris, D. 1991. Schizophrenic syndromes and frontal lobe performance. *British Journal of Psychiatry* 158: 340–45.

Lincoln, A. J.; Courchesne, E.; Kilman, B. A.; Elmasian, R.; and Allen, M. 1988. A study of intellectual abilities in high-functioning people with autism. *Journal of Autism and Developmental Disorders* 18: 505–24.

Lipsey, J. R.; Robinson, R. G.; Pearlson, G. D.; Rao, K.; and Price, T. R. 1984. Nortriptyline treatment for post-stroke depression: A double-blind study. *Lancet* 1: 297–300.

Lord, C., and O'Neil, P. 1983. Language and communication needs of adolescents with autism. In E. Schopler and G. Mesibov (eds.), *Autism in Adolescents and Adults* (New York: Plenum Press), pp. 57–77.

Luxenberg, J. S.; Swedo, S. E.; Flament, M. F.; Friedland, R. P.; Rapoport, J.; and Rapoport, S. I. 1988. Neuroanatomical abnormalities in obessive-compulsive disorder detected with quantitative X-ray computed tomography. *American Journal of Psychiatry* 145: 1089–93.

Machlin, S.; Harris, G.; Pearslon, G.; Hoehn-Saric, R.; Jeffery P.; and Camargo, E. 1991. Elevated medial-frontal cerebral blood flow in obsessive-compulsive patients: A SPECT study. *American Journal of Psychiatry* 148: 1240–42.

Marton, P.; Connolly, J.; Kutcher, S.; and Korenblum, M. 1993. Cognitive social skills and social self-appraisal in depressed adolescents. *Journal of the American Academy of Child and Adolescent Psychiatry* 32: 739–44.

Mazziotta, J. C.; Phelps, M. E.; and Carson, R. F. 1982. Tomographic mapping of human cerebral metabolism: Subcortical responses to auditory and visual stimulation. *Neurology* 32: 921–37.

McCauley, E.; Myers, K.; Mitchell, J.; Calderon, R.; Schloredt, K.; and Treder, R.

1993. Depression in young people: Initial presentation and clinical course. *Journal of the American Academy of Child and Adolescent Psychiatry* 32: 714–22.

Meltzer, H. Y., and Stahl, S. M. 1976. The dopamine hypothesis of schizophrenia: A review. *Schizophrenia Bulletin* 2: 19–76.

Merjanian, P. M.; Bachevalier, J.; Crawford, H.; and Mishkin, M. 1986. Socioemotional disturbances in the developing rhesus monkey following neonatal limbic lesions. *Society for Neuroscience Abstracts* 12: 23.

Merjanian, P. M.; Pettigrew, D.; and Mishkin, M. 1988. Developmental time course, as well as nature of socio-emotional disturbances in rhesus monkeys following neontatal limbic lesions resemble those in autism. *Society for Neuroscience Abstracts* 14: 2.

Migliorelli, R.; Starkstein, S. E.; Teson, A.; Quiros, G.; Vazquez, S.; Leiguarda, R.; and Robinson, R. G. 1993. SPECT findings in patients with primary mania. *Journal of Neuropsychiatry and Clinical Neuroscience* 5: 379–83.

Minshew, N. J., and Goldstein, G. 1993. Autism: A distributed neural network deficit? *Journal of Clinical and Experimental Neuropsychology* 15: 56.

Modell, J. G.; Mountz, J. M.; Curtis, G. C.; and Greden, J. F. 1989. Neurophysiologic dysfunction in basal ganglia/limbic striatal and thalamocortical circuits as a pathogenetic mechanism of obsessive-compulsive disorder. *Journal of Neuropsychiatry and Clinical Neuroscience* 1: 27–36.

Mullins, L.; Siegel, L. J.; and Hodges, K. 1985. Cognitive problem-solving and life event correlates of depressive symptoms in children. *Journal of Abnormal Child Psychology* 13: 305–14.

Murakami, J. W.; Courchesne, E.; Press, G. A.; Yeung-Courchesne, R.; and Hesselink, J. R. 1989. Reduced cerebellar hemisphere size and its relationship to vermal hypoplasia in autism. *Archives of Neurology* 46: 689–94.

Nemeroff, C. B.; Krishnan, K. R. R.; Reed, D.; Leder, R.; Beam, C.; and Dunnick, N. R. 1992. Adrenal gland enlargement in major depression: A computed tomographic study. *Archives of General Psychiatry* 49: 384–87.

Nieman, G. W., and Delong, R. 1987. Use of the personality inventory for children as an aid in differentiating children with mania from children with attention deficit disorder with hyperactivity. *Journal of the American Academy of Child Psychiatry* 26: 381–88.

Nordahl, T. E.; Benkelfat, C.; Semple, W.; Gross, M.; King, A. C.; and Cohen, R. M. 1989. Cerebral glucose metabolic rates in obsessive-compulsive disorder. *Neuropsychopharmacology* 2: 23–28.

Nuechterlein, K. H., and Dawson, M. E. 1984. Information processing and attentional functioning in the developmental course of schizophrenic disorders. *Schizophrenia Bulletin* 10: 160–203.

Nyback, H.; Berggren, B. M.; and Hindmarsh, T. 1982. Computed tomography of the brain in patients with acute psychosis and in healthy volunteers. *Acta Psychiatrica Scandanavica* 65: 403–14.

Obeso, J. A.; Rothwell, J. C.; and Marsden, C. D. 1981. Simple tics in Gilles de la Tourette's syndrome are not prefaced by a normal premovement EEG potential. *Journal of Neurology, Neurosurgery and Psychiatry* 44: 735–38.

Olsson, I.; Steffenburg, S.; and Gillberg, C. 1988. Epilepsy in autism and autisticlike conditions: A population-based study. *Archives of Neurology* 45: 666–68.

Ossofsky, H. J. 1974. Endogenous depression in infancy and childhood. *Comprehensive Psychiatry* 15: 19–25.

Pakstis, A.; Heutink, P.; Pauls, D. L.; Kurlan, R.; van de Wetering, B. J. M.; Leckman, J. F.; Sandkuyl, L. A.; Kidd, J. R.; Breedveld, G. J.; Castiglione, C. M.; Weber, J.; Sparkes, R. S.; Cohen, D. J.; Kidd, K. K.; and Oostra, B. A. 1991. Progress in the search for genetic linkage with Tourette syndrome: An exclusion map covering more than 50% of the autosomal genome. *American Journal of Human Genetics* 48: 281–94.

Parnas, J.; Cannon, T. D.; Jacobsen, B.; Schulsinger, H.; Schulsinger, F.; and Mednick, S. A. 1993. Lifetime DSM-III-R diagnostic outcomes in the offspring of schizophrenic mothers. *Archives of General Psychiatry* 50: 707–14.

Pauls, D. L.; Hurst, C. R.; Kruger, S. D.; Leckman, J. F.; Kidd, K. K.; and Cohen, D. J.1986. Gilles de la Tourette's syndrome and attention deficit disorder with hyperactivity: Evidence against a genetic relationship. *Archives of General Psychiatry* 43: 1177–79.

Pauls, D. L., and Leckman, J. F. 1986. The inheritance of Gilles de la Tourette syndrome and associated behaviors: Evidence for autosomal dominant transmission. *New England Journal of Medicine* 315: 993–97.

Pauls, D. L.; Towbin, K. E.; and Leckman, J. F.; Zahner, G.; and Cohen, D. J. 1986. Gilles de la Tourette's syndrome and obsessive-compulsive disorder: Evidence supporting a genetic relationship. *Archives of General Psychiatry* 43: 1180–82.

Paus, T.; Kalina, M.; Patočková, L.; Angerová, Y.; Černý, R.; Merčiř, P.; Bauer, J.; and Krabec, P. 1991. Medial vs. lateral frontal lobe lesions and differential impairment of central-gaze fixation maintenance in man. *Brain* 114: 2051–67.

Peterson, B.; Riddle, M. A.; Cohen, D. J.; Katz, L. D.; Smith, J. C.; Hardin, M. T.; and Leckman, J. F. 1993. Reduced basal ganglia volumes in Tourette's syndrome using three-dimensional reconstruction techniques from magnetic resonance images. *Neurology* 43: 941–49.

Pitman, R. K.; Kolb, B.; Orr, S. P.; and Singh, M. M. 1987. Ethological study of facial behavior in nonparanoid and paranoid schizophrenic patients. *American Journal of Psychiatry* 144: 99–102.

Piven, J.; Berthier, M. L.; Starkstein, S. E.; Nehme, E.; Pearlson, G.; and Folstein, S. 1990. Magnetic resonance imaging evidence for a defect of cerebral cortical development in autism. *American Journal of Psychiatry* 147: 734–39.

Piven, J.; Chase, G. A.; Landa, R.; Wzorek, M.; Gayle, J.; Cloud, D.; and Folstein, S. 1991. Psychiatric disorders in the parents of autistic individuals. *Journal of the American Academy of Child and Adolescent Psychiatry* 30: 471–78.

Puig-Antich, J., and Chambers, W. J. 1986. *Schedule for Affective Disorders and Schizophrenia for School Age Children (6–18) (Kiddie-SADS)*. New York: New York State Psychiatric Institute.

Puig-Antich, J.; Goetz, R.; Hanlon, C.; Davies, M.; Thompson, J.; Chambers, W. J.; Tabrizi, M. A.; and Weitzman, E. D. 1982. Sleep architecture and REM sleep measures in prepubertal children with major depression *Archives of General Psychiatry* 39: 932–39.

Pycock, C. J.; Kerwin, R. W.; and Carter, C. J. 1980. Effect of lesion of cortical dopamine terminals on subcortical dopamine receptors in rats. *Nature* 286: 74–76.

Radant, A. D., and Hommer, D. W. 1992. A quantitative analysis of saccades and smooth pursuit during visual pursuit tracking: A comparison of schizophrenics with normals and substance abusing controls. *Schizophrenia Research* 6: 225–35.

Rapoport, J. 1991. Recent advances in obsessive-compulsive disorder. *Neuropsychopharmacology* 5: 1–10.

Rao, U.; Weissman, M. M.; Martin, J. A.; and Hammond, R. W. 1993. Childhood depression and risk of suicide: A preliminary report of a longitudinal study. *Journal of the American Academy of Child and Adolescent Psychiatry* 32: 21–27.

Reiss, A. L., and Freund, L. 1990. Fragile X syndrome, DSM-III-R, and autism. *Journal of the American Academy of Child and Adolescent Psychiatry* 29: 885–91.

Rettew, D. C.; Swedo, S. E.; Leonard, H. L.; Lenane, M. C.; and Rapoport, J. L. 1992. Obsessions and compulsions across time in 79 children and adolescents with obsessive-compulsive disorder. *Journal of the American Academy of Child and Adolescent Psychiatry* 31: 1050–56.

Richardson, E. P. 1982. Neuropathological studies of Tourette syndrome. In A. J. Friedhoff and T. N. Chase (eds.), *Gilles de la Tourette Syndrome* (New York: Raven Press), pp. 83–87.

Riddle, M. A.; Rasmusson, A. M.; Woods, S. W.; and Hoffer, P. B. 1992. SPECT imaging of cerebral blood flow in Tourette syndrome. In T. N. Chase, A. J. Friedhoff, and D. J. Cohen (eds.), *Advances in Neurology,* vol. 58, *Tourette Syndrome: Genetics, Neurobiology and Treatment* (New York: Raven Press), pp. 207–11.

Ritvo, E. R.; Freeman, B. J.; Scheibel, A. B.; Duong, T.; Robinson, H.; Guthrie, D.; and Ritvo, A. 1986. Lower Purkinje cell counts in the cerebella of four autistic subjects: Initial findings of the UCLA-NSAC autopsy research report. *American Journal of Psychiatry* 143: 862–66.

Ritvo, E. R., and Garber, H. 1988. Cerebellar hypoplasia and autism. *New England Journal of Medicine* 319: 1152–53.

Ritvo, E. R.; Mason-Brothers, A.; Freeman, B. J.; Pingree, C.; Jenson, W. R.; McMahon, W. M.; Petersen, P. B.; Jorde, L. G.; Mo, A.; and Ritvo, A. 1990. The UCLA-University of Utah epidemiology survey of autism: The etiologic role of rare diseases. *American Journal of Psychiatry* 147: 1614–21.

Robinson, R. G.; Kubos, K. L.; Starr, L. B.; Rao, K.; and Price, T. R. 1984. Mood disorders in stroke patients: Importance of location of lesion. *Brain* 107: 81–93.

Ross, R. G.; Radant, A. D.; and Hommer, D. W. (1993) A developmental study of smooth pursuit eye movements in normal children from 7 to 15 years of age. *Journal of the American Academy of Child and Adolescent Psychiatry* 32: 783–91.

Rubin, R. T.; Villanueva-Meyer, J.; Ananth, J.; Trajmar, P. G.; and Mena, I. 1992. Regional xenon 133 cerebral blood flow and cerebral technetium 99m HMPAO uptake in unmedicated patients with obsessive-compulsive disorder and matched normal control subjects: Determination by high-resolution single-photon emission computed tomography. *Archives of General Psychiatry* 49: 695–702.

Rubinow, D. R.; Post, R. M.; Savard, R.; and Gold, P. W. 1984. Cortisol hypersecretion and cognitive impairment in depression. *Archives of General Psychiatry* 41: 279–83.

Rumsey, J. M.; Andreasen, N. C.; and Rapoport, J. L. 1986. Thought, language, communication, and affective flattening in autistic adults. *Archives of General Psychiatry* 43: 771–77.

Rumsey, J. M.; Creasey, H.; Stepanek, J. S.; Dorwart, R.; Patronas, N.; Hamburger, S. D.; and Duara, R. 1988. Hemispheric asymmetries, fourth ventricular size, and cerebellar morphology in autism. *Journal of Autism and Developmental Disorders* 18: 127–37.

Rumsey, J. M.; Duara, R.; Grady, C.; Rapoport, J. L.; Margolin, R. A.; Rapoport,

S. I.; and Cutler, N. R. 1985. Brain metabolism in autism: Resting cerebral glucose utilization rates as measured with positron emission tomography. *Archives of General Psychiatry* 42: 448–55.

Rumsey, J. M.; Grimes, A. M.; Pikus, A. M.; Duara, R.; and Ismond, D. R. 1984. Auditory brainstem responses in pervasive developmental disorders. *Biological Psychiatry* 19: 1403–18.

Rumsey, J. M., and Hamburger, S. D. 1988. Neuropsychological findings in high-functioning men with infantile autism, residual state. *Journal of Clinical and Experimental Neuropsychology* 10: 201–21.

———. 1990. Neuropsychological divergence of high-level autism and severe dyslexia. *Journal of Autism and Developmental Disorders* 20: 155–68.

Rumsey, J. M.; Rapoport, J.; and Sceery, W. R. 1985. Autistic children as adults: Psychiatric, social, and behavioral outcomes. *Journal of the American Academy of Child Psychiatry* 24: 465–73.

Rutschmann, J.; Cornblatt, B.; and Erlenmeyer-Kimling, L. 1986. Sustained attention in children at risk for schizophrenia: Findings with two visual continuous performance tasks in a new sample. *Journal of Abnormal Child Psychology* 14: 365–85.

Rutter, M., and Schopler, E. 1987. Autism and pervasive developmental disorders: concepts and diagnostic issues. *Journal of Autism and Developmental Disorders* 17: 159–86.

Ryan, N. D.; Birmaher, B.; Perel, J. M.; Dahl, R. E.; Meyer, V.; Al-Shabbout, M.; Iyengar, S.; and Puig-Antich, J. 1992. Neuroendocrine response to L-5-hydroxytryptophan challenge in prepubertal major depression: Depressed vs. normal children. *Archives of General Psychiatry* 49: 843–51.

Ryan, N. D.; Puig-Antich, J.; Ambrosini, P.; Rabinovich, H.; Robinson, D.; Nelson, B.; Iyengar, S.; and Twomey, J. 1987. The clinical picture of major depression in children and adolescents. *Archives of General Psychiatry* 44: 854–61.

Sawle, G.; Hymas, N.; Lees, A.; and Frackowiak, R. 1991. Obsessional slowness: Functional studies with positron emission tomography. *Brain* 114: 2191–2202.

Saykin, A. J.; Gur, R. C.; Gur, R. E.; Mozley, P. D.; Mozley, L. H.; Resnick, S. M.; Kester, D. B.; and Stafiniak, P. 1991. Neuropsychological function in schizophrenia: Selective impairment in memory and learning. *Archives of General Psychiatry* 48: 618–24.

Schilder, P. 1938. The organic background of obsessions and compulsions. *American Journal of Psychiatry* 94: 1397–1414.

Schittecatte, M.; Charles, G.; Machowski, R.; Garcia-Valentin, J.; Mendlewicz, J.; and Wilmotte, J. (1992) Reduced clonidine rapid eye movement sleep suppression in patients with primary major affective illness. *Archives of General Psychiatry* 49: 637–42.

Schmahmann, J. D. 1991. An emerging concept: The cerebellar contribution to higher function. *Archives of Neurology* 48: 1178–87.

Schulz, S. C.; Koller, M. M.; Kishore, P.; Hamer, R.; Gehl, J.; and Friedel, R. 1983. Ventricular enlargement in teenage patients with schizophrenia spectrum disorder. *American Journal of Psychiatry* 140: 1592–95.

Schwartz, M.; Friedman, R.; Lindsay, P.; and Narrol, H. 1982. The relationship between conceptual tempo and depression in children. *Journal of Consulting and Clinical Psychology* 50: 488–90.

Seeman, P.; Bzowej, N. H.; Guan, H.; Bergeron, C.; Reynolds, G. P.; Bird, E. D.; Riederer, P.; Jellinger, K.; and Tourtellotte, W. W. 1987. Human brain D_1

and D_2 receptors in schizophrenia, Alzheimer's, Parkinson's and Huntington's diseases. *Neuropsychopharmacology* 1: 5–15.

Seeman, P.; Guan, H. C.; and Van Tol, H. H. 1993. Dopamine D_4 receptors elevated in schizophrenia. *Nature* 365: 441–45.

Seignot, M. J. N. 1961. Un cas de maladie des tics de Gilles de la Tourette gueri par le R-1625. *Annales Medico-Psychologiques* 119: 578–79.

Shapiro, A. K.; Shapiro, E. S.; Young, J. G.; and Feinberg, T. E. 1988. *Gilles de la Tourette Syndrome*. New York: Raven Press.

Shelton, R. C., and Weinberger, D. R. 1986. X-ray computerized tomography studies in schizophrenia: A review and synthesis. In H. A. Nasrallah and D. R. Weinberger (eds), *The Neurology of Schizophrenia* (Amsterdam: Elsevier Science Publishers), pp. 207–50.

Shukla, S.; Cook, B. L.; Mukherjee, S.; Godwin, C.; and Miller, M. G. 1987. Mania following head trauma. *American Journal of Psychiatry* 144: 93–96.

Siegel, B. V., Jr.; Asarnow, R.; Tanguay, P.; Call, J. D.; Abel, L.; Ho, A.; Lott, I.; and Buchsbaum, M. S. 1992. Regional cerebral glucose metabolism and attention in adults with a history of childhood autism. *Journal of Neuropsychiatry and Clinical Neurosciences* 4: 406–14.

Siever, L. J., and Davis, K. L. 1985. Overview: Toward a dysregulation hypothesis of depression. *American Journal of Psychiatry* 142: 1017–31.

Singer, H. S.; Hahn, I.-H.; and Moran, T. H. 1991. Abnormal dopamine uptake sites in postmortem striatum from patients with Tourette's syndrome. *Annals of Neurology* 30: 558–62.

Singer, H. S.; Reiss, A. L.; Brown, J. E.; Aylward, E. H.; Shih, B.; Chee, E.; Harris, E. L.; Reader, M. J.; Chase, G. A.; Bryan, R.; and Denckla, M. B. 1993. Volumetric MRI changes in basal ganglia of children with Tourette's syndrome. *Neurology* 43: 950–56.

Smucker, M. R.; Craighead, W. E.; Craighead, L. W.; Green, B. J. 1986. Normative and reliability data for the Children's Depression Inventory. *Journal of Abnormal Child Psychology* 14: 25–39.

Starkstein, S. E.; Pearlson, G. D.; Boston, J.; and Robinson, R. G. 1987. Mania after brain injury: A controlled study of causative factors. *Archives of Neurology* 44: 1069–73.

Starkstein, S. E., and Robinson, R. G. 1989. Affective disorders and cerebral vascular disease. *British Journal of Psychiatry* 154: 170–82.

Starkstein, S. E.; Robinson, R. G.; and Price, T. R. 1987. Comparison of cortical and subcortical lesions in the production of post-stroke mood disorders. *Brain* 110: 1045–59.

Staton, R. D.; Wilson, H.; and Brumback, R. A. 1981. Cognitive improvement associated with tricylic antidepressant treatment of childhood major depressive illness. *Perceptual and Motor Skills* 53: 219–34.

Steffenberg, S.; Gillberg, C.; Hellgren, L.; Anderson, L.; Gillberg, I. C.; Jakobssen, G.; and Bohman, M. 1989. A twin study of autism in Denmark, Finland, Iceland, Norway and Sweden. *Journal of Child Psychology and Psychiatry* 30: 405–16.

Stoetter, B.; Braun, A. R.; Randolph, C.; Gernert, J.; and Carson, R. E.; Herscovitch, P.; and Chase, T. N. 1992. Functional neuroanatomy of Tourette syndrome: Limbic-motor interactions studied with FDG PET. In T. N. Chase, A. J. Friedhoff, and D. J. Cohen (eds.), *Advances in Neurology*, vol. 58, *Tourette*

Syndrome: Genetics, Neurobiology, and Treatment (New York: Raven Press), pp. 213–26.

Stroop, J. R. 1935. Studies of interference in serial verbal reactions. *Journal of Experimental Psychology* 18: 643–62.

Stuss, D. T.; Benson, D. F.; Kaplan, E. F.; Weir, W. S.; Naeser, M. A.; Lieberman, I.; and Ferrill, D. 1983. The involvement of orbitofrontal cerebrum in cognitive tasks. *Neuropsychologia* 21: 235–48.

Suddath, R. L.; Casanova, M. F.; Goldberg, T. E.; Daniel, D. G.; Kelsoe, J. R.; and Weinberger, D. R. 1989. Temporal lobe pathology in schizophrenia: A quantitative magnetic resonance inaging study. *American Journal of Psychiatry* 146: 464–72.

Suddath, R. L.; Christison, G. W.; Torrey, E. F.; Casanova, M. F.; and Weinberger, D. R. 1990. Anatomical abnormalties in the brains of monozygotic twins discordant for schizophrenia. *New England Journal of Medicine* 322: 789–94.

Sutherland, R. J.; Kolb, B.; Schoel, W. M.; Whishaw, I. Q.; and Davies, D. 1982. Neuropsychological assessment of children and adults with Tourette syndrome: A comparison with learning disabilities and schizophrenia. In A. J. Friedhoff and T. N. Chase (eds.), *Advances in Neurology*, vol. 35, *Gilles de la Tourette Syndrome* (New York: Raven Press), pp. 311–22.

Swedo, S. 1989. Rituals and releasers: An ethological model of obsessive-compulsive disorder. In J. Rapoport (ed.), *Obsessive-Compulsive Disorder in Children and Adolescents* (Washington: American Psychiatric Press), pp. 269–89.

Swedo, S. E.; Pietrini, P.; Leonard, H. L.; Schapiro, M. B.; Rettew, D. C.; Goldberger, E. L.; Rapoport, S. I.; Rapoport, J. L.; and Grady, C. L. 1992. Cerebral glucose metabolism in childhood-onset obsessive-compulsive disorder: Revisualization during pharmacotherapy. *Archives of General Psychiatry* 49: 690–94.

Swedo, S. E.; Rapoport J. L.; Cheslow, D. L.; Leonard, H. L.; Ayoub, E. M.; Hosier, D. M.; and Wald, E. R. 1989. High prevalance of obsessive-compulsive symptoms in patients with Sydenham's chorea. *American Journal of Psychiatry* 146: 246–49.

Swedo, S. E.; Schapiro, M. B.; Grady, C. L.; Cheslow, D. L.; Leonard, H. L.; Kumar, A.; Friedland, R.; Rapoport, S. I.; and Rapoport, J. L. 1989. Cerebral glucose metabolism in childhood-onset obsessive-compulsive disorder. *Archives of General Psychiatry* 46: 518–23.

Tamminga, C. A.; Thaker, G. K.; Buchanan, R.; Kirkpatrick, B.; Alphs, L. D.; Chase, T. N.; and Carpenter, W. T. 1992. Limbic system abnormalities identified in schizophrenia using positron emission tomography with fluorodeoxyglucose and neocortical alterations with deficit syndrome. *Archives of General Psychiatry* 49: 522–30.

Taub, J. M. 1984. Individual variations in the sleep of depression. *International Journal of Neuroscience* 23: 269–80.

Teicher, M. H.; Glod, C. A.; Harper, D.; Magnus, E.; Brasher, C.; Wren, F.; and Pahlavan, K. 1993. Locomotor activity in depressed children and adolescents: I. Circadian dysregulation. *Journal of the American Academy of Child and Adolescent Psychiatry* 32: 760–69.

Tesiny, E. P.; Lefkowitz, M. M.; and Gordon, N. H. 1980. Childhood depression, locus of control, and school achievement. *Journal of Educational Psychology* 72: 506–10.

Thivierge, J.; Bedard, C.; Cote, R.; and Maziade, M. 1990. Brainstem auditory evoked response and subcortical abnormalities in autism. *American Journal of Psychiatry* 147: 1609–13.

Tourette Syndrome Classification Study Group. 1993. Definitions and classification of tic disorders. *Archives of Neurology* 50: 1013–16.

Tuke, D. 1894. Imperative ideas. *Brain* 17: 179–97.

van de Wetering, B. J., and Heutink, K. P. 1993. The genetics of the Gilles de la Tourette syndrome: A review. *Journal of Laboratory and Clinical Medicine* 121: 638–45.

van Kammen, D. P., and Gelernter, J. 1987. Biochemical instability in schizophrenia: I. The norepinephrine system. In H. Y. Meltzer (ed.), *Psychopharmacology: The Third Generation of Progress* (New York: Raven Press), pp. 745–58.

Vilensky, J. A.; Damasio, A. R.; and Maurer, R. G. 1981. Gait disturbances in patients with autistic behavior. *Archives of Neurology* 38: 646–49.

Volkmar, F. R., and Nelson, D. S. 1990. Seizure disorders in autism. *Journal of the American Academy of Child and Adolescent Psychiatry* 29: 127–29.

Walker, E., and Emory, E. 1983. Infants at risk for psychopathology: Offspring of schizophrenic parents. *Child Development* 54: 1269–85.

Walker, E. F.; Grimes, K. E.; Davis, D. M.; and Smith, A. J. 1993. Childhood precursors of schizophrenia: Facial expressions of emotions. *American Journal of Psychiatry* 150: 1645–48.

Walkup, J. T.; Rosenberg, L. A.; Brown, J.; and Singer, H. S. 1992. The validity of instruments measuring tic severity in Tourette's syndrome. *Journal of the American Academy of Child and Adolescent Psychiatry* 30: 472–77.

Warneke, L. 1975. A case of manic-depressive illness in childhood. *Canadian Psychiatric Association Journal* 20: 195–200.

Weinberg, W. A., and Brumback, R. P. 1976. Mania in childhood. *American Journal of Diseases of Children* 130: 380–85.

Weinberg, W. A., and Emslie, G. J. 1988. Adolescents and school problems: Depression, suicide and learning disorders. In R. A. Feldman and A. R. Stiffman (eds.), *Advances in Adolescent Mental Health,* vol. 3, *Depression and Suicide.* (Greenwich, Conn.: JAI Press), pp. 181–205.

Weinberg, W. A.; Rutman, J.; Sullivan, L.; Penick, E. C.; and Dietz, S. G. 1973. Depression in children referred to an educational diagnostic center: Diagnosis and treatment. *Journal of Pediatrics* 83: 1065–72.

Weinberger, D. R. 1987. Implications of normal brain development for the pathogenesis of schizophrenia. *Archives of General Psychiatry* 44: 660–669.

Weinberger, D. R.; and Berman, K. F.; and Zec, R. F. 1986. Physiologic dysfunction of dorsolateral prefrontal cortex in schizophrenia: I. Regional cerebral blood flow evidence. *Archives of General Psychiatry* 43: 114–25.

Weinberger, D. R.; Cannon-Spoor, E.; Potkin, S. G.; and Wyatt, R. J. 1980. Poor premorbid adjustment and CT scan abnormalities in chronic schizophrenia. *American Journal of Psychiatry* 137: 1410–13.

Weiner, A. S., and Pfeffer, C. R. 1986. Suicidal status, depression, and intellectual functioning in preadolescent psychiatric inpatients. *Comprehensive Psychiatry* 27: 372–80.

Weller, E. B., and Weller, R. A. 1988. Neuroendocrine changes in affectively ill children and adolescents. *Neurological Clinics* 6: 41–54.

Welsh, M. C.; Pennington, B. F.; and Rogers, S. 1987. Word recognition and comprehension skills in hyperlexic children. *Brain and Language* 32: 76–96.

Williams, A. O.; Reveley, M. A.; Kolakowska, T.; Andern, M.; and Mandelbrote,

B. M. 1985. Schizophrenia with good and poor outcome: II. Cerebral ventricular size and its clinical significance. *British Journal of Psychiatry* 146: 239–46.

Wilson, H., and Staton, R. D. 1984. Neuropsychological changes in children associated with tricyclic antidepressant therapy. *International Journal of Neuroscience* 24: 307–12.

Wing, L. 1981. Asperger's syndrome: A clinical account. *Psychological Medicine* 11: 115–29.

Wong, V. 1993. Epilepsy in children with autistic spectrum disorder. *Journal of Child Neurology* 8: 316–22.

Yudofsky, S. C., and Hales, R. E. 1992. *American Psychiatric Association Textbook of Neuropsychiatry,* 2d ed. Washington, D.C.: American Psychiatric Press.

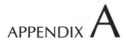

Pediatric Neuropsychology Questionnaire

Child's Name: _____

Date of Birth: _____

Date of Evaluation: _____

Person who referred you for evaluation: _____ _____

Name of person filling out this questionnaire: _____ _____

Child's pediatrician and address: _____

_____

REFERRAL INFORMATION

Reason you are requesting this evaluation: _____

_____

_____

Circumstances/factors you think are important regarding this reason: _____

_____

_____

_____

In my opinion, the major cause of my child's difficulties is _____

_____

_____

Describe some of your child's strengths: _____

_____

_____

Describe some of your child's weaknesses: _____ _____

_____

_____

Do both parents agree about the nature and causes of the problem? _____

FAMILY INFORMATION

Address: _____

_____

Telephone: _____

Names of parents

    Mother: _____ age: _____ education: _____

    Father: _____ age: _____ education: _____

Parents are married _____ separated _____ divorced _____ deceased _____

Child is natural _____ adopted _____ foster _____

    Siblings (name, age): _____

                    _____

                     _____

                     _____

    Others living in home: _____

                     _____

Approximate family income:

    0–15,000   _____

    15,000–35,000   _____

    35,000–55,000   _____

    55,000–75,000   _____

    75,000 or higher _____

Father's occupation: _____

Mother's occupation: _____

Are there any significant family or marital conflicts? _____

PREGNANCY AND BIRTH HISTORY

Age of mother at delivery? _____

Any known health problems of mother during pregnancy? _____

Delivery was vaginal _____ Cesarean _____

Baby was full term _____ premature _____ (_____ weeks gestation)

Birth weight _____ lb. _____ oz.

Was labor prolonged? _____ any complications? _____

Did baby breathe spontaneously? _____

Apgar scores if known: _____

How old was baby at discharge from the hospital after birth? _____

Any medical problems after discharge (e.g., jaundice, fever)?

Any problems in first few months? _____

DEVELOPMENTAL HISTORY

Motor

Age sat alone _____ crawled _____ walked alone _____

Was your child slow to develop motor skills or awkward compared to siblings/
friends (e.g., running, skipping, climbing, biking, playing ball? _____

Handedness: right _____ left _____ both _____

Family history of left-handedness (list relatives)? _____

Was physical therapy ever necessary? _____

Was occupational therapy ever necessary? _____

Language

Age spoke first word _____ put 2–3 words together _____

Speech delays/problems (e.g., stutters, difficult to understand)?

Oralmotor problems (e.g., late drooling, poor sucking, poor chewing)?

(describe) _____

Was speech/language therapy ever necessary? _____

Was child slow to learn the alphabet? _____

name colors? _____ count? _____

Other language spoken at home (besides English)? _____

Toileting

Age when toilet trained _____

Problems with bedwetting?, urine accidents?, soiling? _____

Social Behavior

Does your child get along well with other children? _____ adults? _____
have friends? _____ keep friends? _____
understand gestures? _____ have a good sense of humor? _____ ___
understand social cues well (e.g., knows when others are angry, in
discomfort)? _____
have problems with peer pressure (e.g., alcohol or drug use) _____
_____
_____

MEDICAL HISTORY

Has vision been checked? _____ any problems: _____
Has hearing been checked? _____ any problems: _____

List serious illnesses/injuries/hospitalizations/surgeries

Date   Incident (explain)

_____   _____

_____   _____

_____   _____

_____   _____

_____   _____

Is there a history of:
febrile seizures?   _____
epilepsy?   _____
lead poisoning/toxic ingestion?   _____
asthma or allergies?   _____
loss of consciousness?   _____
abdominal pains/vomiting?   _____
   when do they occur?   _____
headaches?   _____
   when do they occur?   _____

frequent ear infections? _____

sleep difficulties? _____

eating difficulties? _____

tics/twitching? _____

repetitive/stereotyped movements?
  (e.g., hand flapping) _____

impulsivity? _____

temper tantrums? _____

nail biting? _____

clumsiness? _____

head banging? _____

self-injurious behavior? _____

Describe head injuries (e.g., date, type, loss of consciousness?, resulting changes in behavior?):

_____

_____

Current medications and reasons:

_____

Is there a family history of learning difficulty in any family member? _____

_____

Does anyone else in the family have a problem similar to your child's reason for referral? _____

EDUCATIONAL HISTORY

Current school and address:

Grade: _____ Placement: regular _____ resource _____ special education _____ other _____

Any grades that were skipped or repeated? _____

Teachers report problems in:

     reading _____   attention/concentration _____

     spelling _____   behavior _____

     arithmetic _____   social adjustment _____

     writing _____

Grade: **Academic problems?**

Nursery

Kindergarten   _____

First   _____

Second   _____

Third   _____

Fourth   _____

Fifth   _____

Sixth   _____

Seventh   _____

Eighth   _____

Ninth   _____

Tenth   _____

Eleventh   _____

Twelfth   _____

                _____

Was your child unusually hyperactive? _____ inattentive? _____

Specific problems noted: _____

_____

Do teachers report problems that you do not notice? _____

My child's intelligence level is likely:

below average   _____

average   _____

high average   _____

superior   _____

PRIOR PSYCHOLOGICAL HISTORY

Have you previously had direct contact with any social agency, psychologist, psychiatrist, clinic or private agency? _____

Name of professional	Address	Dates

Any other comments you would like to make:

Social-Emotional Questionnaire

NAME: _____

DOB: _____ C.A.: _____ years, _____ months

DOT: _____

Name of Person Completing the Questionnaire: _____

Relationship to Patient: _____

Instructions: Please read each question carefully and answer "yes" or "no" after each statement. Feel free to provide any additional information you think pertinent.

EARLY CHILDHOOD

1. My child achieved developmental milestones (motor, language, social) at an appropriate age.
    If not, list those areas in which there was delay, and indicate when they were achieved.

2. My child was unusually unresponsive to the company of others at an early age; e.g., he/she failed to make an attempt to share interests, toys with parents, siblings, friends.

3. My child made appropriate effort to communicate with others either through babbling while a baby or through gestures and movements with greater maturity.

4. My child engaged in normal imaginative or pretend play.

5. My child's play was generally confined to or revolved about one particular theme with minimal variation.

6. My child was willing to let others join in games and play situations.

7. My child was unusually insistent that others play by his/her rules and follow a similar pattern.

VERBAL

1. My child speaks, or has spoken in the past, in an unusually loud voice, unaware of voice volume in relation to others.

2. My child speaks, or has spoken in the past, in a monotone, flat or exaggerated manner.

3. My child has a lack of inflection when speaking; i.e., it is difficult to discern emotional state through the speech patterns.

4. My child's speech content is often unoriginal or sounds as if it has been learned from a book or mimics another person.

5. My child's tendency, now or in the past, is to become intensely interested in one or two topics to the exclusion of all others.

6. My child's speech content is frequently limited to lengthy statements on a favorite or recurring subject.

7. My child often recites long lists of facts related to a favorite subject without understanding the importance of these facts.

8. My child cannot appreciate subtle verbal jokes.

NONVERBAL

1. My child cannot make and maintain eye contact in interpersonal interactions.

2. My child does not make appropriate use of gestures to communicate.

3. My child's gestures are often awkward, or clumsy.

4. My child is not sensitive to the gestures of others, i.e., unable to discern meaning through the gestures and nonverbal expressions of others.

5. My child often misinterprets or ignores social cues for appropriate behavior.

6. My child does not use appropriate facial expressions.

7. My child has greater difficulty than others understanding nonverbal humorous intent.

MOTOR

1. My child's movements are often clumsy or awkward.

2. My child has an unusual posture or gait.

3. My child has a tendency to stand unusually close to others without recognizing the discomfort of others.

4. My child has difficulty with handwriting or drawing skills.

GENERAL

1. My child expresses intense comfort with familiarity, and is resistant to change.

2. My child often engages in repetitive, stereotyped behaviors.

3. My child tends to become intensely attached to particular possessions.

4. My child had an almost obsessive interest in something.
   If so, what was this and how long was it maintained?

5. My child's sense of humor differs greatly from that of other children.

Hydrocephalus Fact Sheet

Name: _____

Date of Birth: _____ Age: _____

Birth Weight: _____

Etiology: Spina Bifida _____ Obstructive _____

Congenital _____ Communicating _____

Meningitis _____

Tumor _____

Post-trauma _____

Other _____

Age at Diagnosis: _____ _____

Age at First Shunt: _____

		Age	Infection	Blockage
Dates of Revision(s):	_____	_____	_____	_____
	_____	_____	_____	_____
	_____	_____	_____	_____
	_____	_____	_____	_____
	_____	_____	_____	_____

Complications (e.g., hemorrhage, infection): _____

Current Shunt:

Type (e.g., V-P) _____

Side (left or right) _____

Associated Neurological Problems:

Seizures (+ drug Tx) _____

Porencephaly _____

Cerebral Palsy   _____

Other CNS Malformations   _____

Current Status: (circle answer)

    Ventricle Size:

        Normal

        Mildly Enlarged

        Moderately Enlarged

        Severely Enlarged

    Symptoms: (circle if present)

        Headache

        Dizziness

        Lethargy

        Vomiting

        Poor Balance

        Double Vision

    Signs: (circle if present)

        Papilledema

        Decreased Convergence

        Decreased Gaze

    Most Recent Neurodiagnostic Procedures: (type, date, results)

    _____

    _____

    Head Circumference: _____

    Frontal Mantle Measurement: _____

    Ventricular/Brain Ratio: _____

Academic Summary:

    Current Grade: _____

    Failures: (? grade) _____

    Current Placement:

        Regular Class, No Help   _____

        Regular Class, Tutoring   _____

        Regular Class, Resource Help _____

        Special Education

            L.D.   _____

            Level of Special Placement   _____

Problem Areas:

Reading _____

Spelling _____

Arithmetic _____

Writing _____

Memory _____

Perceptual _____

Behavioral _____

Other _____

Recent Cognitive or Behavioral Changes:

Index